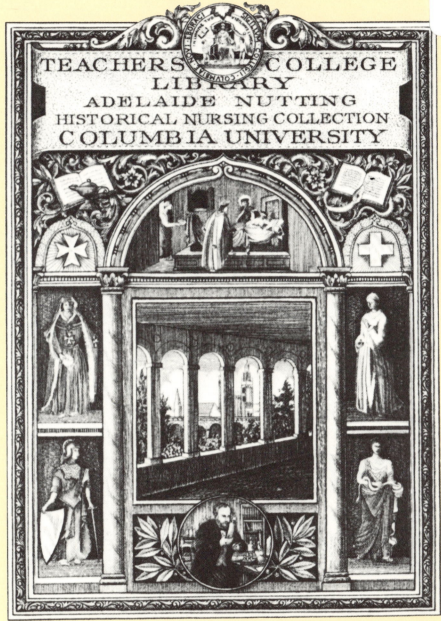

NURSING

The Finest Art

AN ILLUSTRATED HISTORY

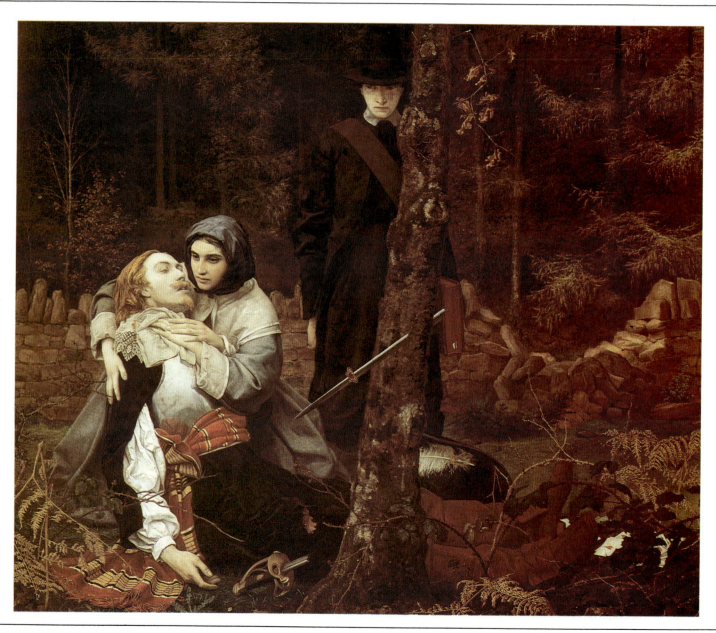

William Shakespeare Burton, THE WOUNDED CAVALIER, *c. 1856. The Bridgeman Art Library, Guildhall Art Gallery, City of London, England.*

NURSING
The Finest Art
AN ILLUSTRATED HISTORY

M. Patricia Donahue, Ph.D., R.N.

Associate Professor
College of Nursing, The University of Iowa,
Iowa City, Iowa

Illustrations edited and compiled by
Patricia A. Russac

with 405 illustrations including 169 in full color

The C. V. Mosby Company

St. Louis   Toronto   Princeton   1985

Editor: Nancy L. Mullins
Developmental editor: Bess Arends
Manuscript editor: Carlotta Seely
Design/Production: The Quarasan Group, Inc.

Publisher: Thomas A. Manning
Editor-in-Chief: Alison Miller

Printed in the United States of America

The C.V. Mosby Company
11830 Westline Industrial Drive, St. Louis, Missouri 63146

Library of Congress Cataloging in Publication Data

Donahue, M. Patricia.
     Nursing, the finest art.

     Dedicated in memory of Dr. Teresa E. Christy.
     Bibliography: p.
     Includes index.
     1. Nursing—History. 2. Nursing—United States—
History. I. Russac, Patricia A. II. Title.
[DNLM: 1. History of Nursing. WY 11.1 D674n]
RT31.D66 1985   610.73′09   84-29450
ISBN 0-8016-1424-4

VT/VH/VH 9 8 7 6 5 4   01/A/096

DEDICATION

I have been given the honor of writing the dedication to this book in memory of the foremost historian and historiographer in nursing, Dr. Teresa E. Christy. For all the students she has taught and for her colleagues, I say that we can still see her gestures in pointing out the nuances in the pictures and we can still hear her words in describing the events recorded in the history of nursing. As Terry's contemporaries, many of us are familiar with her historical anecdotes and how she compared the events of yesterday with those of today. Future generations of nurses will have the great history of nursing preserved in her numerous writings and in this important work.

I will never forget my first meeting with Dr. Christy. It was the beginning of years of dialogue with a colleague and friend about a mutual interest, the history of nursing. At that first meeting a friend had introduced us and had told Terry of my personal search for the historical and philosophical foundations of nursing. I had been told about the doctoral study she had completed, entitled "Cornerstone for Nursing Education" and published in 1969. In our subsequent meetings the air was electrified with ideas and the joy and laughter that accompanied our discussions. I remember one evening after dinner in her home, when we were discussing the problems in nursing education and the various studies, beginning with the 1923 Goldmark Report, which recommended a system of education for nursing. We disagreed on the year that the Ginzberg Report was published, and Terry excused herself, went to her library, checked the primary source, and returned to say that both of us had an incorrect date; and then we laughed about the way we challenged each other.

Dr. Christy was invited to speak on nursing education—past, present, and future—at the College of Nursing's celebration of the twenty-fifth anniversary of the University of South Florida, November 10, 1981. She was my guest, and I noticed her energy level had decreased from that of previous meetings. However, she gave her usual excellent performance. Discussing historical events with Dr. Christy has been described as an experience of intellectual ecstasy and professional joy and pride in our heritage.

Many examples of friendship and colleagueship can be cited, but I will always remember one in particular. Just a few months before Dr. Christy died, I asked her if she would write a letter for me because I was applying for tenure. She wrote a beautiful letter and enclosed a personal note to me that closed with "I want to send this to your dean before I return to the hospital for surgery." Her commitment to principles and to friends and colleagues will be remembered for a lifetime.

Dr. Christy's career demonstrated her active involvement in university life, nursing organizations, and historical societies. Her leadership was seen in nursing research when she reminded us at meetings and through her scholarly writings that the historical method must be promulgated as an essential component in the scientific movement in nursing. In September 1978, when Dr. Christy was admitted as a fellow of the American Academy of Nursing, a major point noted was "her establishing the value of historical research as a creditable and much needed area of research in nursing."

Among Dr. Christy's numerous awards were The Johns Hopkins University Centennial Scholar Award; The DePaul University, Chicago, Illinois Distinguished Alumni Achievement Award; an Honorary Doctorate from McKendree College, Lebanon, Illinois; a Distinguished Achievement Award for Outstanding Contributions to Research in Nursing, Nursing Education Alumnae Association, Teachers College, Columbia University, New York; and the Elizabeth McWilliams Miller Award for Distinguished Research, Sigma Theta Tau. Dr. Christy is listed in several biographies, such as *Who's Who in the Midwest,* and her publications have appeared in many professional journals. She was widely acclaimed for her dinner speeches and keynote addresses for major functions in nursing. During her lifetime Dr. Christy was recognized as a foremost historian and historiographer in nursing.

The legacy that Dr. Teresa Christy has given all of us is recorded in nursing's history and especially in this beautifully illustrated book, which was one of her dreams. This dream was brought to reality by a friend, Dr. M. Patricia Donahue, who not only preserved Terry Christy's hopes and spirit but added her own special skills as an historian to this great publication.

Imogene M. King, Ed.D., R.N.
Professor, College of Nursing,
University of South Florida,
Tampa, Florida

FOREWORD

his remarkable volume is inviting us to a visual celebration of nursing and its history. Therefore it seems only fair to prepare the celebrants, since what follows will alter the traditional perspective of the nurse and the nursing profession.

Through a fascinating array of visual data and the accompanying text, the reader can learn of the complexities inherent in the emergence of nursing as we have come to know it. At the very least, after viewing over four hundred illustrations the reader's view will have been expanded and enhanced.

No single volume can present a comprehensive portrayal of the vanished past. Yet in this engaging book Dr. Donahue has successfully met the challenge in the enormous task of developing the concept of an illustrated history of nursing. In doing so she has given visible evidence of the beauty and the sorrow that encompass the traditions of nursing as it has embraced the human condition over time.

The significance of this book is its achievement in representing the spectrum and diversity of its subject through the multidimensional aspects of photographic and artistic documentation. In addition, as a referenced text with a selected bibliography and a detailed index, this work qualifies as a valuable scholarly resource.

This unprecedented effort is unique in its reliance on art as indicative of nursing's knowable past. Yet the use of art as a framework for appreciating the many facets of nursing history is a natural medium for the expression of the enduring humanitarian ethic that is indispensable to the legacy of nursing. Dr. Donahue's extraordinary chronicle provides a revealing vista of the heritage of nursing as the oldest and finest art and at the same time makes a valuable contribution to an enlightened vision of nursing's future. Come let us celebrate!

Olga Maranjian Church, Ph.D., R.N.
Edgartown, Massachusetts

PREFACE

It is something to be able to paint a picture, or to carve a statue,
and so to make a few objects beautiful. But it is far more glorious
to carve and paint the atmosphere in which we work, to effect
the quality of the day—This is the highest of the arts.

Henry David Thoreau

Nursing has long been defined as both an art and a science.
The primary emphasis, however, has been on the scientific
aspects of nursing with little consideration given to its state
as an art. Nursing is a fine art. According to Florence Nightingale, it is
"the finest of the fine arts." Nursing is not merely a technique but a
process that incorporates the elements of soul, mind, and imagination. Its very essence lies in the creative imagination, the sensitive
spirit, and the intelligent understanding that provide the very foundation for effective nursing care. These have been captured consistently in a wide range of illustrative material that can greatly enhance
the study of nursing history through visual representation. Every art
gallery has its nursing saints, nurturing mothers, healing miracles,
sick beds, and lying-in chambers. Many of the finest paintings and
sculptures dealing with nursing subjects have been done by the
"great masters" and contemporary artists. All of these serve to capture the art of nursing.

Nursing: The Finest Art, An Illustrated History has been a labor
of love and a realization of a dream. It has been a labor because I have
struggled to portray effectively the eloquent beauty of nursing and
nursing care so that all who read the words and see the illustrations
will appreciate its vitality. My love of both history and nursing provided the motivation to demonstrate the historical development of
nursing through an integration of a variety of selected illustrations
and written text. The dream that this book would be written and
published initially belonged to Dr. Teresa E. Christy, who died "too
young and too soon" but not before she had nurtured my interest in
nursing history and had become my mentor as I began my journey
into historical research. The words of this history are mine, but the
spirit is Terry's.

This book is intended to provide an illustrated history of nursing from primitive times to the present. It is written for nurses, other
interested professionals, and the layman. Various forms of art are used
to depict the particular shifts and changes in the roles and functions
of the nurse as they have been created and influenced by major social, political, and historical forces in society. Alterations in the image
of nursing are also portrayed, since nursing has progressed through
an evolutionary process. Although this book is referenced, it is *not a*

comprehensive text of nursing history. It can, however, be used to augment both nursing courses and art courses. Most important is its aesthetic value not only for nurses but for all lovers of art.

It can be argued that some significant events, persons, and places were omitted from the text. Indeed, I have chosen specific occurrences in an attempt to balance the artwork with the text and yet render a fair appraisal of nursing's journey through time. Selected events, topics, and individuals important to the development of nursing have been highlighted. These represent a larger body of information that could be used to demonstrate nursing's struggles, growth, challenges, dilemmas, humanitarianism, and beauty. All would reinforce the recurring themes evident in the text and reaffirm the need to effectively communicate the essence of nursing.

> We need to realize and to affirm anew that nursing is one of the most difficult of arts. Compassion may provide the motive, but knowledge is our only working power. Perhaps, too, we need to remember that growth in our work must be preceded by ideas, and that any conditions which suppress thought, must retard growth. Surely we will not be satisfied in perpetuating methods and traditions. Surely we shall wish to be more and more occupied with creating them.
>
> *M. Adelaide Nutting, 1925*

Many individuals have been involved with this project in different ways. To all of them I extend my sincere appreciation. Those persons who are not identified know of their invaluable assistance and unique contributions.

It is impossible to give adequate thanks to my daughter and my son, Erin and Mark, who freely and unselfishly gave of themselves during this period of writing, when I frequently did not have time to be their mother. Once again they have respected and accepted my need to do what I think I must. To my son Johnny, who throughout his short life provided a living example of unselfishness, patience, love, and a courage to attempt the "impossible," I give thanks. Finally, I acknowledge the interest of my parents, who often did not always understand my excitement about this book or my drive to accomplish but who patiently endured.

My deepest gratitude is extended to my research assistant, Patricia A. Russac, who taught me about the subtleties of art. Her expertise, determination, and precision were a primary factor in the completion of this work. To the many individuals at The C.V. Mosby Company who assisted with this project I extend grateful appreciation, particularly Julie Cardamon, my first Editor, who initiated my contract; Nancy L. Mullins, Editor, Nursing Division, who inherited the project and assisted with the steady progression necessary for completion; and Bess Arends, Developmental Editor, who provided sustained support, encouragement, interest, and understanding throughout all of the difficult phases.

I am deeply indebted to my support network whose members probably do not even recognize their significant contributions in the development of this manuscript. Particular thanks are due to LTC Sarah A. Balkema, U.S. Army (ret.); LTC Joan K. Cotter, U.S. Army (ret.); Karen A. O'Heath; Sandra R. Powell; Dr. Imogene M. King; and Steven Warner. Finally, the support of Dean Geraldene Felton, The University of Iowa College of Nursing, facilitated the progress of the project.

M. Patricia Donahue

CONTENTS

NURSING

The Finest Art

AN ILLUSTRATED HISTORY

Woman is an instinctive nurse, taught by Mother Nature. The nurse has always been a necessity, and thus lacked social status. In primitive times she was a slave, and in the civilized era a domestic. Overlooked in the plans of legislators, and forgotten in the curricula of pedagogues, she was left without protection and remained without education. She was not an artisan who could obtain the help of an hereditary guild; there was no Hanseatic League for nurses. Drawn from the nameless and numberless army of poverty, the nurse worked as a menial and obeyed as a servant. Denied the dignity of a trade, and devoid of professional ethics, she could not rise above the degradation of her environment. It never occurred to the Aristotles of the past that it would be safer for the public welfare if nurses were educated instead of lawyers. The untrained nurse is as old as the human race; the trained nurse is a recent discovery. The distinction between the two is a sharp commentary on the follies and prejudices of mankind.

Victor Robinson

THE ORIGIN
OF NURSING

An adequate identification and description of the exact origin of nursing is difficult because nothing is known about the actual work of the nurse in prehistory. Everything that has been written about nursing during this period is merely inference based on the discoveries of prehistorians, archaeologists, and anthropologists. Yet early records do provide information about the legacy left to civilized man from primitive societies. From the dawn of civilization, evidence prevails to support the premise that *nurturing* has been essential to the preservation of life. Survival of the human race, therefore, is inextricably intertwined with the development of nursing.

■ THE NURSING IMPULSE

It is difficult at times to distinguish nursing from medicine in this evolutionary process, since the early stages of each are so closely interwoven. Although some individuals believe that nursing began with Florence Nightingale, nursing is as old as medicine itself. An interdependence of the two is evident throughout history and has produced a unique and curious relationship. At some periods, such as the Hippocratic era, rational medicine functioned without nursing, whereas at other times, for example, the Middle Ages, nursing was practiced without rational medicine. According to Davison (1943), who identified four main cycles of medicine (primitive, Renaissance, pharmacy, and modern), nursing approached adequacy in three (not pharmacy), and only in these did medicine progress. Davison believes that nursing merits recognition as the "cornerstone of its [medicine's] foundation." Certainly the mother-nurse must have preceded the magician-priest or the medicine man. It is even possible that these two types of service were at first united but eventually divided to produce two practitioners of the healing art—the medicine giver and the caretaker (Stewart and Austin, 1962). Indeed, the modern doctor has the aura of the medicine man, but the seeds of medical knowledge were sown by the natural remedies of the mother.

Nursing has been called the oldest of the arts and the youngest of the professions. As such, it has gone through many stages and has been an integral part of societal movements. Nursing has been involved in the existing culture—shaped by it and yet helping to develop it. The history of nursing has been one of frustration, ignorance, and misunderstanding. It is a great epic involving trials and triumphs, romance and adventure. Most importantly, it is the story of an occupational group whose status has always been affected by the prevalent standards of humanity. The great turning points in world progress have also been important turning points in nursing. Events that give rise to "higher degrees of consideration for those who are helpless or oppressed, kindliness and sympathy for the unfortunate and for those who suffer, tolerance for those of differing religion, race, color, etc.—all tend to promote activities like nursing which are primarily humanitarian" (Dock and Stewart, 1925, p. 3).

In any text concerning the genesis of nursing, there is considerable content that refers to the history of nursing as an episode in the history of woman. In fact, one historian described this phenomenon with a clear and emphatic statement: "The nurse is the mirror in

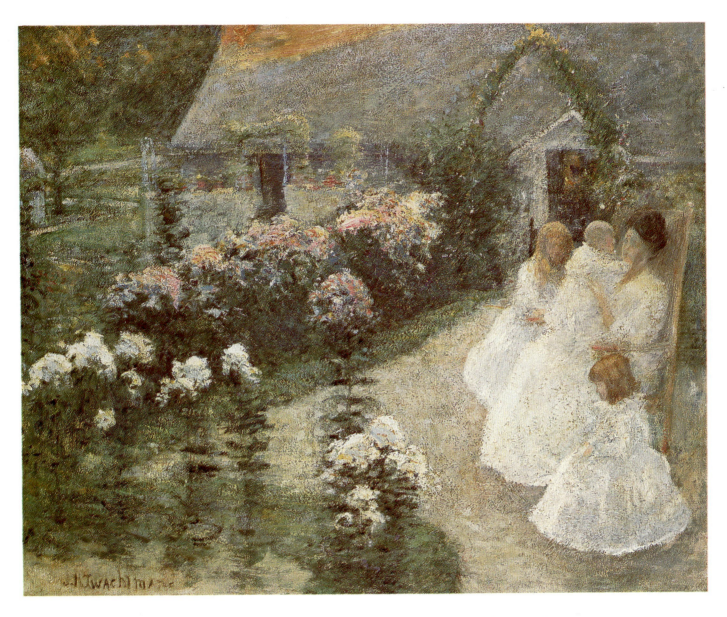

John Henry Twachtman, ON THE TERRACE, *c. 1890–1900. Canvas, approx. 64.8 × 76.2 cm. National Museum of American Art, Smithsonian Institution, Washington, D.C., Gift of John Gellatly.*

which is reflected the position of woman through the ages" (Robinson, 1946, p. vii). During those periods when women were closely restricted to the home by social convention and their energies were limited to family life, nursing must have had the character of a household art. The duties of women, their degree of economic independence, the freedom of women outside the family, and other factors have seriously influenced the progress of nursing. The fullest development of nursing was not possible without emancipation from the conditions of subjection endured by women. Ultimately the full demands of nursing could not be realized without education and knowledge of the social conditions and needs of the day.

Confusion exists regarding the proper role or function of the nurse, since the connotations of the word *nurse* have changed over the course of human history. *Nurse* and *nursing* currently have many meanings, a condition that causes varying interpretations of the appropriate work and function of the nurse. Throughout history the development of nursing has been closely related to the evolution of the word *nurse,* specific definitions of which are dependent upon the major social forces of the day. It is apparent that the meaning of the

3

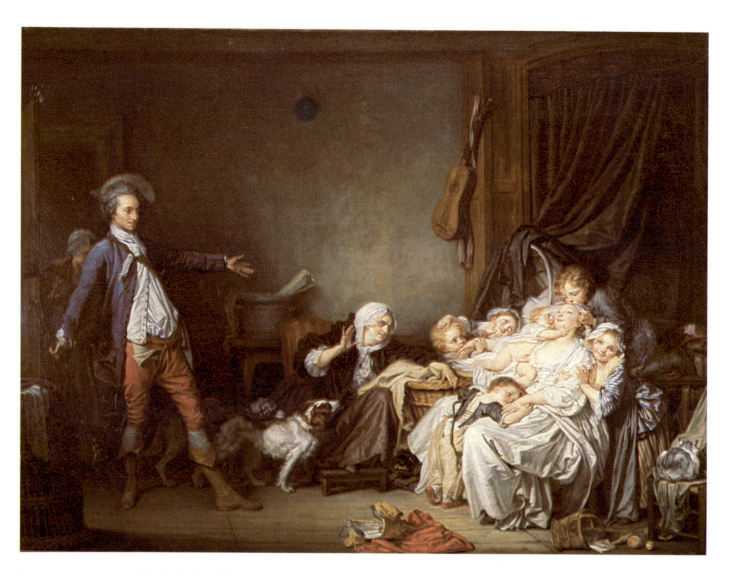

Jean-Baptiste Greuze, THE BELOVED MOTHER,
*late eighteenth century. Le Comte de la
Viñaza–Marquis de Laborde, Madrid, Spain.*

word has progressed from a term indicating the basic unlearned
human activity of suckling an infant to one of a highly learned, sophisticated nature. These shifts in meaning are strongly reflected in
changes in the nursing role.

Nursing has its origin in the mother-care of helpless infants and
must have coexisted with this type of care from earliest times. The
word *nursing* is derived from the Latin *nutrire,* "to nourish." The
word *nurse* also has its roots in Latin in the noun *nutrix,* which
means "nursing mother." Frequently this referred to a woman who
suckled a child who was not her own, that is, a wet nurse. Eventually
the term *nutrix* was used to identify a female who nourished, which
provided a broader yet still gender-related definition. The Latin
words were the basis for the French *nourice,* which also referred to
a woman who suckled a child, particularly the child of another. The
original meaning of the English word was the same, a wet nurse. The
term was first used in English in the thirteenth century, and its spell-
ing underwent many forms, from *norrice, nurice,* or *nourice* to the
present *nurse.* Through this evolution of the word, another dimension was added to its meaning: a woman who cares for and tends
young children.

4

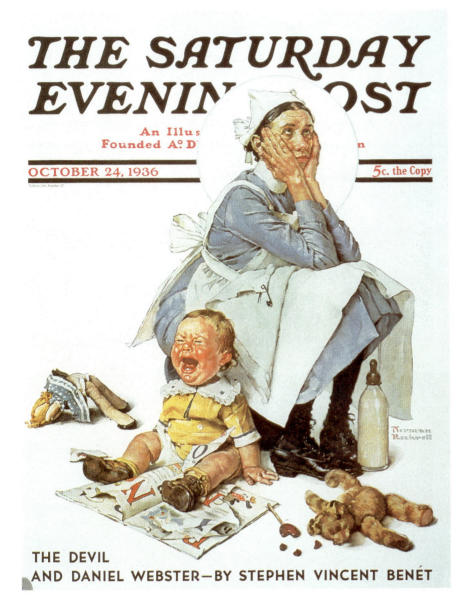

THE SATURDAY EVENING POST

An Illus
Founded A°D

OCTOBER 24, 1936

5c. the Copy

THE DEVIL
AND DANIEL WEBSTER—BY STEPHEN VINCENT BENÉT

Norman Rockwell, THE NANNY, *October 24, 1936, cover of the* SATURDAY EVENING POST. *Courtesy of Curtis Publishing Company, Indianapolis, Indiana.*

The nurse was portrayed in a variety of ways while functioning in different roles. The "child nurse," "nursemaid," or "nanny" fulfilled an important role throughout history. A girl or woman was regularly employed to look after children through sickness and health. Rockwell capitalized on this practice.

Nurse has also been used as a verb, still having its original roots in the Latin *nutrire,* which meant to suckle and to nourish. Again the Latin word transferred into French as *nourir* ("to nourish") and into English as *nurshen, nourishen, norissen.* Abbreviated it became *nursh* and finally led to the present-day usage, to nurse. The meaning of both the noun and the verb continued to broaden to encompass more and more functions related to the care of all humanity. By the sixteenth century, meanings of the noun included "a person, but usually a woman, who waits upon or tends the sick." It was not until the eighteenth century that the meanings of the verb included "to wait upon or tend a person who is sick." During the nineteenth century two more components were added: the training of those who tend the sick and the carrying out of such duties under the supervision of a physician.

Although the aspect of nurturing has long been identified with nursing, it has been even more closely associated with education, particularly with respect to the rearing, training, and general upbringing of the young.

This accounts for the two kinds of helpers who appeared quite early in some households—child-nurses and sick-nurses. Sick-nurses became more closely associated with the healing arts and child-nurses with the teaching and training of children. Often, the two functions were combined.

Stewart and Austin, 1962, p. 4

The words *nursemaid* and *governess* thus emerged and became titles for the young girl or woman who functioned in the role of the child-nurse.

Unfortunately, the origin of the nurse as mother perpetuated the idea that nursing could be done only by women. The maternal instinct provided that strong impulse or motive necessary to care for those who were suffering or helpless. Women, because of their maternal instincts, were considered "born nurses." Consequently, the nurse as a loving mother who intuitively comforts and renders care continues to be a popular image. The parental instinct more accurately describes this strong motive and is present in both sexes of all races and within different age groups. It is, however, generally

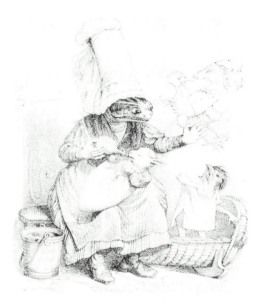

Grandville's illustration, I DID NOT MARRY TO BECOME A WET NURSE, *c. 1830–1840. From the book* GRANDVILLE'S ANIMALS *published by Thames and Hudson.*

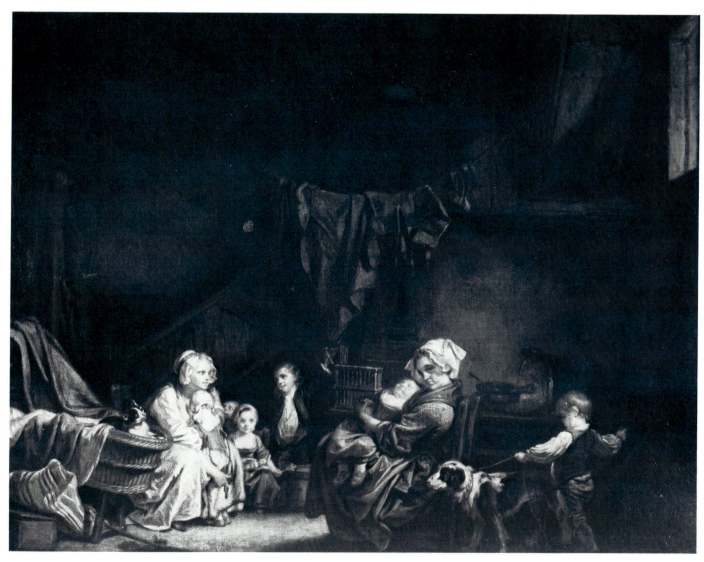

Jean-Baptiste Greuze, THE NURSEMAIDS, *late eighteenth century. Canvas, approx. 31.8 × 39.37 cm. Nelson-Atkins Museum of Art, Kansas City, Missouri (Nelson Fund).*

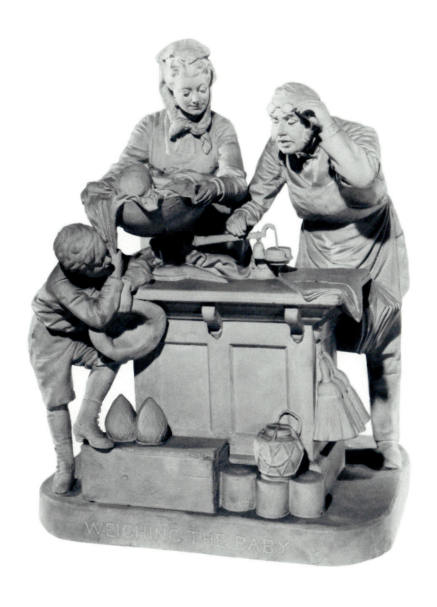

John Rogers, WEIGHING THE BABY, *1876.*
Approx. 50.8 cm high. Courtesy of the
New-York Historical Society, New York.

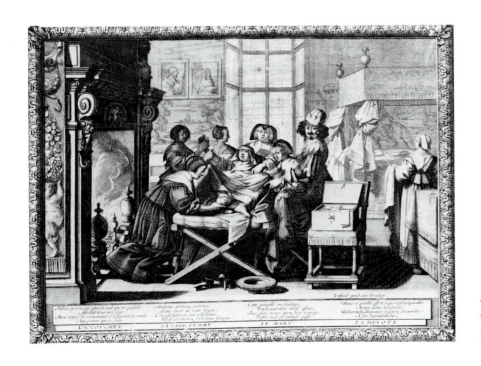

Abraham Bosse, L'ACCOUCHEMENT, *1633.*
Engraving, 26 × 33.7 cm. Philadelphia
Museum of Art: SmithKline Beckman
Corporation Fund.

7

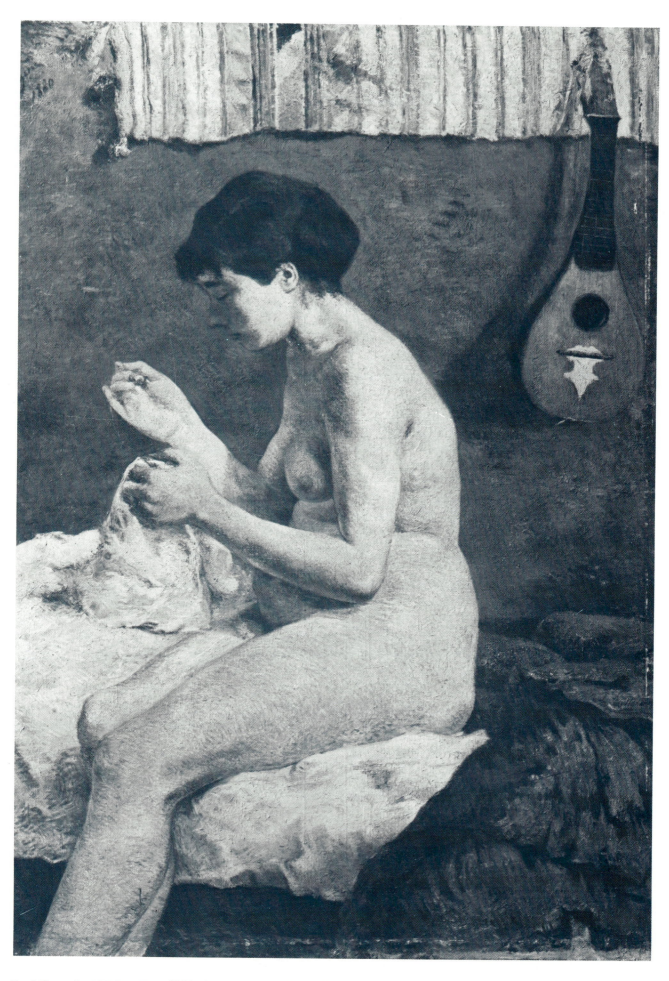

Paul Gauguin, NURSEMAID, *c. 1880. Canvas. Ny Carlsberg Glyptotek, Copenhagen, Denmark.*

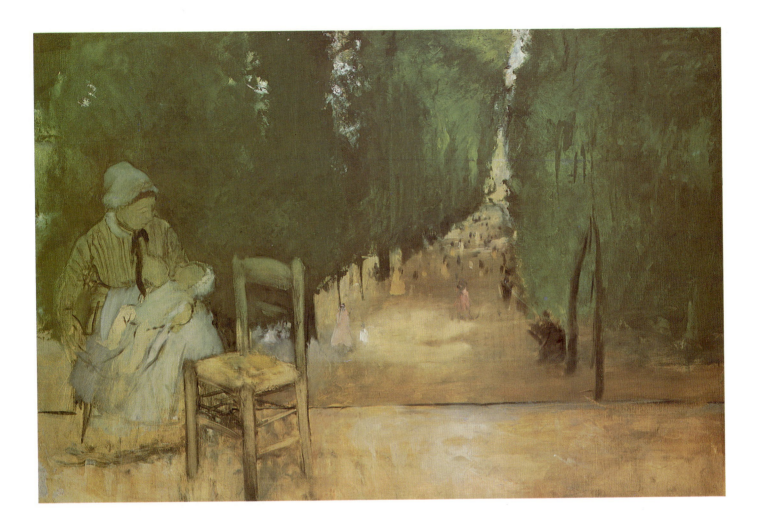

Edgar Degas, NURSEMAID IN THE LUXEMBOURG GARDENS, *c. 1871–72. Canvas. Musée Fabre, Montpellier, France. (Photo Claude O'Sughrue)*

thought that women possess a greater degree of this instinct because of their traditional role in the family, a position that has provided greater experiences in parental activities. Yet the timeless spirit of nursing contains no sexual boundaries. Human beings of both sexes have a natural tendency to respond to helplessness or to a threat to life from disease or injury. Men and women have functioned as nurses throughout various periods in history.

The role of the nurse gradually enlarged from that of a mother whose biological function included the nourishing of infants and the nurturing of young children to one with a much broader scope. Care of the sick, the aged, the helpless, the infirm, and the handicapped as well as promotion of health became vital components of the whole of nursing. In addition, "care" eventually encompassed affection, concern, and solitude, as well as responsibility for individuals in need. In the ancient periods the woman cared for her own kin. As the nursing concept broadened, she also took care of the members of her own tribe. With the development of early civilizations, slaves and servants of households and estates also received care and nursing began to be performed outside the home. As nursing care became more complex, it became apparent that factors other than a strong motive were necessary to do the work of a nurse. Yet this motivation continued to be a vital component of nursing's development and prompted one to care for the suffering or the helpless. In its fullest development it produced altruism or humanitarianism, the noblest forms of love and kindness. Compelling societal forces such as religious fervor reinforced this motive at different historical eras and paved the way for people to lead lives of service and self-sacrifice for the sake of others.

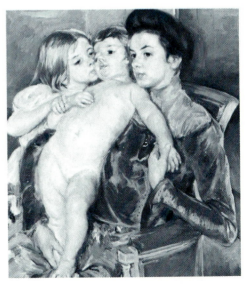

Mary Cassatt, THE CARESS, *1902. Canvas. National Museum of American Art, Smithsonian Institution, Washington, D.C., Gift of William T. Evans.*

9

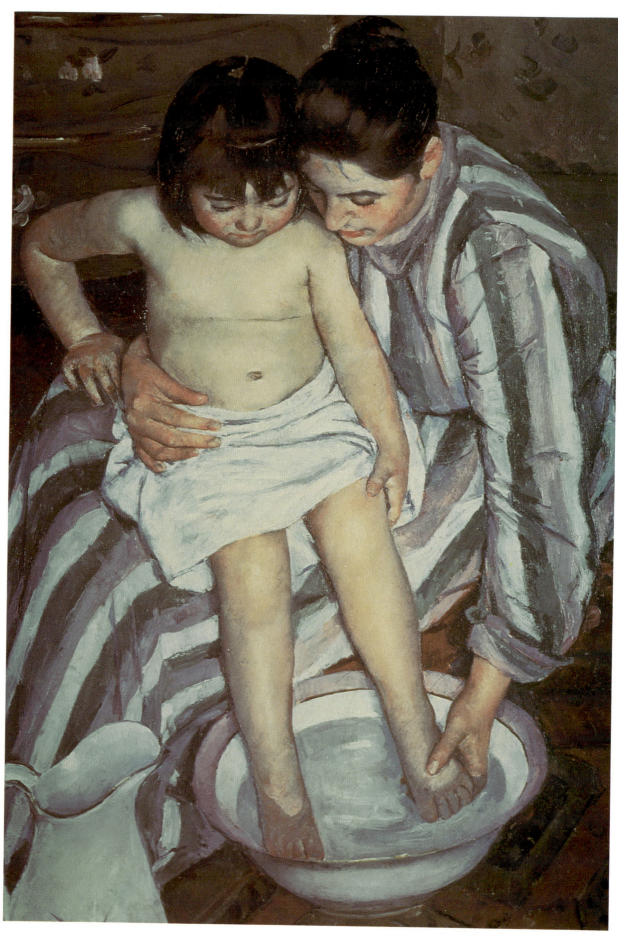

Mary Cassatt, THE BATH, *c. 1891. Canvas, 99.1 × 66 cm. Courtesy of The Art Institute of Chicago, Illinois, Robert A. Waller Fund.*

As time progressed, it became apparent that love and caring alone were not sufficient to nurture health or overcome disease. The development of nursing depended on two additional essential ingredients—skill and expertness, and knowledge. Great manual dexterity in the carrying out of specific procedures was evident even among primitive tribes and continued to be perfected through experience. As more and more information about illness and disease became available, emphasis on the necessity of knowledge began to emerge. Knowledge of facts and principles would provide the initiating force for nursing to become both an art and a science (Dock and Stewart, 1925). The head, the heart, and the hands became truly united to provide the strong foundation for modern-day nursing. These three essentials were also referred to as the science, spirit, and skill of nursing and, at still another point, became synonymous with the theoretical, practical, and moral/ethical aspects of nursing (Stewart, 1918, 1921). The neglect or overemphasis of any one of these would provide for an imbalance in care.

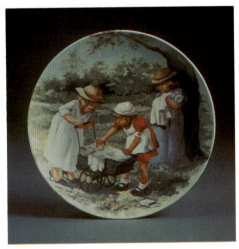

Limited edition collector's plate entitled OFFICE HOURS *in the* FRIENDS I REMEMBER *series by Jeanne Down. The Edwin M. Knowles China Company, Newell, West Virginia.*

The quote on the reverse side of the plate reads: "Playing nurse was one of my favorite games when I was growing up . . . We must have been pretty good at thinking up cures—we never lost a patient!"

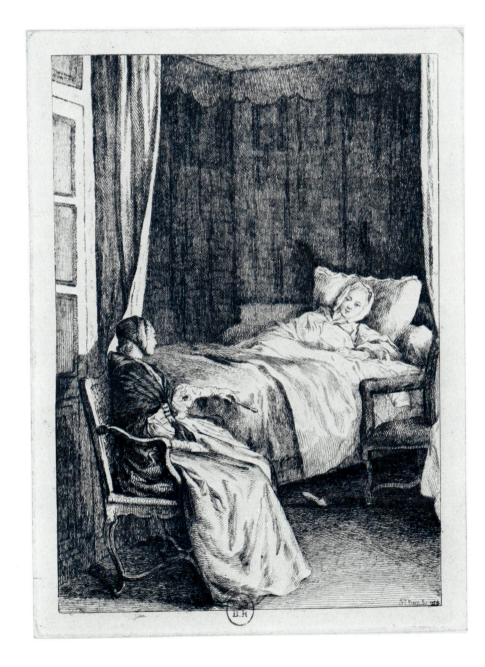

Richard Saint-Non, THE SICK WOMAN. *Bibliothèque Nationale, Paris, France.*

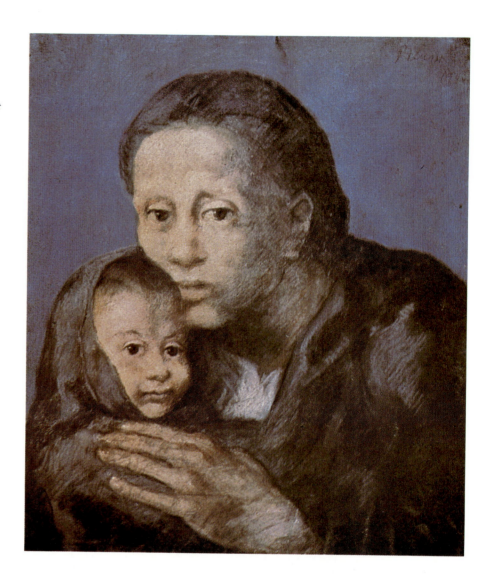

Pablo Picasso, THE SICK CHILD, *1903. Canvas. Museu Picasso, Barcelona, Spain. (c. SPADEM, Paris/VAGA, New York, 1984)*

The woman, and oftentimes mother, nourished and tended the child, the earliest role in nursing.

The concept of nursing that has been evolving throughout the ages has not yet reached its fullest maturity. It continues to grow and develop to include widening spheres of nursing service and practice and expanding functions. It can never, however, "rise higher than the human instruments by which it is administered and the resources they are able to draw upon in the culture of their age and their group" (Stewart and Austin, 1962, p. 10).

■ NURSING: THE SEED OF EARLY COMMUNITY SERVICE

Early in its history, nursing can be distinguished as a form of early community service. This service was originally related to a strong instinct for preservation and protection of the tribe and its members. Love and concern for family and tribe extended to neighbors and strangers. One rudimentary way to assist with this effort was through the nursing of individuals who became ill. As more sophisticated civilizations developed, the care of the sick expanded to include concern for other human conditions. Methods for dealing with problems such as poverty, prevention of disease, and any type of helplessness added a social dimension to the nursing work. Those functions com-

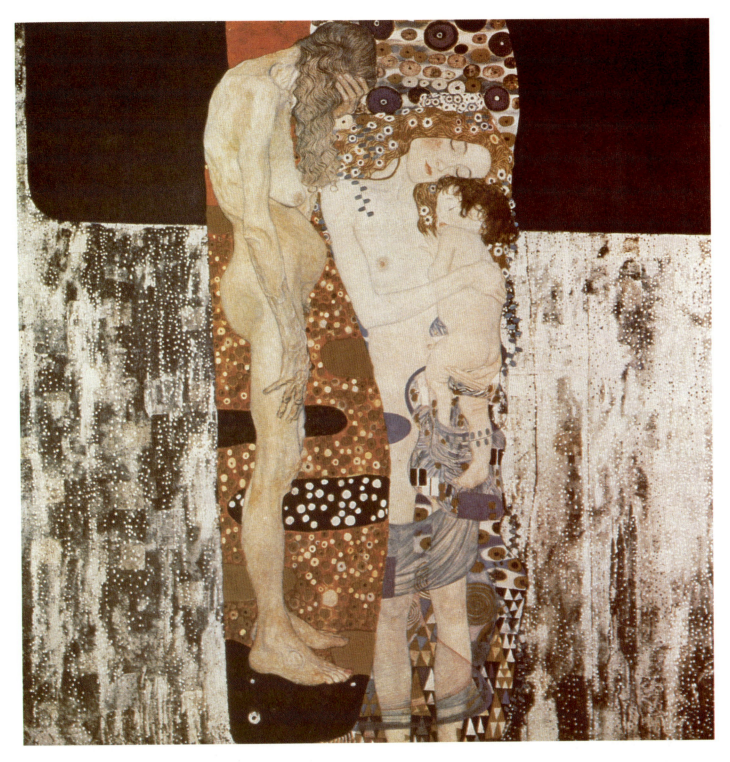

Gustav Klimt, THE THREE AGES OF MAN, *1905. Canvas, 182.9 × 182.9 cm. Galleria Nazionale d'Arte Moderna, Rome, Italy.*

monly associated with present-day social workers were incorporated into the role of the nurse. Historically, the nurse and social worker were one. This phenomenon continued until another group of workers was trained to handle the problems associated with the social ills of society. Even then, as now, nurses were still in a sense true social workers, constantly battling adverse social conditions directly affecting the health and welfare of society.

When we consider the whole movement of social progress—the breaking down of the spirit of hatred and prejudice, the promotion of kindlier and more humane relations between human beings, the organization of practical and effective measures

13

for reducing human suffering and distress—it would be hard to find any group of workers, who have contributed more to the sum total of social effort.

Dock and Stewart, 1925, pp. 374–375

During specific periods this sense of community was influenced by waves of religious awakening, ideals of chivalry, patriotism and democracy, and social and humanitarian efforts. In these instances nursing combined with other available branches of charitable aid and kindness. The religious influence, however, was probably the strongest. For long periods nursing was regarded as a calling that could be done only by those who renounced the world. This intensely religious motive, combined with the element of self-sacrifice, provided an excellent qualification for assuming the nursing role.

Concern for the health of the public or the community was evident in antiquity and continued as civilizations developed. Nearly all primitive tribes fostered some type of sanitary practices in order that the environment would not be tainted. These elementary practices became more sophisticated as technological advances occurred and provided for improvements such as water drainage systems. Eventually concern broadened to include disease and its communicability and an overall emphasis on health.

Jean-Honoré Fragonard, THE HAPPY FAMILY, *after 1769. Canvas, approx. 54 × 64.8 cm. National Gallery of Art, Washington, D.C., Timken Collection 1959.*

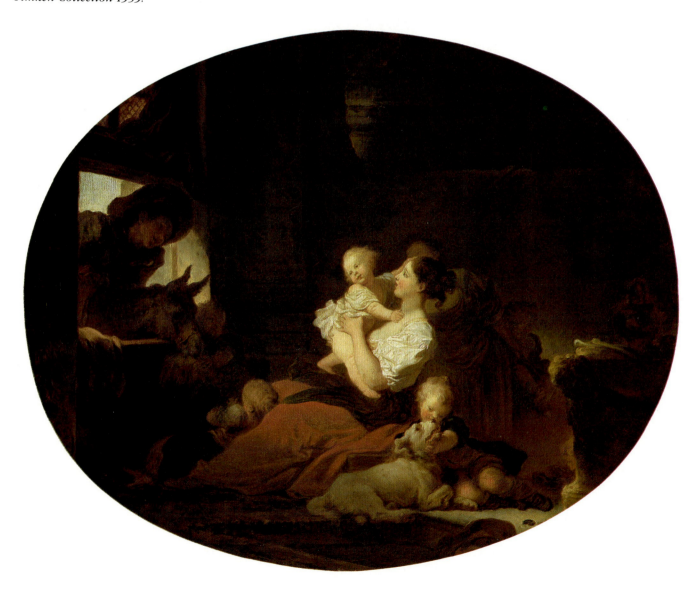

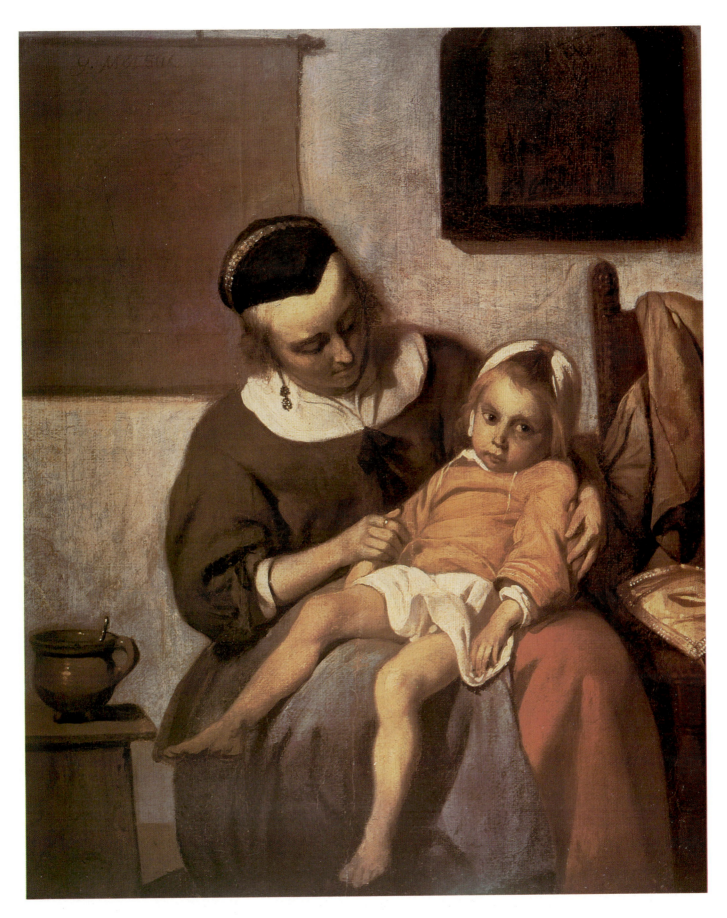

Gabriel Metsu, THE SICK CHILD, *c. 1660. Canvas. Rijksmuseum, Amsterdam, Netherlands.*

Nursing is a development of the mother-care of the young, which has existed from the earliest of times.

15

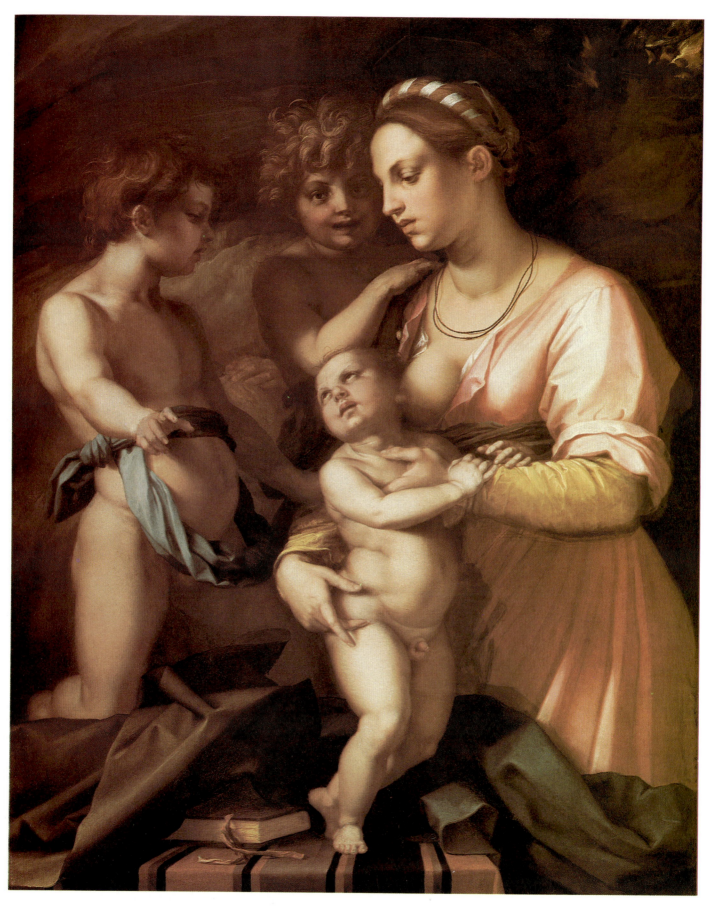

Andrea del Sarto, CHARITY, before 1530. Wood, 120 × 92.7 cm. National Gallery of Art, Washington, D.C., Samuel H. Kress Collection 1957.

From its inception, nursing was involved in this social movement, even in that period when nursing care was integrated as part of the practice of medicine men, priests, wise women, and midwives. Service to the community as well as to the individuals within it was readily incorporated into a basic conception of nursing that included both health and illness. These early roots of public health became a prominent aspect of the nursing role and ultimately provided a variety of community services to achieve this goal. Branches of public service evolved as extensions of nursing and extended into the innermost structures of society. Visiting nurses, school nurses, public health nurses (an older term for community health nurses), nursing settlements, and other facets of community service emerged to become forever a vital and necessary component of nursing.

■ CARE OF THE SICK AMONG PRIMITIVE PEOPLE

It is possible that some of the first ideas related to medical treatment and nursing care were acquired through the observation of animals. Although it may be difficult for some to consider that simple medical and nursing procedures were prehuman in origin, support for this premise exists in natural history. The first traces of parental love, kindness, and mutual aid were exhibited by birds and other animals. The lower animals in particular subjected themselves to appropriate medical and surgical treatment when necessary, treated themselves when injured or ill, and assisted one another (Berdoe, 1893).

Primitive man, in order to escape the ravages of illness and disease, needed to learn to protect himself and find means of treatment and cure. During this period of history man was much closer to nature and moved throughout the animal kingdom with minimal fear. He was able to readily observe and learn the animal practices associated with ailments. Even animals attempted to relieve pain and to remove the causes of infection. Animals cleansed their wounds by licking, ate grasses, leaves, and other plant life, which acted as emetics and purgatives, submerged inflamed wounds in water, and engaged in other practices that had significant effects on their well-being.

It was not possible for primitive man to find a treatment for every illness through this observational process. Nor was he able to detect more than the most obvious natural circumstances leading to illness by using such a system. Yet, instinctively aware that other causal factors of diseases existed, man turned to searching for these additional explanations. Close intimacy with nature, however, colored his ideas about myriad forms of life, of which he had no scientific knowledge. Man ascribed to all such forms those qualities he identified within himself. All natural objects—rocks, rivers, trees, mountains, the wind—were alive, or animate, and possessed a spirit or soul (psyche, anima). Natural phenomena, including those causing disaster or disease, could thus be explained. This basic belief in *animism* unlocked the door to a still greater world in the minds of men, that of imagination.

The introduction of a belief in spirits, good and evil, profoundly affected the development of those practices related to treatments

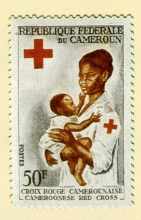

The Federal Republique du Cameroun, on the west coast of Africa, honored its Croix Rouge (Red Cross) with a set of two stamps in 1965. One shows a Red Cross station and ambulance. The companion stamp illustrated here honors Red Cross nurses. Courtesy of Howard B. Hurley.

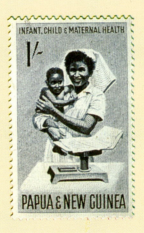

This 1964 stamp issued by Papua & New Guinea pictures nurse and child. Entitled INFANT, CHILD AND MATERNAL HEALTH, the stamp publicizes the territorial health service. Courtesy of Howard B. Hurley.

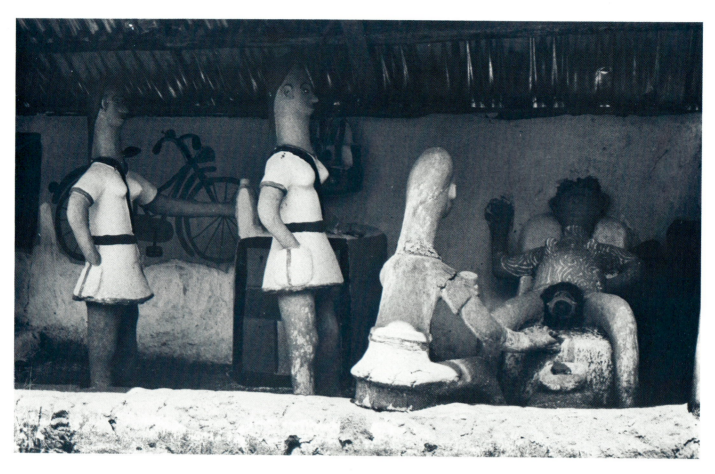

African, Ibo (Near) Oweri, E. Nigeria, Mbari House, MODERN BIRTH SCENE, *1966–67. Courtesy of Herbert M. Cole.*

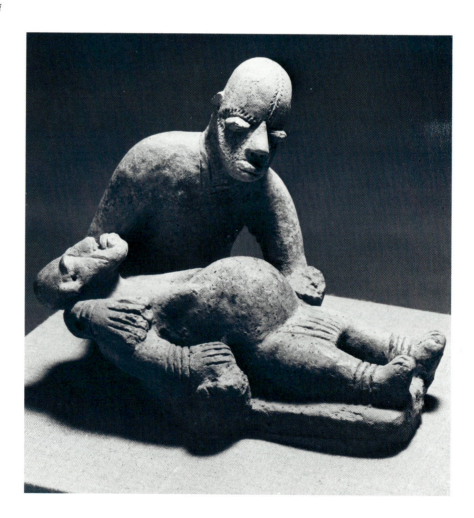

West Africa, Mali, Djenne Culture, MATERNITY SCENE, *c.* AD *1200. Earthenware and paint, approx. 21 cm high. St. Louis Art Museum, St. Louis.*

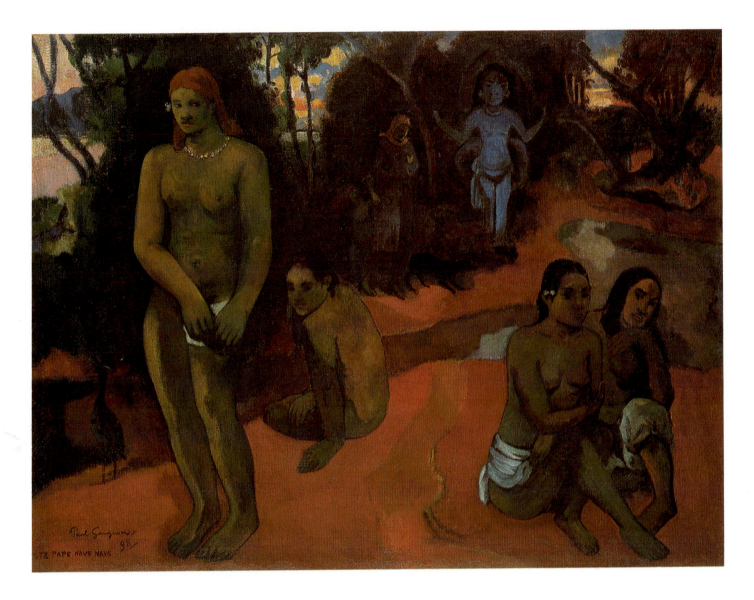

and remedies. Ideas of an occult nature, superstitions, became tightly linked to the etiology of diseases because supernatural origins for most happenings, including illness, were accepted by primitive man. Since man lived in two worlds—the visible and the invisible—a combination of occult practices and empirical ones occurred and provided the necessary climate for the use of magic. The supernatural world could and did affect primitive man.

Since the cause of illness and disease was attributed to evil spirits, cures were attempted through intervention with these spirits. Consequently, a great body of tribal lore arose, which included incantations, rites, rituals, and spells. In time, certain types of symptoms were ascribed to the work of particular spirits and means of driving them away were devised. The primary goal was to make the patient's body an unpleasant dwelling place for the spirit. This was accomplished through the use of various techniques, some of which were the basis for many current practices. Repeated pummeling and pounding of the inhabited area of the body was done to dislodge the evil spirit. (It is possible that the practice of massage originated from this technique.) Plants that had unpleasant effects were used to make concoctions that would be disagreeable to the spirits. Expulsion could occur in two ways, through the intestinal tract or through the mouth, and so appropriate herbs, which acted as either purgatives or

19

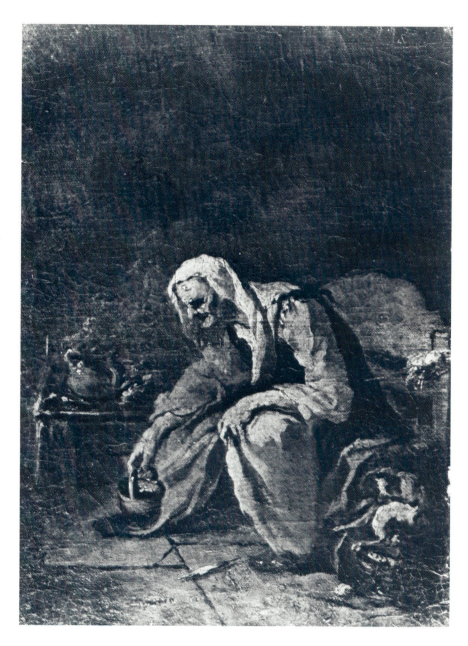

emetics, were chosen and administered. Evil spirits lodged in the head were to be released through holes in the skull. Trephined skulls of primitive peoples give evidence of this extreme measure. Fire, hot instruments, and blistering appliances were used as counterirritants to burn out the spirits. Cold baths, sweating, starvation, bad smells, and hideous noises were all used in the attempt to expel demons from the suffering body.

The magical lore that accumulated became too complex to be understood by the ordinary tribesmen. Chosen individuals who supposedly had special insight or intimate contact with the spirits devoted their time to mastering and interpreting this lore for the benefit of the tribe. These men, and sometimes women, usually went through a long and arduous training period. In addition, they might have lived through some mystical experience, spent weeks alone in fellowship with the spirits, or recovered from a critical illness or injury. In time, these "medicine men," "witch doctors," or "shamans" became the guardians and disseminators of this esoteric knowledge and skill. More importantly, their possession of life-giving powers

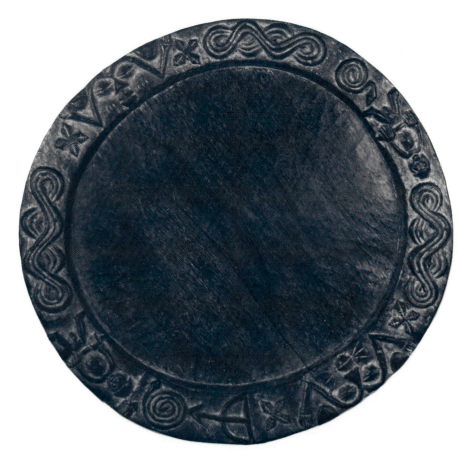

African, Guinea Coast, Yoruba, DIVINA-TION TRAY. *Wood, 3.8 × 54.6 cm in diameter. The University of Iowa Museum of Art, Iowa City, The Stanley Collection.*

Wooden trays called "awua ifa" are used in traditional Yoruba divination cere-monies. The tray, in conjunction with the divination tapper, is used to summon the god Ifa.

granted them a place of prestige, and they were set apart from and above the rest of the tribe. "Here was the beginning of specialization in the art of healing" (Shryock, 1959).

The healer was primarily concerned with occult lore and pro-cedures, although he undoubtedly became an authority on tribal folk medicine. In most instances the problem was not to give the illness a name but to find a cure. Consequently, this required that a magical cause be identified in order to overcome the malady. The healer was also faced with another aspect of the occult related to the cure of disease or dispelling of misfortune. He had to develop the ability to use his magic in an evil or a good way. The use of these two separate functions gave rise to a system of black magic and white magic. White magic invoked the help of good spirits to drive off evil ones and was practiced for benevolent purposes. Black magic, hostile and destruc-tive in its aims, was used to bring disaster or disease upon enemies. This was accomplished with the aid of evil spirits, poisons, and malice.

These practices were organized into ritualistic ceremonies that eventually assumed a religious tone. The result of this union was the labeling of the medicine man as a "holy person." Primitive medicine became a mixture of magic, religion, and naturalistic remedies. Ac-cording to some sources, the medicine man became the priest-phy-sician (Jamieson and Sewall, 1950; Dolan, Fitzpatrick, and Hermann, 1983). Other authors subscribe to a belief in the development of higher and lower ranks among healers, with the priest-physician being the highest (Dock and Stewart, 1925; Stewart and Austin, 1962), or to the idea that it is unclear whether primitives made dis-

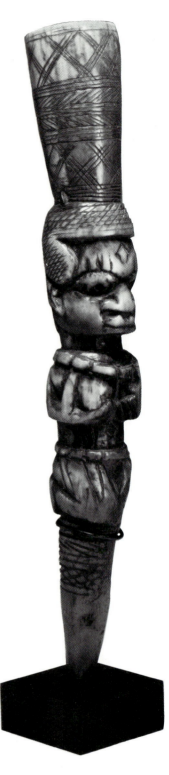

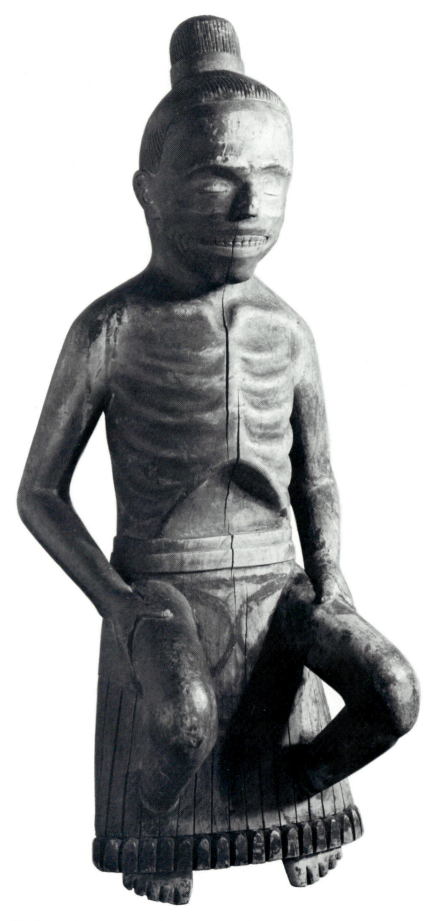

African, Guinea Coast, Yoruba, DIVINA-
TION TAPPER. *Ivory, approx. 25.4 cm high.
The University of Iowa Museum of Art,
Iowa City, The Stanley Collection.*

*The divination tappers are used by the
diviner priest to attract the attention
of the god Ifa. The fecundity symbols of
kneeling women holding their breasts are
the most common ornamentations on
the tappers. The Yoruba have no fertility
god, and many of the clients of the
diviner priest are women seeking to bear
children.*

Northwest Coast Indian, British Columbia, Haida Tribe, SHAMAN CARVING,
*c. 1880. Alder wood and paint, approx. 54.6 cm high. St. Louis Art
Museum, St. Louis, Purchase Fund.*

22

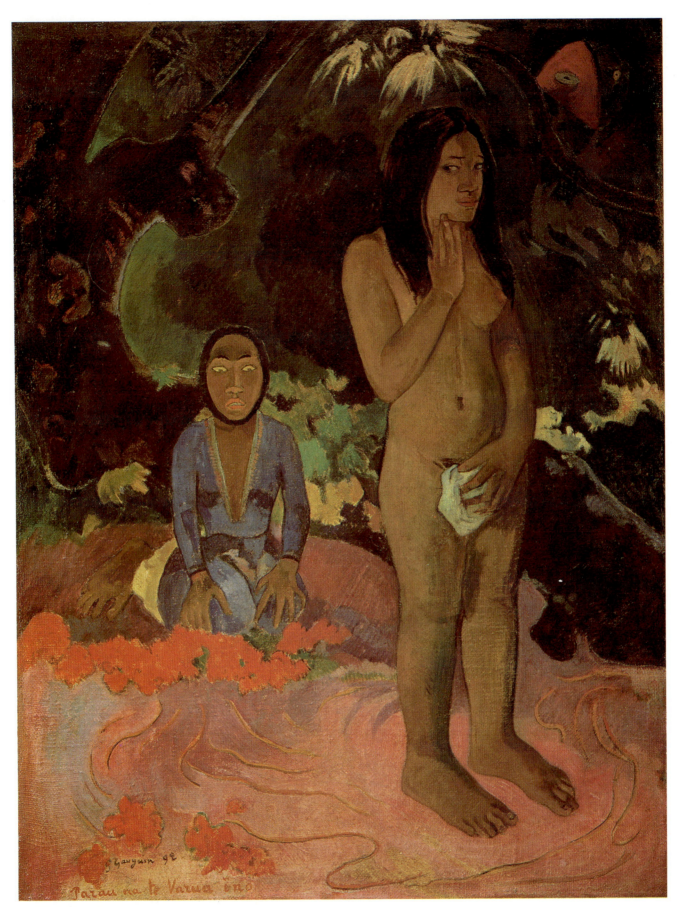

Paul Gauguin, WORDS OF THE DEVIL, *c. 1892. Canvas, approx. 91.4 × 68.6 cm. National Gallery of Art, Washington, D.C., Gift of the W. Averell Harriman Foundation in memory of Marie N. Harriman 1972.*

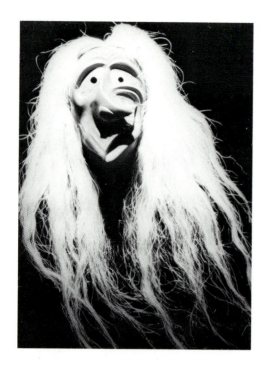

Elon Webster, FALSE FACE MASK, *1957. Wood. Cranbrook Academy of Science, Bloomfield Hills, Michigan.*

Iroquois peoples carved expressionistic masks for use by the False Face Society, whose ceremonies healed physical and psychological sickness and cleansed whole communities of destructive impurities.

tinctions between priests and medicine men (Shryock, 1959). What is clear, however, is that both types of healers dealt with problems of life and death and were authorities on traditional lore.

The omnipotence of these early healers was supported by the use of strange disguises, elaborate ceremonies, mystical signs, charms (amulets and talismen), and fetishes. Skins, hoofs of animals, feathers, grasses, horns, and other objects adorned the ceremonial garb. Extreme drama and mystery kept the observers in awe of the medicine man. The ceremonies might last for hours or days and often included dancing, singing, and playing of instruments. The medicine man's ability to frighten off evil spirits was demonstrated by these props. As late as the 1830s, an account of a medicine man's actual procedures was rendered:

> . . . his body and head were entirely covered with the skin of a yellow bear, the head of which (his own head being inside of it) served as a mask; the huge claws of which also, were dangling on his wrists and ankles; in one hand he shook a frightful rattle, and in the other brandished his medicine spear or magic wand; to the rattling din and discord of all of which, he added the wild and startling jumps and yelps of the Indian, and the horrid and appalling grunts, and snarls, and growls of the grizzly bear, in ejaculatory and gutteral incantations to the Good and Bad Spirits, in behalf of his patient; who was rolling and groaning in the agonies of death, whilst he was dancing around him, jumping over him, and pawing him about, and rolling him in every direction.
>
> *Catlin, 1926, p. 46*

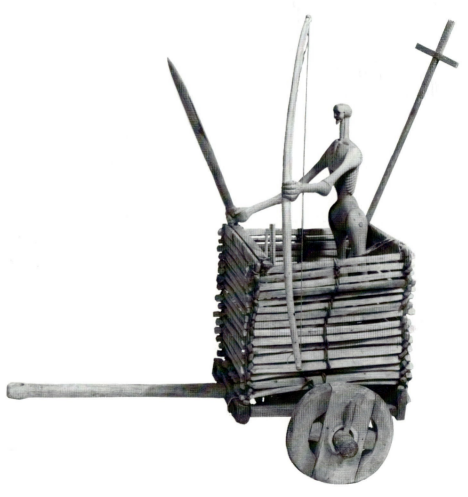

José Dolores Lopez, Cordova, New Mexico, DEATH CART, *c. 1930. Carved cottonwood. St. Louis Art Museum, St. Louis, Gift of the May Department Stores Company.*

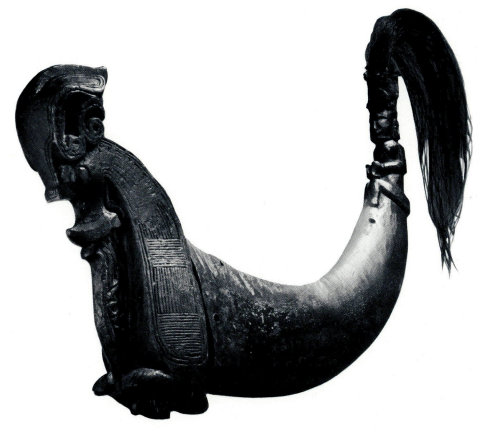

As the caste of medicine men developed, a class of practitioners became associated with them. These individuals, most often the women of the tribe, applied the treatments, ascertained the qualities of drugs, became skillful in dressing wounds, and learned to reduce fevers. Theirs was a practical knowledge of appliances and drugs. These tribal women were the discoverers of medical herbs; they were the first empirical physicians who learned to prepare different potions to be used as remedies (Mason, 1894). Some of these women, particularly the elderly, must have been the earliest prototypes of the so-called witch. These "wise women," who were extremely knowledgeable about medicinal secrets, and who went out early and late to gather herbs, became prominent as caretakers for the sick through prehistoric ages (Alexander, 1782). In time, as a result of superstitious feelings, wise women, or witches, were credited with uncanny powers that were both good and evil, particularly the ability to cause illness and wasting diseases. Eventually, this belief led to the persecution of perhaps the first rivals of the medicine men (Dock and Stewart, 1925). Many similar superstitions still exist today in isolated communities.

The exact relationship between the practical attendants (nurses) and the medicine men or priest-physicians is not clearly understood. If the attendant received orders for the treatment of the patient from the medicine man, the relationship was probably that of physician and nurse. If the attendant prescribed the simple treatments and herbs and the medicine man limited his work to incantations, the relationship could have been the symbolic representation of the combination of the theory and practice of medicine. The latter would be indicative of the yet unspecialized department of nursing (Nutting and Dock, 1937). It is also possible that some rivalry began to occur as the struggle for a monopoly of power began to emerge.

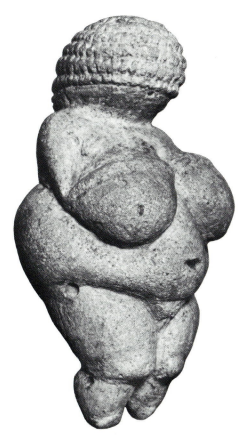

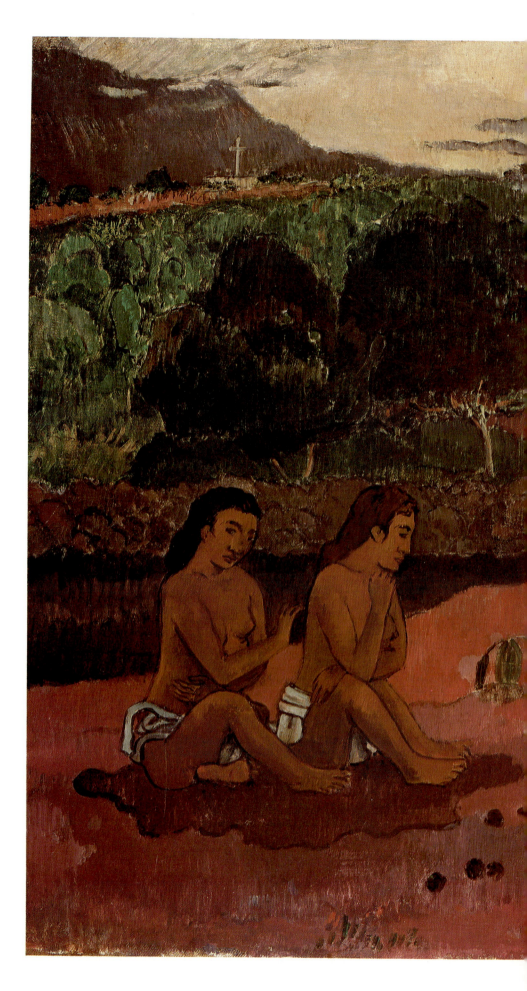

Paul Gauguin, THE INVOCATION, *1903. Canvas, approx. 66 × 76.2 cm. National Gallery of Art, Washington, D.C., Gift from the Collection of John and Louise Booth in memory of their daughter, Winkie, 1976.*

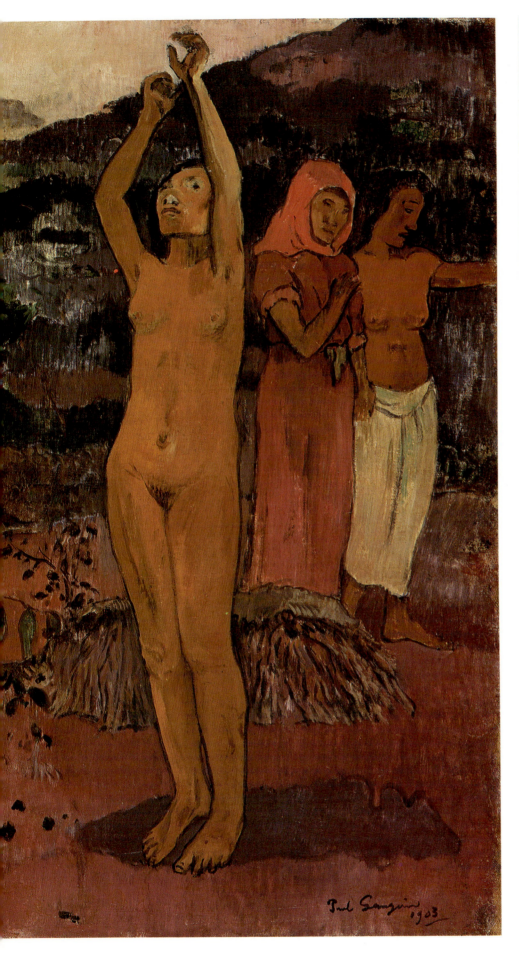

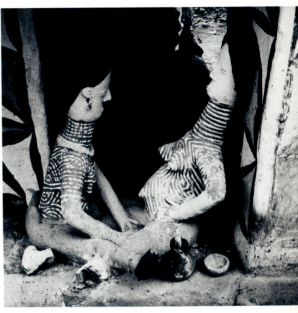

African, Ibo (Near) Oweri, E. Nigeria, Mbari House, TRADITIONAL BIRTH SCENE, *1966–67. Courtesy of Herbert M. Cole.*

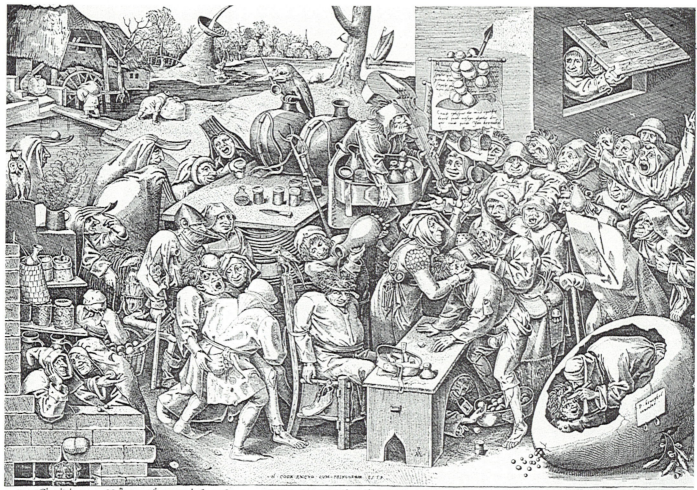

Ghy lieden van Mallegem wilt nu wel fyn gesint
Ick Vrou Hexe wil hier oock wel worden bemint

Om v te genesen ben ick gecomen hier
Tuwen dienste, met myn onder meesterssen fier

Compt vry den meesten met den minsten sonder verbeyen
Hebdy de wesp int hooft, oft loteren v de keyen.

Pieter Bruegel the Elder, WITCHES OF
MALLEGHEM, *1559. Engraving. From the*
GRAPHIC WORLDS OF PETER BRUEGEL THE
ELDER *by H.A. Klein, 1963 Dover Publica-*
tions, New York.

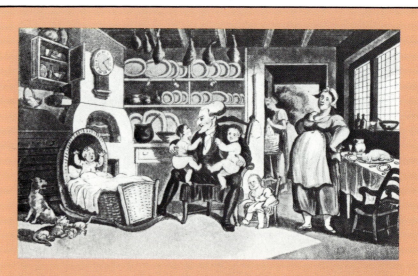

DR. SYNTAX TURNED NURSE, *c. 1820. Aquatint after a drawing by Thomas*
Rowlandson. From the THIRD TOUR OF DR. SYNTAX: IN SEARCH OF A WIFE.
British Library, London, England. Scene when Dr. Syntax sheltered from
a coming storm

"*within the comfortable farm*",
"*Himself and the good dame to please,*
He took the children on his knees;
Then danc'd the urchins to and fro, And sung as nurses often do."

28

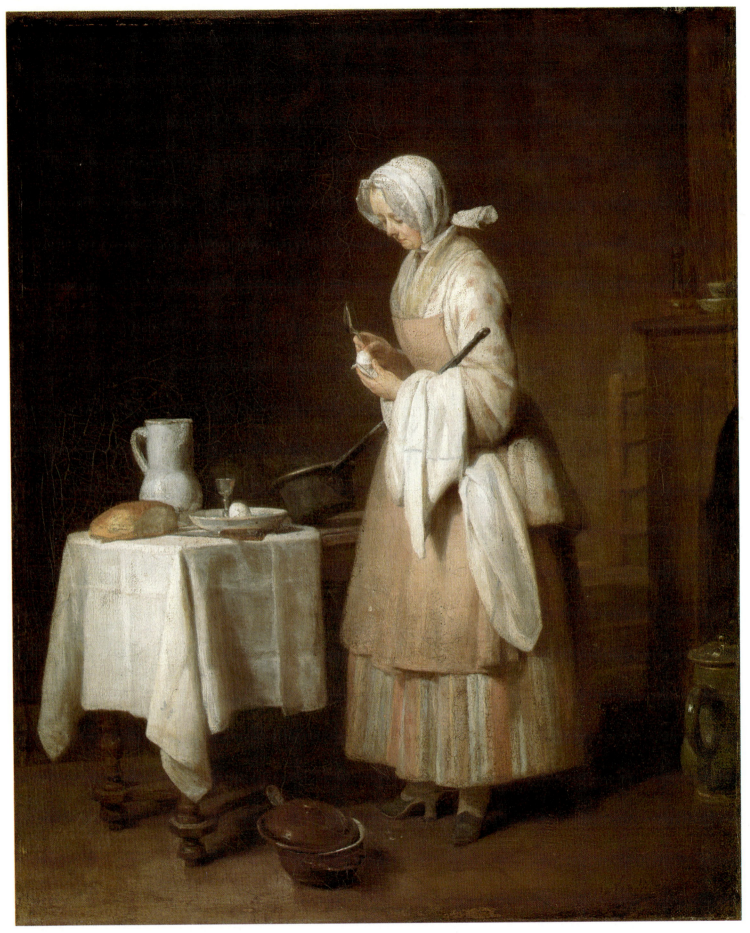

Jean-Baptiste-Siméon Chardin, THE ATTENTIVE NURSE, *c. 1738. Canvas. National Gallery of Art, Washington, D.C., Samuel H. Kress Collection 1952.*

The attentive nurse gives special consideration to the needs, desires, and comfort of patients. The nurse is mindful, observant, and receptive in the process of caring.

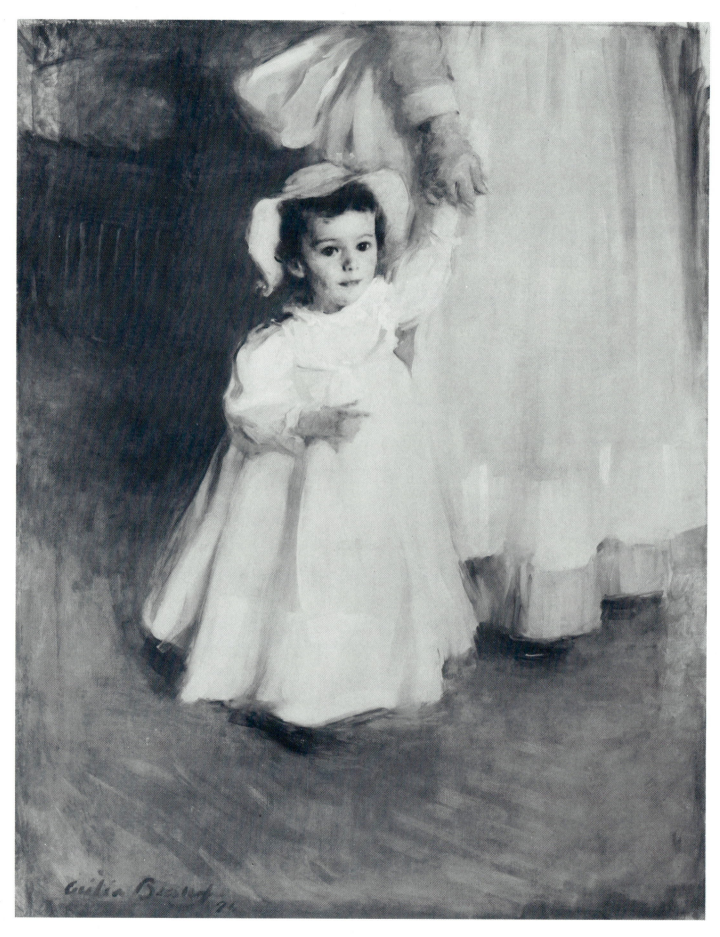

Cecilia Beaux, ERNESTA *(Child with Nurse), 1894. Canvas, approx. 128.3 × 96.5 cm.* *The Metropolitan Museum of Art, New York, Maria DeWitt Jesup Fund, 1965.*

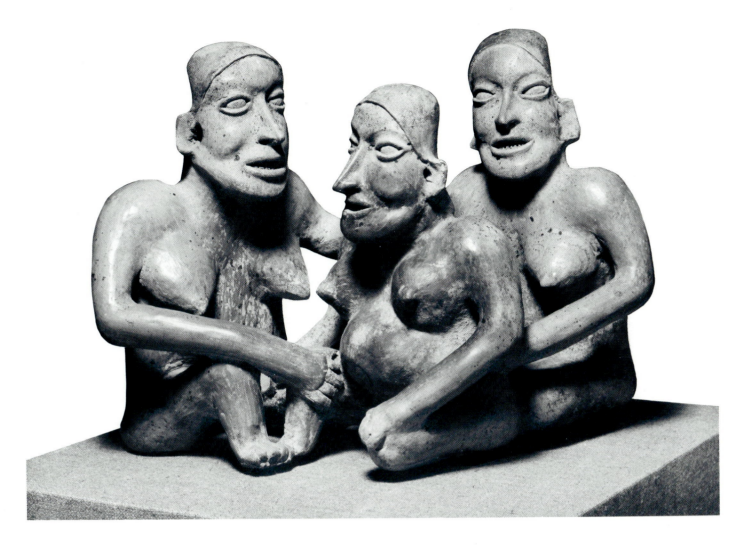

The individuals who provided rudimentary nursing probably varied with the customs of each group or tribe. These practical tasks were first, however, the work of mothers and wives. This naturally occurred as a result of the division of labor: men hunted for the food and provided the defense for the tribe; women cared for the children and eventually for those individuals afflicted by disease, age, injury, or other incapacitating conditions. As knowledge increased, others became specialists in specific areas of medical work.

Primitive societies sowed the seeds of hygiene, sanitation, and public health as well as medicine, surgery, psychiatry, midwifery, nursing, and other branches of the healing arts. Within this structure, nursing's heritage was derived. The role of the nurse as mother, the concept of nursing as a feminine occupation, and the expansion of nursing to include people who were not related emerged and became a vital part of society. The interrelationship, yet separation, of the medical practitioner and the nursing practitioner was established.

West Mexico, Jalisco, PREGNANT WOMAN AND MIDWIFE GROUP, *Terminal Preclassic 200 BC–AD 300. Polished gray earthenware, 21.6 cm high, 20.3 cm in length. St. Louis Art Museum, St. Louis, Gift of Morton D. May.*

31

Human history has moved in a series of stages as we have tried to understand the world around us. The first views we know about attributed to invisible spirits all the inexplicable things that happened. The spirits could not be dominated; they had to be placated. Later, the idea of a multitude of animate spirits was transformed into a vision of gods and goddesses with more-or-less human forms and superhuman attributes. They were not indifferent to people. They could reward and punish. Then came the idea of a single godhead, a unity of man and nature.

Flora Lewis

ANCIENT CIVILIZATIONS

The earliest thoughts of primitive man were simple yet complex. Primitive man personified all that he saw in nature, believed that the phenomena of nature were his greatest mysteries, developed mystic rites around the treatment and cure of illnesses and the preservation of health. These historic facts and the intimate and universal connection between religion and medicine led to a logical belief that was to permeate the majority of the ancient civilizations.

Nature worship became the basic principle upon which the mythologies and religions of the ancient civilizations were founded. The belief in evil spirits as causes of disease progressed to a belief that disease was caused by a failure to do things that the gods wished or by some moral transgression (Goodnow, 1942). Thus illness was a curse, a punishment set forth by the gods and directed at individuals, families and their descendants, and sinners. The many gods of ancient times "were all originally nature gods, or simply external forces of nature or attributes of the physical and intellectual man symbolised and personified" (Nutting and Dock, 1937, p. 26). Legends and myths of deities who watched over health and had powers over life and death were composed and cultivated by nations. This served to bring some order out of the old confusion about innumerable demons associated with the earlier magical medicine. Fewer beings now needed to be appeased. Furthermore, traditions of worship and methods for requesting divine aid for the sick were established. Frequently temples were built to these gods, and they became temples for healing and, ultimately, sanctuaries for the sick.

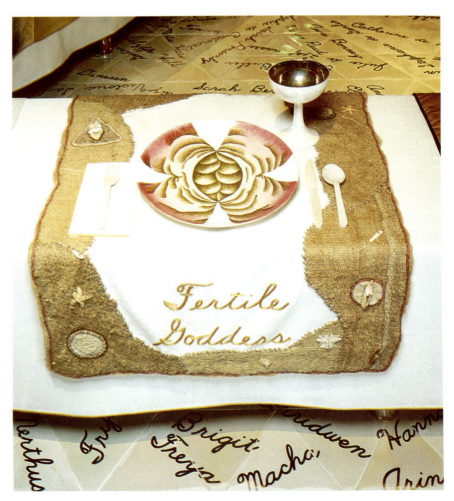

Judy Chicago, "Fertile Goddess," plate from THE DINNER PARTY, *1979. China-painted porcelain, 35.6 cm diameter. Through the Flower, Benicia, California.*

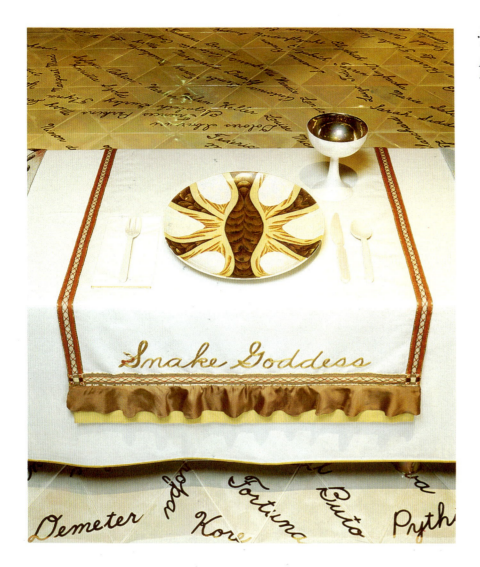

Judy Chicago, "Snake Goddess," plate from
THE DINNER PARTY, *1979. China-painted*
porcelain, 35.6 cm diameter. Through the
Flower, Benicia, California.

The manner of life followed by primitive tribes led to constant changes in their location. These nomadic people naturally followed the presence of food, tending to migrate toward the south, where warmth, rich soil, and vegetative growth made it possible to live with less effort and a greater degree of comfort. Evolutionary improvements such as the development of tools (Stone Age) followed by the incorporation of the use of several metals (Iron Age) occurred along with the domestication of plants and animals. These advances paved the way for tribesmen to settle down as herdsmen and farmers and to supplant the roving life with village life. Slowly, in certain fertile areas, civilization began to develop.

It is generally believed that the movement of these tribes radiated from the interior of Europe and Asia toward the warm shores of the Mediterranean Sea, India, and China. Migration of a much lesser degree evolved in the direction of western Europe and the British Isles. In most instances movement followed the shores of great rivers.

> The early civilizations on which that of the modern western world is based, were those of the eastern Mediterranean area. In Egypt, Syria, Mesopotamia, and even further east in India, oriental peoples developed cultures of a high order long before anything similar appeared in most parts of the world.
>
> *Shryock, 1959, p. 19*

35

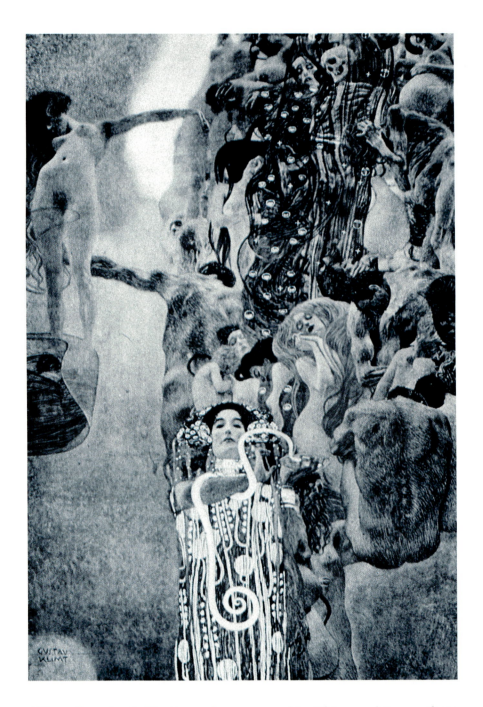

Although early civilizations also appeared in China and Japan, these exerted little influence upon the Western world as a result of limited contact.

Regions bordering on the Mediterranean Sea came to form the greater part of the known world. This body of water was believed to occupy the center of the earth, as its name implies. Consequently, all areas to the east of the Mediterranean Sea became known as "eastern"; those to the west became known as "western" (Jamieson and Sewall, 1950).

The cultural patterns in these early centers of civilization exhibited an interdependence of religion, government, social welfare, and health. As in primitive tribal societies, magic, superstition, and early forms of religion were used to control the forces of nature when other measures were ineffectual. Through the use of magic and superstition government authority was enforced, property disputes were settled, woman's place was determined, social welfare was secured, and disease and injury were cured. Justice and charity toward the poor, the weak, and the sick were taught in some cultures. Human sacrifices might be demanded and mutilation of the body was not encouraged.

By 3000 BC or soon thereafter an advanced civilization had developed in the Near East. Buildings were constructed in brick and stone; the arch, wheel, and plow were in use; a calendar had been invented; and writing made possible the preservation of records. From this time until the fall of Rome, conventionally dated as AD 476, great kingdoms and vast empires were established, extended, and overthrown in constant shifts of power from one people to another. At different periods and in different areas many forms of government appeared. In some, the ruler's control was absolute; in others, it was restricted by custom or by the religion of the people.

Sellew and Nuesse, 1946, p. 32

Religious beliefs and myths were the foundations for medical practice in early civilizations. Thus religious leaders were originally given the responsibility for curing and treating the sick and the in-

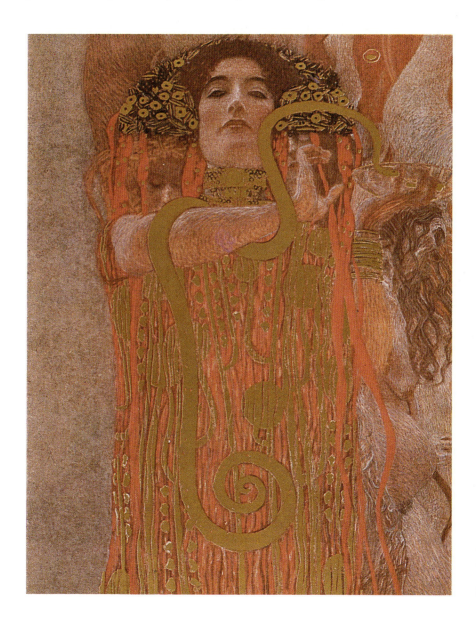

Gustav Klimt, "Hygeia," detail from MEDICINE, *c. 1907. From* ART IN VIENNA 1898–1918 *by Peter Vergo, 1975 Phaidon Press Limited Publication, Oxford, England.*

37

jured. As time progressed, two ideas regarding the cause of illness became accepted: illness was caused by the displeasure of the gods; all illnesses were the result of natural causes. A dualism, the first step in the transition that medicine needed to make from the magical to the rational, was thus exhibited. Rational observations and treatments were preceded and followed by religious chants and rites to ensure a cure. With the development of empirical knowledge, health care was delegated to priest-physicians and eventually to secular physicians. The latter development occurred primarily in Greek and Roman civilizations. This evolution resulted in the development of significant medical contributions (special procedures, biological sciences, diagnostic measures, classification of diseases, and observation recording) that began to transform medicine from magic into a science.

A search throughout ancient history reveals little, however, about attendants to the sick—nurses. This may be so because of the fact that unusual or striking events rather than ordinary ones are generally recorded in history. People have always nursed their sick as a matter of course. It was not until cities became large and problems became acute that the matter of care in illness warranted specific mention. Yet one can be reasonably sure that nurses, male or female, functioned in early civilization. From earliest times the midwife has been accepted in her role during childbirth, as has the child's nurse. Slaves, attendants, and women of good character probably cared for those with curable conditions.

> Priestesses are believed to have performed many functions now recognized as those of the nurse, for, in the temple, man's first center of community thought and activity, is disclosed the nucleus of his religious education, medicine, and nursing.
>
> *Jamieson and Sewall, 1950, p. 52*

Indeed, the beliefs, mores, and culture of each civilization directly influenced the way in which nursing care was given. In addition, who rendered nursing care and what constituted nursing care were reflections of the prevailing society.

■ THE NEAR EAST

Egypt

One of the first civilizations to emerge clearly from barbarism was that of Egypt. The very long, narrow valley on either side of the Nile River comprised its boundaries. The people who settled on this fertile strip built a civilization that far exceeded that of other groups who settled elsewhere. Signs of prosperity became increasingly evident in Egypt: systems of irrigation were devised; roads and ships were built; trade was established; practical arts were developed; architecture became dignified; family and other social relationships were maintained through the use of accepted moral codes; and the entire society was held together by an absolute monarchy headed by the pharaoh or king. Egypt is well remembered; impressive and enduring monuments still exist to herald its glory. Pyramids, tombs, temples, and other edifices are among the wonders of the contemporary world.

More is known about Egypt than any other ancient culture. Surviving Egyptian records are related to periods as distant as 3000 BC. A system of writing was introduced, at first in the form of pictures, and later as signs or *hieroglyphics*. Formal records were carved in stone or written in inks on paper scrolls called *papyri* (writing materials made from the pith of the tall sedge plant). The papyri and the stone carvings have yielded the greatest information on certain Egyptian periods. In the dry sands of Egypt these papyri, which contained the most complete examples of ancient medical literature, were preserved. They were named after their discoverers or owners, for example, the Brugsch, Ebers, Smith, Hearst, Berlin, and London scrolls (Frank, 1953). The Ebers papyrus is known as the oldest complete medical book in the world.

> No less than five medical papyri have come down to our time, the finest being the celebrated Ebers papyrus, bought at Thebes by Dr. Ebers in 1874. The papyrus contains one hundred and ten pages, each page consisting of about twenty-two lines of bold hieratic writing. It may be described as an Encyclopedia of Medicine as known and practised by the Egyptians of the eighteenth dynasty, and it contains prescriptions for all kinds of diseases—some borrowed from Syrian medical lore, and some of such great antiquity that they are ascribed to the mythologic ages, when the gods yet reigned personally upon earth.
>
> *Edwards, 1892, p. 219*

The Smith papyrus revealed a high level of Egyptian surgical practice arranged according to the general parts of the body (only the section relating to the upper parts survives). The Hearst, London, and Berlin papyri, which focus almost entirely on the treatment of diseases of the anus, may have been practical handbooks. The Ebers papyrus outlined many of the diseases known to modern science and minutely described their symptoms. In addition, over 700 substances from the vegetable, mineral, and animal kingdom were given as drugs along with descriptions for their preparation. The complexity of these prescriptions suggests the need for specialists to compound them. The Ebers papyrus also, however, contained incantations and verbal charms.

Three elements are present in these manuscripts: religion, magic, and accounts of illness and treatments (Shryock, 1959). This is consistent with Berdoe's description:

> The art of medicine in ancient Egypt consisted of two branches, the higher, which was the theurgic part, and the lower, which was the art of the physician proper. The theurgic class devoted themselves to magic, counteracting charms by prayers, and to the interpretation of the dreams of the sick who had sought aid in the temples. The inferior class were practitioners who simply used natural means in their profession.
>
> *Berdoe, 1893, p. 61*

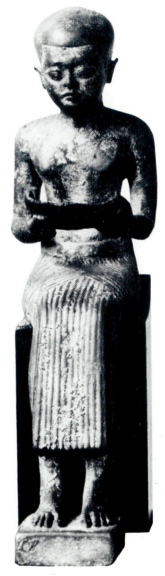

Seated figure of IMHOTEP, *6th Dynasty. Museum of Egyptian Antiquities, Staatliche Museen Preussischer Kulturbesitz, Berlin, Federal Republic of Germany. (Marburg/Art Resource, NY).*

It is possible, however, that the word *magic* did not convey the true medical state, since the Egyptians practiced hypnotism and were aware of how to control the mind and imagination. It is not clear who gave the orders for the practical treatment of the patient, the priest-magician (priests) or the priest-physician (doctors). What is clear is that two professions dealt with the sick at the same time but in different ways. In some instances the two combined to become one, commonly known as the priest-physician.

Out of this structure emerged the first physician known to history. Sometime in the Third Dynasty, c. 2900–2800 BC, Imhotep is identified as the greatest priest-physician of Egypt. His stature as a historic personage grew according to his deeds. He was recognized as a surgeon and architect to one of the Pharaohs, as a temple priest, a learned scribe, and a successful magician (priest-physician). Imhotep was noted for his great wisdom and learning in the field of health, magic, and religion. He was so successful in healing the sick that statues and temples were erected in his honor. After Imhotep's death the Egyptian people elevated him to the rank of Egyptian God of Medicine, the god of healing.

The philosophy of the Egyptians was a form of nature worship that included some aspects of animism. Diseases were believed to have partly natural, partly supernatural causes. The development of astrology also led to the belief that disease, as well as destiny, was influenced by changes in celestial phenomena, such as the movement of sun and stars and the passage of seasons. Astrological medicine arose and functioned harmoniously with mythical premises.

Stepped Pyramid of King Zoser, c. 2610 BC, Saqqara, Egypt. (Hirmer Verlag, Munich).

This structure, with its temples, complex of chambered terraces, and great courtyard, is now thought to be a medical shrine built under the direction of Imhotep.

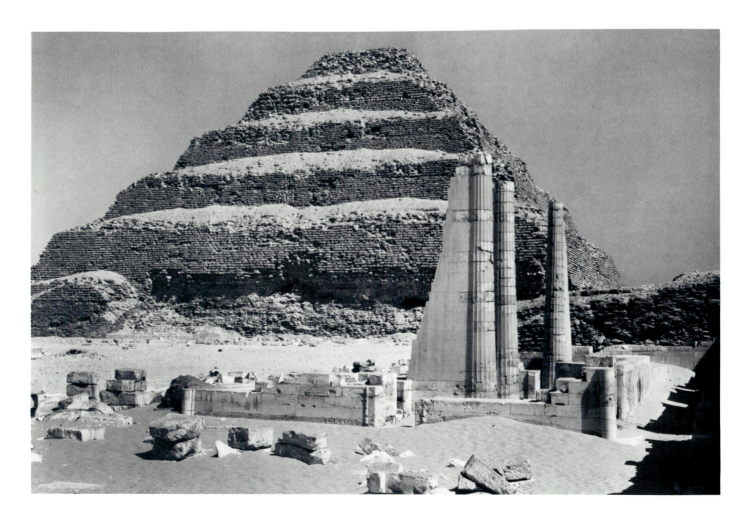

A spirit world inhabited by many gods developed in the Nile valley. Ultimately a trinity assumed control of bodily and spiritual welfare: Isis, Osiris, and Horus, their son. Isis (Mother Earth) and Osiris (Day or Light or Sun God) were regarded as the creators of agriculture and the medical arts. Isis gave her help to the sick most often through the medium of dreams. From his mother, Horus learned medicine as well as the gift of prophecy. Osiris sat in judgment of the souls of those who died, and immortality became an established belief. Magnificent temples emerged and became significant as molding influences in the civilization. Originally built as meager shelters to protect the gods, the temples became centers of community and national life. Priest-physicians functioned in those temples, which were frequented by individuals in search of health.

Concern for the question of life after death was especially prevalent in Egyptian society. The people hoped for personal survival beyond the grave. Therefore symbols of immortality, the pyramids, were erected. Bodies were skillfully embalmed so that souls could remain within or return when the afterlife began. Aromatics, resins, and other preservatives were employed in this process. The custom of embalming enabled the Egyptians to become familiar with the organs of the human body. Over 250 different diseases were identified from clinical observations. Treatments were developed that incorporated the use of drugs and procedures, including surgery. Specialization became a reality, perhaps because of the large quantity of writings that may have necessitated concentration on a limited area of knowledge. Herodotus, the Greek historian, explained:

> Medicine is practiced among them on a plan of separation; each physician treats a single disorder and no more: thus the country swarms with medical practitioners, some undertaking to cure diseases of the eye, others of the teeth, others of the head, others of the intestines, and some of those which are invisible.
>
> *Herodotus*

Splendid examples of the art of bandaging emerged as thousands of yards of linen in various widths and patterns were used on one mummy. These bandages were hardened with a gluey substance to form an impenetrable case for an aseptically cleansed body. Safe repositories in the form of elaborate tombs were constructed to ensure the preservation of body and soul for all time.

The ancient Egyptians also established public hygiene and sanitation at a relatively high level. They appear to have had a corps of sanitary inspectors or health officers (Nutting and Dock, 1937). The Egyptians recognized the importance of an adequate drainage system, a good water supply, and the inspection of slaughter houses. They were very particular about the cleanliness of their bodies and their dress, which was always of linen. They practiced circumcision from earliest times. Strict rules were developed to regulate such matters as cleanliness, food, drink, exercise, and sexual relations. Some sources indicate that the rigid hygienic regulation of the Jews originated from these Egyptian practices (Seymer, 1932).

Modern researchers have yet to disclose evidence regarding the existence of any building identifiable as a hospital. However, according to Caton, "There is reason to believe that institutions closely

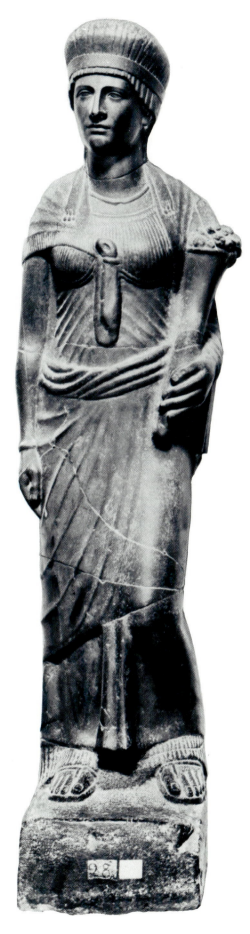

FIGURE OF THE HEALING GODDESS ISIS. *Vatican Museum, Rome. (Alinari/Art Resource, NY).*

41

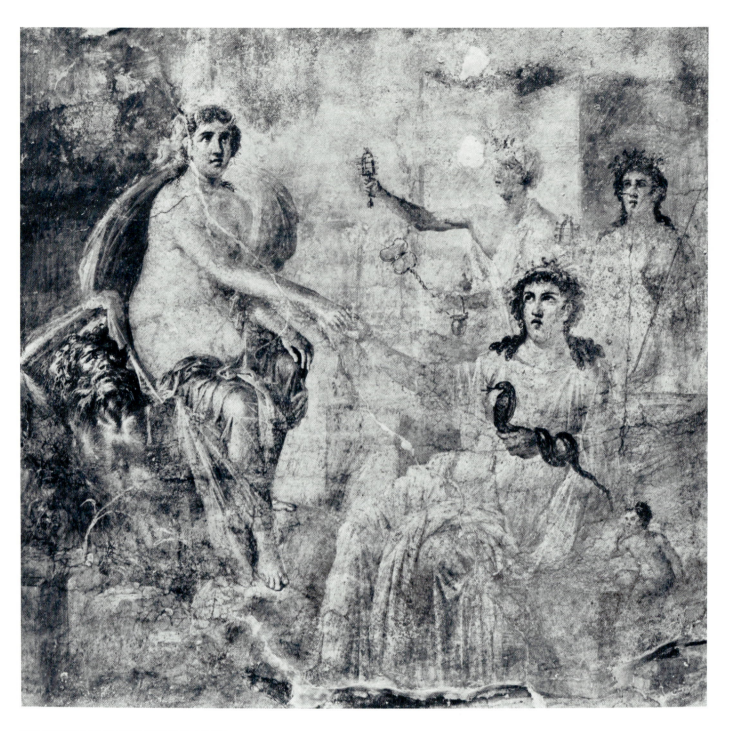

THE COMING OF IO INTO EGYPT. *From the Temple of Isis in Pompeii. Museo Archeological Nazionale, Naples, Italy. (Alinari/Art Resource, NY).*

related to infirmaries or hospitals existed in Egypt many centuries earlier than the Hieron of Epidauros, but no structural trace of such building has been discovered" (Nutting and Dock, 1937, p. 54). Whether there were or were not hospitals, the temples had some type of housing for the sick. In those temples frequented by individuals in search of health, priest-physicians engaged in medical practice. The existence of priestesses or "temple women" is also certain; what their duties were is not clear, although it is assumed that they performed some type of nursing functions.

The position of women in ancient Egypt was higher than in other Eastern countries. In general, women enjoyed considerable freedom and dignity. Within their own households they held a position of authority and importance. It is probable that nursing care was

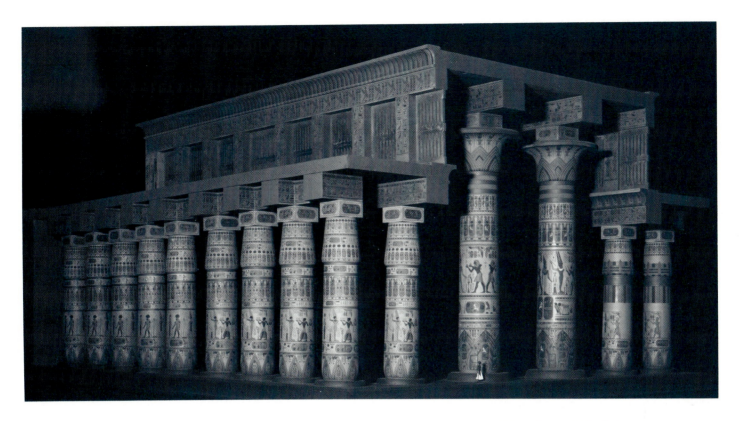

Model of Hypostyle Hall, Temple of Amen-Re, Karnak, c. 1280 BC. The Metropolitan Museum of Art, New York, Purchase 1890, Bequest of Levi Hale Willard.

the chief responsibility of the mother or daughters in the home. In addition, physicians in ancient Egypt did not practice obstetrics; this field was left entirely to midwives. Wet nurses were engaged on contract to breast-feed infants for approximately six months.

In a nation as sophisticated in medicine, pharmacy, and sanitation as ancient Egypt, it is almost impossible to believe that there were no persons, male or female, who engaged in the work of nurses and nursing. History, however, fails to make this point clear.

Persia (Iran)

Persia is presently called Iran, a form of the word *Aryan*. This name indicates that the Persians spoke an Aryan or so-called Indo-European language; the Persians were related to European peoples (Shryock, 1959). The Plateau of Iran was positioned to the east of the Fertile Crescent and between the Persian Gulf and the Caspian Sea. In ancient times the land was occupied by the Medes and the Persians. However, by 500 BC the Persians had conquered the Medes, moved their borders eastward to the Indus River in India, and conquered all of the Fertile Crescent and Egypt. The energies of Persia were directed toward war, tyranny, and the acquisition of wealth and power. The result of these efforts was the founding of the most extensive empire that appeared in the Near East. Fortunately, this empire, which exerted an almost totally destructive influence, existed for only about 200 years.

The religion of the Persians, Zoroastrianism, revolved around Zoroaster, who lived about 600 BC. This prophet wrote the sacred books of Persia, the Zendavesta, which introduced a world ruled by two creators, one producing light and good, the other darkness and evil. Although good and evil were constantly at war, good always

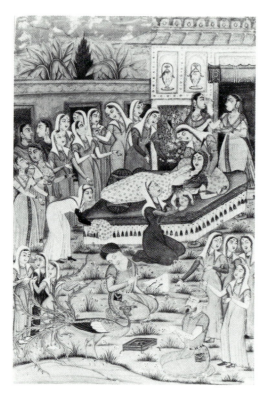

Shah Nameh, BIRTH OF ROUSTEUR BY CAESARIAN. *Musée Condé, Chantilly, France. (Giraudon/Art Resource, NY).*

triumphed. In addition, sacred elements were identified: fire, earth, and water, with fire described as the purest. According to the sacred books, immortality was a mental rather than a physical state. The principal virtues of veracity, virility, and hard work would enable men to achieve happiness. Thus happiness or unhappiness depended on the righteousness or evil of men on earth with the promise of rewards after death (Jamieson and Sewall, 1950).

The Persians absorbed much of the culture of their conquered land, including the medicine and surgery of Egypt. They had great confidence in Egyptian medicine, demonstrated by the Emperor Darius, who renovated an old school to be used for the training of priest-physicians. This is thought to be the first case of a medical center established as a royal or government foundation.

Three types of physicians evolved from the medical center: those who healed by the knife, those who used plants, and those who healed by exorcism and incantations (Nutting and Dock, 1937). No mention is made of nurses, although descriptions of various surgical and medical procedures are given, some of which could well have belonged to the province of nursing. In retrospect, little attention has been given to the medical history of the Persian Empire. It may be that Persia contributed little to medicine in comparison with other countries.

The Fertile Crescent

A series of civilizations developed in the Fertile Crescent, an area that stretched from the Isthmus of Suez, up through Palestine and Syria, east through the region of Damascus, and down the Euphrates Valley. This land has also been called the Cradle of Civilization. In this region thousands of years ago the first cities in the world were built and the first attempt at developing a system of writing occurred. Three great rivers—the Tigris, the Euphrates, and the Jordan—were situated in the area. The combination of well-watered soil and a warm climate encouraged habitation. Successive peoples came and conquered their predecessors in the fertile valleys. Most of them spoke the Semitic languages.

> Sumerians, Assyrians, Babylonians, and Persians followed one another as the dominant people, in that chronological order. Conquerors took over the earlier civilizations, however, so that there was an accumulation of culture from the ancient Sumerian period about 3,000 BC down to the flowering of Persian life more than two thousand years later.
>
> *Shryock, 1959, p. 26*

Agriculture flourished in this area, and wealth and economic changes led to the building of memorable cities. Progress was similar to that of Egypt, with one significant difference: structures were built with clay or bricks instead of stone. Therefore natural phenomena and time crumbled these ancient cities into dust. Fortunately, records were kept on hardened clay tablets, and from these tablets information about religion, business, and medical practice has been deciphered. These cuneiform (wedge-shaped) writings frequently referred to practices performed by royal physicians that today would be carried out by nurses.

44

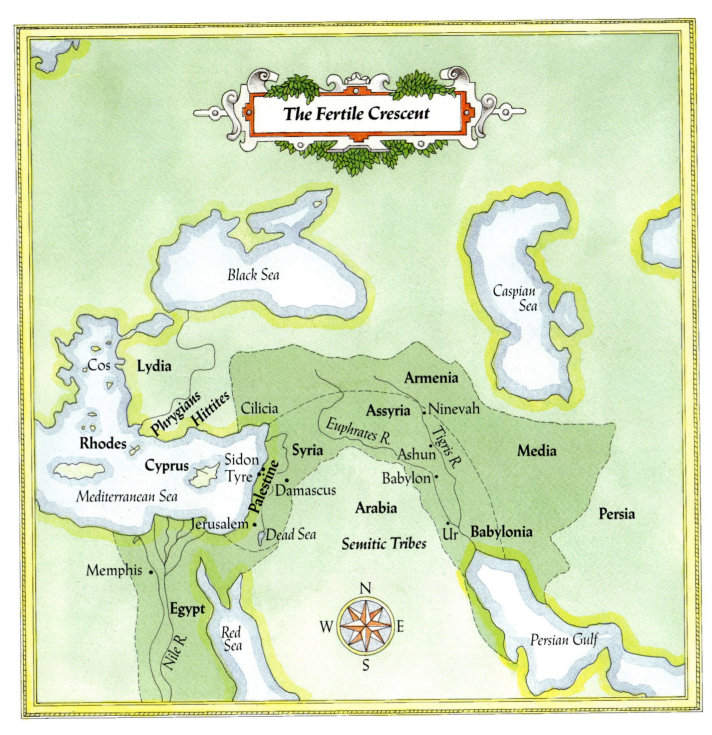

Map of the FERTILE CRESCENT OF THE
PRE-CHRISTIAN ERA.

Babylonia. As Egyptian civilization was developing in the Nile Valley, a comparable advance was occurring in the region between the Tigris and Euphrates valleys, now known as Iraq. This area was originally known as Mesopotamia, a Greek word meaning "between the rivers." City states that developed in southern Mesopotamia were dominated by temples where priests represented the patron deities of the city. Each ancient city was a community center with schools, libraries, granaries, and workshops. Each was governed by a divine ruler and a priest-king who was the actual ruler. The most prominent of these city states was Sumer, regarded as the finest and earliest civilization of mankind. The Sumerians made significant contributions to human civilization in the development of morals,

45

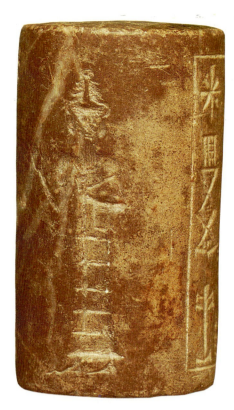

THE SEAL OF MALE MIDWIFE URLUGALEDINNA, *Sumerian, 2200 BC. Musée National du Louvre, Paris, France.*

learning, and the arts. They were eventually conquered by the Babylonians, a Semitic people. The conquered lands ultimately became known as the Babylonian Empire, which was established by about 2100 BC.

Magical and superstitious principles and a strong astral influence comprised the religion of the Babylonians. These people believed in polytheism, a plurality of gods, the majority of whom were nature gods.

> The three greatest were the gods of the sky, the earth, and the sea. Next in rank were the moon god, the sun god, the god of thunder, lightning, wind, rain, and storm: of the planet Venus; Marduk or Merodak (light), (who is also called Bel), the quickener of the dead, who fought and vanquished the dragon or "Chaos" (darkness); Nebo, the god of arts, science, and letters, and others.
>
> *Nutting and Dock, 1937, p. 57*

Local deities were also numerous. Disease was believed to be evoked by the wrath of the gods and by evil spirits; this resulted in the creation of hierarchies of good and evil spirits. Survival was dependent on securing aid from the good spirits. Ceremonies incorporating the use of fire, water, and incantations became important in this process, and various occult practices were cultivated.

The Babylonians were learned mathematicians and astronomers. They originated the division of time into months, days, and minutes, used a system of weights and measures, and followed the signs of the zodiac. Their study of sun, moon, and planets became the basis for scientific astronomy. Astrological interpretation became closely connected with physiological phenomena; the position of the stars and the motions of the planets and the moon were believed to directly affect men. "As their lore accumulated, they began to 'cast horoscopes' in terms of an individual's birth, for the position of the planets at this time was supposed to cast a spell over a man thereafter" (Shryock, 1959, p. 28). Eventually medicine became interwoven with astrology, and the result was the practice of a magic medicine carried out by astrologer-priests. These individuals practiced medicine by using a combination of magic, religion, and science. Sources of epidemics were ascribed to inauspicious astral influences. Human ailments were diagnosed through examination of the livers of dead animals. The art of *divination* (foretelling events or discovering hidden knowledge by the interpretation of omens or by the aid of supernatural powers) was practiced through a variety of methods, including palmistry, crystal gazing, and communication with the dead.

A very primitive stage in Babylonian medicine was recorded in which the sick were brought out into the marketplace. Passers-by were required to stop and render advice based on their own personal experiences. It is difficult to determine how long this empirical stage lasted and whether it occurred before or after there were physicians. What becomes clear, however, is that lay physicians were also prominent in Babylonia. The practice of medicine by these physicians was divided into two basic areas, surgery and internal medicine. Surgery was considered to be the more advanced field. "Their surgeons understood nasal tamponing for bleeding, cataract couching, the use of facial applications in cases of erysipelas, and blood-letting. Bodies of

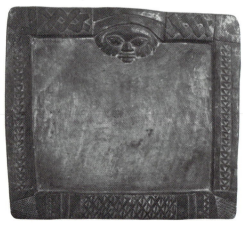

African, Guinea Coast, Yoruba, DIVINATION TRAY. *Wood. The University of Iowa Museum of Art, Iowa City, The Stanley Collection.*

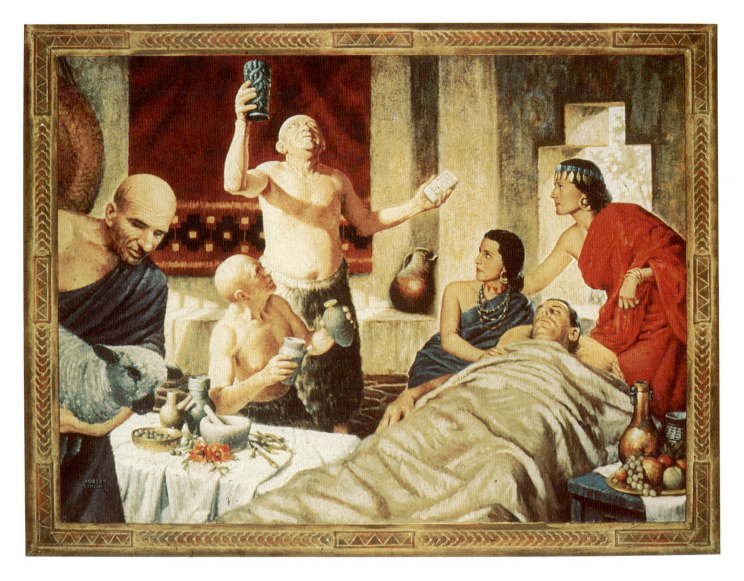

BABYLONIAN SICKROOM, *Parke-Davis Division of Warner-Lambert Co., Morris Plains, New Jersey.*

sacrificed animals supplied the only opportunity for anatomical research" (Jamieson and Sewall, 1950, p. 26). Circumcision is known to have been performed by Abraham, a native of Babylonia.

Internal medicine remained primarily in the magical realm and was concerned with magical formulas to banish demons, the gods of evil spirits. Since illness was thought to be caused by sin and displeasure of the gods, methods of treatment consisted of ridding the human body of these demons through incantations and other remedies. Vile-tasting plant and mineral concoctions, powders, enemas, and human and animal excreta were used. Yet the clinical observations of the physicians were fairly accurate portrayals of symptoms, as reported in vivid descriptions such as the following:

> The sick one coughs frequently, his sputum is thick and sometimes contains blood, his respirations give a sound like a flute, his skin is cold but his feet are hot, he sweats greatly and his heart muscle is disturbed. When his disease is extremely grave his intestines are frequently opened.
>
> *Castiglioni, 1947, p. 39*

Numerous diseases were described, including fevers, plague, abscesses, heart and skin diseases, tuberculosis, tumors, jaundice, and venereal disease.

47

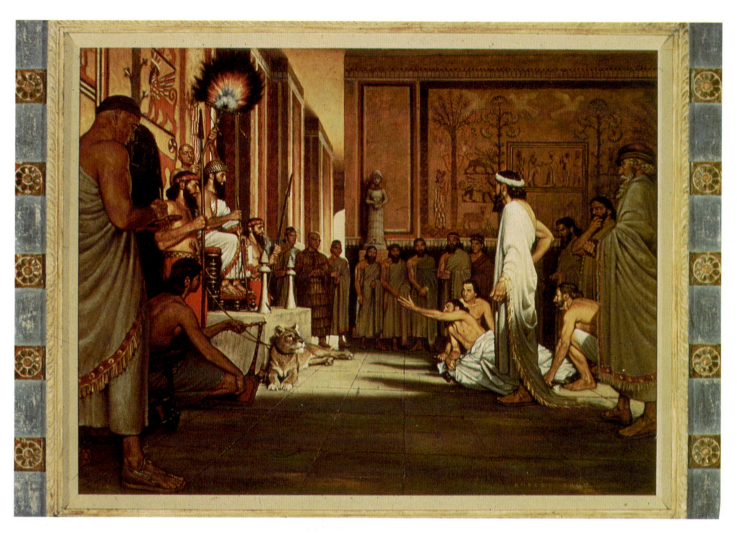

THE CODE OF HAMMURABI, *Parke-Davis Division of Warner-Lambert Co., Morris Plains, New Jersey.*

The lay physicians and surgeons of Babylonia needed to be careful about their practice. The legal codes of this country were more advanced than those of any other ancient culture and held individuals and groups responsible for their actions. Particularly significant was the Code of Hammurabi, inscribed about 1900 BC on a single great shaft of black stone and placed in one of the temples of Babylon. This code was developed by Hammurabi, sixth king of Babylonia, who was considered to be the greatest king and statesman during his reign of approximately sixty years. Hammurabi collected older laws and customs and systematically arranged these into a comprehensive code of law. Justice and consideration for the poor and defenseless classes were evident in this document, which was intended to be humanitarian. The code dealt with both civil and criminal law and contained regulations for various circumstances; for example, business contracts, theft, rents, loans, property rights, doweries, adoption of children, employment policies, sanitation, and public health. In addition, the Code of Hammurabi contained provisions for the veterinarian, a clear indication that the two specialists (physician and veterinarian) were distinct. More importantly, it addressed medical and surgical practice, with control of the surgeon the most severe aspect. Fees due practitioners, severe penalties for failures in treatments, and compensations to patients injured during treatment were outlined. In essence the physician's conduct was regulated by the government, and penalties could result in cruel physical punishment:

> If a physician has treated a free-born man for a severe wound
> with a lancet of bronze and has caused the man to die, or
> has opened a tumour of the man with a lancet of bronze and
> has destroyed his eyes, his hands one shall cut off.
>
> *Code of Hammurabi*

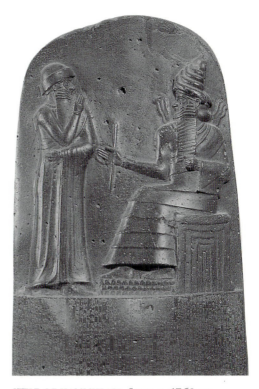

STELE OF HAMMURABI, *Susa, c. 1760 BC.
Basalt, approx. 220 cm high. Musée
National du Louvre, Paris, France.*

This "eye for an eye and tooth for a tooth" philosophy presumably deterred unnecessary surgeries and fostered precautionary measures among the practitioners.

A table of fees for operations was also set and varied from two shekels for surgery on a slave to ten shekels for operating on a freeman:

> If a doctor has treated a freeman with a metal knife for a
> severe wound, and has cured the freeman or has opened a
> freeman's tumour with a metal knife, and cured a freeman's eye,
> then he shall receive ten shekels of silver.
> If the son of a plebeian, he shall receive five shekels of silver.
> If a man's slave, the owner of the slave shall give two shekels
> of silver to the doctor.
> [For the veterinarian] If a doctor of oxen or asses has treated
> either ox or ass for a severe wound, and cured it, the owner of
> the ox or ass shall give to the doctor one sixth of a shekel of
> silver as his fee.
>
> *Code of Hammurabi*

The Code of Hammurabi was the greatest legal masterpiece of ancient civilization. It advanced the common good of Babylonia, and for nearly three centuries this country experienced increasing prosperity.

The history of Babylonia gives little mention of nursing as a separate occupation. The writings, however, frequently refer to practices that are currently performed by nurses. The Babylonian nurse was probably a domestic servant or a slave, either male or female. Accounts of wet nurses, midwives, and children's nurses, who often had great affection for their charges, have been rendered. In addition, in some pictorial scenes the role of the nurse in assisting the patient has been portrayed.

Assyria. The Assyrians, who succeeded the Babylonians, were a hardened, warlike Semitic race who held the balance of power in the Near East from approximately 745 to 635 BC. Their little kingdom of Assur arose in the middle of the Fertile Crescent. Its location afforded protection of its boundaries, with mountain ranges on three sides and a river on the fourth. Nineveh, the capital city, eventually became the center of art and commerce in the Near East. Its walls, which stretched about two and one half miles along the Tigris River, provided the setting for the ruling king.

The Assyrian laws were severe. Mutilation was inflicted as a punishment for many offenses, and the death penalty was frequently used. Absorbed in war, the Assyrians made the "god of the battlefield" their supreme god. Their intensity in military tactics resulted in the introduction of stronger weapons (the Assyrians were the first to use weapons made of bronze) and new techniques of warfare. However, Assyrian power was short lived; it suddenly lost vitality, and Nineveh fell to a coalition of powers about 612 BC. "Denounced by the prophets, its name [Nineveh] has survived as a symbol of luxury for the rich and destitution for the poor, a symbol of vice and of sin" (Sellew and Nuesse, 1946, p. 34).

Assyria preserved the theory of demonology, which held that the sick person's body was possessed by evil spirits. Even further, the Assyrians fostered the belief that illness was a punishment for sin and could be cured only be repentance, magic, or a combination of magic and religion. The aspects of sin and repentance, however, may have been another way of stating that those who broke physiological laws would become ill and could be cured only by resuming the practice of hygienic rules (Nutting and Dock, 1937). The entire theory thus would have been predicated on the natural laws of health. Whatever is accepted as the basis for their belief, the fact remains that the Assyrians practiced only magic and empirical medicine, which was consistent with their superstitious nature. They believed in the influence of lunar changes, and charms and amulets were used extensively. Numbers were regarded as lucky and unlucky; for example, the number seven was so sacred that the seventh day was reserved for rest. Many regulations existed about the gathering of medicinal herbs: some should be gathered by night, some at dawn, and others at a certain time of the moon. Ceremonies were adopted whereby one could be purified by fire and water. Sacrifices involving the offering of human life were sometimes also required.

Medical texts were handed down by the Assyrians on clay tablets with cuneiform script. The greatest number came from Nineveh and were supposedly from the library of King Asurbanipal (668–628 BC). These texts exhibit a mixture of rational therapeutic remedies with purely magical devices:

> If a man's head is full of scabies and itch thou shalt bray sulphur, mix it in cedar oil, anoint him.
> . . . a thread thou shalt spin, double it twice, tie 7 knots. As thou tiest (them) thou shalt recite the charm, bind on his temples and he shall recover.
> If a man has a burning headache affecting his eyes, which are bloodshot, take one third of a measure of *sikhli* crushed and powdered, and knead with cassia juice; wrap it around his head, attach it (with a bandage) and do not remove it for 3 days.
>
> *Seymer, 1932, p. 6*

Nothing about nursing is revealed in the history of Assyria. Nor is there any evidence that buildings were used as hospitals. In regard to women in Assyria, it can be assumed that they did not achieve a very high status.

Palestine. As tribes of the Semitic race were moving into Babylonia and Assyria, other tribes were moving into the region of Palestine at the western side of the Fertile Crescent. The geographical position of the latter tribes, between Egypt on one side and Assyria and Mesopotamia on the other, significantly affected the development of their own culture. These people were given the name *Hebrews* by the natives whom they eventually dominated. The literal translation of the word *Hebrews* is "the people from beyond" (Reinach, 1930). The Hebrews were well established in their towns by the time Hammurabi was king of Babylonia (c. 1955 BC). Agriculture became their chief endeavor, although the mountainous character of this portion of the Fertile Crescent provided less than desirable conditions. The terrain was comprised of narrow, gorgelike valleys; the soil was lacking in minerals; and rainfall was inadequate, causing an insufficient water supply. The industrious Hebrew people, however, overcame these obstacles. They built towns, raised sheep, collected water in cisterns, and patiently cultivated olives and grapes. The country flourished and the city of Jerusalem became the center of religious and political activities.

The Jews (Hebrews, or Israelites) were the first to develop the art of writing historical narratives, and their early histories are preserved in the Old Testament.

> In Genesis, Exodus and other books, we are told how Abraham (Israel) first came into Palestine, how his descendants (the "Children of Israel") were made captives in Egypt, how they escaped therefrom into Palestine, how they were then conquered and taken into exile "by the waters of Babylon," and how the Persians finally restored them to Jerusalem. In the course of these adventures they absorbed much of the culture of both Egypt and Babylon, and the Bible is full of accounts of those two civilizations.
>
> *Shryock, 1959, p. 30*

Thus the Jews traced their descent from Abraham, who was born in Ur, Chaldea, and migrated to Palestine with his family. In the eighteenth century BC famine drove the Jews into Egypt, where they lived for a time in prosperity. Ultimately, they were taken into captivity, where they remained as slaves for more than 400 years. It was not until the fifteenth century BC that the Jews left Egypt under the leadership of Moses. Their reentry into Palestine took place after forty years of wandering. At that time the people were divided into twelve tribes, with the thirteenth, the tribe of Levi, comprising the priesthood. State and church were under the same head, a theocratic government. The chiefs of the tribes and the elders possessed the power of civil authority. A tribal assembly approved or rejected decisions.

From approximately 1095 BC, Palestine was ruled by kings. Saul was its first king, followed by David, under whom the country flourished. David's successor was Solomon, who financed his love for luxury by burdening the people with taxes. Yet Solomon earned respect for wisdom and justice in administration. After his death the kingdom was split into two, and each of these new kingdoms fell to invading powers. Israel was conquered by Assyria in 722 BC; Jerusalem fell to Babylonia in 587 BC. From this time forward the Jews became a people without a country, since rising empires constantly seized Palestine. By 1 AD, Palestine was under the rule of Rome.

The Hebrews embraced a theocentric philosophy, a belief in a personal God. This philosophy held that man has free will, an immortal soul created by God, and is a body-mind-spirit unity. Hebrew religious belief was theocratic and monotheistic. The Hebrew people abhorred the innumerable deities of other nations. They denounced superstitious and magical practices to the extent that death was the penalty for performing them. Yet they held the extreme view that disease is a punishment for one's own sins. Their strength was derived from belief in the one true God. According to Shryock (1959), this monotheistic conception had been formed in Egypt earlier but had exerted only temporary influence there. All power over life and death was in the hands of Jehovah. God became the source of health, and its preservation was to be found in "keeping pure before the Lord." A way of living emerged that did not necessitate specific medical practices.

Religion and medicine were combined, and responsibility for the public health centered on the priest-physicians drawn from the priestly tribe of Levites. These men were held in high esteem:

> Honor the physician for the need thou hast of him: for the most
> High created him.
> For all healing is from God: and he shall receive gifts of the king.
> The skill of the physician shall lift up his head: and in the sight
> of men he shall be praised.
>
> *Ecclesiasticus 36: 1–4*

It is possible that much of the knowledge of the Hebrew people was borrowed from the Egyptians. Moses, the adopted son of the Pharaoh's daughter, had led the enslaved people out of Egypt. Undoubtedly, he was well acquainted with Egyptian wisdom and received a sophisticated education, most likely at the University of Heliopolis (now Cairo). Although Moses' learning took place in a pagan atmosphere, he was taught the religious beliefs and traditions of his Hebrew heritage by his mother, who had been selected as his nursemaid. Mosaic Law was given to the Hebrew nation by Moses upon God's command. It contained civil specifications similar to those of the Code of Hammurabi. Yet the Mosaic Law exhibited consideration for the poor and the weak. As a result, justice became one of the most important characteristics of Hebrew social thought.

The laws ascribed to Moses, although expressed in religious terms, had definite hygienic significance. Regulations were provided for the general public health. Every detail of personal, family, and national hygiene were specified and directed toward the maintenance of health and the prolongation of life. A method for prevention of disease included personal hygiene, cleanliness, rest, sleep, and hours for work. Definite provisions were ascribed for women during menstruation, pregnancy, and childbirth. Other provisions dealt with inspection and selection of food, disposal of excreta, notification of authorities in cases of communicable disease, quarantine, and disinfection. It is interesting to note that the health regulations were planned to improve the endurance of the race, which was in keeping with the thought that the Israelites were the chosen people (Deuteronomy 14: 2).

The priest-physicians also functioned as health inspectors. Contagious diseases had to be reported and isolation was compulsory. The orders for treatment and isolation came from the priest, who also initiated the disinfection of the body, clothing, and environment. Permission had to be secured from the priest to reenter the camp after being quarantined. The acceptance of these practices demonstrates the ancient Jewish belief in infection by contact (contagion), the idea that epidemic diseases were spread from one individual to the next.

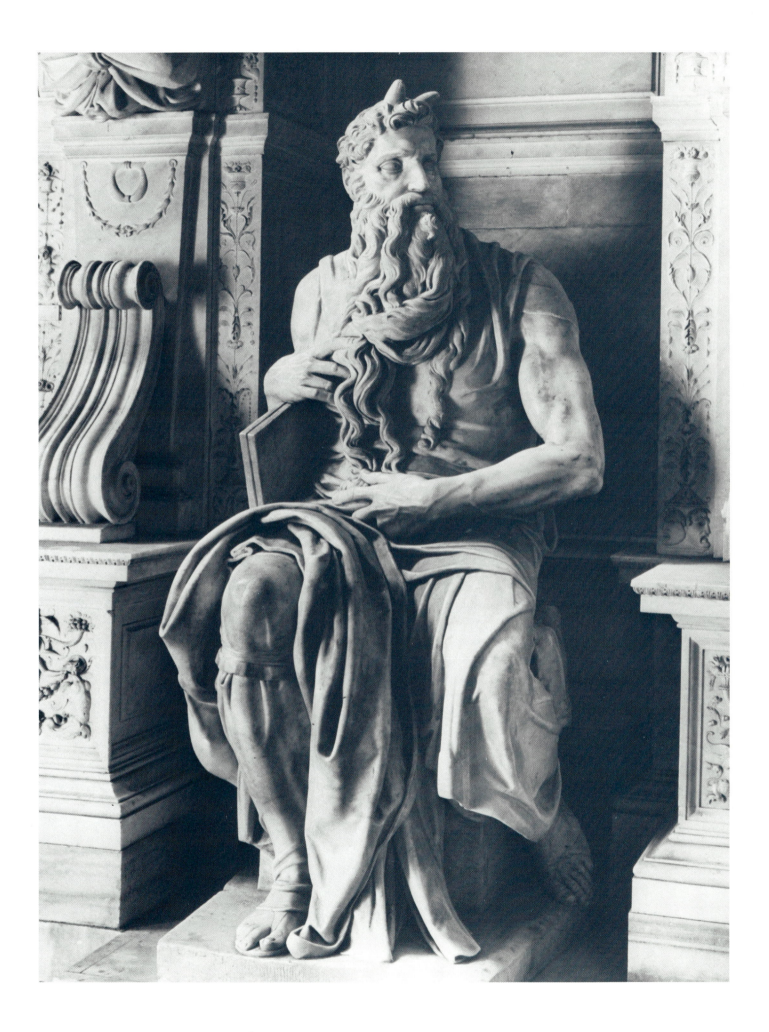

Joachim Uytewael, MOSES STRIKING THE
ROCK, *1624. Wood, 44.5 × 66.7 cm.
National Gallery of Art, Washington, D.C.,
Ailsa Mellon Bruce Fund 1972.*

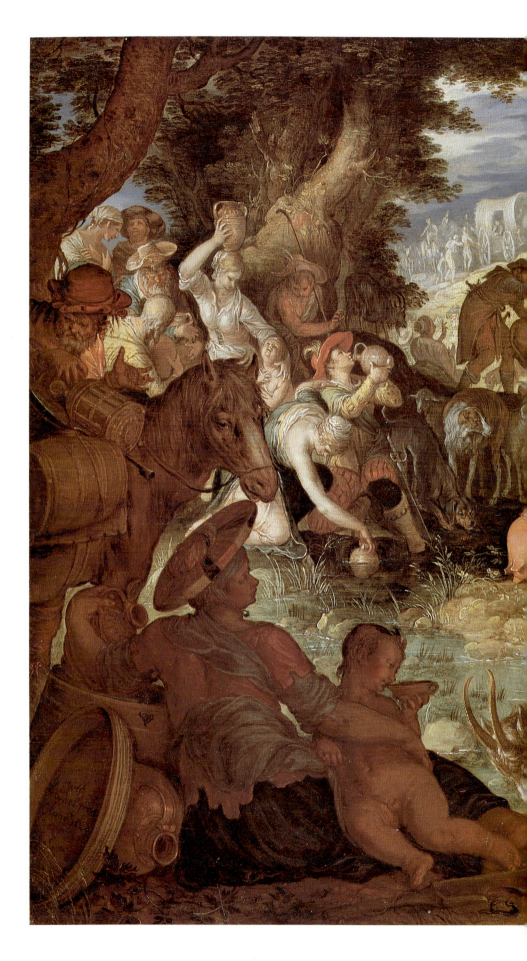

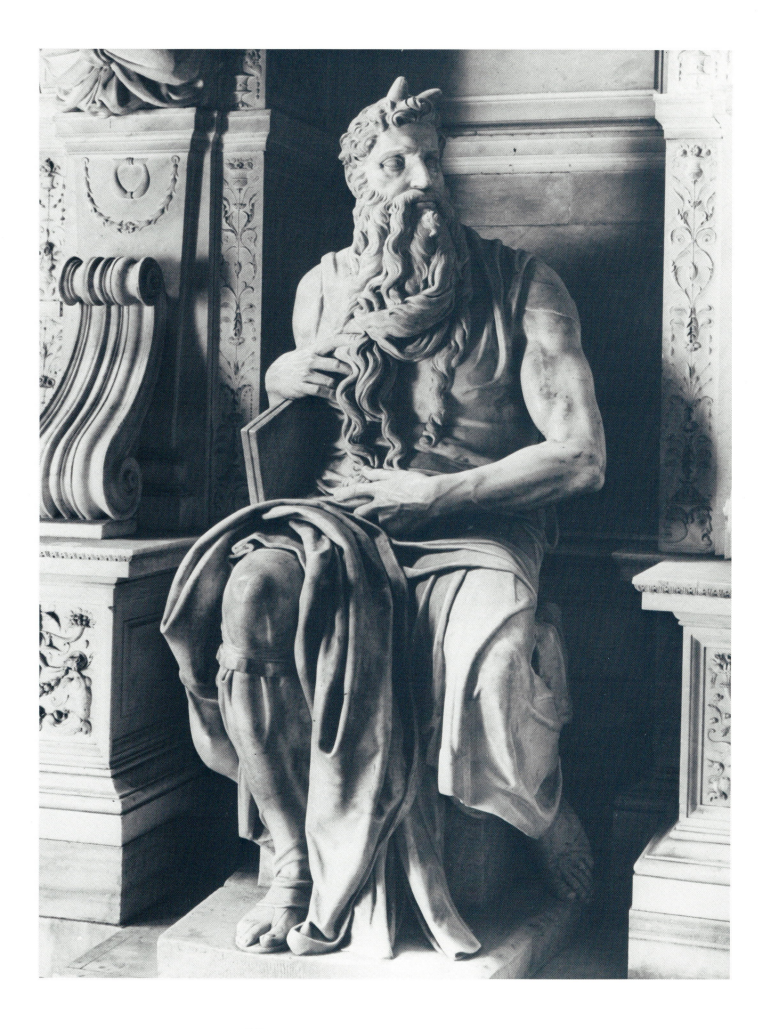

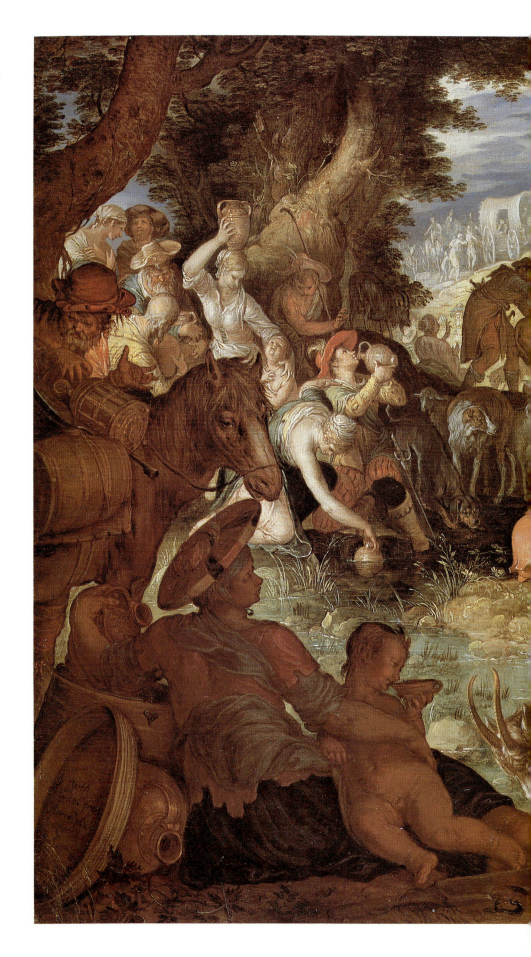

Joachim Uytewael, MOSES STRIKING THE
ROCK, *1624. Wood, 44.5 × 66.7 cm.
National Gallery of Art, Washington, D.C.,
Ailsa Mellon Bruce Fund 1972.*

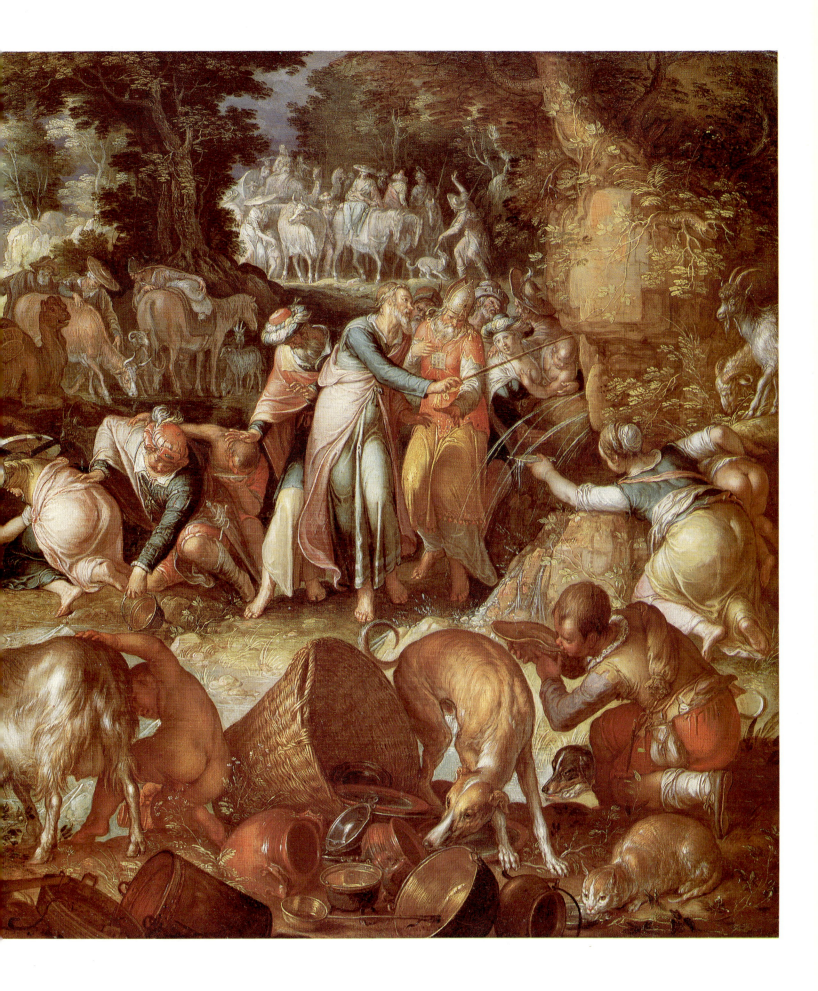

Thus the Jews not only pioneered in establishing the concept of contagion but also in those measures of notification and isolation which were based upon it. This approach to public health control, however, made little impression on other ancient races, and it remained for European Christians to revive it during the Middle Ages.

Shryock, 1959, p. 32

Dietary laws were a significant part of the Mosaic Law. Four cardinal points were to be observed about animal food. First, blood was forbidden as food. Meats were to be drained of their blood before cooking (animals were scientifically bled). Second, animals torn by wild beasts or accidentally killed were not to be used as food. Third, animals that died naturally were not to be used as food. Fourth, the pig was forbidden as unclean. Cloven-hoofed animals that chew their cud and are not scavengers, birds that are not birds of prey, and fish that have fins and scales were permitted in the diet. According to Lyons, there may have been explanations for food prohibitions other than those with a medical basis. He renders this account:

One recent suggestion is that the taboo against pigs was originally related to their competition with humans for water and grain (scarce commodities in a barren land), in contrast to cattle and sheep which consume relatively little water and graze on forage inedible to man. Since transmissible parasitic diseases and infestations such as tapeworm are also found in sheep and cows, singling out trichinosis in pigs would not be wholly logical. However, to discourage the raising of swine so as to conserve water and grain resources for human consumption, a strict religious taboo may have been necessary—considering man's nearly universal agreement on the delectableness of pork. Medical observations may indeed have been at the core of hygienic codes, but the Biblical listing of seemingly unrelated creatures prohibited as food is difficult to associate with purposes entirely hygienic.

Lyons, 1978, p. 71

Knowledge of ancient Jewish medicine is derived almost entirely from the Old Testament of the Bible and the later Talmud, the authoritative compilation of Jewish tradition. The two Talmuds, the Jerusalem and the Babylonian, were written approximately over the second to the sixth century AD. In addition to exhibiting remarkable medical observations, they incorporate the attitudes, influences, and methods of the various peoples with whom the Jews lived. References to nurses in the Talmud and the Old Testament suggest wet nurses or children's nurses rather than nurses who were caretakers of the sick. The Jewish midwife was important, but more attention was given to the hygiene of pregnancy than to the actual assistance of the mother at the time of delivery. A woman was usually delivered while sitting on a stool designed in a circular fashion; the midwife sat on a lower stool before her. If complications arose and all known methods failed to improve the situation, religion dictated that she be cared for and comforted until she died (Sellew and Nuesse, 1946). Deborah was the first nurse to be recorded in history, as shown in the twenty-fourth chapter of Genesis. She is included in the story of Rebekah, who sets out by camel train with her nurse (Deborah) to meet her future husband, Issac. Deborah was a child's nurse and a com-

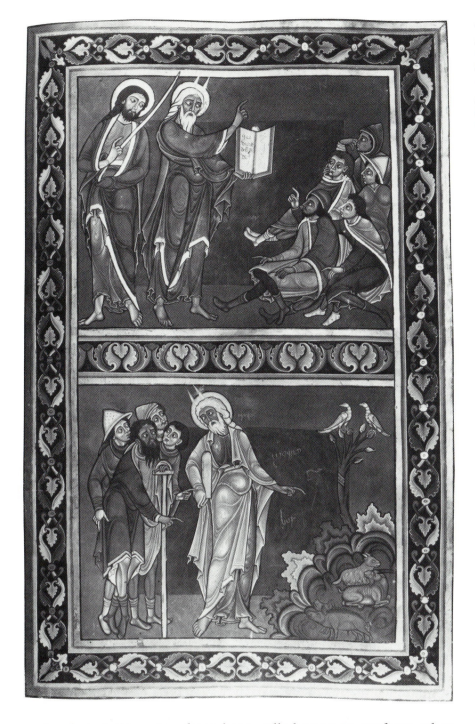

Master Hugo, MOSES EXPOUNDING THE LAW, *frontispiece of the Book of Deuteronomy of the Bury Bible, the abbey of Bury St. Edmunds, early twelfth century. Illuminated manuscript, approx. 50.8 × 35.6 cm. Reproduced by permission of the Master and Fellows of Corpus Christi College, Cambridge, England.*

panion but at times may have been called upon to perform other nursing duties.

Ancient Jews believed that all men should have access to medical care, regardless of their social status. With an emphasis on human brotherhood and social justice, the duties of hospitality to the stranger and relief for widows, orphans, the aged, and the poor were constantly urged as righteous. Visiting the sick was a prominent feature of everyday life and a designated duty. Houses for strangers, called xenodochia, were instituted and later expanded to include the care of the sick. These xenodochia were supported financially through a system of tithing. Whether these institutions had nurses is unknown. They did, however, become predecessors of the modern inn and the modern hospital. Overall, the Hebrews recorded achievement in the practice of hygiene, sanitation, and the systematic and organized prevention of disease.

■ THE FAR EAST

As the great civilizations of ancient times were developing in the Near East, others were developing on a vast continent that eventually became known as Asia. This region included current-day India, China, and Japan, an area usually distinguished by modern historians as the Far East or Orient. Little evidence of human progress in primitive times is available from this area. It is believed, however, that the stages of development were similar to those experienced by other cultures.

India

India lay in the southern part of the Far Eastern continent. This triangular region was almost completely isolated from the rest of the world by two chains of mountains (Himalayas) along its northern border and waters (Arabian Sea, Bay of Bengal, Indian Ocean) on its other three borders. It is thought that an advanced civilization existed in the Indus Valley by approximately 3000 BC. Migration from central Asia occurred through the mountain passes on the north by Aryan peoples of Indo-European stock. This group found in India a warm climate, an extremely rich vegetation, and a race darker-skinned than themselves. The difference in skin color may have been the basis for the formation of a caste system that developed gradually and had far-reaching consequences for health and well-being. The immigration continued over a long period with the descendants, Indo-Aryans, a vigorous people whose wealth consisted of cattle and amusements included hunting, gambling, and chariot racing. Eventually the native peoples of this area were conquered by the Aryans. An advanced culture developed that had direct access to Persia on the west and indirect contact with China to the east.

Excavated remains indicate that in the first civilization in India (2500–1500 BC) there were large cities and a highly developed culture. Within the carefully planned cities were baths, shops, multi-room buildings, and temples built with burnt brick. An exceptional feature of this pre-Aryan culture was its system of public sanitation. Drainage systems, wells, bathrooms, public baths, and collection chutes for trash were in evidence. Practical arts included cultivation of soil, domestication of animals, and smelting of metals. The script from the writings left by this civilization is yet to be totally deciphered.

The Vedic Age, beginning after 1500 BC, produced the classical Indian civilization and Brahmanism (also known as Hinduism). Agriculture became the principal occupation at this time, although crafts were also practiced. Organized labor appeared in the form of guilds. The territory of the Jumna and Ganges rivers became sacred to the Hindus. India became a home of architectural beauty with a people who were well versed in war and politics, inventors of the decimal system, and discoverers in geometry and trigonometry. A priesthood was established, and the population was divided into tribes ruled by elected chiefs. In time the state replaced the tribes and kings replaced the chiefs.

India was known as the Land of the Temples. Its temples were masterpieces of artistry and were vitally important to the Hindu people. The idols, however, were usually hideous. Worship was directed to one or more of the prominent deities. Uppermost was the Trimurti, or divine triad of gods: Brahma, the power and spirit of the universe; Vishnu, the preserver of the world; and Shiva, the destroyer and conqueror of death. The other principal deities included Lakshmi, goddess of life, beauty, and good fortune; Soma, personification of the hallucinatory plant used in Aryan rituals; Indra, god of war and weather; Agni, god of sacrifice and fire; Varuna, god of justice and cosmic order; and Dhanvantari, patron god of medicine. The twin Ashvins were also medical gods, patrons of eyesight, who acted as physicians to the gods themselves.

Two philosophical systems greatly influenced the lives of the people of India: Brahmanism and Buddhism. Both were closely connected with strong religious beliefs, and both were pantheistic and nihilistic. Pantheism is the belief that reality is a single being of which everything else is a part. (The deities were parts of the eternal whole because Brahman permeated everything in the universe.) Nihilism is the belief that conditions in the social organization are so poor as to make destruction desirable. It holds that existence is senseless and progress involves destruction for its own sake.

Brahmanism, the religion of the Aryan conquerors, provided religious development during thirty centuries. It revolved about Brahma, the eternal spirit, who permeated everything in the universe. The ideal of perfection rested in absolute unity with Brahma. This was attained by sacrifice, penance, and contemplation. Transmigration of the living soul, the doctrine of reincarnation, was affirmed. Man might be reborn into a lower or higher rank of human being, or even into the form of lower animals after death. Ancestor worship was encouraged, and reverence for animals, especially cows and monkeys, was advocated. Consequently, consumption of products from these animals was forbidden. Inherent in Brahmanism was stratification of the society into four distinct castes: Brahmins (priests and their descendants); Kshatrityas (warriors); Vaishyas (merchants, farmers, and artisans); and Shudras (menial workers).

The religious and moral codes within Brahmanism were written in the Vedas (Vedic, the parent language of Sanskrit, was used), which served as the sacred books or scripture and were the historical documents of India. These doctrines, presented in the form of hymns, prayers, and teachings, were administered by the priestly class. The priests retained a very high position and were responsible for interpretation, enforcement, and preservation of the dogma.

The Vedas, usually dated about 1600 BC, consisted of four books. The Rig-Veda, the Yajur-Veda, and the Sama-Veda were almost entirely religious. In the Rig-Veda, disease was regarded as the result of divine wrath. The Atharva-Veda contained innumerable incantations and charms for the practice of magic; disease, injuries, sanity, health, and fertility were mentioned.

> In India, as in all other countries curative spells and healing mantras (charms) preceded medicine; and the first man of medicine in India was a priest, a Bhisag Atharvan (i.e., *magic doctor*), who held a superior position to a surgeon in society.
>
> *Sushruta-Samhita, Introduction, p. xiv*

59

Supplemental Vedas (Upavedas) were also developed. Of these the Ayur-Veda or Science of Life was supposed to have been derived from Brahma himself. It contained eight parts that dealt with subjects such as medicine, surgery, and children's diseases and stressed hygiene and prevention of illness. From these writings various authors made Samhitas or compendiums for which they claimed divine origin. Two of these contributors were regarded as the most influential: Sushruta and Charaka. The dates of origin of these documents vary widely from the fourth century BC to the fifth century AD.

> The surgical treatise (Sushruta-Samhita) is probably the older, though some critics have assigned the two works to the same period, the fourth century BC. The question of date is chiefly important as involving a doubt whether the Hindu medical system is primitive and entirely indigenous, or was influenced by Greece and through Greece by Egypt.
>
> *Seymer, 1932, p. 9*

Sushruta represented the surgical aspect of Indian medicine; Charaka symbolized the medical aspect. Charaka was believed to have inherited wisdom from a serpent-god with a thousand heads who was the caretaker of all the sciences, especially medicine (Stewart and Austin, 1962). Both authors reveal a highly developed medicine and surgery, which no doubt evolved slowly after the writing of the Vedas and was incidentally influenced by contacts with the cultures of the Near East.

Indian surgery was the most skilled of any ancient culture. Operations such as tonsillectomies, which were unknown to the later Greeks and Romans, were performed in India. Furthermore, Hindu surgeons performed amputations, excised tumors, repaired hernias and harelips, removed bladder stones, couched cataracts (displaced the opacifying lens down and away from the line of vision), reconstructed noses, and delivered by Cesarean section. In addition to the procedures related to surgery, about 125 different surgical instruments were described. Hindu physicians drugged their patients with hyoscyamus, henbane, and *Cannabis Indica* and used hypnosis in an attempt to provide anesthesia. Great care was taken in the washing and bandaging of wounds (fifteen principal varieties of bandage were available). The Ideal Doctor was identified in the following way:

> He should be cleanly in his habits and well shaved, and should not allow his nails to grow. He should wear white garments, put on a pair of shoes, carry a stick and an umbrella in his hands, and walk about with a mild and benignant look as a friend of all created beings. . . . A physician should abjure the company of women, nor should he speak in private to them or joke with them.
>
> *Bhishagratna, 1907, p. 74*

Many illnesses, such as tuberculosis, typhoid fever, leprosy, hepatitis, neurological disorders, and cholera were described. The epithet "mellitus" (honeylike) was applied to diabetes, and its symptoms were identified as languor, thirst, and foul breath. Variolation was practiced. About fifteen scarifications were made with a needle on the upper arm of a person to be immunized; the area was then covered with cotton dipped in pock material. Transmitters of specific diseases, such as mosquitoes in connection with malaria, were described. It was believed that prevention of disease was more important than the cure. Indian medicine also displayed ideas about pathology, the most notable being that disease might be caused by impurities in the body fluids or humors. This humoral pathology later was emphasized by Greek physicians and ultimately became a basic concept for European medicine.

An interesting portrayal of a team concept of medical care was presented in one Indian document:

> The Physician, the Drugs, the Nurse, and the Patient constitute an aggregate of four. Of what virtues each of these should be possessed, so as to become causes for the cure of the disease, should be known.
>
> *Physician.* Thorough mastery of the scriptures, large experience, cleverness, and purity (of body and mind) are the principal qualities of the physician.
>
> *Drugs.* Abundance of virtue, adaptability to the disease under treatment, the capacity of being used in diverse ways, and undeterioration are attributes of drugs.
>
> *Nurse.* Knowledge of the manner in which drugs should be prepared or compounded for administration, cleverness, devotedness to the patient waited upon, and purity (both of mind and body) are the four qualifications of the attending nurse.
>
> *Patient.* Memory, obedience to direction, fearlessness, and communicativeness (with respect to all that is experienced internally and done by him during the intervals between visits) are the qualities of the patient.
>
> As in the task of cooking, a vessel, fuel, and fire are the means in the hands of the cook; as field, army, and weapons are means in the victor's hands for achieving victory in battles; even the patient, the nurse, and drugs are the objects that are regarded as the physician's means in the matter of achieving a cure.
>
> Like clay, stick, wheel, threads, in the absence of the potter, failing to produce anything by their combination, the three others, viz., drugs, nurse, and patient cannot work out a cure in the absence of the physician.
>
> *Kaviratna, n.d., pp. 102–103*

As time passed, the people of India became dissatisfied with the religion of the Vedas. There had long been those who had chosen the life of a recluse to attain a more intimate relationship with the spiritual. Among them was Siddhartha Gautama (560–480 BC?), from the caste of princes, who left home, wife, and child at the age of twenty-nine to find salvation. After wandering and speculation, he announced himself as Buddha, the Enlightened, and offered a new religious philosophy that came to be known as Buddhism. The major premise of Buddhism was based on the idea that perfection consisted of attaining nothingness, which was to be accomplished by severe penances.

"The long period of India's Golden Age was that in which the religion of Buddha prevailed. It was a religion of mercy, compassion, and justice which enjoined humane treatment for animals as well as man" (Stewart and Austin, 1962, p. 24). Buddhism was, however, more of a moral discipline than an organized religion and encouraged the development of social institutions. India's greatest convert to Buddhism was King Asoka (269–237 BC), but he was unsuccessful in instituting its acceptance on a permanent basis. During Asoka's reign the greatest advances in charitable and sanitary work were made. Among his many generous works, he established hospitals that are considered to be the first in world history. The exact number of hospitals he developed is not known. According to Shryock (1959), there was difficulty with the Sanskrit word for "hospital," since it could also be interpreted as "pharmacy" or "dispensary." However, there is no question that hospitals of some type were built during this period. These hospitals were constructed periodically by government order, serviced by government-paid physicians, and supplied by government stores. Consequently, state medicine had become a reality in India.

The early physicians came from the priestly or Brahmin caste. Later, physicians were drawn from the upper castes, and eventually all practitioners came to be known as Vaidya. High moral standards were expected of those who chose the care of the sick as a life's work. Permission to practice was obtained from the king, a procedure similar to the current licensing system. Appearance, dress, speech, and manners had to be above reproach. Rules for ritual and daily life were dictated by the Laws of Manu, which were compiled between 200 BC and 200 AD. These laws have been compared to the Mosaic Laws because they include ordinances for regulation of family and personal hygiene and dietary practices. According to the Laws of Manu, physicians could be penalized for improper treatment of patients.

The history of India reveals a more complete description of nursing principles and practice than that of any other ancient civilization. Throughout the historical documents of India frequent references are made to nurses. In most instances these nurses were male; however, in rare cases they were old women. Three main qualities of character—high standards, skill, and trustworthiness—were also required of these attendants. The specific requirements are described in the following passages:

> After this should be secured a body of attendants of good behaviour, distinguished for purity or cleanliness of habits, attached to the person for whose service they are engaged, possessed of cleverness and skill, endued with kindness, skilled in every kind of service that a patient may require, endued with general cleverness, competent to cook food and curries, clever in bathing or washing a patient, well conversant in rubbing or pressing the limbs, or raising the patient or assisting him in walking or moving about, well skilled in making or cleaning beds, competent to pound drugs, or ready, patient, and skilful in waiting upon one that is ailing, and never unwilling to do any act that they may be commanded (by the physician or patient) to do.
>
> *Charaka-Samhita, vol. 1, pp. 168–169*

Nurse. That person alone is fit to nurse or to attend the bedside of a patient who is cool-headed and pleasant in his demeanour, does not speak ill of anybody, is strong and attentive to the requirements of the sick, and strictly and indefatigably follows the instructions of the physician.

Sushruta-Samhita, vol. 1, chap. 34, pp. 305–307

It was apparently the existence of hospitals that created a need for this special group. Although it is certain that nurses were employed in the hospitals of India, it is unclear whether they were viewed as glorified servants or as professional personnel. Women were midwives and in some cases the experts of drug lore. They held a high position in India, and their activities centered about the management of the home. It is assumed that women functioned as nurses when members of their family became ill.

China

Ancient China was cut off from the Mediterranean world by the great range of the Himalaya Mountains. It lay far to the northeast of India and remains somewhat a mystery, since accurate records are not available before the Shang Dynasty (c. 1776–1122 BC). The inhabitants of China are believed to have come from central Asia about 3000 BC, settling along the banks of the Yellow River. The land of this region was very fertile. Grain became the staple crop, fruit trees were prevalent, and vegetation was so luxurious that the title of The Flowery Kingdom was conferred upon China.

Information about this early civilization is primarily legendary, yet it emerged in possession of social, religious, and political institutions. China's history became authentic with the appearance of the second Chou Dynasty (1122–249 BC), a rule that lasted almost 900 years. Civilization spread south from the Yellow River to the Yangtse River during this time. The people belonged to the Mongoloid race and had great respect for social order. A creative people, they carved in wood and ivory, produced works of art in bronze and lacquer, and used irrigation systems for their fields. Poetry and history were written, although the Chinese writing was slow, complicated, and difficult. It contained symbols that represented objects (pictograms), ideas (ideograms), and sounds (phonograms). Sacred books were also written, and these were comparable to the papyri of Egypt and the Vedas of India.

The Chinese form of government was a patriarchal rule. Since the family was the fundamental unit of the society, the government was concerned with the social group rather than the individual. Local government was comprised of a group of elders who were representatives of various families making up a particular village. The elders, who met in the local temple to manage the village affairs, were the liaison between the people and the monarch. Shang, the first known dynasty, was followed by the Chous with a feudal form of government. These were succeeded by the Ch'in in the third century BC, when various feudal states were united into one empire.

Four social classes were recognized in China: scholars, farmers, artisans, and traders. In reality, however, two classes functioned; these were the officials (mandarins) and the nonofficials. The officials were selected on a talent basis rather than by class, since civil service, an ancient institution in China, opened examinations to all who could qualify.

Three religious systems influenced China: Taoism and Confucianism, which were indigenous, and Buddhism, which was imported from India. "Taoism was characterized by freedom from desire within one's self and an absence of self-determined actions for particular ends in things exterior to one's self" (Frank, 1953, p. 26). It was a religion concerned with obtaining long life and good fortune, often through magical means. The value of charms was emphasized as a method to combat the demons of disease. These charms were written on paper that was burned; the ashes were administered in a liquid such as tea. The study of alchemy arose from the practice of searching for the elixir of life, the transmutation of base metals into gold. Taoism ultimately yielded to Confucianism and Buddhism.

Confucius entered the life of China about 500 BC. He studied the sacred books as a child and later emerged as one of the greatest reformers and teachers the world has ever known. Confucius was a political reformer rather than a religious originator. His political reforms were based on moral principles, and he sought to relieve oppression by returning to ancient customs as a basis for government. Confucius stressed family cohesion, the value of knowledge, right conduct (etiquette), and ancestor worship, which prevented dissections of bodies. (No worship was accorded to female ancestors.) Confucius' philosophy was the negative version of the Golden Rule: What you do not wish done to yourself, do not do unto others. On the whole, Confucianism did not promote progress, since it failed to stimulate ambition for better things. Yet some progress was achieved in China. By 200 BC Buddhism became the religion of the land, having been brought from India into the Far East.

The religious practices of China were polytheistic, animistic, and idolatrous. Images of painted wood were adored and sacrifices were offered to these images because the people believed them to be inhabited by souls. The evil spirits responsible for disease and disaster were frightened off by loud noises. It is interesting to note that sacrifice to the gods was an official state function. Only distinguished social groups were permitted to participate in the ceremonies; the people could participate only in those ceremonies for worship of their own ancestors.

Chinese medicine was focused on prevention. Health was considered to be a state of harmony or equilibrium within the individual and the universe. This state was accomplished through the interplay of nature's basic duality: the yang (male principle), which was positive, warm, dry, light, full of life, and the yin (female principle), which was negative, passive, dark, cold, moist, weak, and lifeless. An improper balance of these energies resulted in discomfort and disease. Illness could also be caused by evil spirits and animistic forces.

The works of three legendary emperors provided the basic foundation for Chinese medicine. Fu Hsi (c. 2900 BC) created the *pa kua,* a symbol with yang and yin lines combined in eight separate trigrams. These could represent all yin-yang conditions. Shen Nung (Hung Ti), the Red Emperor, wrote the *Pen Tsao* (*Herbal*), which

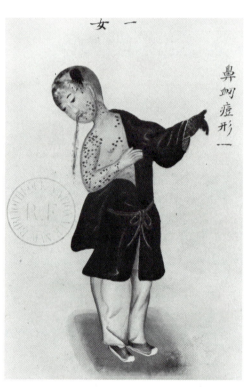

INFANTILE ERUPTION. *Chinese silk, eighteenth century. Bibliothèque Nationale, Paris, France.*

was the result of his investigations of medicinal herbs. The effects of 365 drugs personally tested were reported. Shen Nung is also thought to have drawn the first charts on acupuncture. Huang Ti (Yu Hsiung), the Yellow Emperor, was credited with writing the great medical compendium titled *Nei Ching* (*Canon of Medicine*). According to this work, four steps in examination were necessary to determine a diagnosis: Look, Listen, Ask, Feel (observation, auscultation, interrogation, and palpation). All phases of health and illness, including prevention and treatment, were recorded in this canon of medicine.

Medical knowledge in early China included dissection techniques, studies of the circulatory system, massage, the therapeutic use of baths, and the significance of pulse rates. Diagnoses were often made on the basis of a complicated pulse theory in which the pulse of the patient was studied over a period of several hours. Some 200 types of pulse beat were listed.

> The physician felt the right wrist and then the left. He compared the beats with his own, noting precise time as well as day and season since each hour affected the nature of the pulsations. Each pulse had three distinct divisions, each associated with a specific organ, and each division had a separate quality, of which there were dozens of varieties. Moreover, each division or zone of the pulse had a superficial and deep projection. Thus literally hundreds of possible characteristics were obtainable. In one treatise, *Muo-Ching,* ten volumes were necessary to cover all the intricacies of the pulse.
>
> *Lyons, 1978, p. 127*

Five methods of treatment were identified in the *Nei Ching:* cure the spirit, nourish the body, give medications, treat the whole body, and use acupuncture and moxibustion. Acupuncture consisted of inserting needles an inch or so into areas along the twelve meridians that traverse the body and using a twisting motion. Moxibustion used the same meridians. However, this treatment used a powdered plant substance (cones of mugwort), which was fashioned into a mound on the patient's skin and burned slowly. This method of counterirritation caused blisters to form on the area.

Smallpox was a widely known disease in China. A more primitive form of variolation than that used in India was performed by the Chinese. Crusts of diseased pustules were ground into a powder and blown into the nostril with a bamboo tube. Surgery was limited to castration of males seeking advancement at court and to treatment of wounds. The limited development of surgery may have been a result of the belief that mutilation of the body would remain in evidence in life after death. Chinese medicine spread into Korea, Japan, and Tibet, where superstition mixed with these practices.

Little mention is made of hospitals in ancient China, although Halls of Healing are described. These were adjuncts to the temples where the sick prayed for recovery. Berdoe (1893) correlates the absence of hospitals with the duty of the Chinese people to care for their families at home. Even more striking is the lack of reference to nursing in the literature of the ancient Chinese. If there were nurses, they were probably not women, since the woman's position, as

65

defined by Confucius, was inferior. A woman's work was confined to the keeping of the home and the building of families. Her value was greatest when she produced a son. It is also possible that the belief that disease could be caused by evil spirits taking up residence in the patient's body had a distinct impact on care of the sick. The fear that these spirits could enter anyone who touched a sick person would make nursing almost nonexistent.

■ THE MEDITERRANEAN WORLD

Greece

Ancient Greece was a peninsula that jutted out into the Mediterranean Sea from the southeastern part of Europe. Surrounded by gulfs and ocean, its indented coastline provided good harbors, which led to the establishment of trade. The interior of the country was mountainous; the climate was warm and sunny. This topography led to a particular political organization in which small groups of people settled in the plains and valleys between the mountains. Cities were built within a 200- to 300-square-mile area. A location with a commanding view was chosen in each city for use during an attack by enemies. Temples and other buildings were also erected on this site. Eventually government functions were assumed by these cities, which became the ruling authorities in areas with a radius of approximately ten miles. Each area was designated as an independent "city state" with a king, a council, and an assembly.

Civilization entered Greece through the island of Crete by way of Egypt and Phoenicia. It was not unlike that of the peoples of the Near East. Its growth was nourished partly by the inhabitants of the Crete and Aegean islands and the mainland and also by communication with the ancient civilizations of Egypt and Mesopotamia. The Greek people or Hellenes, as the Greeks called themselves, who migrated into the area were of Indo-European stock. They assimilated the preexisting civilization. The Greeks were unlike other ancient peoples because they were keen observers, not experimenters; they were philosophers, not scientists. Their sense of beauty encompassed proportion and spatial relationships, resulting in architecture and temples of the highest artistic caliber. The scattered nation was unified by language, literature, and religious worship. The Panhellenic or Olympic Games, held every four years dating from 776 BC, brought the people together to compete for prizes. In addition, every family aimed to produce participants with healthy bodies.

Recorded Greek history begins with the Homeric Age or Age of Heroes. The writings of Homer, *The Iliad* and *The Odyssey,* became the sacred books of Greece. Through mythology the origins of the peoples were traced and health, illness, and medical practice were discussed. "In the Homeric poems, one gets a glimpse of common-sense remedies and of simple wound surgery, of charms against sickness, and of appeals to this god or that to protect a warrior against injury" (Shryock, 1959, p. 41).

The Greeks had the ancient gods of the earth and the underworld as well as special healing agents such as snakes and moles.

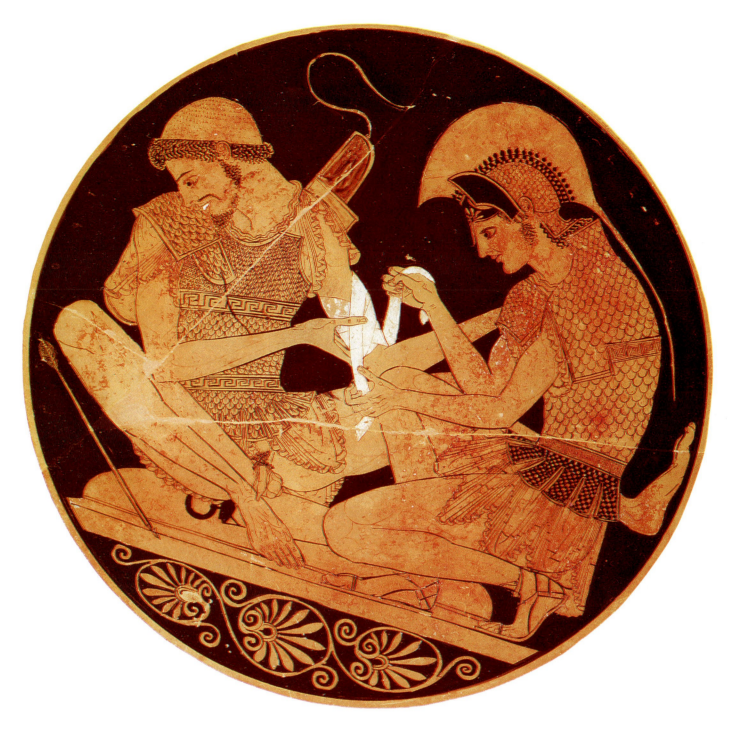

Apollo, the sun god, was the god of health and medicine. Asklepios (in Rome called Aesculapius), son of Apollo and a human mother, was the chief healer of Greek mythology. His fame may have been created from a mortal of fame and skill, for it is traced to about thirteen centuries before Christ. According to Frank (1953), this mortal was a Greek physician who was raised to the rank of a god. In addition, two of his sons accompanied the Greek army to the Trojan War. Machaon was a surgeon with "skilled hands to draw out darts and heal sores"; Podalirius was an internist who was "given cunning to find out things impossible and cure that which healed not." Asklepios was represented holding the wand of Mercury, a wayfarer's staff entwined with the sacred serpents of wisdom. The medical caduceus is derived from this portrayal.

ACHILLES BANDAGING THE WOUNDS OF PATROCLUS, *detail from the bowl of Sosias, c. 50 BC. Museum of Greek and Roman Antiquities, Staatliche Museen Preussischer Kulturbesitz, Berlin, Federal Republic of Germany.*

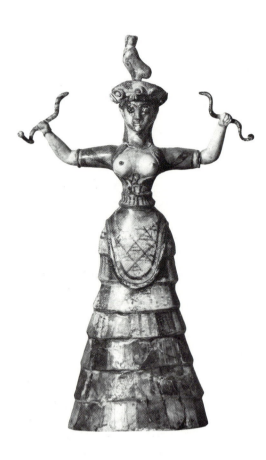

THE SNAKE GODDESS, *from the Palace of Knossos, c. 1600 BC. Faience, approx. 34.3 cm high. Archaeological Museum, Herakleion, Greece. (Hirmer Verlag, Munich).*

The women also shared the work of health conservation in the myth of Asklepios. Epigone, the wife, was revered as "the soothing one." The six daughters included Hygeia, the "goddess of health"; Panacea, the "restorer of health," who personified miraculous all-healing herbs; Aegle, the "light of the sun"; Meditrina, the "preserver of health" (supposedly the ancient forerunner of the public health nurse); and Iaso, who personified the "recovery from illness."

> The whole family of Asklepios has significance for the medical and nursing arts, for if its members were only symbolic, they must have been meant to depict those arts as they existed at that time, and if they were actual persons they combined in their careers all the main lines of specialism that we consider modern.
>
> *Stewart and Austin, 1962, p. 28*

The myth of Asklepios became highly complex. Temples were built to him on sites of great natural beauty with pure spring water (often this water had already been noted for its medicinal properties) and refreshing breezes. The buildings, masterpieces of architecture, were exquisitely decorated. Those temples that became famous for cures would emerge as great social and intellectual centers. Theaters, gymnasiums, a stadium, places for worship, a hospital, living quarters for patients, baths, lodgings for visitors and attendants, housing for priests and physicians, and libraries were built nearby and surrounded by gardens and park lands. These health resorts were frequented not only by people who were ill but also by those who enjoyed the beauty and contentment of the surroundings and the brilliance of cultural life and entertainment. The most famous of these centers was Epidauros, situated a few miles from Athens. It accommodated about 500 patients and was serviced by a chief administrator and various grades of attendants, including priestesses.

Upon arrival, patients offered sacrifices of animals to Asklepios and underwent a cleansing or purifying process consisting of a series of baths and a period of abstinence from certain foods and wines. After several days in the outer courts, the patient was admitted to the inner court to participate in religious ceremonies that included elaborate rites and rituals. Finally, the patient was admitted to the abaton to sleep in full sight of a great statue to the god. This incubation or temple sleep would reveal through a dream or hypnotic state the treatment to be administered. Votive tablets were left behind that attested to innumerable cures. Yet maternity patients and the incurably ill were not admitted to the temples for medical assistance.

Two other institutions offered care to the sick: the xenodochium and the iatrion. The xenodochium was similar in function to the Hebrew xenodochium and first provided care for travelers, then for people who were sick or injured. In the later centuries of Greek history, it was placed under municipal management and may have been the forerunner of the modern city and county hospital. The iatrion was a facility where ambulatory care was received. It corresponds most closely with the dispensary or outpatient clinics of present-day hospitals.

The cult of Asklepios, which evolved from Greek mythology, provided religious healing and offered a blend of natural and supernatural remedies. Eventually the priests of Asklepios branched into

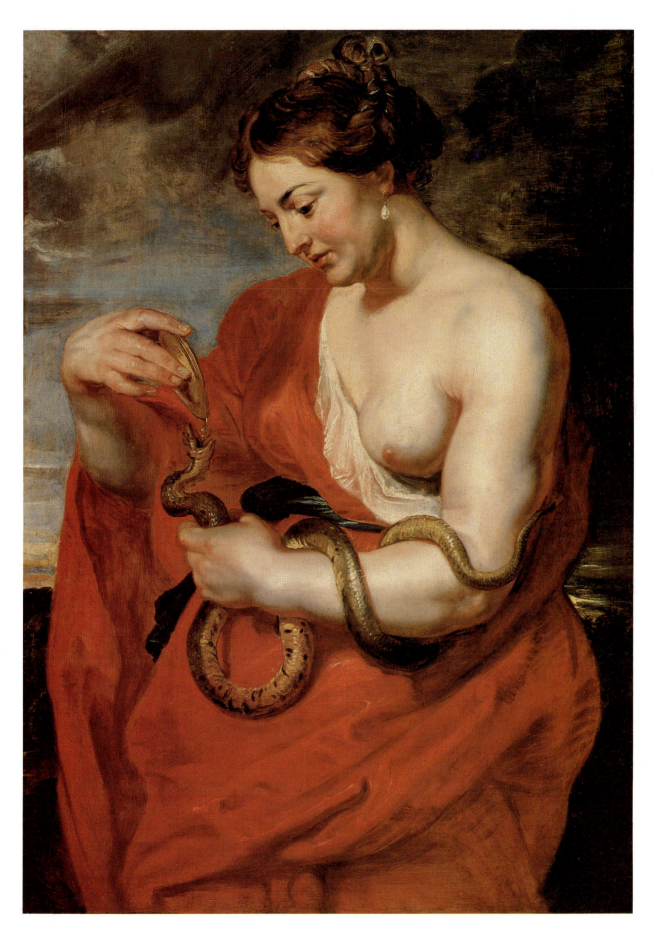

Peter Paul Rubens, HYGEIA, GODDESS OF HEALTH, *c. 1615. Oil on panel, 106.7 × 74.3 cm. Detroit Institute of Arts, Michigan, Gift of Mr. and Mrs. Henry Reicchold.*

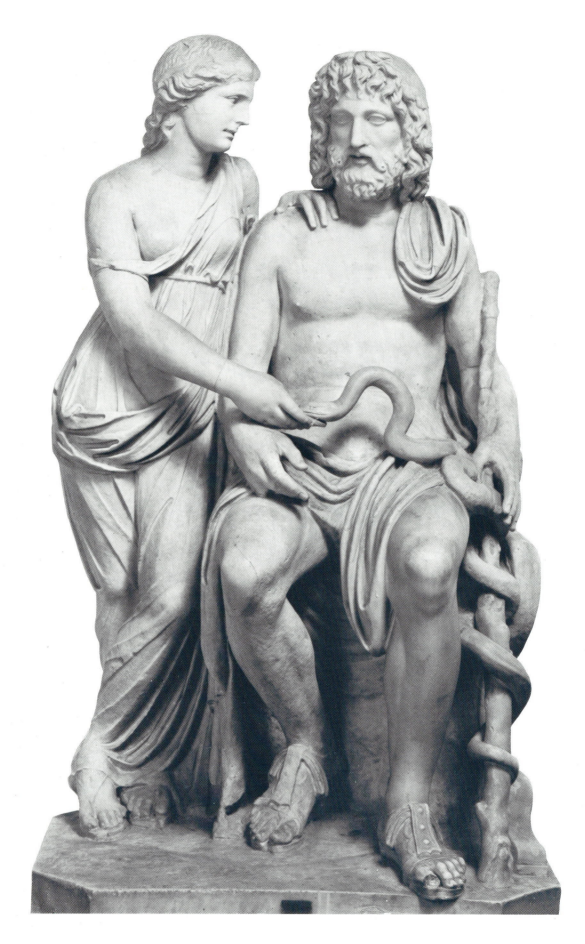

ASKLEPIOS AND HIS DAUGHTER HYGEIA, *Vatican Museum, Rome, Italy.*

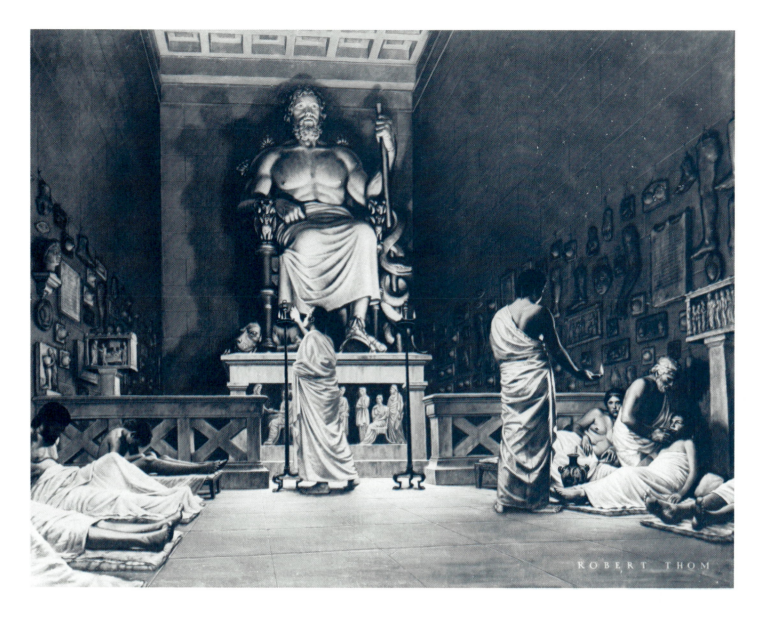

two specialized areas, one strictly medical and the other purely occult. From the medical branch a group of lay physicians developed.

TEMPLE AND CULT OF ASKLEPIOS, *Parke-Davis Division of Warner-Lambert Co., Morris Plains, New Jersey.*

> While the shrines of Aesculapius continued to offer religious
> healing, lay physicians accumulated factual knowledge about
> common illnesses and how to handle them. These men moved
> from one town to another as skilled artisans and learned much
> from the bedside. They practiced both general medicine and
> surgery, and the experience of a number of them was finally
> incorporated in a collection of writings ascribed to Hippocrates.
> Although there probably was a physician of that name, he did not
> write all these works; as his name became legendary, it was
> applied to the whole collection. This became the first general
> text on medicine and was long viewed as a sort of Bible by the
> medical profession.
>
> *Shryock, 1959, pp. 46–47*

As Greek civilization progressed, many changes took place. The
healing arts were particularly affected during the Golden Age of
Greece between the sixth and fourth centuries before Christ. This

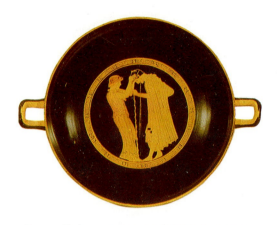

Brygos Painter, WOMAN ATTENDING A MAN VOMITING, *detail from the interior of a kylix, c. 490 BC. Martin V. Wagner Museum der Universität, Würzburg, Federal Republic of Germany.*

was "the birth or age of reason," which culminated in the classical philosophy of Socrates, Plato, Aristotle, and others. These days of the philosopher-scientists were devoted to an attempt to attribute natural rather than supernatural explanations to phenomena. Truth was sought through clear thinking and close observation of physical and social phenomena. This study of nature was eventually called "natural philosophy," the first clear expression of what is now known as science. The results of these scientific and philosophical investigations provided the fundamentals of good living.

Thales (640?–546 BC) was the first of the Greek scientist-philosophers. He made many contributions to navigation, astronomy, mathematics, and geometry but was known best for his explanations of phenomena. Thales did not use religious means to prove the natural processes of the universe; he did not rely on the supernatural. He proposed that the underlying principles of solutions to problems must be found in addition to the solutions themselves. Socrates and Plato laid the foundation for philosophy and government. It was Aristotle (384–322 BC), however, who had a profound influence on medicine. He was credited with laying the foundation of biology as well as comparative anatomy. His contributions in the field of both plant and animal biology greatly aided the development of medical thought. In addition, Aristotle dealt with ethical matters in a scientific manner.

Despite the fact that rational medicine had been developing before him and magical medicine persisted long after his time, Hippocrates of Cos (460–370 BC?) was given credit for the establishment of rational or scientific medicine. He belonged to the order of Asklepiades and was believed to have been a direct descendant of Asklepios himself. Hippocrates is considered to have been one of the greatest physicians who ever lived and became known as the Father of Medicine. He taught that disease was not the work of spirits, demons, or deities but the result of the breaking of natural laws. The true art of the physician, therefore, was to assist Nature to bring about a cure. The writings attributed to Hippocrates relate to nearly all aspects of medicine—pathology, anatomy, physiology, diagnosis, prognosis, mental illness, gynecology, obstetrics, surgery, therapy, bedside observations, hygiene, and professional ethics. Epilepsy, tuberculosis, malarial fever, ulcers, and other diseases were described. Perhaps the most interesting and significant portions of these writings were the "case histories," which were preserved in the *Epidemics.* These included a compilation of the details of the patient who was ill, the patient's environment, and the complete examination. Even today, these case histories could serve as models for succinct clinical records, since they are comprehensive, concise, and direct.

The practice of hygiene was more than a medical specialty. It was a way of life depicted in part by Hippocrates' discussion of diet, the avoidance of sexual excesses, and the importance of exercise. His emphasis on the role of environment in the spread of disease, as presented in *Airs, Waters and Places,* provided a basic epidemiological text in which the concepts of endemic diseases (those always present) and epidemic diseases (those that broke out at certain periods and involved large numbers of people) were illuminated (Rosen,

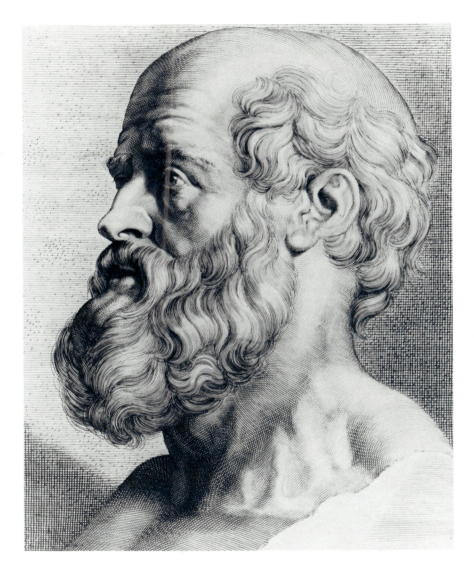

Paulus Pontius, HIPPOCRATES, *early seventeenth century. Engraving after a drawing by Peter Paul Rubens from an ancient marble bust. National Library of Medicine, Bethesda, Maryland.*

1958). Therapy was related to the elements of fire, air, earth, and water. In different combinations these exhibited the four basic qualities of heat, cold, dryness, and moisture. Everything, including the body, was composed of one or more of these elements. This led to the classic four humors (blood, phlegm, yellow bile, and black bile) theory of disease. When these humors were in balance, the result was a healthy body; excess or deficiency of one or more caused illness.

The Hippocratic method rested on the following four principles (Lyons, 1978):

1. Observe all.
2. Study the patient rather than the disease.
3. Evaluate honestly.
4. Assist nature.

These principles were to be combined with the professional spirit, or ethical conduct. The true physician needed to be devoted to his profession and his patients and was to abstain from all that would dishonor one and injure the other.

The literature of the Greeks contains many references to nurses. However, these were primarily children's nurses, wet nurses, and midwives. (Midwives provided most of the obstetrical care; physi-

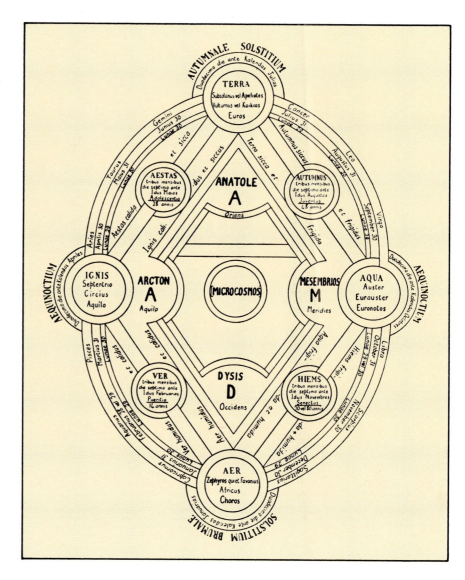

cians assisted with difficult or abnormal childbirth.) In historical accounts discrepancies exist about who performed the other nursing functions because the activities of a Greek woman were confined to the home unless she was a priestess, a slave, or a harlot. According to Shryock (1959), Greek women could not be admitted to the "mysteries" of any art. Thus, even if the Greeks had nurses, they would probably have been men. Even Hippocrates, the master of medical art, left no direct reference to nurses.

> A most remarkable feature of the ancient medical writings is the scant attention paid to that very important factor in modern treatment—the nurse. Professional nurses were, apparently, unknown, (Note: midwives were common enough) and the general impression that the reader forms is that the physician did not consider the work of the attendant to be of great value. In some cases, doubtless, the household slaves acted as nurses.... But the burden of nursing fell chiefly upon the wife.... It is clear then that in ordinary cases it was the duty of the wife to nurse the whole household, with the help no doubt of her daughters and maid servants.
>
> *Jones, 1909, pp. 123–126*

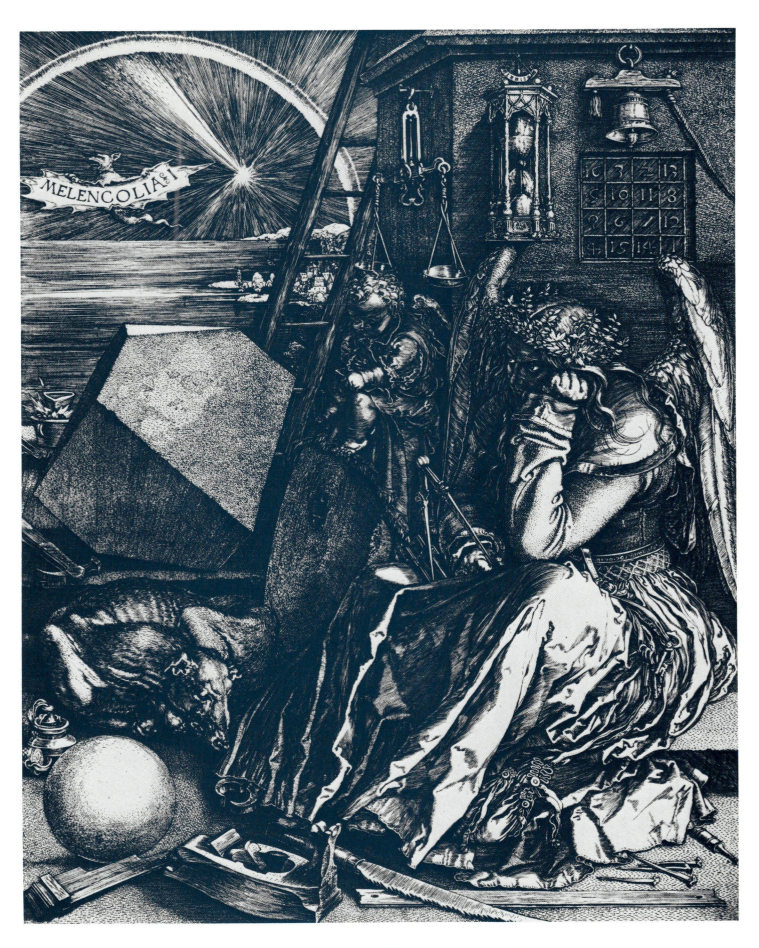

Albrecht Dürer, MELENCOLIA, 1514. Engraving, approx. 24.1 × 16.5 cm. Wallnaf-Richartz-Museum, Cologne, Federal Republic of Germany.

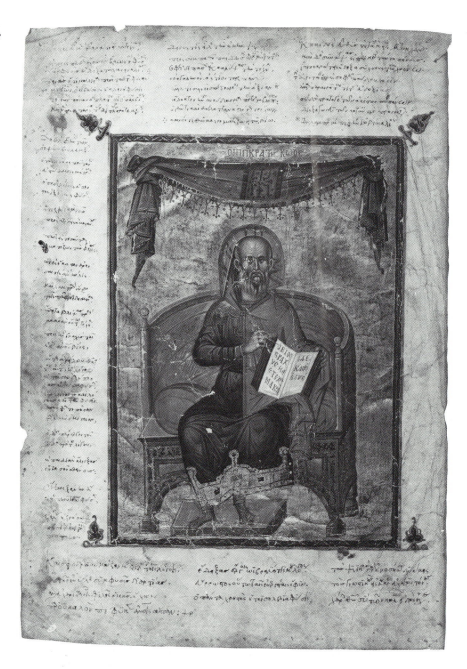

HIPPOCRATES *as envisioned by a Byzantine artist, c. 1342. Illuminated Greek Manuscript 2144, f. 10v. Bibliothèque Nationale, Paris, France.*

Yet in the Hippocratic writings what we now call nursing is taught in minute detail and the assistant or attendant is indicated as the co-worker of the physician. Specific directions about poultices, cold sponging, fluid diets, warm baths, light and regular nourishment for heart cases, large amounts of fluid for kidney cases, the use of mouth-washes, and clean, smooth bed linen are given. It is clear from these writings that nursing care existed in ancient Greece. However, what nursing care was actually like is left to the imagination.

Rome

While civilization was progressing in the East and Greece was emerging in the realms of art and thinking, a new power began to form in the West. This occurred in the peninsula we now know as Italy, where an agricultural people known as Latins resided. Italy was separated from Greece by water and divided into two sections by a chain of mountains. The level plains on the western side were initially chosen by the Latins for the location of their homes. This area was occupied in ancient times by various peoples, the oldest of whom were the Etruscans, who had migrated from Asia Minor. The Etruscans achieved a higher degree of culture than other tribes of this area. They were later conquered and absorbed by the Romans.

The Gauls, or Celts, from Western Europe originally occupied the northern part of Italy. The Greeks began to settle in southern Italy about the eighth century BC in an area that became known as Magna Graecia (Greater Greece). Eventually the Romans, who were excellent warriors, conquered and absorbed them all. This Latin tribe had occupied the central and northern portions of Italy. In time, they succeeded in bringing unity to the country under their rule. As a result, the village of Rome passed from a simple farming community to a thriving commercial center.

Legend places the birth of Rome at 753 BC. Located at the mouth of the Tiber, Rome progressed through the stages of a kingdom, a republic, an empire and a city. The event of its founding is

Baburen, ROMAN CHARITY, c. 1620. Canvas. York City Art Gallery, England.

This painting illustrates the story of Cimon and Pero. Cimon, an aged man, was in prison awaiting execution, and was therefore given no food. The jailer allowed his daughter, Pero, to visit; she secretly nursed him by giving him her breast.

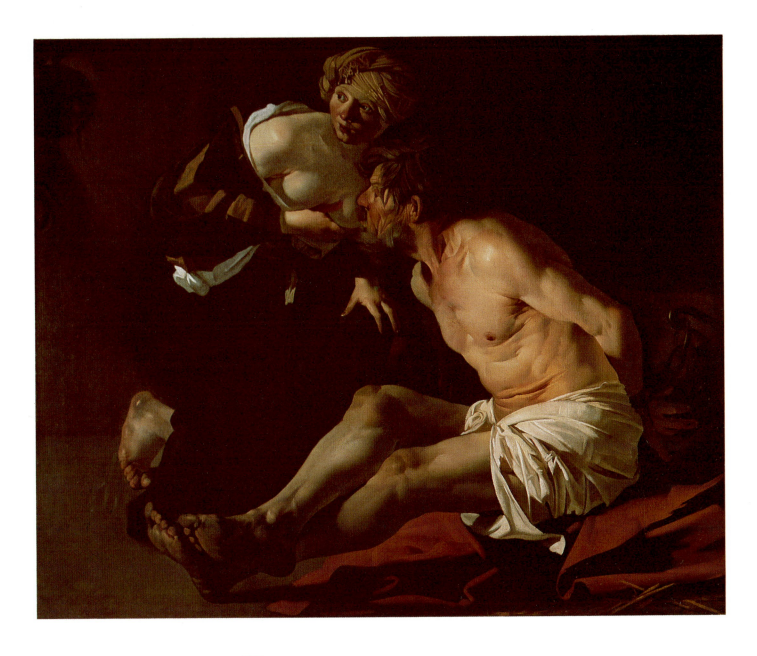

intertwined with a variety of mythological interpretations. One account is told by Virgil in his great epic poem, *The Aeneid*, which describes the wanderings of Aeneas and his companions in the period from the fall of Troy to the founding of Rome. It is also said that the site of Rome on seven hills "appears to have been the choice of twin brothers, Romulus and Remus, themselves indebted for life to the nourishment and care given them by a kindly wolf who found them on a mountain top, abandoned by a goddess mother" (Jamieson and Sewall, 1950, p. 74).

The Romans did not develop a religion, a medical system, or an art of their own. These were borrowed from their conquests, from other peoples and nations. From Greece, which was under Roman control by 146 BC, tangible things such as money, textiles, and sailing ships were acquired. Eventually Greek ideas were also absorbed, as well as art and religion. The Greek alphabet was adapted to the Latin tongue.

Early Romans possessed gods whose functions were highly practical. Jupiter guarded the welfare of the city, Juno was the woman's patroness, Mars was the god of war, and Janus was the god of openings or beginnings. Prosperity occurred if one pleased the gods; failure resulted if the wrath of the gods was incurred. During this early period no distinctive gods of healing were identified. However,

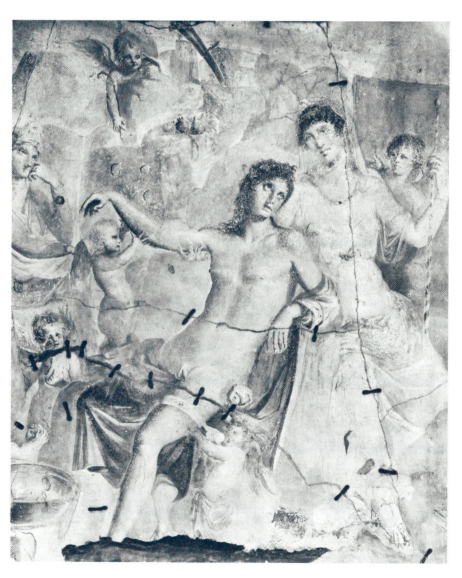

THE WOUNDED ADONIS ASSISTED BY VENUS AND BANDAGED BY CUPID. *Pompeiian fresco. Casa di Adone, Rome, Italy. (Alinari/Art Resource, NY).*

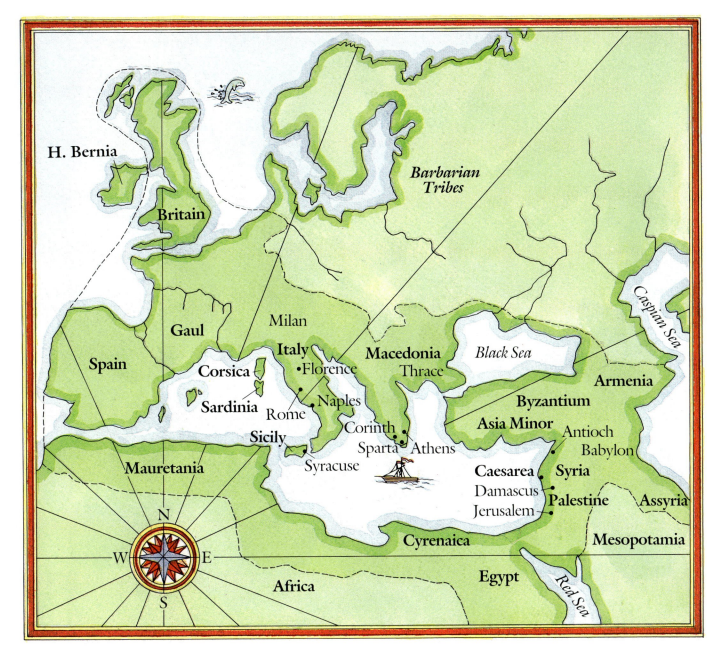

H. Bernia

Britain

Gaul

Spain

Milan

Italy

Corsica

Florence

Sardinia

Rome

Naples

Sicily

Mauretania

Syracuse

N

W

E

S

Barbarian
Tribes

Macedonia

Thrace

Black Sea

Caspian Sea

Armenia

Byzantium

Asia Minor

Antioch

Babylon

Corinth

Sparta

Athens

Caesarea

Syria

Damascus

Jerusalem

Palestine

Assyria

Cyrenaica

Mesopotamia

Africa

Egypt

Red Sea

Map of the ROMAN EMPIRE AT ITS GREATEST
EXTENT.

in a later period gods were borrowed from the Greeks and polytheism prevailed. These gods included Hygeia and Asklepios. It is
also said that there was a god or goddess for almost every known
physiological function or disease process, for example, Scabies, Ange-
ronia, Fluonia, Uterina, and Febris. Febris became particularly significant to Rome for the power of reducing fevers associated with
malaria (Frank, 1953). Yet the ancient Romans were free from the
superstition that the sick and insane were possessed by demons.

The Roman population was divided into two classes: the patri-
cians (wealthy or privileged group), who were given civil and legal
privileges and whose right to citizenship was hereditary, and the
plebeians (poor or lower class), who were denied the right of citizenship. Work was given over to home slaves who were brought
from conquered countries. Homes became luxurious, dress elaborate, and social functions extravagant. The demarcation line between
the rich and the poor broadened. Internal decay emerged and con-

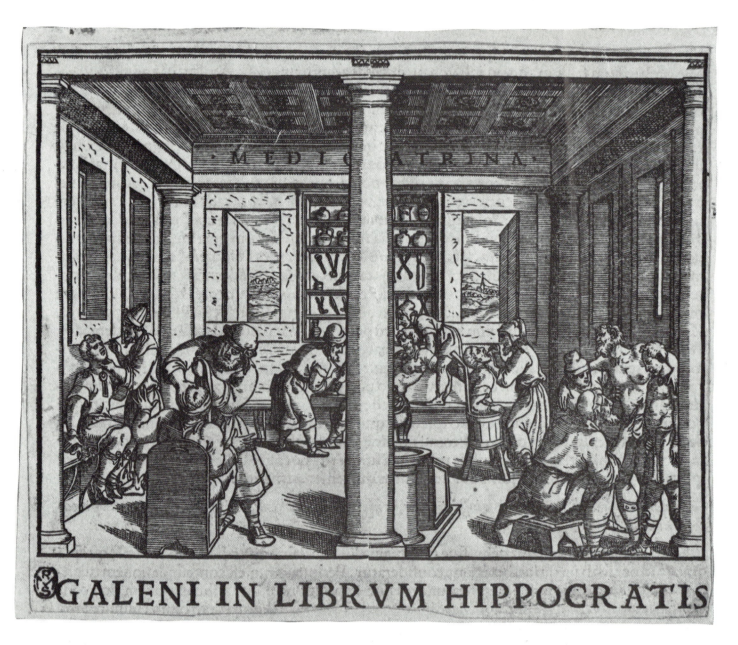

GALENI IN LIBRVM HIPPOCRATIS

CLINIC SCENE FROM THE WORKS OF GALEN.
Printed in Venice 1550. Achille Bertarelli Collection, Milan, Italy.

tinued. The Roman Empire lasted about five centuries, from 31 BC to 476 AD. The first two centuries were spent in peace and prosperity; the third century was marked by frequent disorder within the Empire; the last two centuries were characterized by internal rebellion and external attack. The decline and fall of Rome was unavoidable and occurred by 476 AD. The church founded by Jesus Christ was the one institution that remained unshaken during this time.

Before the conquest of Greece, Roman medicine combined folk, magical, and religious practices. After 200 BC the Greek physicians, who were made slaves, did the medical work and their practices filtered throughout Rome. The most skillful of these were given Roman citizenship during the rule of Julius Caesar. Legend, however, indicates that Greek medicine was introduced to Rome in a year when pestilence was devastating the city (293 BC). Sibylline books were consulted, and the oracle replied that Asklepios be brought from Greece to Rome. A galley was sent and returned with a staff of physicians and attendants. As it came up the Tiber, a sacred serpent sprang out on the little island in the river and established itself there.

Since this was a divinely chosen spot, a temple was erected there to Asklepios (Aesculapius).

Several medical practitioners achieved fame during the rise of the Roman Empire: Dioscorides Pedanius, Aretaeus, Asclepiades, and Galen. Dioscorides Pedanius was a Greek physician and a surgeon in the army under Nero. His *De Materia Medica* contained descriptions of over 600 preparations from medicinal herbs. He observed these herbs as he accompanied the armies.

Aretaeus refocused the study of medicine on the methods of clinical observation used by Hippocrates. His writings rendered vivid descriptions of such diseases as pneumonia, empyema, epilepsy, tetanus, diphtheria, and a type of diabetes.

Asclepiades of Bithynia was a Greek physician from Asia Minor who assisted with the establishment of Greek medicine in Rome. He repudiated the teachings of Hippocrates, for he believed that the physician, not nature, cured disease. Asclepiades proposed an atomistic theory in which disease resulted from a disturbance of the movement of atoms in the body. Treatment consisted of diet, baths, exercise, massage, soothing medications, music and singing. Tracheostomies were frequently performed for respiratory distress. Asclepiades' theory paved the way for the development of the system of methodism, which was founded about 50 BC.

Galen (130–201 AD), a Greek physician from Asia Minor, was probably the most renowned and influential medical writer of all time. He became a physician to the gladiators and athletes in Rome and was also connected with the army. Consequently, he developed great skill in surgery, which is reflected in his writings based on physiological functions. Galen's knowledge was acquired through personal observations and experiences. His system for the use of drugs lasted through the medieval period in history. Galen is considered to be the great experimental physiologist of ancient times. His volumes of writings contributed greatly to medical knowledge and represent a preservative amalgamation of Aristotle's teaching and the Hippocratic tradition with additions by Galen himself (Taylor, 1922).

Two other individuals recorded much of the information available on the medical practice of Alexandria and Rome: Cornelius Celsus and Caius Pliny. Known as encyclopedists, they lived during the first century AD.

Celsus wrote the first organized medical history, translated works from Greek into Latin, and described the characteristics of inflammation as redness and swelling with heat and pain ("rubor et tumor cum calore et dolore"). These are still considered to be the four cardinal symptoms of inflammation. According to most scholars, Celsus was not a physician. Yet he provided detailed accounts of surgical procedures and the ligation of blood vessels. The *De Medicina* of Celsus included topics such as the history of medicine, pharmacy, dietetics, psychiatry, the preservation of health, and surgery. Celsus also recognized the importance of basic research and fostered anatomical knowledge through animal dissections.

Pliny wrote extensively in the areas of history, biology, chemistry, physics, philosophy, magic, folklore, plants, food, and medicine. Some of this information is regarded as superstitious or inaccurate. Pliny's *Historia Naturalis* contained every piece of information he could gather from the past or the present (Lyons, 1978).

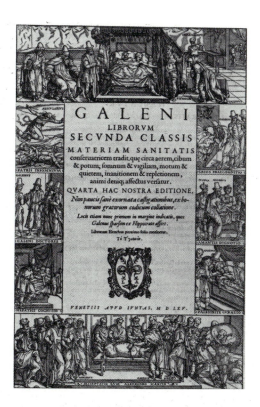

TITLE PAGE OF AN EDITION OF THE WORKS OF GALEN. *Printed in Venice 1565. Achille Bertarelli Collection, Milan, Italy.*

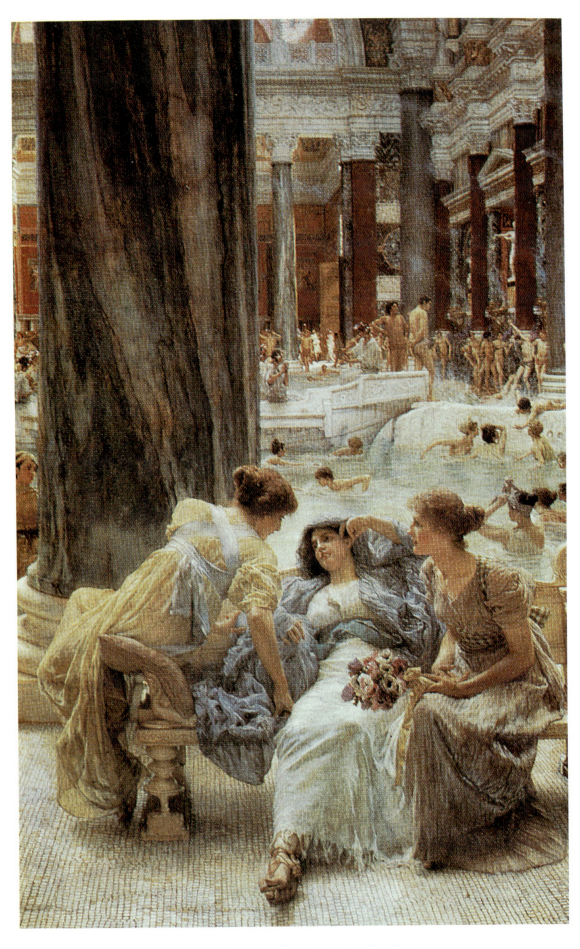

Alma-Tadema, THE BATHS OF CARACALLA, *1899. Sotheby's, London, England.*

The genius of the Romans found its expression not in medical achievement but in works of public hygiene. It is quite possible that public health had its beginning in Rome. Of greatest importance were the colossal engineering feats accomplished by the Romans: the creation of drains, aqueducts, good roads, a system of central heating, proper cemeteries, and the draining of marshes. Massage and baths reached perfection among the Romans. "Rubbing and washing, warm and cold baths, both for cleanliness and for therapeutic uses, steam, oil, hot sand, steambox baths, and sitz baths were all in use, and there was a class of professional masseurs, the *iatralepta*" (Nutting and Dock, 1937, p. 88). Public and private bath houses were developed and assumed the character of clubs or social centers. Roman cities were cleaner than those of any other ancient civilization. Yet Rome had many epidemics, probably because of a number of factors related to conquests and modernization (for example, tenements were introduced by Rome to assist with the rapid growth of the city).

The Romans were advanced in military medicine and provided excellent care for their soldiers. First aid was rendered on the battlefield and a field ambulance service was devised. Originally, wounded soldiers were carried to private homes. Later they were cared for in

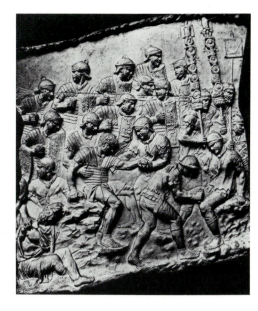

Detail from the COLUMN OF TRAJAN, AD *113. Marble, approx. 39 meters high. Rome, Italy (Bettmann Archive, New York).*

The detail of this commemorative monument shows Roman soldiers helping the wounded.

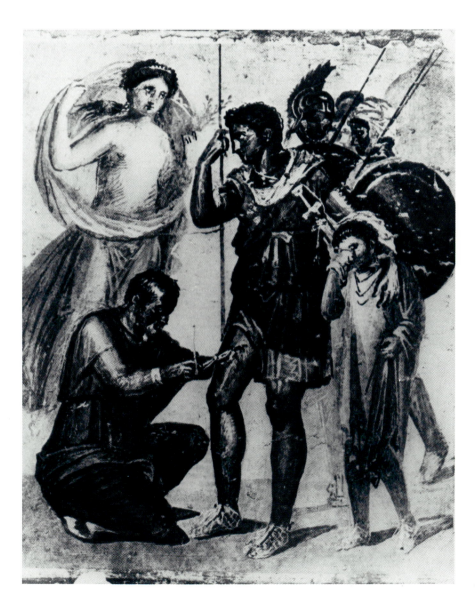

PHYSICIAN TREATS WOUNDED SOLDIER, *first century* AD. *Pompeiian fresco. The Bettmann Archive, New York.*

tents or separate buildings and nursed by women and old men of upstanding character. Eventually many military hospitals (valetudinaria) were erected, some of which could accommodate 200 sick or wounded soldiers.

> A few years ago, several of the original military hospitals of about 100 AD were unearthed in the Rhine and Danube valleys. As such border areas had to be constantly defended against barbarians, these buildings probably served as base hospitals for frontier forces. The ground plans reveal long corridors from which opened a series of suites—each of the latter containing two private rooms connected by a small hall. In addition there were central courts for kitchens, dining rooms, pharmacies, and so on. Apparently there were no wards, so it may be assumed that each soldier-patient enjoyed considerable privacy. Many surgical instruments have been found in the ruins, indicating that advanced Roman wound-surgery was here placed at the service of the troops.
>
> *Shryock, 1959, p. 76*

A class of orderlies, the nosocomi, acted as nurses. Valetudinaria were also established for sick slaves of rich homes or estates, since slaves were considered to be a most valuable commodity. It is probable that slaves functioned as nurses in these institutions.

Roman women were very independent and became involved in many activities outside the home. The care of the sick was no doubt

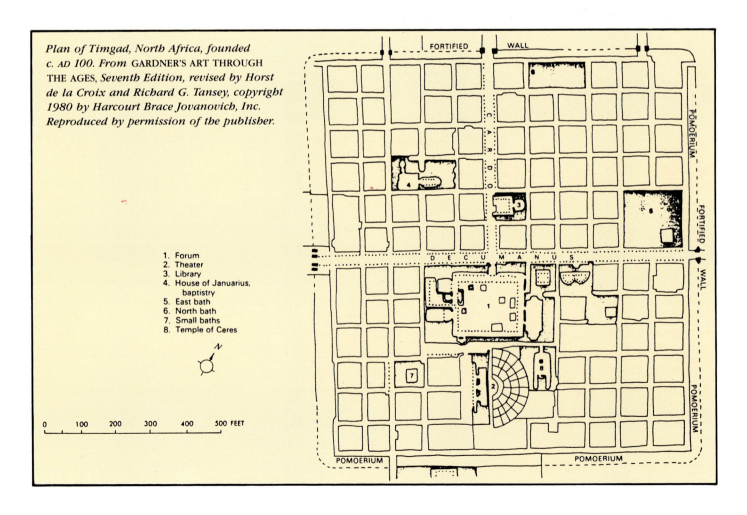

Plan of Timgad, North Africa, founded c. AD 100. From GARDNER'S ART THROUGH THE AGES, *Seventh Edition, revised by Horst de la Croix and Richard G. Tansey, copyright 1980 by Harcourt Brace Jovanovich, Inc. Reproduced by permission of the publisher.*

1. Forum
2. Theater
3. Library
4. House of Januarius, baptistry
5. East bath
6. North bath
7. Small baths
8. Temple of Ceres

0   100   200   300   400   500 FEET

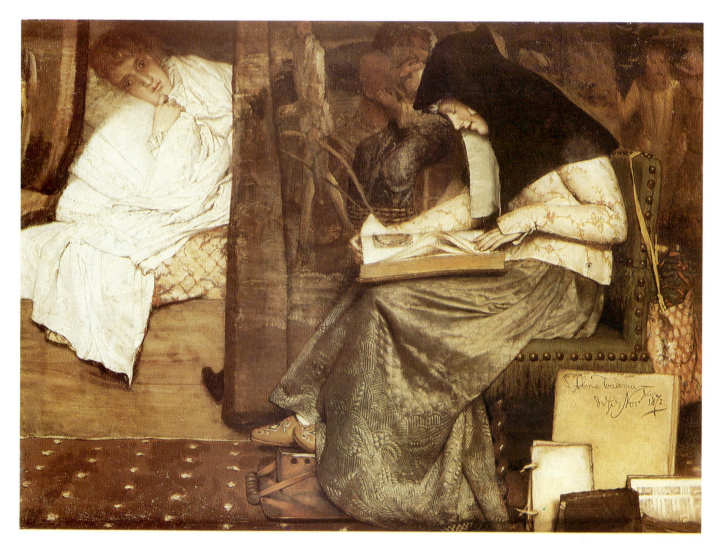

Alma-Tadema, THE NURSE, *1872. Sotheby's, London, England.*

undertaken by the mistress and by the male and female slaves of the household. Children's nurses and midwives were still the chief nursing roles for women.

■ THE FAR WEST

The Americas

The New World, as the Americas were titled by historians, was really an old world in which highly developed cultures had thrived. It may even be that some cultures within the Near East, the Far East, and the Mediterranean had begun and ended before it became known that a rich land lay across the endless sea. It may be that civilization was reached earlier in the Americas than in Egypt. Although the exact date for the habitation of this area is not agreed upon, "it may be assumed with some certainty that highly evolved cultures flourished on the soil of the New World from 2000 to 1000 BC" (Hermann, 1954, p. 188). Some individuals believe it began 10,000 or even 20,000 years ago.

It is thought that the earliest inhabitants of the American continents came from Central Asia. Access was gained by crossing the Bering Strait into the territory currently known as Alaska. The people

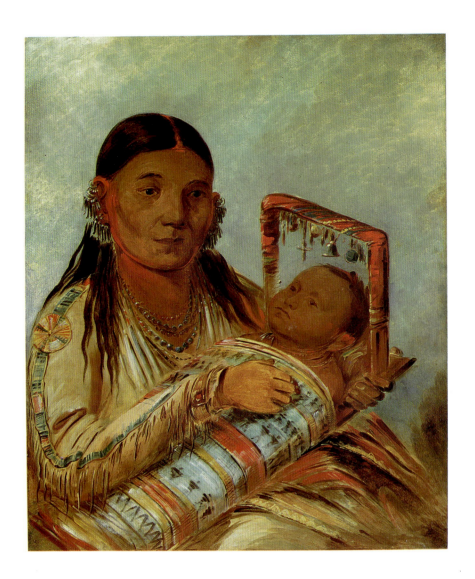

(Indians) followed the pattern of other primitive tribes by migrating toward food, water, and acceptable climates. They tended to move in the direction of east and south, and traces of their occupancy have been found as far east as the Atlantic coast. Mexico, Central America, and Peru eventually became the primary sites for their settlements. Hunting and agriculture became a way of life. In addition, the originality of these tribes resulted in the development of various processes such as basket weaving, the tanning of leather with oak bark, and the manufacture of cleaning powder from wood ashes and of glue from fish. The numerous American Indian nations in North and South America eventually decreased, the consequence of tragic events.

Several tribes attained a high degree of civilization: the Mayas, the Incas, the Aztecs, and the Toltecs. Religion, magic, medicine, nursing, and pharmacy were frequently combined in these tribes; these activities were carried out by one individual who was set apart from the rest of the tribe. The medicine men (or shamans and later priests) attempted to cure the ills of both mind and body. As in other ancient cultures, it was believed that disease was caused by displeasure of the gods. The sun god in particular was recognized and worshiped by many of these groups.

Health was simply a matter of balance among man, nature, and the supernatural. Although the systems of healing might vary from

86

tribe to tribe, rituals or ceremonies, prayers, chants, herbal therapy, plans for prevention of disease, and the use of protective devices such as charms and fetishes were an integral part of the process. In some tribes human sacrifice was a viable part of the religious ceremony; in others transference of disease to animals was a magical ritual. Various other practices emerged that were significant to Indian health care and therapy.

Sweat baths or sweat huts were used to purify the body and maintain health. Various methods were used to achieve this goal. Water might be poured or sprinkled over hot stones, aromatic substances were used, and the body was sometimes beaten with bunches of twigs to stimulate circulation and hasten the sweating process (Dolan, Fitzpatrick, and Hermann, 1983).

Sand painting was another form of therapy. Intricate designs were created by the medicine man for a specific individual and a certain occasion. These designs took form through a process whereby the medicine man trickled varieties of colored sand and crushed minerals through his thumb and forefinger onto a pattern drawn on the ground. The natural colored sand provided the background. These paintings were done on the floors of hogans, or specially built medicine huts, and were believed to promote healing.

As in other ancient civilizations, many types of treatments were used. These included massage, tooth extractions, bloodletting, trepanning, bandaging, suturing, and amputation. In addition, herbal therapy was used extensively.

Significant contributions were made by American Indians to modern-day medicine and medical practice. Little mention, however, is given to nursing as a separate entity. Yet the position of Indian women was unusually good. It is said that they held complete authority over the home, took part in a women's council, and declared war after it was agreed upon. One may assume that their role included the nursing of children, assistance with childbirth, and some type of involvement with the care of the sick and the elderly.

*T*he care of the sick was only one of many forms of charity undertaken by the Church, but it was always given a place of honor because of the emphasis put on it by the founder of the Christian faith. In the first and second centuries, the visiting of the sick was a part of the duty of all Christians but especially the deacons and deaconesses, who took the poor and homeless members of the group into their own homes and cared for them there. No technical preparation was considered necessary for such service. All that was asked was devotion to the faith, brotherly love, and obedience to the Christian law of hospitality and service. Later, much of this charitable work was centered in hospitals or guest houses requiring full-time staffs. Such institutional workers were chosen, as a rule, from among the widows and virgins and other members of the Church most free from domestic ties. With the rapid growth of the monastic movement, after the sixth century, large numbers of voluntary celibates—men and women—joined religious orders, and the care of the sick, helpless, and infirm became in many cases their permanent vocation.

Isabel Maitland Stewart

NURSING IN A CHRISTIAN WORLD

The beginning of the Christian era revealed a Roman Empire that extended over the greater part of Europe, a part of Britain, and areas of Asia Minor and Northern Africa. In essence, Rome was an eminent power over nearly all the peoples of the known world. This empire continued for approximately five centuries after it replaced the republic (about 31 BC to 476 AD). During this time the Roman Empire became distinguished for its political, legal, and administrative organization, as well as for advances in sanitation and hygiene. Its pagan religion was, in general, tolerant and free from ignorant superstitions. The fact remains, however, that it was superior as a conquering military empire. Conquered freemen were permitted freedom of thought and action except in two areas, politics and economics. Slavery, which ultimately undermined the empire, became the basis for the political economy of Rome.

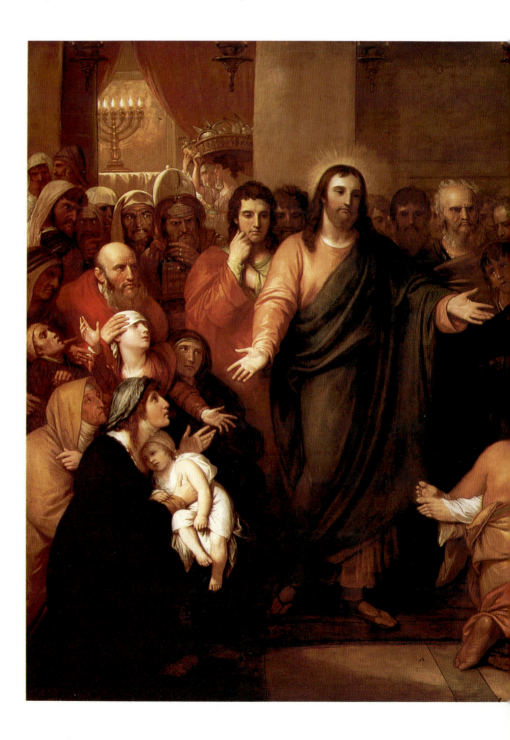

■ THE DAWN OF CHRISTIANITY

The first two centuries of the Roman Empire, known as the *pax Romana,* were marked by relative peace and prosperity. This interval included the period between the accession of Augustus, the first emperor, to the death of Marcus Aurelius in 180 AD. Order was achieved through power, which served to conceal the emerging basic weaknesses in the Roman social order. A minority of men became rich and powerful and enjoyed control of the lands. Theirs was a life of luxury, extravagance, and idleness. The masses were either poverty stricken or indentured slaves. A middle class was nonexistent, and the division between rich and poor was evident. The value of life was lessened by slavery. Exhaustion, misery, and corruption added to the gradual erosion of the empire.

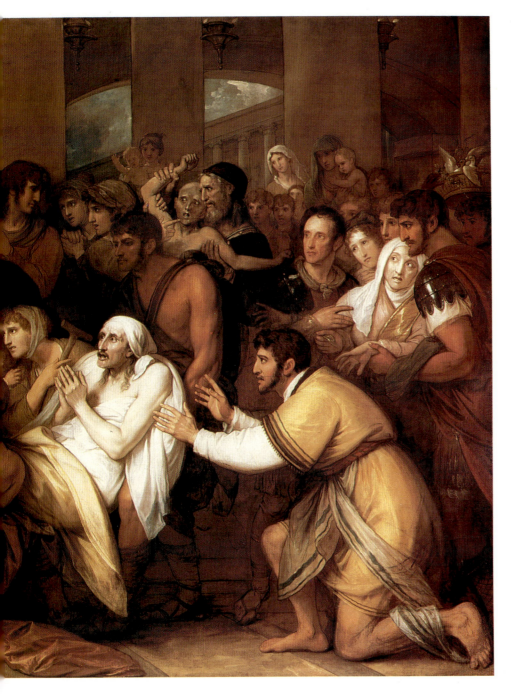

Benjamin West, CHRIST HEALING THE SICK, *late eighteenth century. Canvas. Courtesy of Pennsylvania Hospital, Philadelphia.*

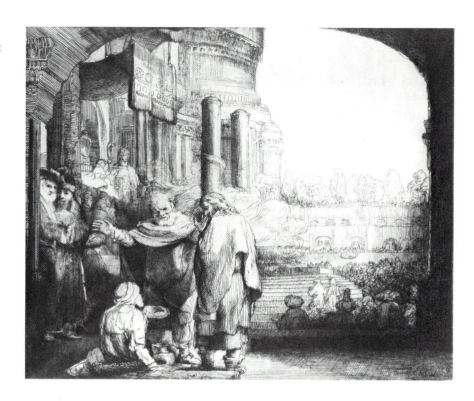

Rembrandt Harmenszoon van Rijn, PETER AND JOHN HEALING THE CRIPPLE AT THE GATE OF THE TEMPLE, *c. 1659. Etching. British Museum, London, England.*

After the death of Marcus Aurelius, frequent disorder prevailed within the empire. Economic crises occurred frequently and taxation became oppressive. The government was often overthrown and its power declined. "Religion had come to represent formal duties imposed upon worshipers who had other religions" (Jamieson and Sewall, 1950, pp. 88–89). Rebellions threatened the city of Rome itself. Invasions occurred and took their toll on an already declining society. The fourth and fifth centuries gave way to increased plagues and pestilences, which may well have been the final ingredient necessary for the collapse of Roman power.

It was during this period of social change and confusion that Christianity spread throughout the European world. Christianity was based on the teachings of Jesus Christ, who was born in Judea when Rome was at the height of her power under Augustus Caesar. With the culmination of his public life, his crucifixion, resurrection, and ascension, Christ's teachings were spread throughout the Empire by his apostles. The concept of a loving god of all mankind was the basis of the teachings of Jesus as preached in the first century of this era, and it became one of the principal tenets of Christianity.

Contrary to popular belief, the idea of one God as the loving father of all men can actually be attributed to Ikhnaton, an Egyptian pharaoh who ruled about 1375 BC. He labeled this god Aton, to whom temples were erected and worship was directed throughout Egypt. This religion eventually faded, perhaps because the Egyptian army had a vested interest in the old gods. This decline occurred, however, only after it had profoundly influenced the captive Israelites who nourished and carried the idea to Canaan. Important changes took place over time: Jehovah evolved from a god of wrath and retribution to a god of love and mercy; this loving god became the god of all mankind, not just the god of the Jews.

Christianity ultimately prevailed over the other religions and philosophies of the world. It embraced the customs, rituals, ideals, and ideas that were closest to the hearts of the people. Consequently, what began as a simple religion with minimal ceremony, ritual, or doctrine expanded into a complex religion with many sacraments and a complicated and rigid hierarchical structure. Initially forbidden by law, Christianity became the state religion into which men were born. In 313 AD, one year after his own conversion to the faith, the Emperor Constantine proclaimed freedom for the Church. By 400 AD it was probably as dangerous *not to be* a Christian as it had been *to be* one in 100 AD. Thus, as the Roman Empire declined, Christianity was bringing Christ into the personal and community life of the people.

■ THE CHRISTIAN MOTIVE AND NURSING

The history of nursing first becomes continuous with the beginning of Christianity. Pre-Christian records of nursing are fragmentary and scattered; however, records of nursing from the days of the early Christian workers to the present day are continuous. Christ's teachings of love and brotherhood transformed not only society at large but also the development of nursing. "Organized nursing" was a direct response to these teachings and epitomized the concept of pure altruism initiated by the early Christians. The term *altruism* was derived from the Latin *alter,* meaning "other"; hence, altruism means thought for and interest in others. Altruism at this time was not a new idea but an old idea with a new motive:

> Animism had advocated good works as a charm, to prevent misfortune. Judaism urged justice and mercy in order to secure prosperity in this world. Buddhism taught that helpfulness and kindness to others would secure merit in the hereafter. Even in the deteriorated Christianity of the Middle Ages we find the same thing taught, that kindness and service to others stored up merit in heaven.
>
> *Goodnow, 1942, p. 23*

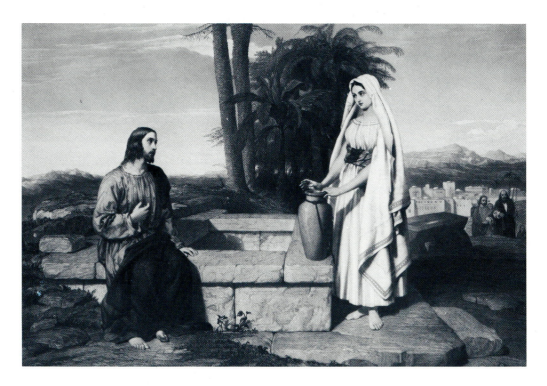

Samuel Bellin, CHRIST AND THE WOMAN OF SAMARIA, *nineteenth century. Engraving. British Museum, London, England.*

93

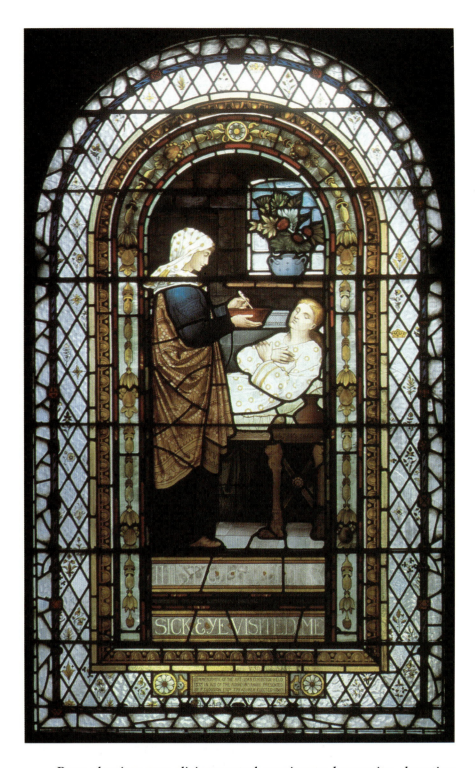

Pure altruism was disinterested service to humanity, devotion to others without hope of any sort of reward (material or spiritual) but done for the love of God and desire to be like Him. From this development of the concept of altruism evolved the care of the sick or disabled as a corporal act of mercy:

To feed the hungry.
To give water to the thirsty.
To clothe the naked.
To visit the imprisoned.
To shelter the homeless.
To care for the sick.
To bury the dead.

The Corporal Works of Mercy encompassed basic human needs, recognized the needs of a variety of groups within the society, and reflected the desire for human compassion. A spiritual meaning became deeply attached to the care of the sick and the suffering. This flowering of Christian idealism was to forever have a deep and significant impact on the practice of nursing.

The original inspiration of Christians to care for the sick stemmed directly from the teachings of Christ himself. Many instances are cited of Christ's healing the sick and raising the dead by direct intervention and without the use of any medicine or treatment. Faith healing, therefore, was a part of the Christian belief. In addition, those conditions that would promote natural healing were added and eventually supplied the impetus for the establishment of centers for nursing care. Caring for the sick became an activity especially pleasing to God and through which an individual might inherit "eternal life." Inherent in such a philosophy was a life of charity in a world of selfishness and hatred: "A new commandment I give you, that you love one another: That as I have loved you, you also love one another. By this will all men know that you are my disciples, if you have love for one another" (John 13: 34–35). As explained in the epistles of St. Paul, "There is neither Jew nor Greek; there is neither slave nor freeman; there is neither male nor female. For you are all one in Christ Jesus" (Galatians 3: 28).

Charity was love in action, taught most significantly in the para-

Rembrandt Harmenszoon van Rijn, CHRIST HEALING THE SICK, *or "The Hundred Guilder Print," c. 1649. Etching and drypoint, 29.8 × 41 cm. The Norton Simon Foundation, Pasadena, California.*

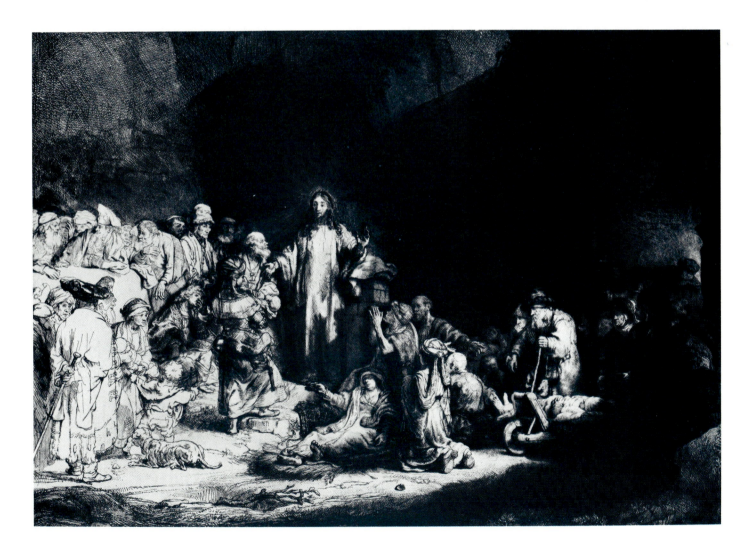

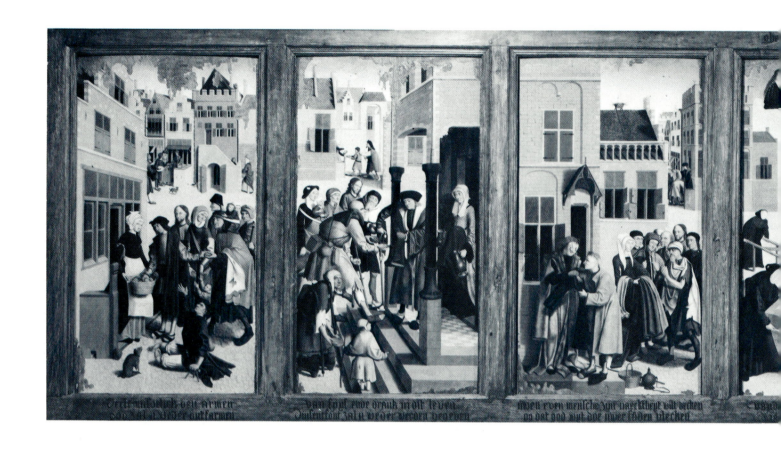

ble of the Good Samaritan. This parable was a plea for sympathy, generosity, kindliness, brotherly love, and dignity for all human life. It taught character development and purification of the soul as an aim for the givers of care.

> A certain man was going down from Jerusalem to Jericho; and he fell among robbers, who both stripped him and beat him, and departed, leaving him half dead. And by chance a certain priest was going down that way: and when he saw him, he passed by on the other side. And in like manner a Levite also, when he came to the place, and saw him, passed by on the other side. But a certain Samaritan, as he journeyed, came where he was: and when he saw him, he was moved to compassion, and came to him, and bound up his wounds, pouring on them oil and wine, and he set him on his own beast, and brought him to an inn, and took care of him. And on the morrow he took out two shillings, and gave them to the host, and said, "Take care of him; and whatsoever thou spendest more, I, when I come back again, will repay thee."

> *Luke 10: 30–36*

The practical test of the new faith was "not to be ministered unto, but to minister." This golden rule later often appeared on the seats of benches in hospitals. The care of the sick was lifted to a higher plane; what had once been an occupation primarily of slaves, or a necessary service of any household, became a sacred vocation. Service to others was an avowed duty of all Christian men and women.

The entry of women into nursing after 300 AD was affected by at least three factors: "First, the improvement in the social position of

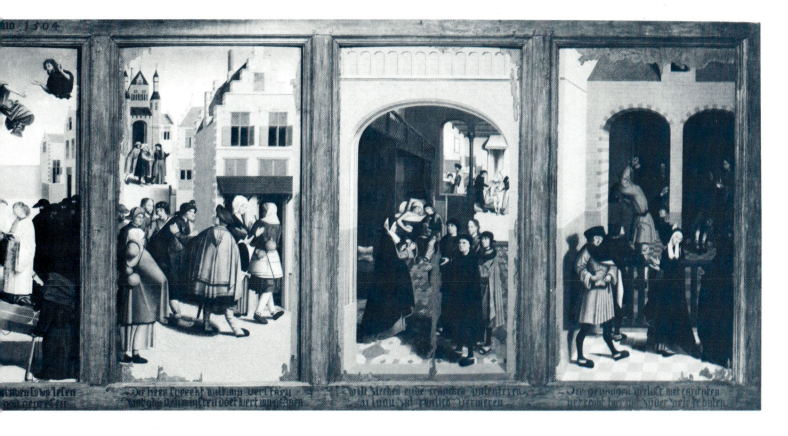

Master of Alkmaar, SEVEN ACTS OF MERCY, *1504. Panel, 101 × 54 cm. Rijksmuseum, Amsterdam, Netherlands.*

The theme of the seven acts is developed by the appearance of Christ as both witness and member of the groups receiving the benefits of the works of mercy and charity.

Roman women; second, the Christian teaching of the equality of men and women before God—and therefore in God's work; and, third, the Christian appeal to carry on His work in behalf of all who were in distress" (Shryock, 1959, p. 77). The position of women was indeed an extremely important factor. Yet discrepancies exist in writings that refer to this matter. Some writers indicate that the status of women was strikingly elevated by Christianity (Dolan, Fitzpatrick, and Hermann, 1983). Others (Nutting and Dock, 1937; Dock and Stewart, 1925) caution that one cannot assume this to be true, stating that the position of women, socially and legally, was not always low under the old religions. All agree, however, that the essential element was that Christianity vastly enlarged women's opportunities for useful social service by opening the door to honorable and active careers, particularly for unmarried women. In addition, Christ's teachings tended to place men and women on an equal plane, which led to the assumption of leadership positions by women engaged in charitable and social endeavors. Finally, the freedom to engage in humanitarian efforts led many men to the field of nursing. Caring activities were shared by men and women and at times included the carry-over of magic, empirical remedies, and home treatments of the earlier periods of history.

From a chronological point of view, there was a vast difference between nursing in the Christian era and that of the ages that preceded it. A superior type of care was given by those who understood the best medical and surgical techniques of the times. The rich and the powerful who converted to Christianity and engaged in charitable works were socially, culturally, and intellectually endowed. Some were recognized scholars. The educationally prepared in-

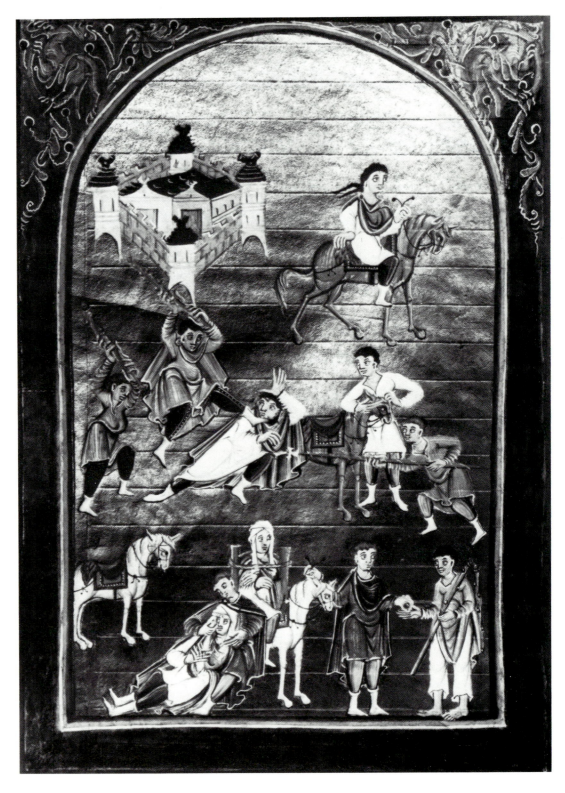

"Parable of the Good Samaritan," from the GOSPEL BOOK OF THE EMPEROR OTTO III, *late tenth century. Manuscript illumination. Bayerisches Staatsbibliothek, Munich, Federal Republic of Germany. (Marburg/Art Resource, NY).*

cluded members of the clergy, who for several centuries were the only group that was exposed to any type of formal training. Furthermore, a true integration of services was in evidence because medical and nursing care was seldom separated from other forms of charity for the poor (Sellew and Nuesse, 1946).

Many benefits were derived from the Christian effort. Chief among these were a distinctly humanitarian approach to the care of the sick and the poor and the development of organized nursing services. The positive aspects of nursing's heritage from the Christian teachings are evident and have been specifically identified. Yet this religious thought also handicapped progress in nursing. As nursing

98

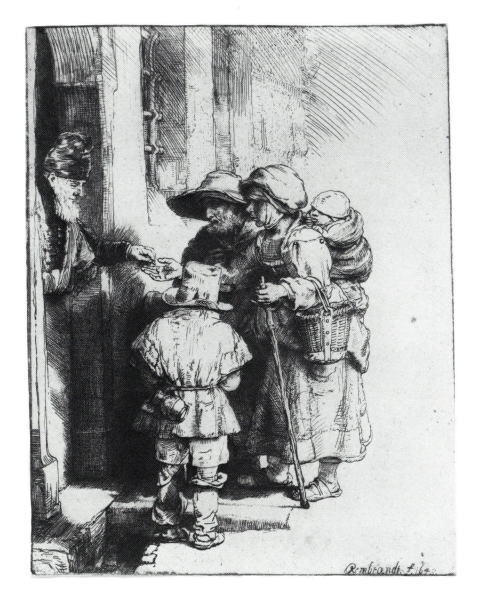

Rembrandt Harmenszoon van Rijn, BEGGARS RECEIVING ALMS AT THE DOOR OF A HOUSE, *1648. Etching and drypoint. The Art Institute of Chicago, Illinois, Clarence Buckingham Collection.*

became closely identified with religion and religious orders, strict discipline became a way of life. Those engaged in the nursing work were eventually trained in docility, passivity, humility, and total disregard for self. Unquestioning obedience to the decisions of others higher in rank, usually the priest or physician, was promulgated. An individual nurse's accountability, the personal responsibility for decision making in regard to patient care, was thus bypassed and totally alien in nursing for many years to come.

> It is not difficult to see the parallels to the training schools for nurses of the late nineteenth and early twentieth centuries. Indeed, one need only read some of the very early writings of our own American nursing educators who advocated a zealous dedication to the work, a selfless denial of personal comfort, and an unquestioning loyalty to the physician (Robb, 1901). Nursing as an occupation was likened to a religious vocation by many and was often referred to as a special "calling," which required selfless service to man and God. The essential characteristic of the "good" nurse was that of obedience, and the rigor with which this quality was developed is common knowledge among those nurses who graduated from nursing schools prior to the last decade.... The "good" student was the student who did as she was told, and she soon learned that the classmate who ques-

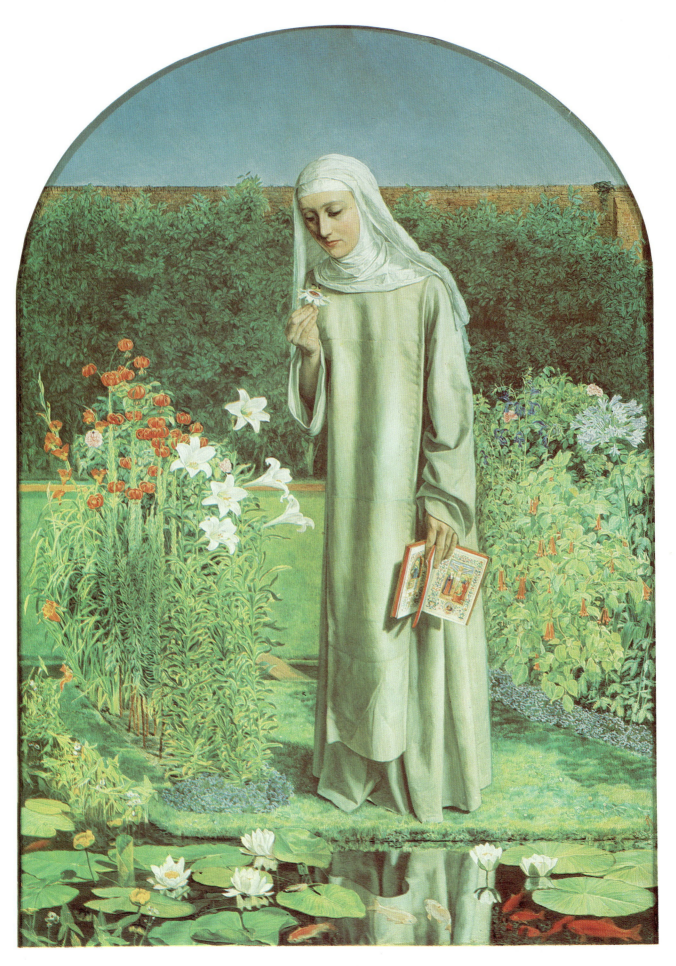

Charles Allsten Collins, CONVENT THOUGHTS, *1851. Ashmolean Museum, Oxford, England.*

tioned too much often fell into a general category termed "personality unsuitable to nursing," a category that usually led to dismissal from the school. The greatest proponents of the concept of unquestioning obedience were physicians, but faculty members aided and abetted this attitude since they too had been indoctrinated with these ideas.

Christy, 1976, p. 3

■ THE EARLY CHRISTIAN ERA: 1–500 AD

The first five centuries of the Christian era witnessed the rise of a religious and social movement that enabled the systematic development of organized nursing. This marvelous activity of love and mercy was embraced by many men and women who responded to the teachings of Christ. More importantly, the right of the single woman to acquire a position of usefulness and responsibility was established, thereby opening the door to respected careers, particularly in the area of social service. Indeed, the foundations of the "nurses' calling" and of all modern works of charity were laid and perpetuated.

VISITING THE SICK. *Fresco. Church of San Martino, Florence, Italy. (Archivi Alinari, Florence).*

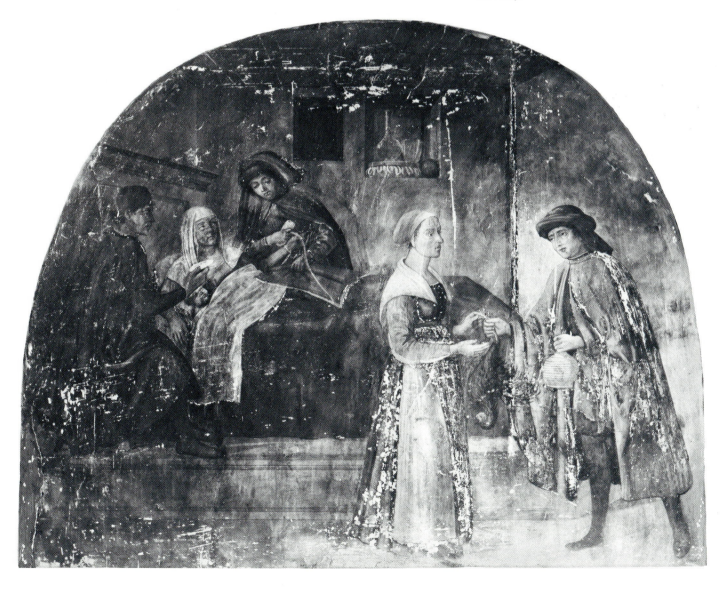

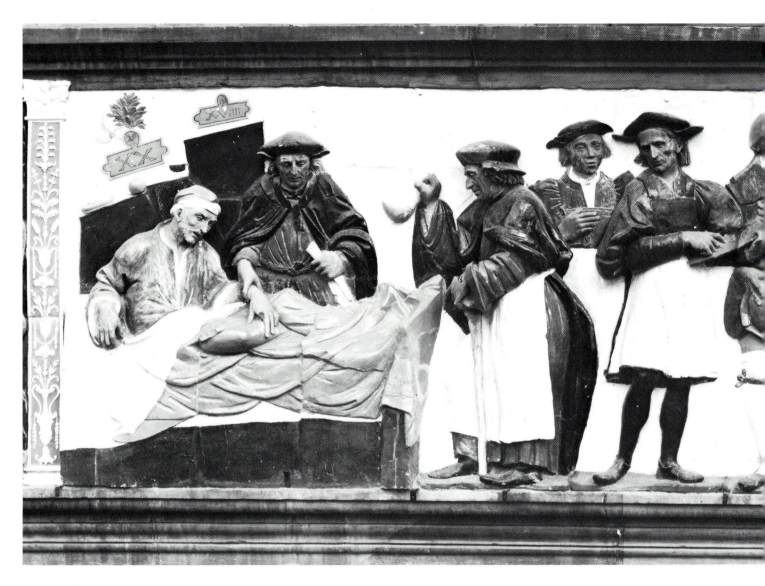

Giovanni della Robbia, VISITING THE SICK, *c. 1525. Glazed terracotta. From the facade of the Ospedale del Ceppo, Pistoria, Italy. (Archivi Alinari, Florence).*

From the earliest point in its history, the Christian Church assumed the care of the sick, the poor, and the helpless. This activity was in keeping with Christ's refusal to accept human suffering. Other religions had viewed suffering as deserved, as something to be left alone; Christ specialized in relieving it. Thus spiritual meaning became attached to the care given to humanity as well as to the suffering endured by it. The care of the sick and distressed became an avowed duty of all Christian men and women.

The women of this early church shared activities with men in all works of the community. Chief among these was the care of the ill and infirm. Information about the various groups of women that developed, however, is confusing and contradictory; at times it is difficult to distinguish between what is actually known and what is surmised (Dock and Stewart, 1925; Seymer, 1932; Nutting and Dock, 1937; Sellew and Nuesse, 1946; Frank, 1953; Shryock, 1959). What is definitely known is that women in these groups concentrated on social work and nursing, which paved the way for the present role of the public health/community health nurse. These nursing groups (orders) flourished and became expressions of philanthropic desires

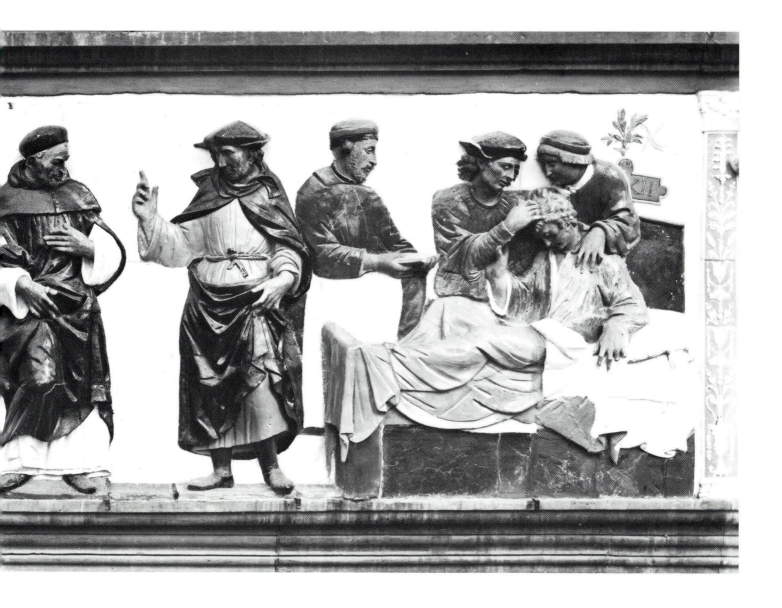

for some and a kind of security for others. They were to be hospitable, pious, and committed to the relief of the afflicted. According to Tuker and Malleson (1900), the earliest orders of women workers were the Deaconesses and Widows. Later, the Virgin, Presbyteress, Canoness, and Nun appeared. Only deaconesses, widows, and nuns were involved with nursing (Nutting and Dock, 1937). It is apparent that the titles of these groups in themselves presented some difficulty, since the primitive deaconess could be married, a widow, or a virgin.

> The terms "Widow," "Deaconess," and sometimes also "Virgin"
> are used with bewildering inexactitude by all the ancient
> authors, and pages of learned controversy have been written as
> to whether the Deaconess was the same as the Widow, or above
> her, or subordinate to her.
>
> *Seymer, 1932, pp. 23–24*

What is important here is that organized nursing became a reality within society.

Deaconesses

It is difficult to trace the origin of the deaconesses because the Greek word *diakonos* could refer to either a special group, a Christian who served his brothers in Christ, or those who served their masters. The verb *diakonein*, "to serve," was used to refer to serving tables or distributing alms. The noun, according to some writers, was also used by Christ to infer a "minister." Consequently, confusion exists regarding what the term actually meant, but it would appear that the word was used in its generic sense of "one who ministers to the needs of another."

Phebe (Phoebe, 60 AD), a friend of St. Paul, is the only woman called a deaconess in the New Testament:

> I commend unto you our sister Phoebe, a deaconess of the church at Cenchrae, that you may receive her in the Lord as befits the saints, and help her in whatever she may require from you, for she has been a helper of many and of myself as well.
>
> *Romans 16: 1–2*

Jacopo Tintoretto, THE CONVERSION OF ST. PAUL, *c. 1545. Canvas, approx. 152.4 × 236.2 cm. National Gallery of Art, Washington, D.C., Samuel H. Kress Collection 1961.*

Phebe was thus credited with being the "first deaconess" and the "first district or visiting nurse." The latter referred to the thought that she nursed the poor in their homes, which eventually became a major part of the work of deaconesses. Documents are sometimes contradictory with reference to the status of these individuals. According to the Bible, Phebe was entrusted with the letters of St. Paul

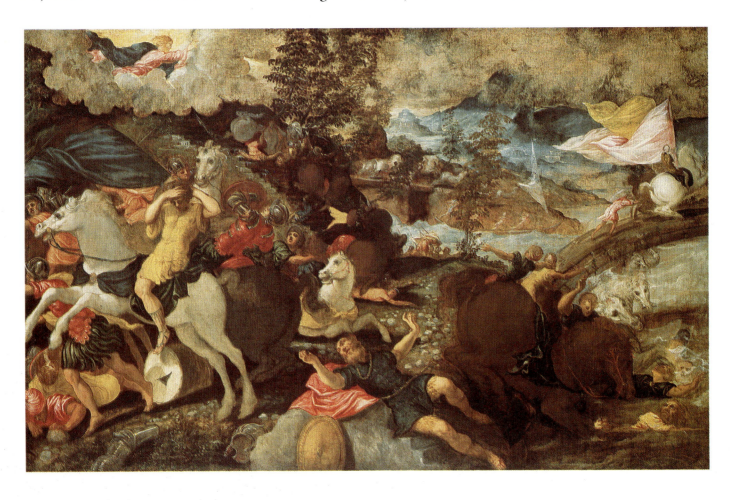

and was considered to be a woman of importance and dignity. Mention is made of her education, wealth, position, and the fact that her travels to Rome were associated with her work.

Very early the Church, in accordance with Christ's teachings, created officers to carry out acts of service for the members of the Church community. Bishops and other officers were empowered with the allocation of church funds for charitable purposes. Ministration to the sick was a vital component of the personal service that was emphasized. Men and women who became involved rapidly developed into ecclesiastical orders in a very definite hierarchy. The deaconesses were made popular during this time by the type of women who joined—daughters of the rich, the able and the well born, who frequently were the sisters of bishops, or the wives and daughters of emperors. Nursing as such was not their chief occupation; nursing was a way to assist with the salvation of the soul.

The deaconesses were usually ordained to service, worked on an equal basis with the deacon, and were required to be unmarried or a widow. They were usually mature women who could make judgments based on life experiences. The primary function of deaconesses was to attend the female catechumens at their baptism by immersion and to anoint them with oil. Their visiting and charitable duties appear to have been a secondary function in which they carried the Church into the home by visiting the poor and caring for the sick. Deaconesses provided food, money, clothing, medicines, and physical and spiritual care to those in need.

Ecclesiastical histories have provided knowledge of the nursing carried out by these early workers of the church. Letters have included the names of many deaconesses. St. John Chrysostom gave the names of five: Olympias, Sabiniana, Pentadia, Amprucla, and Procla. Olympias (or St. Olympias, as she is frequently called), the most famous, was a daughter of a count of the Roman Empire who inherited a fortune from her parents. She became the wife of the prefect of Constantinople, a widow at eighteen, and an ordained deaconess at the age of twenty. Eventually, Olympias became the head of a community of deaconesses who resided in a convent strengthening their religious life as well as tending the needs of the community.

The deaconess orders held a position of importance for many years. However, as adult baptisms became uncommon and deaconesses were no longer needed to assist women catechumens, gradually this group faded. The growing importance of the monastic movement may have also contributed to this occurrence. Yet these orders never did entirely die out. Periods of revival occurred throughout history in connection with religious movements, particularly in the nineteenth century when the order became active in the Lutheran and other Protestant churches.

Widows and Virgins

Characteristics and duties of the widows and virgins, who were early Church officers, were frequently identified. At certain periods they wore distinctive dress, lived either in their own homes or in monasteries, and took the vow of chastity. They were closely related to

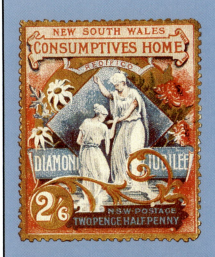

Philatelists specializing in the fields of medicine, nursing, and health are generally agreed upon the 1897 stamp issued by New South Wales, now part of Australia, to be the earliest emission pertaining to nursing. It depicts the nurse as symbolic of charity and mercy. The stamp was issued for Queen Victoria's Jubilee. Courtesy of Howard B. Hurley.

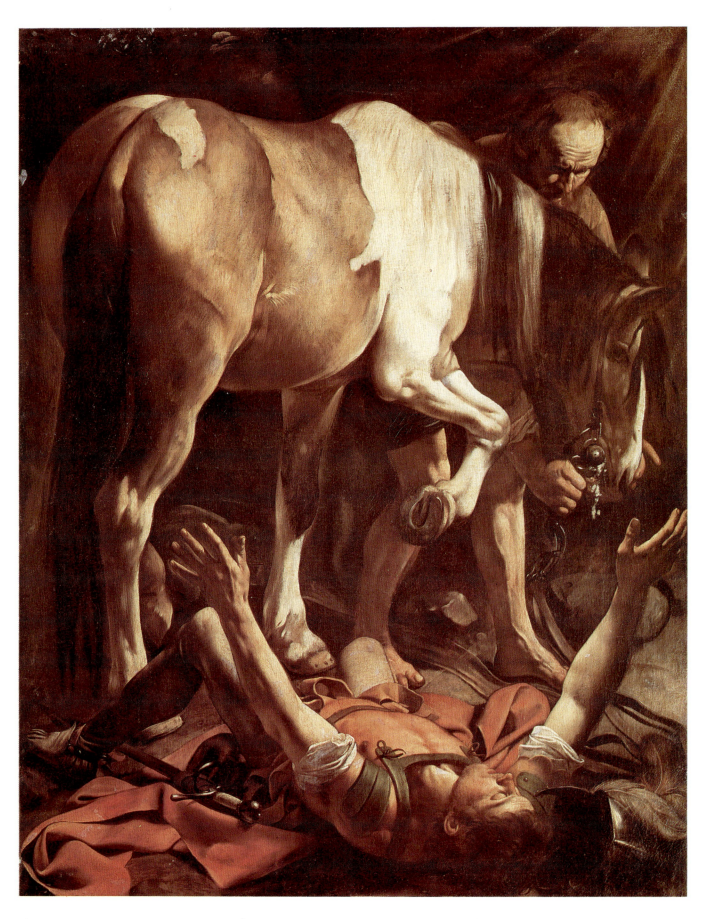

Caravaggio, CONVERSION OF ST. PAUL, *c. 1600. Cerasi Chapel, S. Maria del Popolo, Rome, Italy. (SCALA/Art Resource, NY).*

deaconesses in duties, and they shared in the work of relief and in nursing. In addition, they were not always clearly distinguished from deaconesses, since the appointments to the diaconate were often made from the groups of widows and virgins.

The widows were the second classification of women recognized as having special functions among the poor in the early Church. They were not necessarily women whose husbands had died; the title of *widow* was also used as a designation of respect for age. If the woman had been a widow, however, she had to vow never to marry again. Qualifications were explicitly defined by St. Paul in his first epistle to Timothy (5: 6): the woman must be pious, devoted in hospitality to strangers and saints, anxious to relieve the afflicted; the age requirement was sixty. Younger widows, in the opinion of St. Paul, were too anxious to marry and were inclined to be idle, indulged in gossip, and talked too much! Considerable numbers of women joined in spite of the restrictions and engaged in work among the sick and the poor, eventually taking an important part in the development of hospitals. In the third century the widows' work was greatly curtailed as a result of jealous disapproval on the part of men (Stewart and Austin, 1962; Nutting and Dock, 1937). The vow of chastity, which originally had been spoken in private, became a public function and led to the absorption of the widows into the community life of the *monastriae,* or nuns.

There are discrepancies in the literature regarding the duties and responsibilities of the virgins. In some instances they are credited with responsibility for religious exercises and church duties rather than with charitable work. In others they are ascribed with the visiting or nursing of the sick or the pursuit of missionary labors. It is clear that the virgins were highly respected and ranked with the clergy. This rank, originally shared by both men and women, was comparable to that of the consecrated nun, the lineal descendant of the virgin. The virgin was ". . . distinguished by a white veil, but in Rome the earliest distinguishing mark of her dress was a gold fillet, the symbol of virginity. At a much later date a ring and bracelet were added" (Tuker and Malleson, 1900, vol. 3, p. 34). In this way virginity began to be interpreted as essential to purity of life. The virgins were also eventually absorbed into community life as nuns (*non nuptae,* "not married").

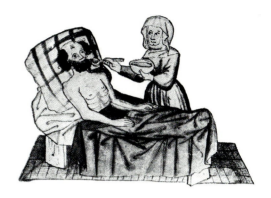

"Nurse Feeding a Sick Man," from a rare Medieval manuscript, the SIXTH WORK OF CHARITY, *Alsatian, c. 1450. The New York Academy of Medicine, New York. Reproduced with permission from the J.B. Lippincott Co.*

Roman Matrons

Deaconesses were rarely mentioned in the Western or Roman church. Yet illustrious women of Rome devoted themselves to the care of the sick and other charitable works. The noble Roman matrons were active during the fourth and fifth centuries after converting to Christianity. Roman women of the upper classes had, by this time, attained considerable social and legal freedom. They had proven themselves to be successful managers of their wealthy husbands' estates and had participated in public affairs. The names and histories of these matrons, some fifteen in number, have been preserved in the writings of St. Jerome. Their independent positions and great wealth were used to establish community life and to initiate the groundwork for charity and nursing work. The ascetic lives of these

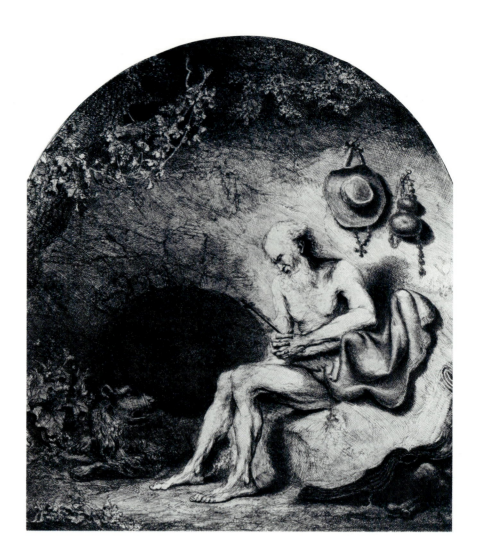

Ferdinand Bol, ST. JEROME, *1644. Etching. The Art Institute of Chicago, Illinois, a Gift from Marie Louise Pritchard.*

women were held in high regard. Three of these matrons, Marcella, Fabiola, and Paula, were particularly significant to continued progress in nursing.

The most famous of the Roman matrons was Marcella, who was considered to be the leader of this group of notable women. She converted her palace, located in a most exclusive part of Rome on the Aventine, into a monastery (the prototype of the later convent), which led to her titles of Mother of Nuns and Founder of Convents in the West. She encouraged other intelligent and spiritually inclined Roman matrons to join her. One of the chief interests of this religious community of women was the care of the sick poor. Marcella was considered to be extremely intelligent and possessed of great virtue and purity. She devoted herself to the study of the scriptures, and the clergy often consulted with her about scriptural passages. Marcella instructed her followers in the care of the sick, while also devoting her time to charitable works, prayer, and study. She was attacked during the raid on Rome by the Visigoths under Alaric in 410 AD and died soon after. She is referred to as St. Marcella by some authors (Sellew and Nuesse, 1946; Dolan, Fitzpatrick, and Hermann, 1983); others identify her simply as Marcella (Nutting and Dock, 1937; Jamieson and Sewall, 1950).

One of the most charming, and perhaps the most worldly, of the

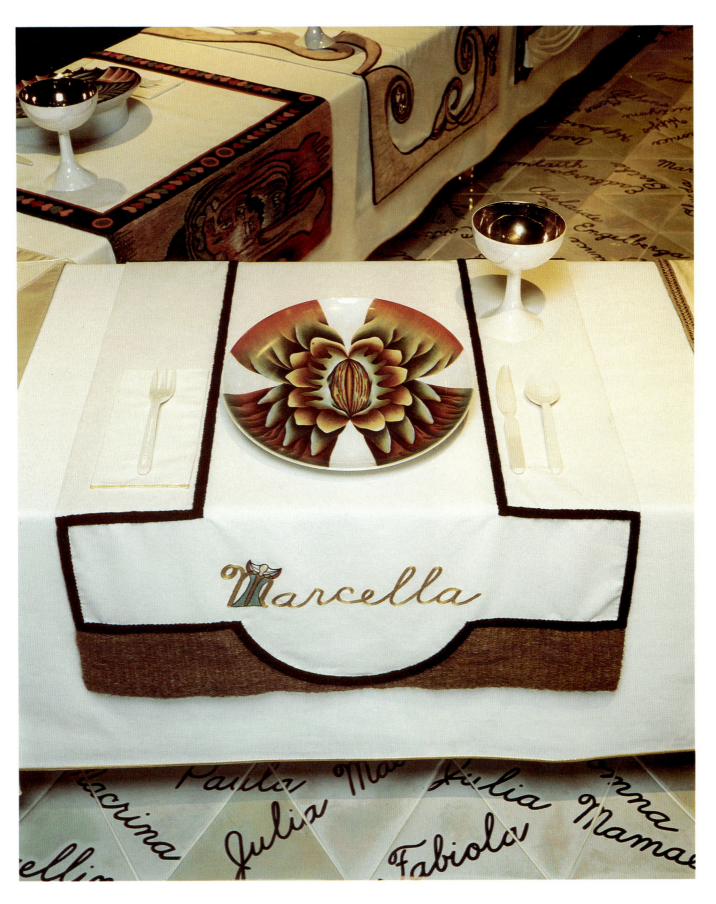

Judy Chicago, "Marcella," plate from THE DINNER PARTY, *1979. China-painted porcelain, 35.6 cm diameter. Through the Flower, Benicia, California.*

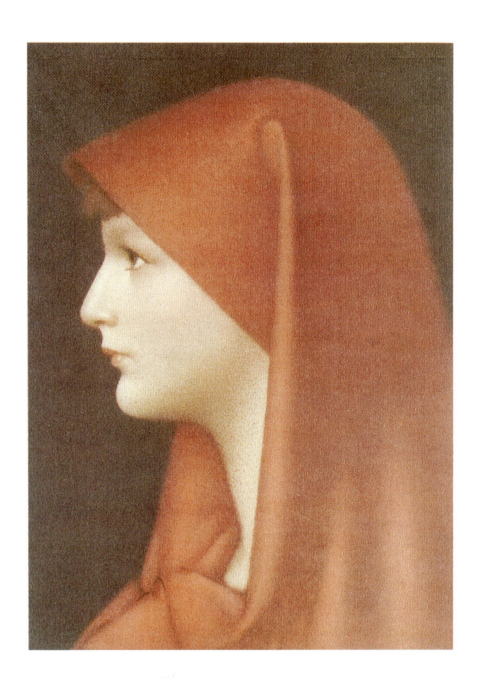

J.J. Henner, FABIOLA, *nineteenth century.*
Donahue Collection.

Roman matrons was Fabiola. A member of the patrician Fabian family, she married, divorced, and remarried, again unhappily. After the death of her second husband and her conversion to Christianity, Fabiola acknowledged her "evil ways" and joined the ranks of penitents. She renounced her earthly pleasures and bestowed her immense fortune on the sick and the poor. The first free Christian hospital in Rome was founded by Fabiola in her own palace in 390 AD. It was described by St. Jerome as a *nosocomium,* a place for the sick as distinguished from objects of charity who were simply poor. Fabiola sought out the poor and the sick in the streets of Rome and cared for them herself. It is said that she was particularly skilled with the dressing of wounds and sores that were ugly and repugnant. She has been viewed almost as the patron saint of early nursing, and her idealized portrait is well known. Fabiola not only nursed but shared in the poverty of her patients. Some reports also indicate that she helped to establish a great hospice for pilgrims and strangers at Ostia, a seaport of Rome. Some writers have made the supposition that this hospice was a home for convalescent patients (Haeser, 1857). The entire life and works of Fabiola were related in a famous eulogy by St. Jerome upon her death in 399 AD:

> There she gathered together all the sick from the highways and streets, and herself nursed the unhappy, emaciated victims of hunger and disease. Can I describe here the varied scourges which afflict human beings? — the mutilated, blinded counte- nances, the partially destroyed limbs, the livid hands, swollen bodies, and wasted extremities? . . . How often have I seen her carrying in her arms these piteous, dirty, and revolting vic- tims of a frightful malady! How often have I seen her wash

Joachim Patinir (active 1515, died before 1524), ST. JEROME IN A ROCKY LANDSCAPE. *Wood, approx. 35.6 × 34.3 cm. The National Gallery, London, England.*

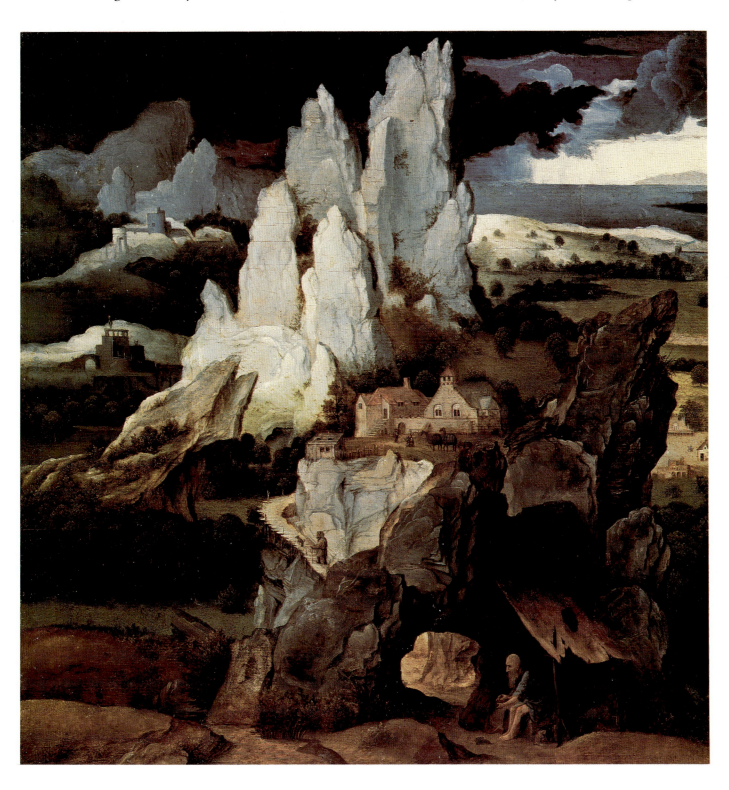

111

wounds whose fetid odour prevented every one else from even looking at them! She fed the sick with her own hands, and revived the dying with small and frequent portions of nourishment. I know that many wealthy persons cannot overcome the repugnance caused by such works of charity; ... I do not judge them, ... but, if I had a hundred tongues and a clarion voice I could not enumerate the number of patients for whom Fabiola provided solace and care. The poor who were well envied those who were sick.

St. Jerome, Letter to Oceanus

Paula traced her descent to some of the oldest and noblest families, and her husband, Toxotius, was of the Julian family, who claimed descent from Aeneas. Her family was immensely wealthy and owned, among other things, the entire town of Actin. Paula was the wife of a pagan and the mother of five children, four daughters and one son. Her worldly life ended with the death of her husband, when she

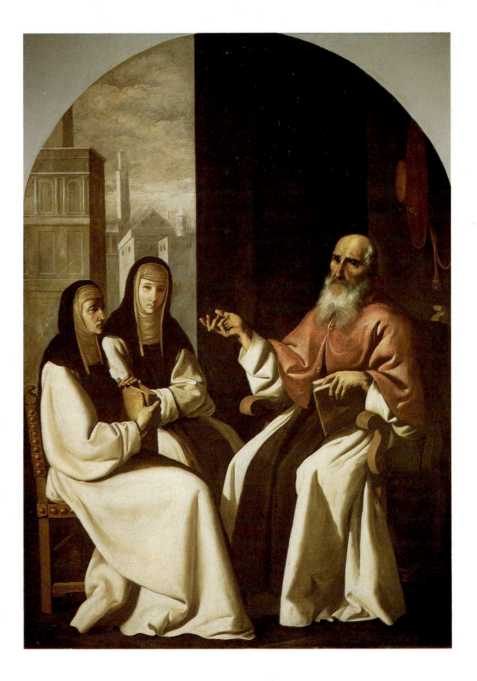

Francisco de Zurbaran, ST. JEROME WITH ST. PAULA AND ST. EUSTOCHIUM, *c. 1640. Canvas, approx. 245.1 × 172.7 cm. National Gallery of Art, Washington, D.C., Samuel H. Kress Collection 1952.*

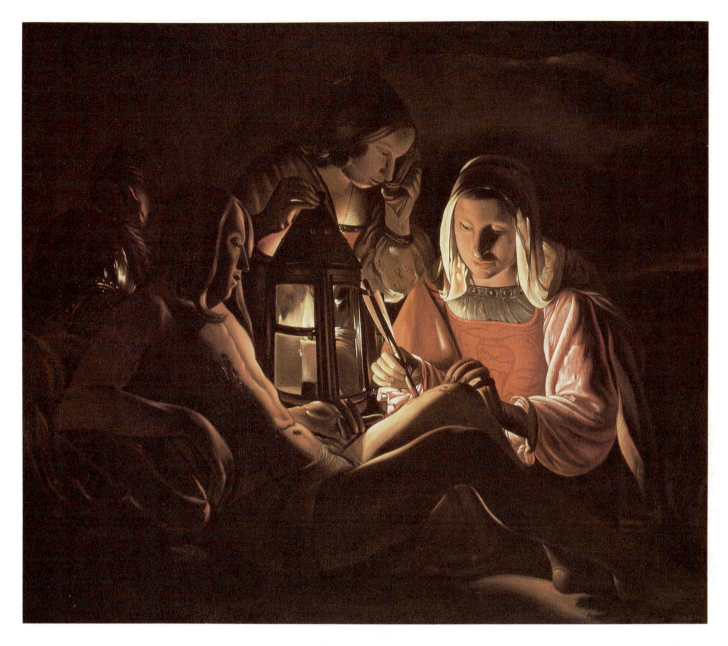

Georges de La Tour, ST. SEBASTIAN TENDED BY THE HOLY WOMEN, *c. 1638. Canvas. Detroit Institute of Arts, Michigan, Founders Society Purchase, Ralph Harman Booth Bequest Fund.*

began to devote herself to strict asceticism. Paula and her daughter Eustochium adopted Christianity, shared in charitable work, and studied with Marcella. Paula was particularly respected for her intellectual ability, which enabled her to develop a relationship with the recognized scholars of the day. This example of colleagueship between the sexes was described by Lord as an important advent of Christianity:

> If to her [Paula] we do not date the first great change in the social relations of man with woman, yet she is the most memorable example that I can find of that exalted sentiment which Christianity called out in the [relationship] of the sexes, and which has done more for the elevation of society than any other sentiment except that of religion itself.
>
> *Lord, 1885, p. 63*

Paula was one of the most learned women of this period of history. She studied Hebrew and Greek and assisted St. Jerome with his

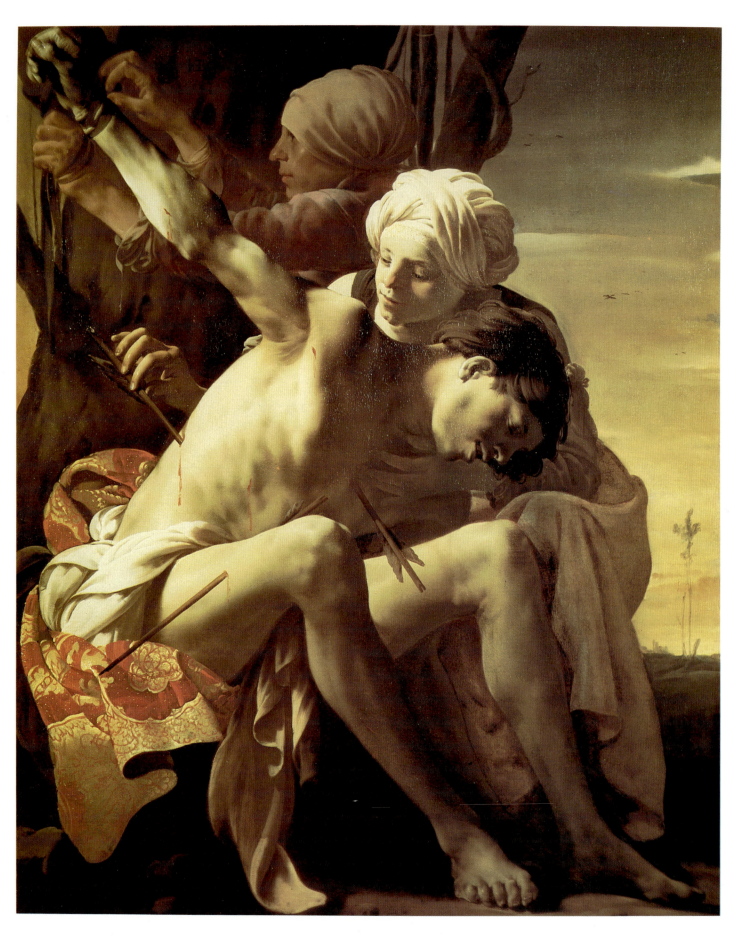

Hendrick Terbrugghen, ST. SEBASTIAN ATTENDED BY ST. IRENE, *c. 1625. Canvas. Allen Memorial Art Museum, Oberlin, Ohio.*

Latin translations of the Scriptures, known as the Vulgate. In 385 AD Paula and Eustochium sailed for Palestine. Eventually they settled in Bethlehem, where they attracted a following of devout women and founded a monastery. In addition, Paula built hospices for pilgrims and hospitals for the sick along the road to Bethlehem. The design and construction of the buildings were the plainest, which demonstrated the philosophy that it was better to spend money on the poor than on fine buildings. For approximately twenty years, Paula managed the institutions and personally nursed the weary travelers and the sick. It is thought that she was the first to train nurses in a systematic way, to teach nursing as a distinct art rather than as a generalized service to the poor. The following description of nurses at work is thought to explain the origin of the tradition of hard manual labor as an expression of good nursing: "They trim lamps, light fires, sweep floors, clean vegetables, put heads of cabbage in the pot to boil, lay table cloths and set tables, hand cups, help to wash dishes, and run to and fro to wait on others" (St. Jerome, Letter to Pammachius).

In the late fourth century in Rome the place in good works was taken by this notable group of women, all friends of St. Jerome. All

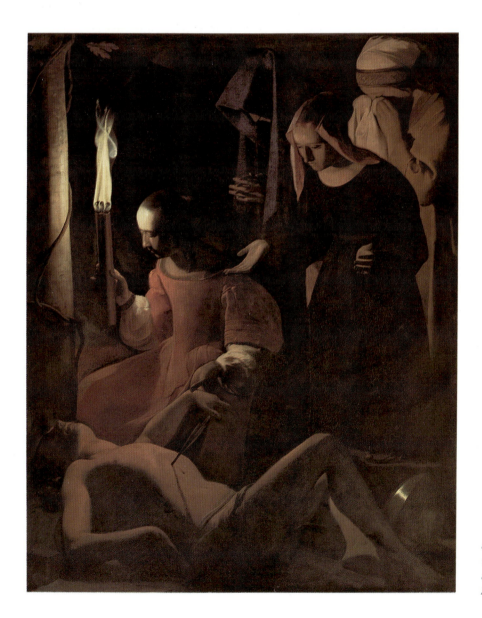

Georges de La Tour, ST. IRENE CURING ST. SEBASTIAN, *c. 1648. Approx. 157.50 × 127.50 cm. Musée National du Louvre, Paris, France.*

115

were Christian converts and lived not too many years after Constantine gave freedom to the Church. Probably no group of women has surpassed them in intellectual powers and commanding characters. Many individuals benefited from their services, including St. Sebastian. Sebastian was company commander in the Praetorian Guards during the reign of Emperor Diocletian (284–305 AD). The public declaration of his faith in Christianity and his affiliation with the Christian Church resulted in his being fastened to a stake and shot by arrows. Later that night, St. Irene, the widow of his martyred friend St. Castulus, found him still alive. She and her associates provided the nursing care that has been documented and portrayed through the years by many artists. Consequently, St. Sebastian became a popular subject of medieval art. The idea that contagious or infectious diseases were shot into the body by invisible arrows fostered the practice of praying to St. Sebastian for prevention or cure.

Men in Nursing

An early organization of men in Rome was the *Parabolani* brotherhood. The name referred literally to those who risked their lives by coming in contact with the sick. It is believed that this group originated during the third century, when the Black Plague depleted the population of the entire Mediterranean area. When this dreaded disease was at its peak in Alexandria, the Parabolani reportedly organized a hospital and traveled throughout the city nursing the sick. These several hundred men and their nursing work were vividly described in *Hypatia,* a novel written by Charles Kingsley (n.d.).

Physicians and Medicine

In the early centuries of Christianity approximately sixteen Christian physicians reached distinction. The majority of them came from Syria and included Aetius of Amida, Paul of Aegineta, and Alexander of Tralles (Frank, 1953). Two of the most prominent ones, St. Cosmas and St. Damian, were twin brothers who were born in Arabia and educated in Syria. They became known as the "moneyless ones," since they did not charge for professional services. It was their hope that this practice would gain converts to Christianity. Although they specialized in both medicine and pharmacy in Asia Minor, St. Cosmas and St. Damian were chosen as the "patrons of the medical profession." They suffered martyrdom in 278 AD during the reign of Diocletian and soon achieved a following for numerous miraculous cures in life and after death.

Perhaps the best known of physicians of this era was St. Luke, the Evangelist. St. Paul called him the "beloved physician." It has been suggested by several writers that Luke had some type of medical preparation, that he may have studied at the famous school at Tarsus. His writings demonstrate an interest in medical subjects.

St. Pantaleon, like Luke, Cosmas, and Damian, practiced free medicine among the sick poor. This, as well as the fact that he was a Christian, created hostility among his pagan friends. Eventually he was put to death and regarded as a healing saint. Later, Pantaleon was associated with the image of the comic in Venetian commedia dell'arte, and his name provided the term *pantaloon* for men's trousers (Petrucelli, 1978).

Aetius wrote of treatments for varicose veins, hypertrophied tonsils, hydrophobia, goiter, and aneurysm of the brachial artery (ligation is described). Paul discussed dietary regimens, pathology, pharmacology, surgery, and medicine; his writings include discussions of cancer, particularly of the uterus and breast. Alexander wrote of internal medicine and pathology. His excellent powers of observation led to accurate deductions about diseases such as ascites, the origin of epilepsy in the brain, and the detection of an enlarged spleen by palpation. Alexander made a study of diseases of the nervous system and described melancholia ". . . as a condition that could terminate in mania which he classed as an advanced state of dementia" (Frank, 1953, p. 67).

During the period of the Roman Empire and the early centuries of Christianity, medicine experienced a gradual loss of the scientific knowledge that had been attained by the Greeks. In addition, the idea that work with the hands was degrading was applied to medicine.

Hospitals

The development and construction of early Christian hospitals was not left entirely to the charity of individual women. As the Church became freely established, the bishops also assumed responsibility for the expansion of charitable facilities as well as responsibility for the care of the sick. Consequently, one reads of houses for the sick, for strangers, for the poor, and for the aged that existed in the fourth century. The original rooms in homes for hospitality and the care of the sick were called *diakonia*. The title was indicative of the close association of the nursing care of the sick poor in private homes with the activities of the diaconate. The term *diakonos* later became synonymous with hospital or nursing director.

An expectation of Christianity was that all who needed help would be received. As the congregations grew, it thus became necessary to expand the social services of the Church. As a result, the original diakonia became too small and new rooms, wings, and buildings were added. "Usually it seemed more economical to gather all classes of unfortunates into one institution known as a *xenodocheion*, which was the ancestor of the modern hospital as well as of most other types of charitable institutions" (Shryock, 1959, p. 79). Inns for strangers (hospitality centers); hospitals for the sick, the insane, and lepers; homes for the aged; almshouses; asylums for foundlings, orphans, the maimed, and the deformed; dwellings for nurses and physicians; and offices were included in these institutions. As early as the First Council of Nicaea (325 AD), it was decided that each bishop should establish a xenodocheion. These institutions were administered by deaconesses and visited by widows of the Church. They were financed by Church alms and direct gifts from wealthy Christians. Eventually names for the various special divisions that were found in these charitable institutions arose: *xenodochia*, inns for strangers or travelers; *nosocomia*, wards or rooms for the sick; *brephotrophia*, foundling asylums; *orphanotrophia*, orphan asylums; *gerontokomia*, homes for the aged; *cherotrophia*, homes for widows;

117

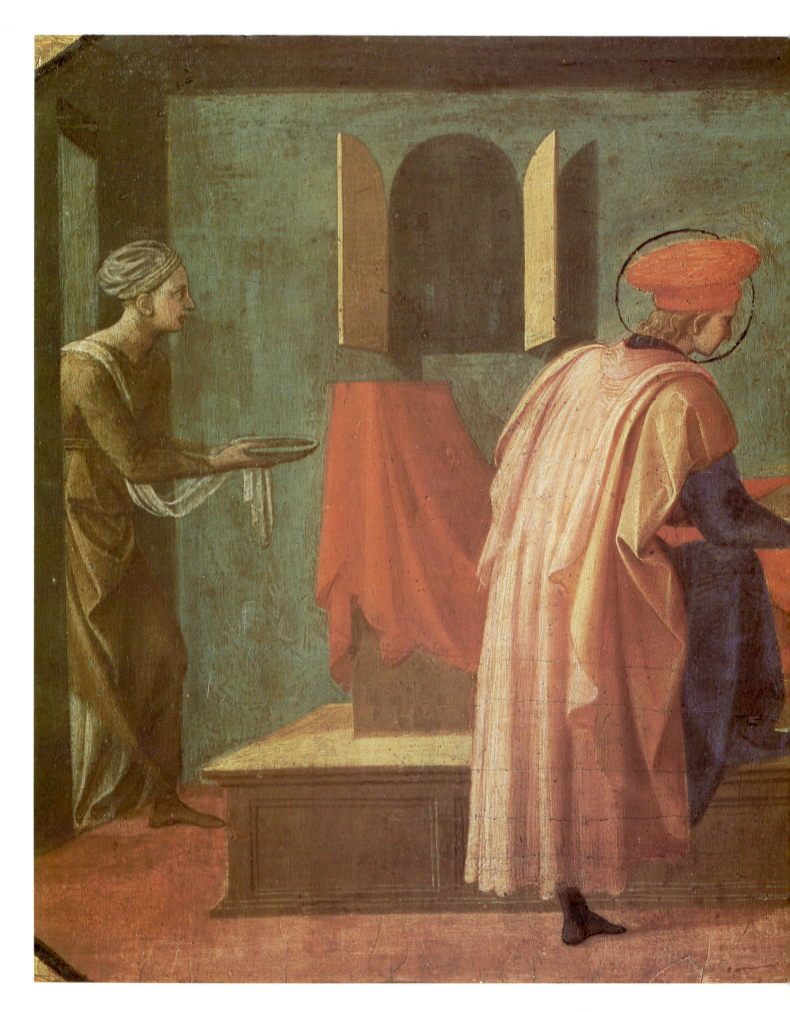

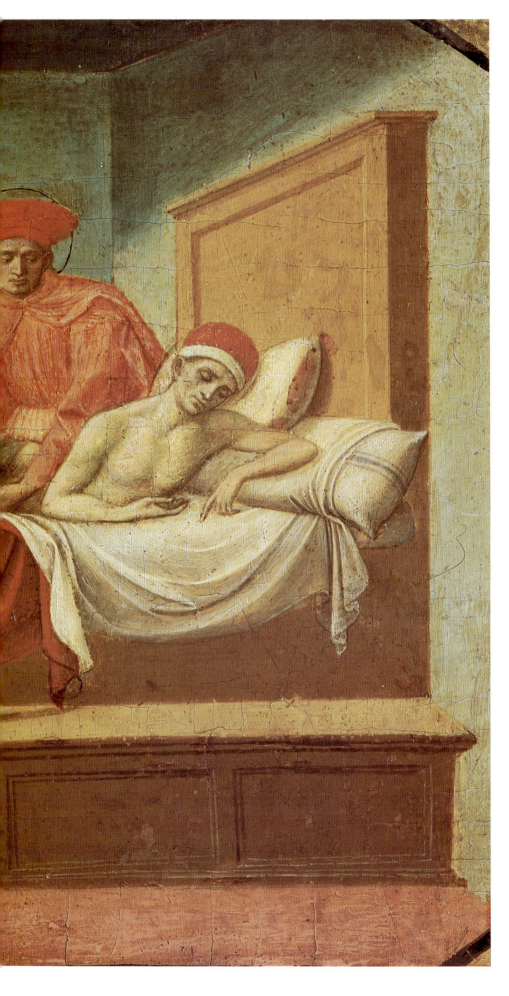

Francesco Pesellino, ST. COSMAS AND ST. DAMIAN VISITING A SICK MAN, *early fifteenth century. Wood. Musée National du Louvre, Paris, France.*

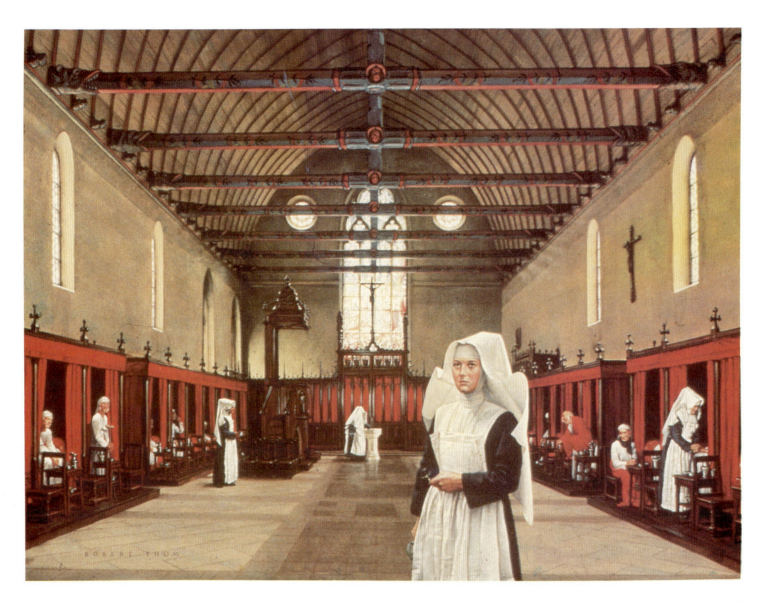

A MEDIEVAL HOSPITAL, *Parke-Davis Division of Warner-Lambert Co., Morris Plains, New Jersey.*

ptochotrophia, almshouses for the poor. According to Nutting and Dock, the evolution of the earliest forms of Christian care of the sick proceeded in the following manner:

> . . . diakonia, or rooms in private houses; xenodochia, amplifications of the diakonia; and finally, hospitals; while the forms of the earliest nursing organizations, beginning in the congregation, passed through the diaconate, the widows' sisterhoods, the parabolani, to monks and nuns.
>
> *Nutting and Dock, 1937, p. 119*

Controversy exists regarding the exact date of the earliest xenodocheion. It is said, for instance, that one was built in Constantinople in the reign of Constantine but also that those built during the time of Julian the Apostate were the earliest. What is certain is that the most famous of these is the one founded by St. Basil the Great in Caesarea (370 AD), often referred to as the "Basilias." St. Basil's institution was almost a "second city" and was as self-sufficient and self-supporting as possible. All individuals who were able to work were given employment in blacksmith shops, in the foundry, the laundry, the dairy, in shoe and clothing shops, and in the kitchen. Out of gratitude the

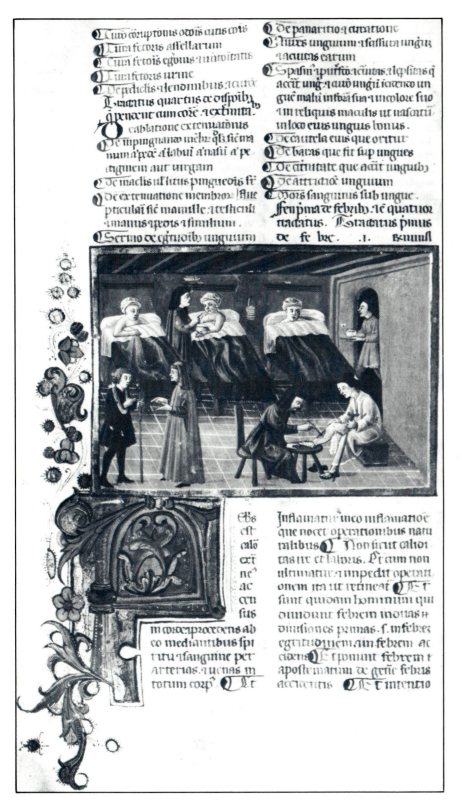

THREE BED HOSPITAL, *fifteenth century manuscript from Ferra: Florence, Laurentian, Gaddian, Ms 24, folio 247 v. Avicenna, "Canon," beginning of book IV. Biblioteca Medicea Laurenziana, Florence, Italy.*

public officials of the city of Caesarea remitted taxes on the property. "This was an important instance in the development of the precedent which has exempted from taxation properties used for religious or charitable purposes" (Sellew and Nuesse, 1946, p. 67).

The Basilias was an outstanding example of Christian charity that embraced total hospital care—prevention, treatment, and social service. In the hospital were resident physicians, resident nurses, and

Jean Pucelle, "St. Louis Administers to the Sick," from the HOURS OF JEANNE D'EVREUX, *1325–28. Illumination, grisaille and colors on vellum, approx. 8.9 × 6.4 cm. The Metropolitan Museum of Art, Cloisters Collection, 1954.*

Jean Pucelle, "St. Louis Feeds a Leprous Monk," from the HOURS OF JEANNE D'EVREUX, *1325–28. Illumination, grisaille and colors on vellum, approx. 8.9 × 6.4 cm. The Metropolitan Museum of Art, Cloisters Collection, 1954.*

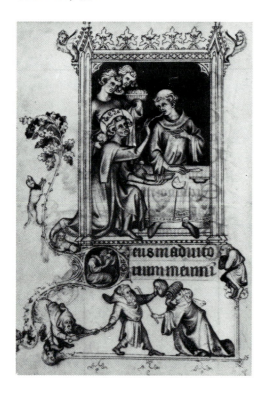

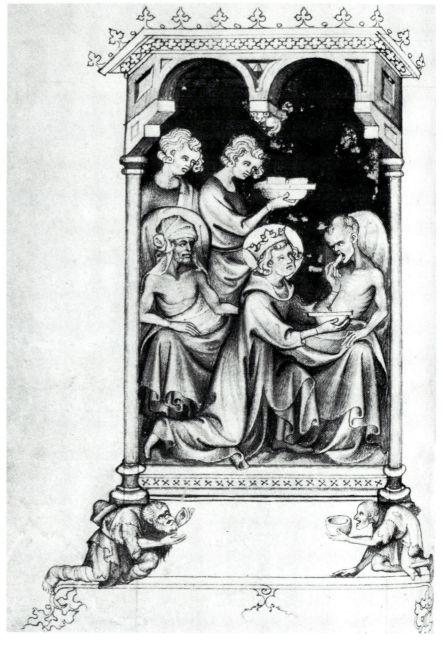

carriers of the sick (Walsh, 1929). There was an orphanage, a place of hospitality for strangers, an asylum for infants and children, a building for the aged, lepers, and those with contagious diseases, a trade school for the physically impaired, and a hospital that cared for the sick, the crippled, and the poor. In addition, Basil's hospital had a special department for the insane.

The early Christians combined the sacred custom of hospitality with loving service. This resulted in an effective system for the care of the sick and the destitute. Little, however, is known of the specific nursing service that was provided in these hospitals. It is reasonable to assume that deaconesses may have served as nurses. It is also possible that servants did the ordinary labor under the direction of Church authorities. Certainly, no indication is given of any type of formal training for the women or men who did participate in the nursing work. Eventually, nursing orders were formed in the Church to serve in the hospitals. The practice of clustering buildings was adopted by monasteries and continued until the twelfth century, when it became customary to separate hospitals from other branches of relief service and build them separately. This intimate connection between the Church and the care of the sick during this period in history is an important factor in an understanding of the organization and functions of the hospital:

> At the outset it will be well to make clear what the hospital was, and what it was not. It was an ecclesiastical, not a medical, institution. It was for care rather than cure; for the relief of the body, when possible, but pre-eminently for the refreshment of the soul.... Faith and love were more predominant features in hospital life than were skill and science.
>
> *Seymer, 1932, p. 36*

■ THE EARLY MIDDLE AGES (DARK AGES): 500–1000 AD

The term *Middle Ages* is used by historians to denote the period of time that occurred between the middle of the fifth century (fall of Rome, 476 AD) and the middle of the fifteenth century (fall of Constantinople, 1453 AD). The thousand-year period that followed the collapse of the Roman Empire is also referred to as the medieval period of history, the division between ancient and modern times. Although this is a useful term because it is fairly well understood, it must be remembered that no period in history has hard and fast boundaries. In addition, this period can be subdivided into the early and later Middle Ages. The early centuries are collectively known as the Dark Ages, a title that clearly demonstrates the prevalent social destruction of the times, the deteriorating world.

During the Dark Ages the domination of society by the Church was practically unchallenged. As the Roman Empire was slowly disintegrating, the Church had been developing into a well integrated and highly organized institution. Its organization followed a pattern similar to that of the Roman government. Each ecclesiastical province paralleled a civil province. Dioceses were formed under bishops, and these corresponded to a Roman governmental unit. Over all was the bishop of Rome, the Pope, who corresponded to the Emperor. Finally, when the Emperor removed himself to Constantinople in 330 AD, the Pope was left the most powerful figure in the West. The bishops emerged as the natural leaders of the people and the Empire was perpetuated through the Church. All of these events contributed to the evolution of the image of the nurse as a saint. The activity of nursing itself became honored as many royal, noble, and distinguished people engaged in it and regarded it as the work of God. Nursing became a penitential activity used as a means of purgation and purification. It was a work calling for unceasing toil without expectation of earthly reward.

Three large classes of people dominated society in the early Middle Ages. The majority were serfs, who were farmers living under primitive conditions. Above them were the aristocratic and warlike lords. Finally, there was the clergy, both secular and monastic, who were bound by celibacy in order to give undivided devotion to the religious life. Women had again fallen into a subordinate position, but positions in religious orders were open to them as well as to men. It was possible to acquire dignity as a nun.

There were even joint monasteries of men and women, living in separate houses but ruled over by a woman superior. Certain of the orders, both for men and for women, came to devote themselves to nursing; and it was this trend that brought women into such service for the first time on a large scale. By the modern period, indeed, nursing began to be viewed as primarily a woman's field.

Shryock, 1959, p. 89

The early Middle Ages revealed a crumbling world. Chaos reigned supreme as a result of the impact of the onslaughts of barbarian tribes and extreme moral decay. The middle class disappeared because of exorbitant taxes, widespread epidemics, natural disasters, and wars. Money and cities disappeared along with trade, commerce, and industry. The population declined, crime waves occurred, poverty was abysmal, torture and imprisonment became prominent as civilization seemed to slip back into semibarbarianism. In essence, the Graeco-Roman culture stumbled to a halt.

"The fate of civilization rested upon health protection, a different form of government, the education of thousands of barbarians to civilized standards, and many changes in Roman outlook and attitudes" (Jamieson and Sewall, 1950, p. 128). Medieval life became increasingly dangerous and necessitated the formation of protective groups by the populace. The people had lost their sense of security and gathered together in search of safety. This phenomenon was characterized by three great movements that arose during this early period of the Middle Ages: feudalism, monasticism, and Islamism. These movements developed simultaneously and were thought to be possible solutions to the chaos of the time.

Feudalism

Feudalism was a new system of land tenure with complex social arrangements in which self-sustaining groups prepared themselves to resist attacks from bands of fighting men sworn to uphold the might of their leaders. It involved cooperative farming units, isolated from each other, and governed by individuals known as knights, counts, earls, barons, or lords. Feudalism was a type of patriarchal rule that provided men with homes for their families, food, and bodily protection. In return for these services, the tenants worked the land as farmers and became soldiers in the case of war. Political, economic, and social life were based on the holding of land. The typical edifice was the rural manor or estate owned by the lord. It was usually set high in an inaccessible location, and massive turreted walls enclosed the manor, which was also encircled by a moat.

Feudalism acted as a cohesive force in the new society and demanded a strong bond of loyalty between lord and tenant. It offered a temporary solution to the land problem and provided an armed force for Europe against Frankish and Islamic invasions. Feudalism did, however, have drawbacks that eventually led to many abuses within the society. Although protection was indeed provided, constant warfare prevented progress.

Most women were forced to marry young, often without their consent. Their chief value to society was their breeding power and

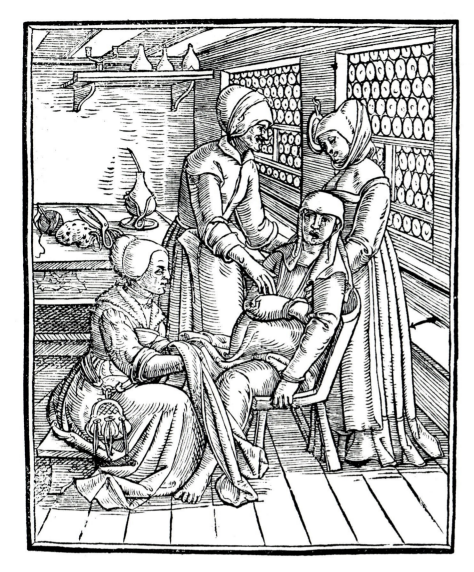

the ability to manage a home. The lord's wife, the lady of the manor, was faced with a difficult life. She was responsible for the supervision of the entire establishment, for bearing and caring for children, for riding and hunting, for whatever needed to be done. She was frequently called upon to nurse family guests or villagers. The lady was in charge of the care of the sick of the manor and was a combination of doctor and nurse. She applied first aid, faced surgical emergencies, and had an extensive knowledge of home remedies for all types of illnesses. Empirical medicine was almost entirely in the hands of such women. The number of doctors was small, and only a few of them were located in the manors.

> The lady was thus obliged not only to be housewife in her own capacity, but also amateur soldier and man of the house in her husband's absence and amateur physician when no skilled doctor could be had. She was supposed to be manager of the household and know how to choose and treat servants, to air and mend and keep moths out of clothes and furs, to know the best recipes for catching flies and other "familiar beasts to man," and for keeping bedrooms free of mosquitoes and barns of rats. There is even an injunction to his [the lord's] wife "If one of your servants fall ill, do you yourself lay aside all other cares, very lovingly and charitably care for him or her."
>
> *Walsh, 1929, p. 35*

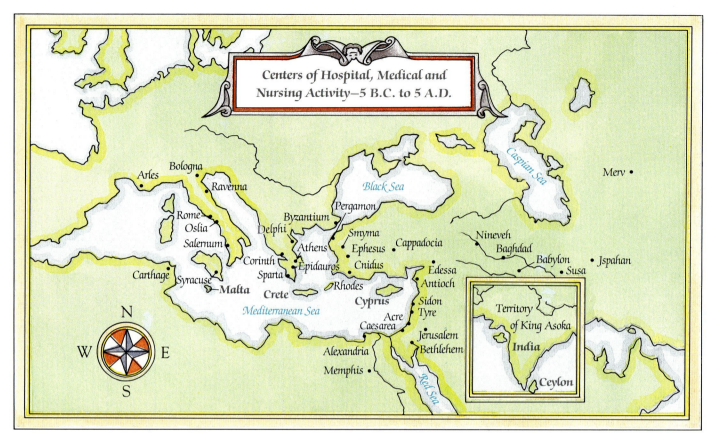

Map of the CENTERS OF HOSPITAL, MEDICAL,
AND NURSING ACTIVITY–5 BC TO 5 AD.

Monasticism

The idea of finding the ineffable love of God by renouncing the world
found a practical outlet in monasticism. The dangers of medieval life
led many men and women who were spiritually minded to the
monasteries to escape worldly chaos. Others probably entered the
monasteries to obtain security and protection. From the efforts of St.
Basil in the fourth century, the monastic movement spread to the
West and assumed prominence in the social structure of the early
Middle Ages. Through the fifth century the movement spread slowly
because the majority of monasteries were weak, poor, and disorganized. The monks tended to be idle and dissolute, often wandering
from one monastery to another in search of the easiest path. By the
sixth century, however, monasticism provided great practical and
spiritual value to concerned individuals as well as to society at large.

The basic concept of monasticism was withdrawal from society
for the sanctification of one's soul. Ascetism was also a marked feature of this religious life, particularly in the earlier periods. All
degrees of self-mortification, self-denial, and strict discipline were
observed. The monks and nuns were governed by a rule—the constitutions, bylaws, and directives by which they were to live. Four
rules were recognized by the Church for the government of monastic
orders, those of Basil, Augustine, Benedict, and Francis. Monasteries
were not established to care for orphans or to educate children or
even to nurse the sick. These were secondary works that arose
serendipitously and were done well by the monks and nuns who
performed them; they were not an essential part of their calling.

The credit for the organization of many of these institutions is
given to St. Benedict of Nursia (480–543 AD), who founded the

126

order of Benedictines in the sixth century. St. Benedict began life as a hermit who practiced the most excessive and excruciating asceticism, which led to his ultimate fame. His followers were formed into twelve communities of twelve monks. St. Benedict established the most influential monastery in western Christendom at Monte Cassino. This monastery became a Nazi stronghold during World War II and was bombed by the Allied forces. About the year 529 AD, St. Benedict composed his rule, the Benedictine Rule, which had a great influence on Western civilization. The success of the Benedictine Rule lay in its moderation, an adaptation of monastic tradition to Western conditions. It helped to bring stability and organization out of chaos, to bring calm out of panic. The rule provided for reasonable and moderate conditions, which included adequate sleep, rest, diet, and clothing, and a balance of study, prayer, and manual labor both indoors and out. It was, therefore, possible for persons of ordinary spiritual gifts to follow it. Communities were able to retain monks, to be physically, spiritually, and socially healthy and, most important, to be effective.

The Benedictine monasteries became centers of influence, learning, and culture. The monks revived agriculture through labor in the fields, orchards, and vineyards. They improved the plow and invented the windmill, the waterwheel, and the horse collar. They labored not only for souls but tilled the soil and made barren lands bountiful. The excess food produced was used to feed the poor. The monks increased the available knowledge in many ways. They were scholars, librarians, and teachers and opened schools so that all, not only their own members, could read and write. They laboriously copied, clarified, and illustrated precious manuscripts. They used their knowledge of medicine and herbs to care for the sick. The monasteries offered hospitality and shelter to the homeless and refuge to the persecuted.

> The work of the Benedictine monasteries manifested itself in several directions: in the conversion of the Teutons, in civilizing northwestern Europe, and in extending the works of education: literature, arts, sciences, libraries. It is to the monasteries that we are indebted today for practically everything extant in ancient secular and religious literature. The monks were not only the official copyists of manuscripts, they were also the official chroniclers of the history of their times.
>
> *Frank, 1953, p. 84*

Nursing of the sick eventually became a chief function and duty of the community life. This command was stated in the rule: "Before all things and above all things care must be taken of the sick." Every monastery provided an *infirmarium* for its members and a *hospitalarius* just inside or outside the gates for the needy of the community. These were at first hospices rather than hospitals, since they were refuges for the poor, devoted more to shelter and comfort than to cure. More affluent monasteries later sought to divide the sick from the poor and to offer more than food and shelter to those who needed help. As time elapsed, it was not only the sick poor who requested assistance. Monks were called from their monasteries to the courts of kings and nobles and to the homes of the wealthy. From the original refuges city hospitals grew and became the responsibility

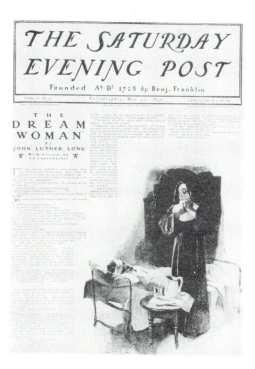

J.C. Leyendecker, Illustration for "The Dream Woman," cover for THE SATURDAY EVENING POST, *May 20, 1899.*

of a monastic order. In most instances the nursing in these institutions was done by a monastic sisterhood.

Information about the nursing personnel of these earliest monastic hospitals is scanty. It is possible that deaconesses were still active as nurses. In some cases religious societies were instituted to meet the needs of specific situations. It was also the custom for the monks and nuns of related orders to serve the hospitals. Monastic orders for women had developed concurrently with those for men and followed the same pattern. Monks did nursing in the men's wards and nuns in the women's wards, an arrangement that became common toward the middle of the thirteenth century. In some cases the nuns were in charge of an entire hospital and the monks of the same order acted as priests. It is doubtful, however, that all the nursing work was done by them, since they had many lay attendants and perhaps volunteers.

Little is known about the actual care given the sick during the Dark Ages. Secular medicine was almost completely extinguished, and there was little impetus toward advancement in the science and art of nursing or of medicine. In fact, little distinction was made between medicine and nursing. The monks and the nuns practiced medicine as well as nursing and for long periods seemed to have been the only practitioners. Medical historians report that the medical practice was almost entirely confined to the members of these monastic orders. Considerable folk and drug lore, mysticism, religious faith, and, at times, superstition crept into the care of the sick. Bloodletting, diet, and baths were common treatments of the day along with the application of cups and leeches and the use of blisters, cautery, scarification, and enemas. "The main advancement in nursing during this period probably came through the internal organization and operation of monastic institutions and the discipline and training of large groups of sisters and brothers in their cooperative undertakings" (Stewart and Austin, 1962, p. 50). The nursing of the times was done partly by monks and nuns and partly by servants. It is difficult, however, to determine the division of labor between the two and whether either received much formal training.

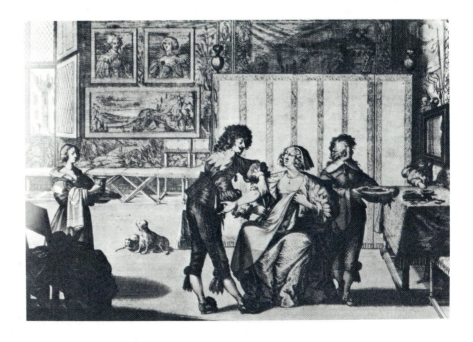

After Abraham Bosse, INTERIOR SCENE WITH WOMAN BEING PHLEBOTEMISED BY A BARBER SURGEON, *c. 1635. Engraving. National Library of Medicine, Bethesda, Maryland.*

Monastic Nurses

Monastic houses for women grew in number in the sixth and seventh centuries. Many of the women who entered these houses were wealthy and had great influence in the community. The two primary reasons given for women's entry into these orders were the prevailing need for protection and the opportunity to lead the occupational career of one's choice. The women in these monasteries were sheltered by a rule, granted by the Church, that afforded freedom and safety to pursue intellectual studies or practical interests. Many famous women of the early Middle Ages were connected to the monastic life. They included Hrotswitha, who knew the Latin classics and wrote dramas; Lisba, Walburga, and Berthgythe, who went from Ireland and England to evangelize Germany; and Hildegarde, whose medical knowledge and political insight were remarkable (Dock and Stewart, 1925). Other women carried on hospital nursing and medical work.

Large twin communities, or double monasteries, of men and women were also a feature of early monastic life. These were under the direct control of an abbess, who held a position of great importance. The two related houses, one of monks, the other of nuns, were usually kept rigidly apart. It is interesting to note that the opposite system of the rule of women's orders by an abbot met with failure; the groups did not flourish or survive (Tuker and Malleson, 1900). A sense of joint ownership united the members of these religious settlements and resulted in the emergence of centers of culture and of art. Famous abbesses who ruled the twin communities were Radegunde at Poitiers; Hilda at Whitby in England, who had some of the great bishops as her scholars and taught Caedmon, the first English poet; and Hersende at Frontevrault, who ruled a vast establishment of 3000 members. Each abbess administered the property of the monastery and maintained discipline. The monks and the nuns swore obedience to her.

The most famous double establishment was founded and ruled by St. Radegunde (519–587 AD) at Poitiers in 559 AD. Radegunde, the daughter of a Thuringian king and a descendant of Theodoric, experienced numerous tragedies in her young life. Her father was murdered by her uncle; she was captured and forced to marry Clotaire, the Frankish king of Neustria, becoming one of his six wives; she fled to Noyan after her husband murdered her brother. Eventually Radegunde made her way to Poitiers, where she took refuge in the Christian Church. She founded the Holy Cross Monastery, a religious settlement of about 200 nuns.

Scripture reading, the study of ancient literature, the transcription of manuscripts, and the performance of dramas (mystery plays of the Middle Ages) were important activities of this community. The care of the sick, however, was the chief function. Radegunde nursed the patients herself in the hospital she established. She was particularly sensitive to the lepers, who were social outcasts, and was seen giving a kiss to their diseased bodies. There is no indication that physicians were connected with this hospital. Nursing care seems to have been the key to the restoration of health. Baths were built at the instigation of Radegunde. This was particularly significant because Christian monasticism had destroyed the cult of the Roman bath. Stimulation of the skin was condemned as a provocative sexual desire

129

in an age of asceticism. In a sense Radegunde carried on the forgotten tradition of the Baths of Caracalla (Robinson, 1946).

The monastic ideal of humility led to the use of plain coarse materials for clothing. This ideal was perpetuated by the poverty of many of the earliest convents. Yet abbesses and nuns of royal birth wore beautiful clothing, as depicted by the following description:

> A vest of fine linen of a violet colour is worn, above it a scarlet tunic with a hood, sleeves striped with silk and trimmed with red fur; the locks on the forehead and temples are curled with a crisping iron, the dark head-veil is given up for white and coloured head-dresses which, with bows of ribbon sewn on, reach down to the ground; the nails, like those of a falcon or sparrow-hawk, are pared to resemble talons.
>
> *Putnam, 1921, p. 85*

Criticism of this costume as incongruous with monasticism paved the way for a clothing reform that ended in uniformity. A distinctive dress for religious women became a custom. The veil as part of convent dress symbolized humility, obedience, and service. Regulations were developed that governed the use of the veils. They came to be a part of the prescribed habit and were always white during the probationary period of the novice. Various forms of the veil were worn by women to distinguish social position. The cap of the modern nurse is a modification of the religious veil and has been associated with humility and the rendering of service to mankind.

St. Brigid (452–523 AD) introduced female monasteries into Ireland as early as the fifth century. She was the daughter of an Ulster prince and a disciple of St. Patrick. Brigid became a famous abbess in Ireland and was respected as a scholar, educator, counselor, and an expert in the healing arts. References are made to the miracles of Brigid, who was also known for her healing of the lepers and her care of the sick. She was labeled as "the patroness of healing."

St. Scholastica, the twin sister of St. Benedict, founded a Benedictine community for women. This order was established near Monte Cassino, and Scholastica became its abbess.

Islamism

During the early centuries of the Christian era and into part of the Middle Ages, Arab kingdoms extended from Spain, through northern Africa, and into western Asia. The Arab influence was felt as far away as India and China. The conquests of the Arab people exposed them to a variety of native cultures, and they developed a certain tolerance for different beliefs and ways of living. They learned from the achievements of the Egyptians and the Greeks. They built universities where experimental research and scientific studies in astronomy, mathematics, and chemistry were conducted.

Mohammed (570–632 AD) was born at Mecca, the religious and commercial center of Arabia. His tribe was one of the most influential and guarded the sacred Kaaba, the idolatrous shrine where heathen Arabs made an annual religious pilgrimmage. He was considered to be the first and only prophet of a new world religion: "There is no God but Allah, and Mohammed is his prophet." At Mohammed's command primitive gods and native animism were abandoned. Submission was the core of the religion and the basic ideal that led to the name of *Islam* ("surrender to the will of Allah"). The followers of the monotheistic religion were called Moslems. The teachings of Mohammed were written down and incorporated in the *Koran*. Both the civil and religious lives of Moslems were directed by the tenets of this new religion. Mohammedanism has been called a "religion of the sword," since the followers of Islam were inspired by the creed to spread their conquests throughout the Mediterranean and to threaten the gates of Europe.

Medicine was an interest of the Arabians, and they strongly encouraged its study. They translated many Hellenic works into Arabic, particularly those related to medicine and including the works of Hippocrates and Galen. They studied hygiene and developed an extensive materia medica. Their belief in the uncleanliness of the dead forbade dissection. Thus knowledge of anatomy and physiology was hampered. Surgery, however, was practiced, and the Moslems are credited with the use of catgut. Physicians were held in high esteem and were required to pass qualifying examinations.

The Arabs built large well-constructed hospitals and introduced new methods of caring for the sick. The hospital at Cairo had chief physicians who held clinics for medical students. Some of the unusual features of this hospital included classified wards, male and female nurses, streams of running water in some of the wards, and fever wards cooled by fountains.

> The great Al-Mansur hospital of Cairo was a huge triangular
> structure with fountains playing in the four courtyards, separate
> wards for important diseases, wards for women and convales-
> cents, lecture rooms, an extensive library, out-patient clinics, diet
> kitchens, an orphan asylum and a chapel. It employed male and
> female nurses, had an income of about $100,000, and disbursed
> a suitable sum to each convalescent on his departure, so that he
> might not have to go to work at once. The patients were nour-
> ished upon a rich and attractive diet, and the sleepless were
> provided with soft music or, as in the Arabian Nights, with
> accomplished tellers of tales.
>
> *Garrison, 1913, pp. 92–93*

Alexandria and Damascus also had well-equipped hospitals under the control of expert physicians. The latter gave free treatment and drugs for over three centuries. The hospital at Bagdad employed sixty salaried physicians on its staff, probably the earliest instance of a paid staff. A system of care of the patient incorporated spiritual and mental aspects as well as attention to the body. Yet the care of a woman during childbirth and in the case of gynecological disease remained in the hands of untaught midwives.

Among the many outstanding physicians, three in particular are remembered: Rhazes, Avicenna, and Maimonides. Rhazes (Razi-abu-Bakr Muhammad ibn-Zakarīyā al-Rāzi, 850–932 AD) was one of the greatest of the Arabic physicians. He was especially known for his writings on measles and smallpox and contributed material to an encyclopedia of medicine. Rhazes was respected for his clinical descriptions of illness, his observations, and his pragmatic approach to treatment.

Avicenna (abu-Ali al-Husayn ibn-Sīna, 980–1037 AD) was considered to be both a philosopher and a scientist. Although he may have practiced medicine, his principal contribution in this area was his writings. The *Canon of Medicine* in use for centuries after his death was considered to be one of the most important textbooks in the field of medical education. Until the middle of the seventeenth century, medical curricula of the Christian universities were based on his writings.

Maimonides (Moses ben Maimon, 1135–1204 AD) was the most famous Jewish physician in Arabic medicine. He was born in Moslem-controlled Cordova, Spain, but fled with other Jews to Fez in Morocco when nonbelievers began to be harassed. Later he went to Palestine and then to Cairo, where he entered medicine for financial reasons. He finally became court physician to the sultan Saladin. Maimonides aimed at practical therapeutics and gave advice on such things as hygiene, poisons, diet, and first aid. However, he was basically a philosopher who attempted to reconcile scientific reasoning and religious faith. He is remembered specifically for codifying the Talmud. Although attributed by some with composing the Morning Prayer of the Physician, Maimonides probably was not the author (Lyons, 1978). This section of the prayer is often quoted:

> O God, let my mind be ever clear and enlightened. By the bedside of the patient let no alien thought deflect it. Let everything that experience and scholarship have taught it be present in it and hinder it not in its tranquil work. For great and noble are those scientific judgments that serve the purpose of preserving the health and lives of Thy creatures.
>
> Keep far from me the delusion that I can accomplish all things. Give me the strength, the will, and the opportunity to amplify my knowledge more and more. Today I can disclose things in my knowledge which yesterday I would not yet have dreamt of, for the Art is great, but the human mind presses on untiringly.
>
> In the patient let me ever see only the man. Thou, All-Bountiful One, hast chosen me to watch over the life and death of Thy creatures. I prepare myself now for my calling. Stand Thou by me in this great task, so that it may prosper. For without Thine aid man prospers not even in the smallest things.
>
> *Morning Prayer of the Physician*

School of Salerno

The earliest universities were established at Salerno, Bologna, Paris, and Oxford. The circumstances of the founding of each remain obscure. Their growth, however, was gradual. Salerno began as a medical center and served a vital role in the transition from monastic to lay medicine. The date of its founding as well as its origins are unclear. Legend states that the school was started by four physicians, one Jew, one Greek, one Latin, and one Arab.

Salerno became an important center of medical learning and assisted with the revival of medicine in Europe. It was open to female students and women physicians were on the faculty. Trotula and Abella were the two most famous women of this school. Trotula was supposedly the author of a treatise on obstetrics and gynecology and the head of the department of diseases of women. Throughout the early Middle Ages, however, midwifery was the province of women, and other medical concerns were generally forbidden to them. Women physicians usually specialized in diseases of women and children, even though they were licensed for general practice.

Standard requirements of the school of Salerno included three years of premedicine at the college level in the study of logic, philosophy, and literature, five years of medicine and surgery, and one year's practice with a reputable physician. A law was enacted about 1140 AD to prohibit anyone from practicing medicine without a license. *Regimen Sanitatis Salernitanum* was the most famous work of the Salernitan school. This Latin poem, which consisted of rational dietetic and hygienic precepts, underwent many versions and more than 300 editions.

Medieval Hospitals

Three famous medieval hospitals, the Hôtel Dieu of Lyons, the Hôtel Dieu of Paris, and the Santo Spirito Hospital of Rome, were built outside monastic walls and are still in existence. The most complete records dealing with the nursing arrangements are available for the Hôtel Dieu of Lyons and of Paris. The name *Hôtel Dieu,* meaning "God's house," was generally used to indicate the principal hospital in a French town or city (Nutting and Dock, 1937). The original hospitals were established as xenodochia or almshouses and attended to the needy and infirm as well as to the sick.

Miniature of the "Reception of Patients in the Hôtel Dieu," from the BOOK OF THE VERY ACTIVE LIFE OF THE NUNS OF THE HÔTEL DIEU IN PARIS, *fifteenth century. Musée de l'Assistance Publique, Paris, France.*

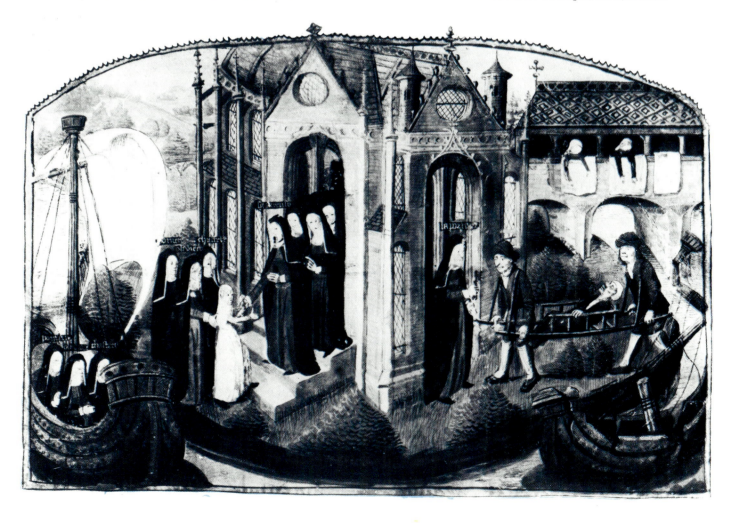

133

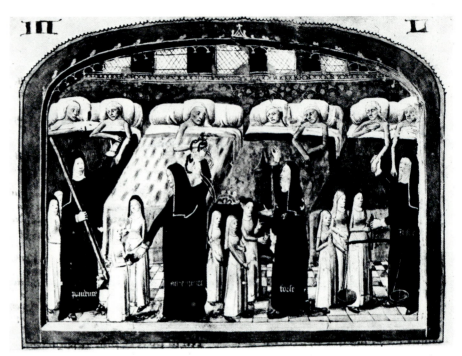

The Hôtel Dieu of Lyons was founded in 542 AD at the request of Sacerdos, the archbishop of Lyons. It was originated on the almshouse plan and was managed by lay groups. Including other charitable works besides nursing, it was designed to shelter pilgrims, orphans, the poor, the infirm, and the sick. Its earliest nurses were laywomen who were recruited from penitents (fallen women) and widows. Eventually, men who were originally called *servants,* and later *brothers,* assisted with the nursing work. This particular hospital provided a striking contrast to other institutions of the time in that it was free from clerical control.

The Hôtel Dieu of Paris dates from 650 or 651 AD. It was founded by Bishop Landry (Landericus), whose statue stands in its courtyard. This "house of God" was built with an open door for all who suffered. Also patterned after the almshouse, it was governed by a lay administration. The Hôtel Dieu began as a small hospital and grew to immense proportions. The original group of laywomen who cared for the sick were organized into a religious body by Pope Innocent IV. They became known as the Augustinian Sisters, since they adopted the Rule of St. Augustine. Brothers, too, belonged to this strict order. These Sisters were responsible to the clergy and for all practical purposes were about the same as cloistered nuns. They are considered to be the oldest purely nursing order of Sisters in existence.

The importance of the Hôtel Dieu of Paris is noted in the following description:

> No other ancient hospital has bequeathed to posterity a nursing history so extensive or one that has thrown so much light on internal hospital management. For the publication of these interesting records we have mainly to thank the unremitting and bitter contest which for centuries was carried on by the clerical and civil powers over the administration of the important and extensive institution. In this, as in every similar contest, the nursing service was the chief storm centre, and to gain control

134

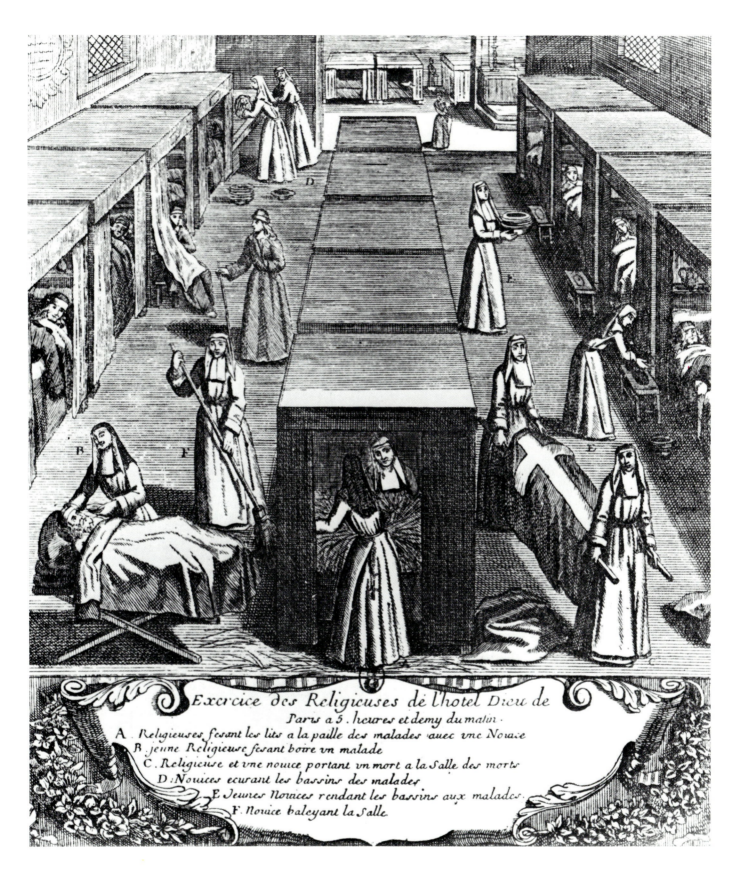

Exercice des Religieuses de l'hôtel Dieu de
Paris a 5. heures et demy du matin.
A. Religieuses fesant les lits a la paille des malades auec vne Nouice
B. jeune Religieuse fesant boire vn malade
C. Religieuse et vne nouice portant vn mort a la Salle des morts
D. Nouices ecurant les bassins des malades
E. Jeunes Nouices rendant les bassins aux malades
F. Nouice baleyant la Salle

NUNS AT WORK ON A WARD AT THE HÔTEL DIEU, PARIS, *c. 1650. Wood engraving. From Casimir Tollet's* LES EDIFICES HOSPITA-
LIERS, *1892. National Library of Medicine, Bethesda, Maryland.*

135

A WARD OF THE HÔTEL DIEU, *c. 1500. Wood engraving. Bibliothèque Nationale, Paris, France.*

The nuns at the Hôtel Dieu not only cared for the sick; they are shown here wrapping the bodies of those who have died.

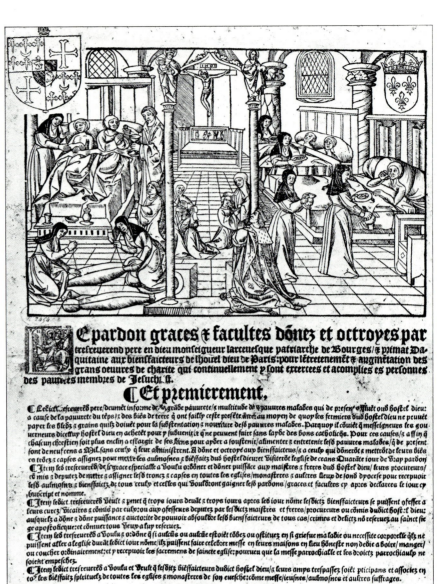

of the nursing staff the main point of vantage sought. The story of this struggle points anew to the elemental importance of the nursing factor in the composition of hospitals, and many useful lessons may be taken therefrom.

Nutting and Dock, 1937, p. 294

Both the Brothers and the Sisters were assigned specific activities that fell into the categories of exterior work, hospital administration, care of the sick, and religious services. Some nursing was done by the Brothers in the general wards, but in the women's wards only Sisters did the nursing care. The Augustinians went through three stages of training. Their nursing role included the admission and discharge of patients, responsibility for the kitchens and the laundry (all the washing was done on the banks of the nearby Seine), and the burying of the dead. In addition, religious rites were an essential part of the hospital routine with services conducted for both patients and staff.

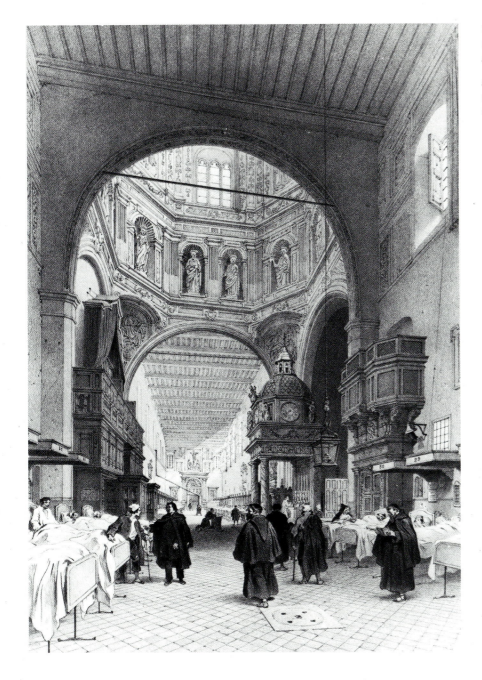

The Santo Spirito Hospital in Rome, established in 717 AD by order of the Pope, was probably the largest of the medieval hospitals. It was built for the primary purpose of care for the sick. By 1500 AD it possessed a main hall that contained nearly 1000 beds. Several distinct wards were included for men, women, and convalescents. As the revival of a lay medical profession in the later medieval period brought physicians into the hospitals, Santo Spirito encouraged this connection. It is said that more than 100 physicians and surgeons were eventually in attendance at this hospital. This institution became a well-known prototype for the development of other medieval hospitals.

*T*he most spectacular product of the feudal system was the Crusader, a man who was supposed to combine a lofty spirit devoted to the service of God with a fierce, belligerent temper, ready to fight the infidel wherever he was to be found, that the holy ground upon which Christ trod might again belong to his followers. He carried the principles and the glory of knighthood to their fullest as he traveled over the continent of Europe and throughout the Mediterranean basin. When he traveled in the Near East, he learned much from the enemy; the idea of the organized hospital was originally borrowed from the Arabs. The natural places for the establishment of hospitals were the outposts, particularly Jerusalem itself, where those wounded in battle sought refuge while they recovered. The hospital had to be staffed by physicians and nurses who were members of the regular orders. The nurses went to battle and then retired to attend the sick. They were called "knight hospitalers."

Gerald Joseph Griffin
Joanne King Griffin

138

NURSING IN A CHANGING WORLD

Aristocratic and Military Influences

The roots of a movement toward the creation of religious orders of men and women with the primary motivation of nursing the sick began to occur in the late Middle Ages. This was accompanied by a marked tendency toward the secularization and commercialization of nursing.

■ THE LATE MIDDLE AGES: 1000–1500 AD

Numerous interacting forces were activated in the period known as the late Middle Ages, the end of the Dark Ages. As a result of these forces, society would never be the same again. By this time many barbarian tribes had settled somewhere in Europe, staked claims to lands, and often been Christianized and civilized. It was a period in history characterized by mobility of the population and eventually with the detachment of individuals from protective units. It was a time in which surprising progress was made, not only in the arts and writing (greatly aided by the invention of printing) but also in architecture and the healing arts. In some ways it was marked by a spirit of optimism and enthusiasm that would become shattered nearly five centuries later by war, plagues, famine, and instability.

Trade promoted the development of inland cities and a middle class of merchants, bankers, shop owners, and shopkeepers; craftsmen arose and became as wealthy and powerful as the land barons. New inventions in crafts and trades occurred in relation to these changes. Learning was revived, and university education became a privilege of the middle class. This middle class grew as social forces freed the serfs from their manor duties and set them adrift into the cities to seek paid employment. The protection that the castle or monastery walls had previously offered was secured by the building of town walls. The gates in the walls were secured at sundown; the bridge was raised in those cities surrounded by moats. In many instances the walled cities were overpopulated. There were limited, if any, facilities for sanitation and for the provision of pure water and food. Slums became hotbeds of disease, crime, violence, and death.

A new spirit challenged the domination of the Catholic Church, which remained the chief influence over the people. This spirit was characterized by an emerging interest in the things of this earth and the life of the present rather than a focus on life after death with its emphasis on the soul. The Church had grown rich and powerful, and this caused criticism of the priesthood and monastic orders as well as the Church itself. Wealth, laxity, and greed failed to exemplify the teachings of Christ. Unrest occurred as the middle class grew more independent, knowledgeable, and sophisticated. Various reform movements, which included new patterns of religious thought and action, tended to divert the unrest, at least for a time. Eventually a new interpretation of the doctrine of the Church was demanded. Individuals such as Peter Abelard (1079–1142 AD) broke from the rigid Augustinian doctrine of predestination. In the Augustinian doctrine the life of the body was held to be of little importance except as an opportunity for the soul to find unity with God. This unity could be achieved through suppressing physical desires and appetites, having faith in Christ, and obeying the commands of Christ. Life in this world was a journey between life and death. Each person would struggle with the forces of good and evil and would be rewarded in the next world on the basis of success. Reason and logical analysis as the means to truth began to be advocated as an alternative. The writings of St. Thomas Aquinas (1225–1274 AD) became a part of this new ideology and the basis of Catholic doctrine for many centuries thereafter. Aquinas, also known as the "angelic doctor," incorporated his interpretation of the whole doctrine of Catholicism in *Summa Theologica.*

A resurgence in religious fervor demonstrated itself in reforms of the monasteries and priesthood, crusades against the heretics of the Near East, and an increase in pilgrimages to the Holy Land. Nursing was affected by these events because crowded living conditions and the resulting increase in the spread of disease created a need for the establishment of new and different types of orders to care for the sick. The redistribution of the population and urban growth brought nursing out of the institutions and back into the home. Those individuals who were drawn to nursing continued to be of high intellec-

William Shakespeare Burton, THE WOUNDED CAVALIER, *c. 1856. The Bridgeman Art Library, Guildhall Art Gallery, City of London, England.*

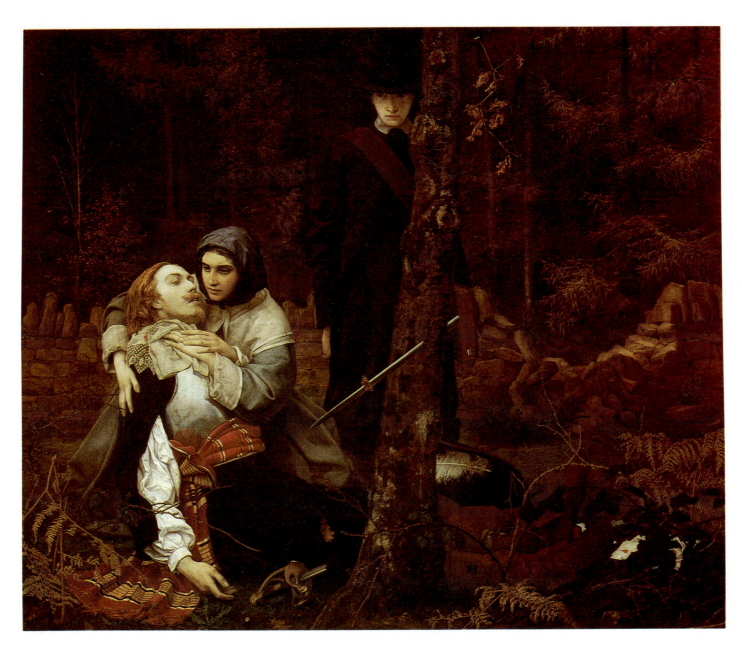

141

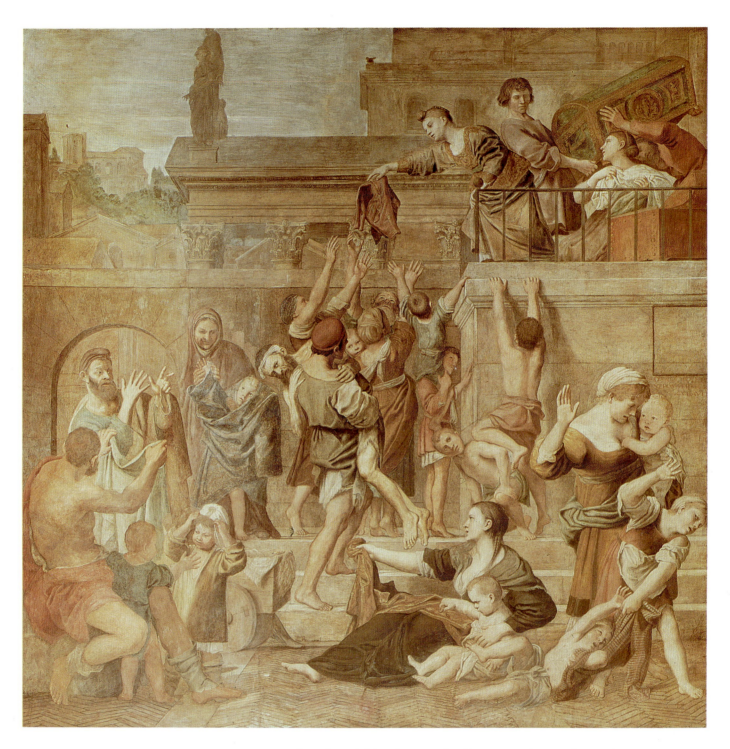

Domenichino, ST. CECILIA DISTRIBUTING ALMS TO THE POOR, *c. 1615–17. Fresco. San Luigi dei Francisi, Rome, Italy. (SCALA/Art Resource, NY).*

tual and social backgrounds. Great numbers of men became nurses, and the military ideal of discipline and order entered nursing. This era was rich in nursing saints, several of whom were widely acclaimed and highly honored.

> Among the momentous forces and developments of this period that in one way or another influenced health practices generally and nursing in particular were the Crusades, the military nursing orders, the institution of chivalry, the guilds, the further development of hospitals and medicine, the decline of monasticism, the rise of the mendicant orders and the devastation of Europe by the great plague. None of these factors in what was a changing world can be considered in isolation from the rest.
>
> *Frank, 1953, p. 96*

Guilds

According to many historians, references to guilds are thought to have first been made in England. Guilds were initially mentioned in the eighth century. In England they were primarily religious in nature and played an important role in English social life as charitable institutions. These social organizations demonstrated a localized system of control that involved self-regulation by the members.

The earliest guilds were specifically religious and social in orientation, an attempt to balance the spiritual and temporal needs of the members. They were often named for a saint whose patronage they sought. Activities included the building of chapels, the founding of schools, and the presentation of mystery plays. Eventually hospitals were maintained and social insurance (distress assistance for sickness, poverty, and death) was provided through dues paid by the members. Other types of guilds also developed. These included the peace guilds for the maintenance of justice in the town and merchant guilds for the purpose of carrying on trade. Frequently the law of the guild became the law of the town, as exemplified in London in the tenth century.

The first associations of workers arose in the form of guilds and were extremely important in the late Middle Ages. These were usually known as craft guilds, which divided workmen into three levels of vocational training: the *apprentice,* who remained under the direction of a master craftsman for three to ten years; the *journeyman* or *craftsman,* who hired his services to another; and the *master craftsman,* who was required to make an original contribution to the craft, pass an examination, and be economically stable in order to achieve this status. The craft guilds were the vocational training schools of the era. Under an apprenticeship method the learner worked with an expert, was motivated to become a master, and recognized the value of his craft. These guilds were also the labor organizations of the day and as such protected and improved the status of the members. Wage scales and prices were fixed, hygienic working conditions were demanded, reasonable hours of labor were established, and quality in workmanship was demanded.

Men in the same crafts and professions thus banded together to promote high standards. Ultimately physician guilds were established and fostered the separation of surgeons from medical practitioners. This was necessary because of the inclination to draw individuals together according to the similarity of their tools and materials rather than a consideration of their purposes. For example, surgeons' guilds admitted barbers, and physicians were joined with apothecaries and artists because of their common use of powders.

In general, the guild system provided an element of stability to the larger social order. It was a viable method of regulating economic life and providing for the discharge of personal responsibility to the community as a whole. It was a system whereby the consumer as well as the worker could be protected and a quality product could be ensured. In addition, the medieval apprenticeship system survived and affected the development of some types of workers throughout various periods in history. The apprenticeship form of nursing prevalent in the United States until the 1940s was probably influenced by the pattern of the craft guilds. Unfortunately, this type of system did not foster a bona fide educational process; rather, it encouraged a

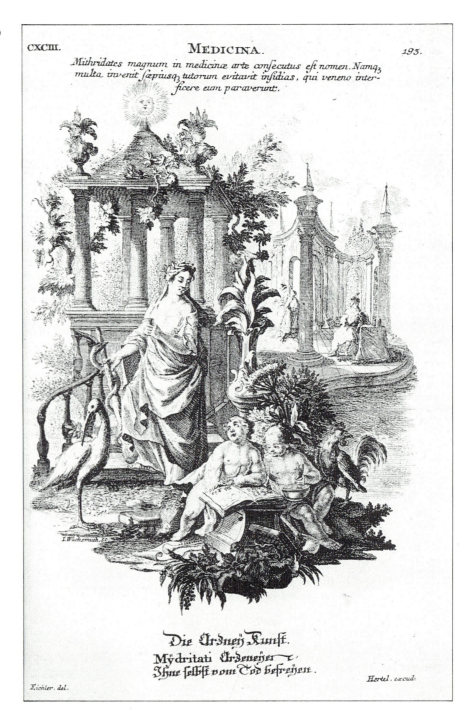

The depiction of MEDICINE *in the 1758–1760 Hertel Edition of Cesare Ripa's* ICONOLOGIA. *From* BAROQUE AND ROCOCO PICTORIAL IMAGERY, *edited by Edward A. Maser, 1971 Dover Publications, New York.*

strong aspect of service, which impeded the progression of nursing for many decades.

The Crusades

The Crusades have been identified as the "supreme folly of the Middle Ages" in one source (Nutting and Dock, 1937). This statement, however, is in direct opposition to the idea that throughout history men have regarded certain places, events, and objects as sacred and have journeyed long distances to revere them. From the fourth century, people had made pilgrimages to shrines and to the Holy Land. By the eleventh century, both the number and size of these pilgrimages had greatly increased, until some were made up of thousands of individuals. There are records of six pilgrimages in the eighth century, twelve in the ninth century, sixteen in the tenth century, and 117 in the eleventh century.

Pilgrim travels to Palestine started soon after the Crucifixion. Initially these journeys were made by the inhabitants of the Holy Land itself but eventually included inhabitants of distant lands. By the late eleventh century, however, a series of military and political changes took place in the Middle East and the Seljuk Turks, who had embraced Islam, captured Jerusalem. Mosques were erected in the Holy City of Jerusalem, and Christians who had been making pilgrimages there were persecuted. Therefore a united effort to stop the actions of the Turks was launched in the form of military expeditions known as *Crusades.* Hundreds of thousands of men answered the call of Pope Urban II to initiate this movement:

> Come forward to the defense of Christ. O ye who have carried
> on feuds, come to the war against the infidels. O ye who have
> been thieves, become soldiers. Fight a just war. Labor for ever-
> lasting reward, ye who were hirelings, serving for a few solidi.
> And more — whosoever shall offer himself to go upon this
> journey and shall make his vow to go, shall wear the sign of the
> cross on his head or breast.
>
> *Lamb, 1930, pp. 39–41*

Each Crusader was identified as a soldier of Christ by a red cross on his head or breast. The first expedition of these crossbearers began in 1096 AD.

Numerous crusades occurred between 1096 and 1291 AD (the dates may vary somewhat according to the reference used). They are generally divided into four major expeditions and four minor ones.

The major expeditions included the First Crusade (1096–1099), led by knights of France and the Normans; the Second Crusade (1147–1149), under the direction of the kings of France and Germany; the Third Crusade (1189–1192) led by the kings of France, England, and Germany; and the Fourth Crusade (1202–1204), led by French nobles and the doge of Venice.

The minor Crusades took place from 1216 to 1220, 1228 to 1229, 1248 to 1254, and 1270 to 1272. Jerusalem was captured dur-

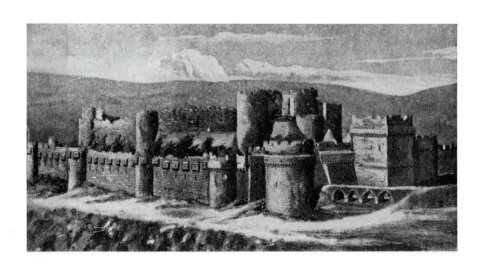

The CRAC DES CHEVALIERS, *a famous stronghold of the Hospitallers in the eleventh century. The Bettmann Archive, New York.*

145

ing the First Crusade but was lost once again to the Turks in 1187. It was never regained by the Western world until the First World War.

Innumerable fanatical efforts also occurred, including the Peasants' Crusade and the Children's Crusade. The former resulted from the preaching of such men as Peter the Hermit and was the first stirring of the serfs against their lot. The latter was organized with the idea that Jerusalem would fall to a band of children so young as to be pure of heart. All the children, who were under twelve years of age, eventually fell ill or were captured and made slaves.

The Crusades were extensive expeditions to conquer the Holy Land, which had been in the hands of the Mohammedans for several centuries. Among the participants were members of the clergy, adventurers, pious individuals, and others who sought an opportunity to satisfy a variety of motives. The Crusades indeed represented many things to many people: aristocratic and military ideals in social life, political ambition, economic gain, the desire for adventure, and the extension of Christianity by means of war, a holy war.

These enterprises extended over a long period of time and increased the need for hospitals along the Crusader and pilgrim routes as well as in Syria and Palestine. An acute demand arose for hospitals and for providers of health care because of the effects of the war, which became more and more deadly as disease was carried wherever armies were sent.

O. Cennl, THE KNIGHTS OF MALTA ENTERING JERUSALEM, *1908. Drawing. The Bettmann Archive, New York.*

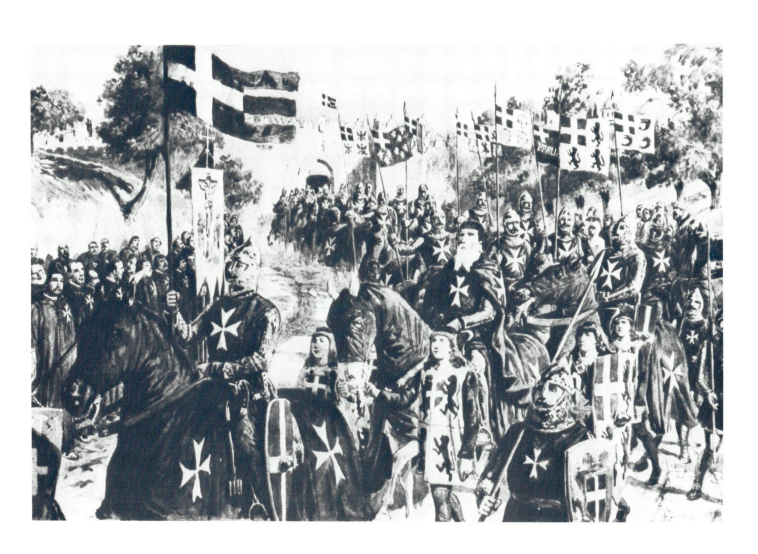

That the Crusades were turned back by epidemics much more effectively than they were by the armed power of the Saracens can hardly be questioned. The history of the Crusades reads like the chronicle of a series of diseases, with scurvy as potent as infections. In 1098, a Christian army of 300,000 men besieged Antioch. Disease and famine killed so many and in such a short time that the dead could not be buried. The cavalry were rendered useless within a few months by the death of 5000 of their 7000 horses. Nevertheless, the city was captured, after a nine months' siege. On the march to Jerusalem, the hosts were accompanied by an enemy more potent than the heathen. When Jerusalem was taken, in 1099, only 60,000 of the original 300,000 were left, and these, by 1101, had melted to 20,000.

The story of the second Crusade, led by Louis VII of France, is sadly similar. Of half a million men, only a handful—most of them without horses—managed to get back to Antioch, and few returned to Europe.

Zinsser, 1934, p. 155

The response to these identified needs resulted in the development of military nursing orders, knighthood, additional hospitals, mendicant orders, and the rise of several great nursing saints. In addition, with the advent of the military order, a harsher element entered nursing. Emphasis was now placed on rank, deference to superior officers, and the vow of unquestioning obedience. All of these would profoundly affect the progress of nursing and nursing education for many years to follow.

Military Nursing Orders

The military nursing orders were an outcome of the Crusades to the Holy Land. They were a special type of nursing order that appeared in the military brotherhoods. These orders combined the attributes of religion and chivalry, as well as militarism and charity, in their dedicated services. Unfortunately, the chronicles and histories of this period contain little information about how the knights cared for the sick and the wounded because the primary emphasis in these documents was the military aspects of the pilgrimages. However, they do indicate that great hospitals were built and equipped and that knights nursed patients (Austin, 1957). So great was the influence of these orders on nursing that Nutting and Dock devoted an entire chapter of the *History of Nursing* to the origin and development of them. There is no doubt that the religious zeal that called forth groups of knights to care for the wounded and the sick was important to the organization and structure of European hospitals and to the pattern of nursing service that was established and standardized by them. The majority of what was written about these orders is good; the members were benevolent, brave, and charitable. Yet the accumulation of vast riches and large land holdings proved to be the eventual downfall of the orders. Soon after the Holy Wars ended, devotion to the calling of nursing diminished, works of mercy dwindled, and warfare against unbelievers became the sole focus. "The pride of riches and power, with the gradual abandonment of the humbler humanitarian duties for a spiritual dominance, had made the once peerless order of serv-

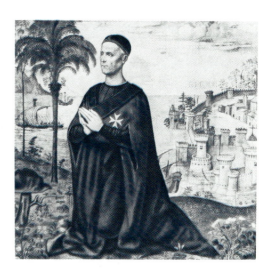

Fr. Alberto Arringhieri, 'IN THE CONVENT' A KNIGHT OF RHODES. *From the fifteenth century painting by Pintoricchio in the Siena Cathedral. The Bettmann Archive, New York.*

147

John Singleton Copley, THE RED CROSS
KNIGHT, *1793. Canvas. National Gallery
of Art, Washington, D.C., Gift of Mrs.
Gordon Dexter.*

*Knights or men-at-arms, whose first duty
was to fight, yet who were expected to serve
in the hospital wards when not engaged in
battle, wore a white cross on their habits.
Frequent references are also made to the Red
Cross Knights (Knights Templars) although
this group was always purely military.*

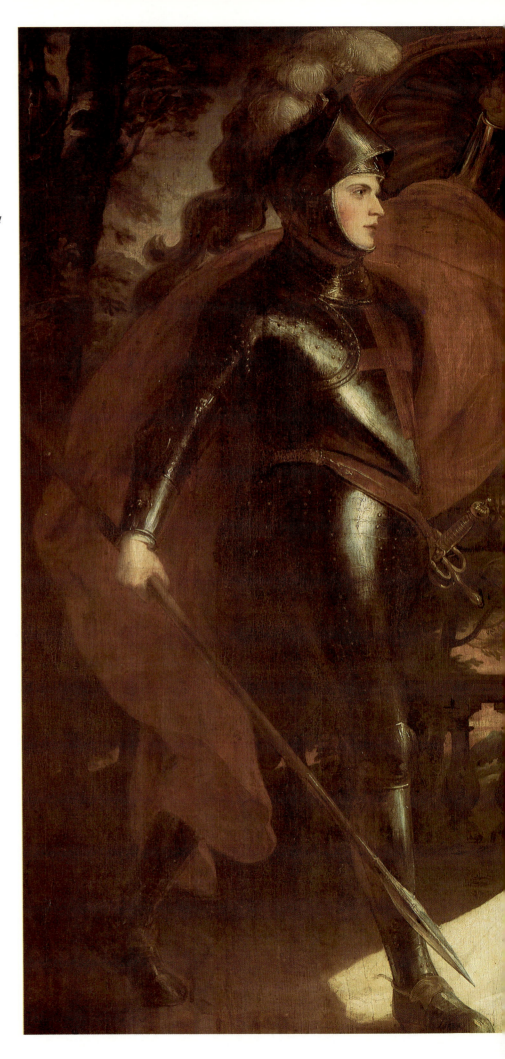

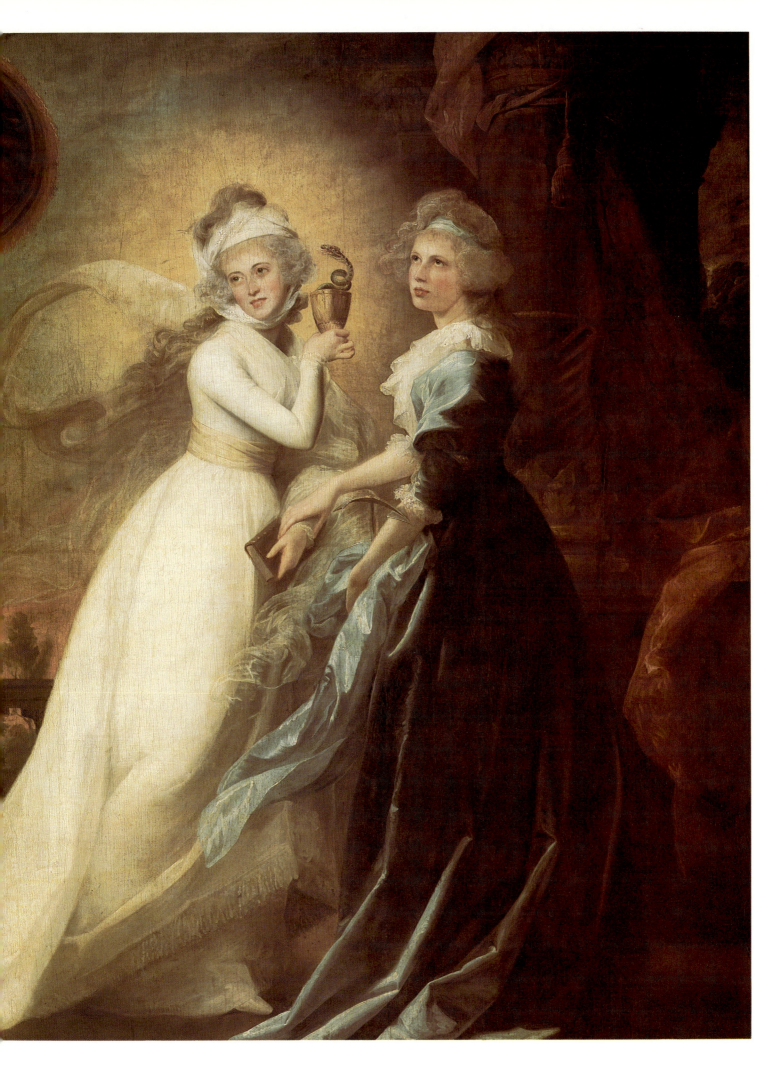

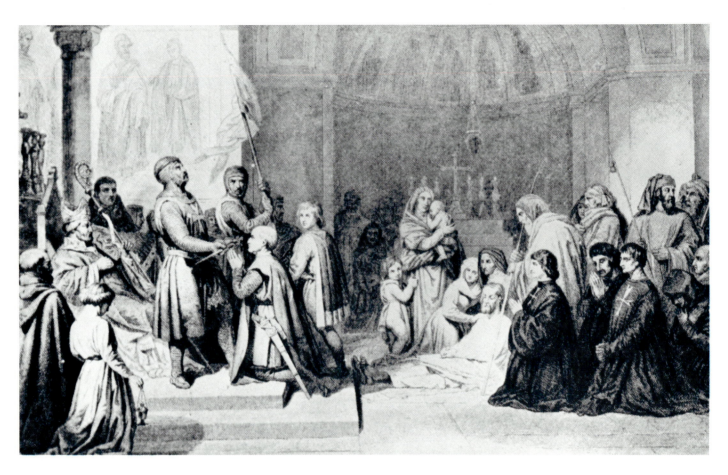

ing brothers a menace to the secular power" (Nutting and Dock, 1937, p. 206).

Great orders were formed, all called by the name *Hospitallers.* The membership of these orders consisted of three classes—knights, priests, and serving brothers. The knights were men of patrician birth who bore arms, protected pilgrims, and fought in the Crusades. When they were not engaged in battle, they helped to nurse the sick. The priests attended to the religious duties in churches, camps, and hospitals. The serving brothers (*serjeus* or half-knights) were primarily responsible for weary travelers and the care of the sick. Three of these nursing orders stand out as being the most famous and the most important in history: the Knights Hospitallers of St. John of Jerusalem, the Teutonic Knights (der Deutsche Orden), and the Knights of St. Lazarus. Both the Hospitallers and the Teutonic Knights formed women's orders that were subordinated to the men's communities, as was often the case. Frequent references are also made to the Knights Templars or Red Cross Knights, although this group was always purely military.

Knights Hospitallers of St. John of Jerusalem.

Rich merchants of Amalfi, Italy, established two hospitals (one for each sex) in Jerusalem about 1050 AD. These were placed under the protection of St. John the Almoner (neither the Evangelist nor the Baptist but a Cypriot) and St. Mary Magdalene. These hospitals originally tended any individual who was sick, including the pilgrims and the insane, but they became crowded with wounded and dying Crusaders during the siege of Antioch and the battle for Jerusalem. Many

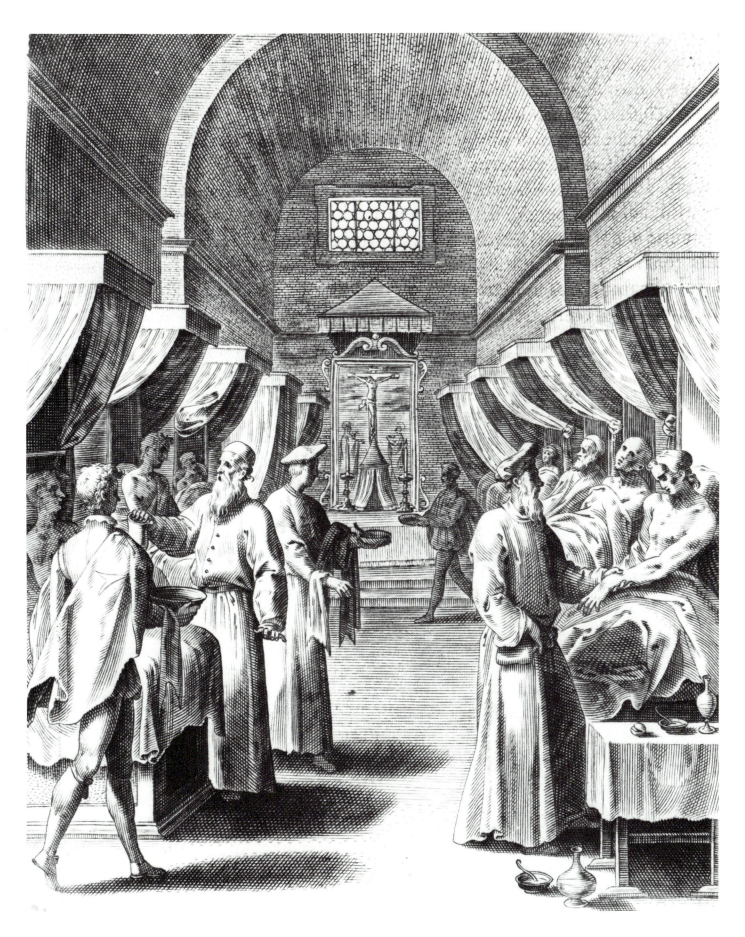

KNIGHT HOSPITALLERS, *1676. Engraving. From* STATUES OF THE ORDER OF ST. JOHN. *Courtesy of the Museum and Library of the Order of St. John, London, England.*

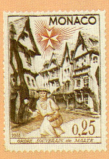

The Monaco 1961 stamp was issued to honor the Sovereign Order of the Knights of Malta (Knights Hospitallers). The Knights Hospitallers traces its origin back to the eleventh century; the Knights of Malta, back to 1530. The hospital at Malta was the equal of any other in Europe. In 1926 an association was established in the United States devoted to the care of the sick and wounded. The stamp depicts a medieval town and a leper beneath the Maltese Cross. Courtesy of Howard B. Hurley.

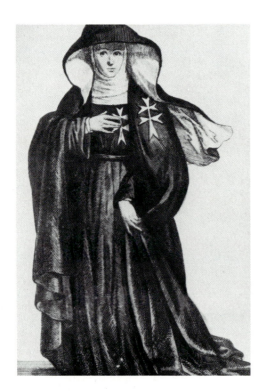

The nuns of this Order distinguished themselves as nurses in the Hospital of St. John of Jerusalem during the Crusades. The Bettmann Archive, New York.

Crusaders of noble birth laid aside their arms to help with the work of tending the sick in the Hospital of St. John. Thus was born the order of the Knights Hospitallers of St. John of Jerusalem.

Until 1099, when Godfrey was made King of Palestine, the order was secular and was directed by Peter Gerard, who was considered to be a pious and saintly man. A female branch of the order served the Hospital of St. Mary Magdalene. The women met at first on terms of equality with the knights; both nursed, ate, and worshiped together. Eventually the men and women formed a religious fraternity and dedicated themselves as servants of the poor and of Christ to function under the rule of St. Augustine. Segregation became total, and the Sisters were subordinated to the Brothers. Solemn vows of poverty, chastity, and obedience were taken, and a black robe with a white linen cross embroidered on the left breast was donned. (Later the Knights of St. John were differentiated from other Hospitallers by a white cross on a red background.) The order became extremely wealthy through gifts of grateful benefactors, which enabled the building of additional hospitals, hostels, and hospices. Rules were drawn up for hospital management, and they were followed by the best city hospitals or *Maisons-Dieu* of Europe for many centuries.

The career of this order was one of distinction in nursing until the expulsion of the Christians from Palestine. Nursing was gradually neglected as the Sisters of St. John disappeared temporarily and the men's order fled to Cyprus and then to the island of Rhodes, where they remained for approximately 200 years. With the conquest of Rhodes the care of the sick became a secondary objective. In 1522 the Knights were forced out of Rhodes and were without a headquarters until Emperor Charles V granted them the isles of Malta, Goza, and Tripolis in 1530. Finally, the Knights were turned out of Malta by Napoleon in 1798. The name of the order changed as its geographical location shifted. The members were successively known as the Knights of St. John of Jerusalem, the Knights of Rhodes, and the Knights of Malta. The significance of this organization in nursing history is great:

> First and foremost, the glamour shed on its activities by what we may call the "Crusading spirit" gave to it such a position that membership was sought after by the flower of knighthood of the day and the prestige thus received caused it to influence and stimulate all subsequent hospital organization.
>
> Secondly, as the Knights were always very rich they could equip and conduct their hospitals far better than any other community of that period.
>
> *Seymer, 1932, p. 38*

The most important and the largest of the many hospitals of the order was established in 1575 at the seaport town of Valetta in Malta. In its early days this hospital was a model for all of Europe, but by the time of John Howard's visit in 1786 it had fallen into a deteriorated state. The hospital, which remains a magnificent monument of architecture, initially accommodated somewhat less than 1000 patients. A well-defined organizational structure provided for department heads, nursing, almsgiving, distribution of food to the poor, mending of clothing, and foundling care. Acute cases and cases of hemorrhage, lithotomy, and insanity were isolated. Chaplains attended spiritual

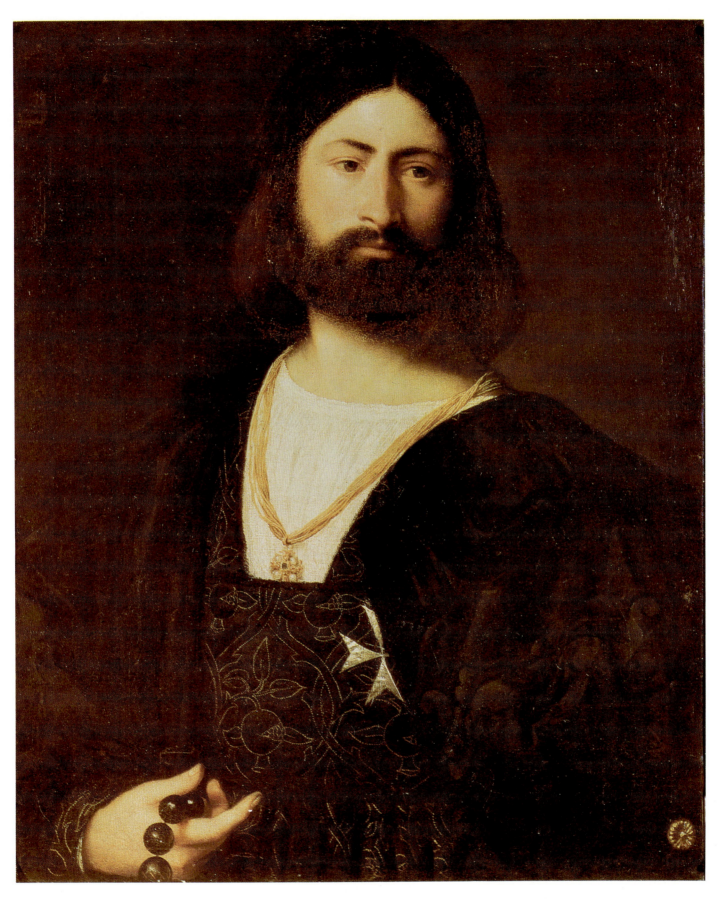

Titian (or Giorgione), PORTRAIT OF A KNIGHT OF MALTA, *c. 1515. Canvas, 80 × 64.1 cm. Uffizi, Florence, Italy. (Giraudon/Art Resource, NY).*

The Knights of St. John of Jerusalem became known as the Knights of Malta when Emperor Charles V granted them the isles of Malta, Gozo, and Tripolis in 1530. The Knights of Malta are famous as the only military order that cared for insane patients.

153

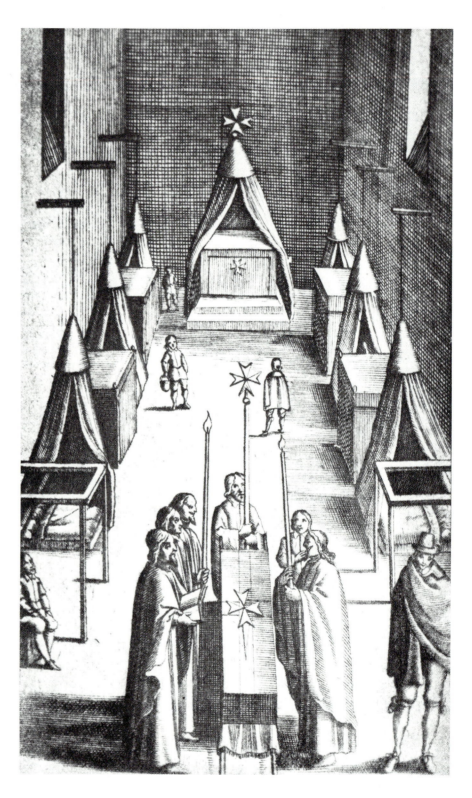

needs; paid physicians assisted knights in anatomy and the care of
disease.

> A peculiar interest attaches itself to this institution because of
> the remarkable splendour of its equipment and service. They were
> unrivalled in their day, and indeed, with all the improvements in
> hospital service which modern progress has brought, we would find
> it hard to better some of these old regulations of 1533. In reading
> them over one is struck with the careful arrangements made for the
> division of labour, and the proper conduct of the work.
>
> *Nutting and Dock, 1937, p. 196*

The Knights of St. John were finally suppressed but later continued their activities in a modified form. Branches were developed in several countries, including England and the United States. Continuing a semimilitary tradition, the Hospitallers functioned as units in Europe, supplying ambulance and other medical services during times of war. "But their original functions have been largely taken over and expanded during the last century by the International Red Cross" (Shryock, 1959, p. 109). The order lives in the St. John's guilds and ambulance corps and first aid to the injured societies. The hospital buildings established by the Knights of St. John can still be seen on Rhodes and Malta.

The Maltese Cross, once worn by the Knights of St. John, survived the Crusades period and became a part of the insignia of many groups caring for the sick. It was on the banner of the United States Cadet Nurse Corps and was worn on the shoulders of the nurse's uniform. The eight points of the cross signify the eight beatitudes that knights were expected to exemplify in the works of charity in their daily lives:

1. Spiritual joy
2. To live without malice
3. To weep over thy sins
4. To humble thyself to those who injure thee
5. To love justice
6. To be merciful
7. To be sincere and pure of heart
8. To suffer persecution

The Teutonic Knights.   The German order of Knights Hospitallers formed in 1191 was called the Deutsche Orden, or Teutonic Knights. German pilgrims during the Third Crusade set up a temporary hospital beside the walls of the Acre, engaged religious knights for defense, and originated this group. The Teutonics followed the hospital rules of the Knights of St. John and the military structure of the Templars. The first members were from noble families. They took the usual vows of poverty, chastity, and obedience but added a fourth vow that required them to care for the sick and defend the faith. They, too, were divided into three classes—warriors, nurses, and spiritual brothers. The Teutonic Knights had from the very beginning both nursing and military duties. They were distinguished by a black habit over which was worn a white cloak with a black cross embroidered in gold on the shoulder.

A women's order was founded in Germany to specifically perform hospital work. The women were not, however, admitted to full membership and were called *consorores* (lay sisters). They took vows but lived outside the monastic precincts. Their nursing duties were perhaps regarded as menial, since "the Rule says that women are to be admitted 'because services to cattle and to sick persons in hospital are better performed by the female sex'" (Seymer, 1932, p. 40).

The Teutonic Knights became very powerful in Germany, and many hospitals were given over into their hands. From different princes they received rich possessions in various countries, particularly in Sicily. According to reference material, their history is similar to that of the Knights of St. John but their nursing service was not as effective. By the fourteenth century they had fulfilled their destiny.

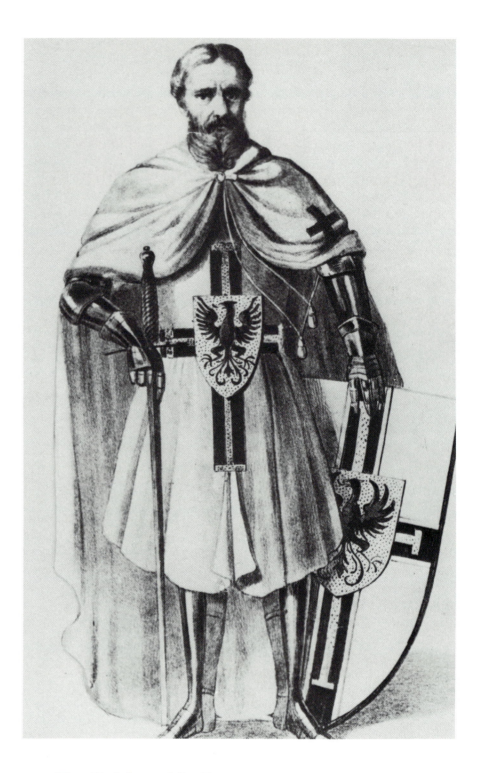

The Knights of St. Lazarus. According to some historians, the Knights of St. Lazarus were the oldest of all the orders of hospitallers. It is speculated that this order originated from the hospital built by St. Basil at Cesarea, which kept a separate house for lepers. Attempts have also been made to trace it back to the days of Christ's raising of Lazarus, the brother of Mary and Martha. Whatever the origins of this order, the fact remains that leprosy, which had always been a problem in society, became its special cause. Lepers had been excluded from society and confined to institutions called *lazarettos* in honor of the leper spoken of in the parable of the rich man. Those who were not confined to institutions were obliged to wear a distinctive dress and carry a wooden clapper to warn of their approach; they

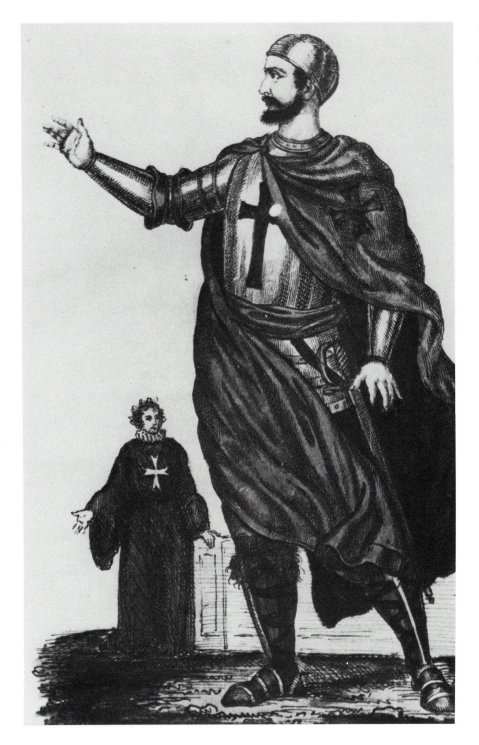

were isolated and considered to be incurables. At this time the term *leprosy* was also applied to syphilis and many chronic skin diseases.

The members of the Knights of St. Lazarus were not only knights who participated in the wars of the Crusades but also those who had been stricken with leprosy. Initially it was a purely nursing order, but by the thirteenth century the order added armed combatants to membership. This action created two categories of knights, the warriors and the hospitallers, who were headed by a grand master of a noble family who was himself a leper. This rule was in effect until 1253, when permission was given by Pope Innocent IV to elect a nonleper to this office. With the addition of the warring aspect, care of the lepers became secondary and the order became purely military. Decay and deterioration set in until Pope Innocent VIII suppressed it in the fifteenth century. The order ceased to exist by 1830.

Details of the work of the order is obscure. There is little information regarding what real service was rendered to the sick poor or to the lepers. After the Crusades, however, the incidence of leprosy began to decrease and the need for the special work of the order diminished. As with the other hospitallers, the Knights of St. Lazarus received lavish gifts and rich possessions. According to Nutting and Dock (1937), there were also Sisters of the order. Yet few sources mention the existence of a female branch.

The first Knights of St. Lazarus varied both their habit and their cross in different countries. The color of the original cross is unknown, but its form was distinguished by four arms of equal length, somewhat flared at the ends. The French cross was an eight-armed golden and green or purple-red cross with tiny golden lilies in the corners. The Italian cross was white and green. The emblem of the order of St. Lazarus was adopted by the German Nurses' Association.

Rise of Mendicant Orders

Social groupings for nursing and neighborhood work occurred with the rapid spread of sickness and disease and the fear associated with the plagues. Religious fervor escalated and led to the development of types of care different from that required when monasteries were the focal points of the communities. Emphasis began to be placed upon the great reward that could be achieved through total withdrawal from the world. Religious missionary bodies thus arose and pledged themselves to literal poverty. These groups exemplified the democratic and secular tendencies that developed along with the military orders. Extension of Christianity, however, in this case would transpire through peaceful means. Many devout individuals took part in this movement.

Success in this endeavor meant taking religion and nursing out among the people. The mendicant orders were founded to accomplish this goal. The members lived as part of the world, owned no property, gave their possessions to the poor, and followed the teachings of Christ. They depended on begging for sustenance, a practice that earned them the name of *mendicants*. The personification of this approach was St. Francis of Assisi (1182–1226), who instituted three religious orders: The first order, Friars Minor (Little Brothers), was for friars; the second, called Poor Clares, was for nuns; the third order, Tertiaries, was for lay men and women who wished to continue to lead secular lives. (St. Dominic also founded three orders and patterned them after these.)

St. Francis of Assisi. St. Francis became one of the best known and best loved saints in history. Born to a life of wealth and ease as the son of a cloth merchant in Assisi, he spent his youth as a gay, carefree cavalier. His style of living changed after Francis suffered from a serious illness in his early twenties. Even before the illness, however, he looked with aversion upon the miseries that were prevalent in the society and was particularly affected by the plight of the lepers. A variety of circumstances, particularly his giving of great

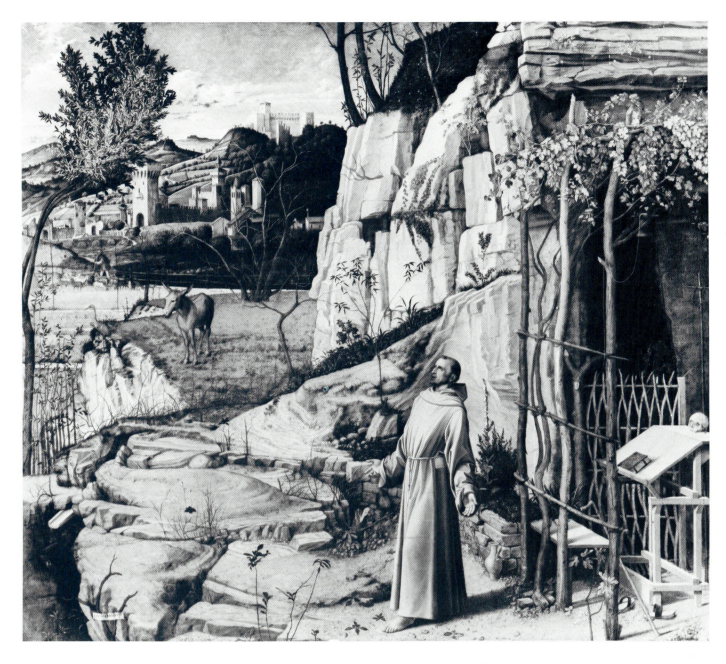

Giovanni Bellini, ST. FRANCIS IN ECSTASY, *c. 1485. Panel, 124.5 × 142 cm. Copyright the Frick Collection, New York.*

amounts of alms to the poor, led to Francis' being disinherited by his father. Rejected by his family, Francis set out alone, barefooted, and clothed with a rough brown tunic tied at the waist with a heavy white rope to travel the countryside. Appalled by the sufferings of the poor and the sick, he devoted his life to their ministrations. Most important, he provided a necessary example of consideration of human beings as individuals:

> What distinguishes this very genuine democrat from any mere demagogue is that he never either deceived or was deceived by the illusion of mass-suggestion. . . . To him a man was always a man and did not disappear in a dense crowd any more than in a desert. He honored all men; that is, he not only loved but respected them all. What gave him his extraordinary personal power was this; that from the Pope to the beggar, from the sultan of Syria in his pavillion to the ragged robbers crawling out of the wood, there was never a man who looked into those brown

159

burning eyes without being certain that Francis Bernardone was really interested in *him*; in his own inner life from the cradle to the grave; that he himself was being valued and taken seriously, and not merely added to the spoils of some social policy or the names in some clerical document.

Chesterton, 1924, pp. 141–142

St. Francis became the champion of lepers. He frequently visited the leper houses and the lepers were always waiting for him, knowing that he brought not only alms but also love. Initially St. Francis became the jest of the town because the people could not understand his close association with the lepers. Adults and children flung mud at him and shouted "Pazzo! Pazzo!" According to Robinson (1946), the pale and gaunt appearance and cadaverous face with the burning eyes probably did make him look like a madman. Francis' work for these sufferers eventually influenced and inspired others to improve their conditions.

Slowly, disciples began to gather around and follow Francis of Assisi. When they numbered twelve, they went to Rome to seek permission of Pope Innocent III to preach and follow an ascetic life. With papal sanction, the Franciscans, or the Order of Friars Minor (Brothers Minor), grew rapidly. The habit of the Franciscans was the same rough tunic with rope girdle that St. Francis himself had worn. The shade of the garment might be brownish or grayish, and the wearers were called Gray Friars. Poverty and humility were emphasized in the Franciscan order; begging was done for the members themselves and for the poor.

St. Francis died in 1226, aware that his order was departing from his original concept of complete poverty and simplicity. Leadership passed into other hands and a new rule was established. The structure of the order became more elaborate and properties were acquired. Some of the Brothers had even established themselves in universities before the death of St. Francis, despite his great opposition to scholarship. Both Francis and Clare were canonized, and the bodies of these two saints repose in their native Assisi. The feast of St. Francis of Assisi is kept on October 4.

While the Franciscans were achieving success, St. Dominic (1170–1221) established the Order of Preachers, the Dominicans. A member of a noble family of Guzman of the village of Castile, Dominic had given up his plan of becoming a monk in a monastery in order to have closer contact with the rich and the poor who needed spiritual assistance. He set forth to restore to the Church those who had fallen away and to convert others. Both men and women gathered about him, and this led to the development of the Dominicans. The followers were sent abroad as traveling preachers in an effort to make Christianity the one religion. The order practiced both individual and corporate poverty. The Dominican robe was made of white wool and topped by a black cape with a hood. The hood could be pulled over the head for warmth. This cape led to the title of Black Friars.

Eminent scholars arose from the Franciscans and the Dominicans. Many of them taught at great universities such as Padua, Cologne, Vienna, Prague, and Paris. Among them were the Dominican Albertus Magnus; the Franciscan Roger Bacon, who stressed the value of observation, experimentation, and inductive reasoning, which as-

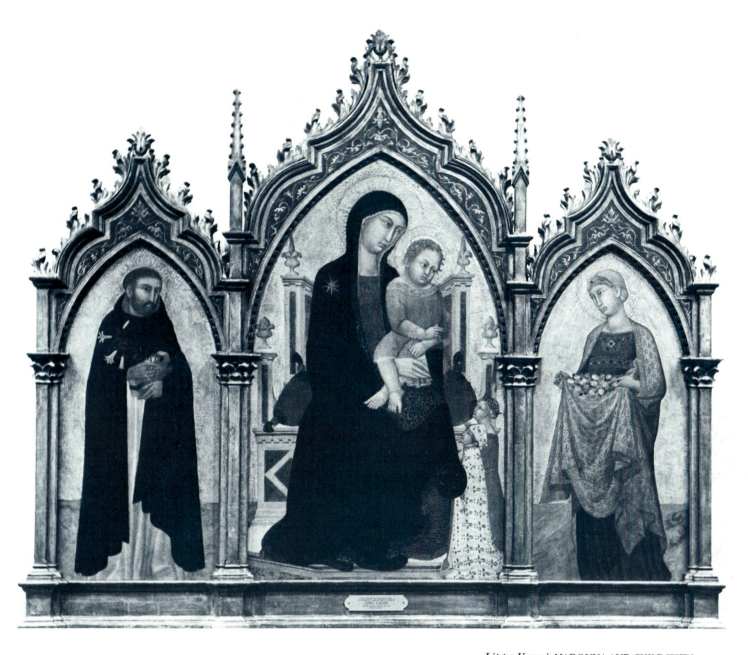

Lippo Vanni, MADONNA AND CHILD WITH DONORS ST. DOMINIC AND ST. ELIZABETH OF HUNGARY, *late fourteenth century. Tempera-gesso on panel, 171.5 × 201 cm. The Lowe Art Museum, University of Miami, Coral Gables, Florida, Samuel H. Kress Collection.*

sisted with the development of experimental science; the Dominican St. Thomas Aquinas, who studied under the Benedictines at Monte Cassino and completed the *Summa Theologica,* his greatest work.

St. Clare of Assisi.   The life of St. Clare of Assisi (1194–1253) was closely interwoven with that of St. Francis. Clare, a beautiful daughter of a knightly family of the Sciffi, at the age of sixteen heard St. Francis preach in the churches of Assisi. She became convinced that his way of life, extreme poverty, was what the Lord wished for her. She believed that the adoption of this type of life would provide her with contentment, peace, and joy. Clare remained in the household of her father until the age of eighteen, then ran away to the chapel of the Franciscans where she exchanged her expensive dress and jewels for a rough woolen robe. Francis cut off her long hair and received her vows of poverty, chastity, and obedience. Clare lived in a Benedictine convent for a brief period until a special convent was established for her. Other women who wished to share this

161

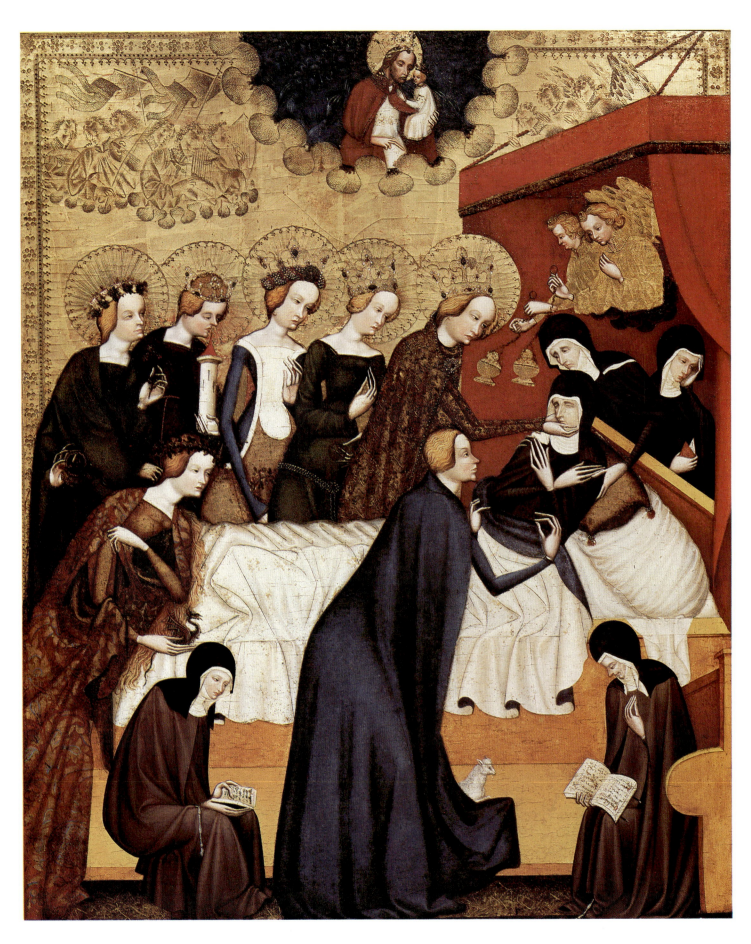

Master of Heiligenkreuz, THE DEATH OF ST. CLARE, *c. 1410. Wood, approx. 66 × 54.6 cm, National Gallery of Art, Washington, D.C., Samuel H. Kress Collection 1952.*

simple life joined her. Thus began the second order of St. Francis, more commonly referred to as the order of Poor Clares (Clarisses), with Clare as its abbess. A short time later Clare was followed by her younger sister Agnes.

It is said that the Poor Clares cared principally for lepers, whom they housed in small mud and wattle huts around their convent in San Damiano. Accounts vary, however, about the actual services they provided. One author (Austin, 1957) suggests: "It would probably be a mistake to ascribe to the Poor Ladies any widespread activity in the care of the sick. Their chief preoccupation seems to have been with the contemplative life" (p. 67). Austin goes on to say that "the Rule of 1253 indicates that the Poor Clares cared for their own members, but whether their care extended to the surrounding community is uncertain" (p. 69). Other authors (Nutting and Dock, 1937; Robinson, 1946; Jamieson and Sewall, 1950; Shryock, 1959) discuss the nursing activities of this order of Franciscan nuns.

Clare outlived St. Francis for over twenty-five years. After her death the order experienced many changes. It has been known at different times and in different countries by a variety of names: Order of Poor Ladies, Clarisses, Minoresses, and Poor Clares. It was a strictly cloistered order. Professed Sisters living under rule did not go outside their walls; nor were they in contact with the outside world until after the Protestant Revolution. Since its original founding, the Poor Clares, and numerous sisterhoods that have adopted Franciscan rule, have founded many hospitals and other institutions for the sick.

Tertiaries: Third Orders of St. Francis and St. Dominic.
The Tertiaries, or Third Orders, were founded for the laity of both sexes who wished to continue their ordinary lives in the world. They were to practice charity and devotion to God in a manner similar to that of the religious orders. Several communities of Tertiaries lived almost the same life as the religious without being cloistered. These orders attracted thousands of people of all classes and were a powerful force for a number of years. Some were later formed into communities (convents arose in different countries) that often undertook nursing as their main work. The idea became so popular that many tertiary orders emerged, and this prompted Gregory at the Council of Lyons (1272) to reduce them to four: the Dominicans, Franciscans, Carmelites, and Augustinians.

The Third Order epitomized the ideals of St. Francis. It represented a revival of the early Christian spirit. Religion was carried into everyday life and unselfish and useful service was rendered to humanity. Many famous nursing saints were enrolled in this order of St. Francis: Elizabeth of Hungary (1207–1231), Louis of France (1214–1270), Elizabeth of Portugal (1271–1336), Isabelle of France, Anne of Bohemia, and Bridget of Sweden (Tuker and Malleson, 1900).

St. Elizabeth of Hungary was probably the most renowned among the women tertiaries of St. Francis. Her virtues have been set forth in prose, poetry, art, and music. Elizabeth, the daughter of the Hungarian king Andreas II, was married at the age of 14 to Ludwig of Thuringia. She became the mother of four children. With her husband's support she built hospitals in Thuringia and humbly ministered to the sick with her own hands. Daily she distributed alms to the poor, fed the hungry, nursed the lepers, bathed newborns and comforted their mothers with special tenderness. Hers was a life of

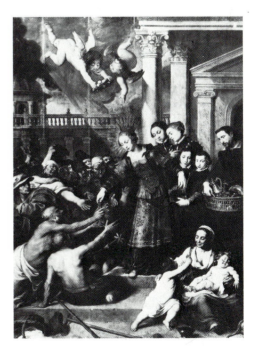

M. Pepijn, ST. ELIZABETH GIVING HER JEWELS TO THE POOR. *Panel. Koninklijk Museum Schone Kunsten, Antwerp, Belgium.*

163

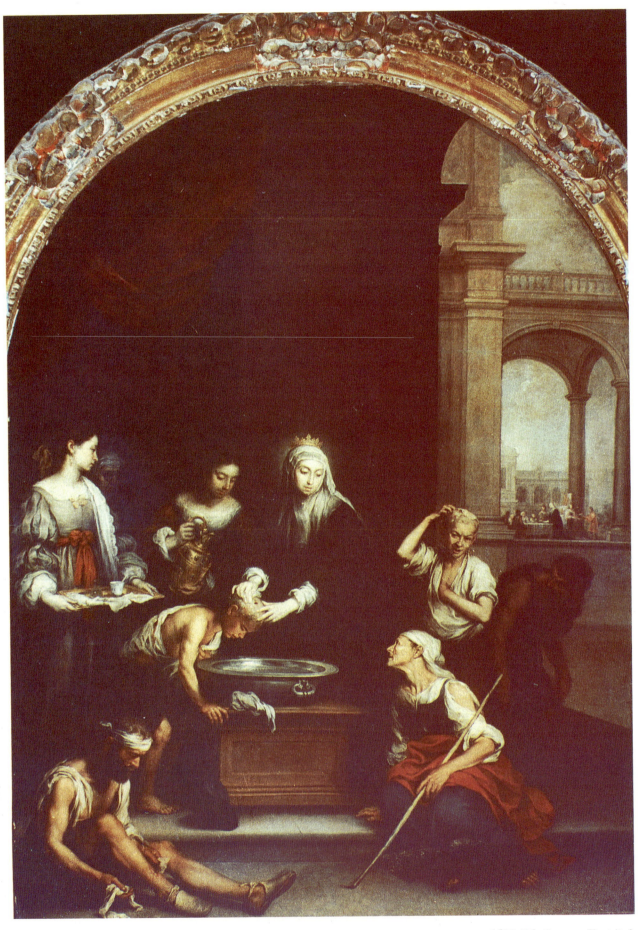

Bartolomé Esteban Murillo, ST. ELIZABETH BATHING PEOPLE AFFLICTED WITH RINGWORM, *c. 1670–74. Canvas. Hospital de la Caridad, Sevilla, Spain.*

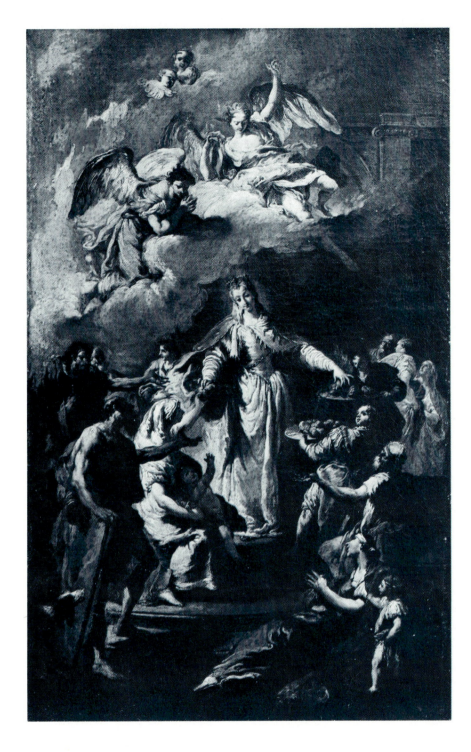

extreme piety, asceticism, and austerity. Elizabeth was the heroine of beautiful tales, which were accepted either as fact or fiction. The story of the miraculous roses is perhaps the most well known. It is said that one winter day while Elizabeth was carrying a basket of food to the poor she met Ludwig (in some accounts it is her father-in-law whom she met). Irritated by complaints against Elizabeth by his family, Ludwig demanded to see what she was carrying. When she opened her cloak, Ludwig saw an armful of blooming white and red roses.

Upon Ludwig's death during the Crusades, Elizabeth was driven from her husband's castle, the Wartburg, by her in-laws. She became a member of the Third Order of St. Francis and built the Franciscan hospital at Marburg, where she spent the remaining years of her short

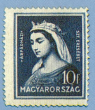

Hungary's 1932 set of four stamps commemorated the 700th anniversary of the death of St. Elizabeth (1207–1231). During the famine of 1226 Elizabeth organized food distribution and devoted her life and strength to helping the sick and poor. She had hospitals built where she cared for lepers and comforted prisoners. When her husband of six years died, she moved to Marburg and spent the rest of her young life nursing the sick. She died at age twenty-four. Courtesy of Howard B. Hurley.

life nursing the sick. Elizabeth was considered to be an excellent organizer, administrator, and nurse. Her conception of social service carried a modern ring, since her service to the needy "was tempered with discretion; and instead of encouraging idleness such as were able to work, she employed them in a way suitable to their strength and capacity" (Butler, 1934, vol. 10, p. 43). Always frail, Elizabeth died at the age of twenty-four. Considered to be the patron saint of nursing, she is honored on November 19. Elizabeth is regarded by some as the forerunner of the visiting and public health nurses of the twentieth century. The Gray Nuns of the thirteenth century, who were also Tertiaries of St. Francis, were often called Sisters of St. Elizabeth, since they had chosen her as their patron saint.

St. Louis IX was another saint whose endeavors with lepers was well known. His special care of their needs was recognized and respected by his subjects, who mourned his death during one of the Crusades. France flourished under Louis' rule and experienced peace and prosperity. Louis personally tended to the sick and devoted his life to humane treatment for all individuals. He was interested in education, particularly for health care workers, and attempted to assist with its provision. His efforts resulted in the establishment of the

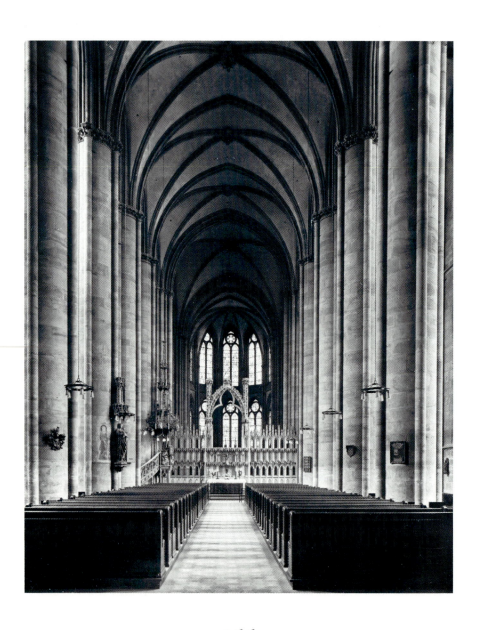

Interior of St. Elizabeth's Church looking east to the choir and altar, c. 1233–83. Marburg, Federal Republic of Germany.

Saint-Chapelle in Paris and the Sorbonne College of the University of Paris. Louis belonged to the Franciscan Tertiaries.

The Third Order of St. Dominic was originally formed to recover Church property. The Tertiaries, however, performed other services and assisted the poor and the ill as a regular function of their religious duty. They were patterned after the Third Order of St. Francis. There are at least hints that some competition existed between the two groups. Robinson presents an interesting account of this rivalry:

> Dominic was the imitator, Francis always the originator; and the story of Dominic lacked the emotional fire of the Francis legend. Moreover, the Franciscans had the inestimable advantage that only upon the body of their founder had been miraculously inflicted the Five Wounds which Christ received at his crucifixion: after the death of Francis, Clara saw the wounds in his feet, but could not extract the nails which had been driven through them. In the contemporary rivalry between the Franciscans and the Dominicans, Catherine came to the rescue of the latter: Christ put a ring on her finger as proof that she was to be his heavenly spouse; and, as she knelt in a church in Pisa, she received the crowning glory of the wounds of the Lord.... The Franciscans coldly denied, while the Dominicans fervently accepted, the stigmatization of St. Catherine.
>
> *Robinson, 1946, pp. 46–47*

The first members of the Third Order of St. Dominic were known as the Mantellate. They wore the Dominican habit—a white tunic bound by a leather belt, a white veil, and a black cloak (mantella). Margaret of Metola was the first young woman to join the Mantellate. She was the daughter of wealthy parents who abandoned her because she was blind and deformed. Margaret gave her life to the needs of others. She had a special affinity for prisoners and visited them daily, giving them food, clothing, medicines, and bedding. Other remarkable personalities joined the Dominican Tertiaries.

St. Catherine of Siena (1347–1380), a favorite subject of painters, is often portrayed in the act of expelling demons or in an ecstatic state with a lily, thorn, or book. She is also frequently pictured carrying a lighted lamp, which she carried on her nightly visits to La Scala hospital. (Her lamp was as famous as the Nightingale lamp of later years.) Catherine Benincasca was the daughter of a wealthy merchant and the last of twenty-five children. Her twin died at birth. At the age of seven, Catherine devoted herself to Christ. She became a member of the Third Order of St. Dominic at eighteen. The literature identifies Catherine as a hospital and visiting nurse, social welfare worker, reformer of society and of the Church, peacemaker, stateswoman, and great mystic.

When the Black Death (bubonic plague) swept over Siena, Catherine personally cared for the victims. For more than a year she rarely went home but spent her nights and days in the La Scala wards tending to the afflicted. She organized groups of young men as stretcher bearers to transport the stricken from all over the city to wards of the hospital, which she supervised. Catherine's prominence, however, lies in her influence in the political affairs of the day. She never hesitated to speak out to the highest and mightiest in the land and had some part in persuading the Pope to end the Babylonian

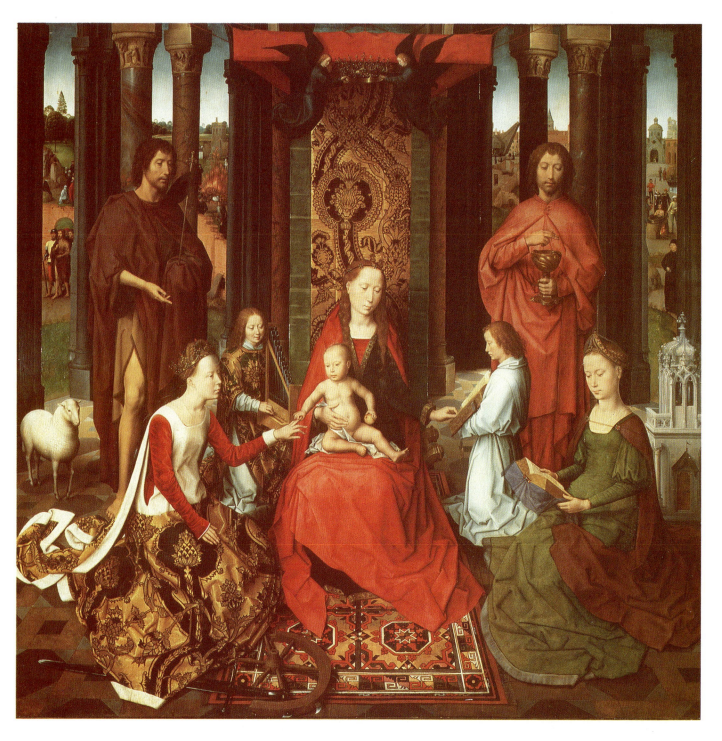

Hans Memling, THE MYSTIC MARRIAGE OF ST. CATHERINE, *1479. Center panel of the* ST. JOHN ALTARPIECE, *approx. 172.5 × 172.5 cm. Hospital Sint Jan, Bruges, Belgium.*

Captivity and to return to Rome from Avignon. Catherine attempted to start another Crusade to rescue Jerusalem from the Muslims. She was also instrumental in healing breaches between members of prominent families in Genoa.

Secular Nursing Orders

At the same time that the military knights and the first, second, and third orders were developing, groups of workers banded together in semireligious orders. These orders were not bound by vows to monastic life and have been referred to as *secular nursing orders.* They made many contributions to nursing and served the sick, the poor, foundlings, and orphans in their own communities. At times

168

they also did hospital nursing. The development of these orders marks a significant step in the secularization of nursing. Their success was in part a result of their "freedom" in the community.

Another order of men in this period was the Antonines (Hospital Brothers of St. Anthony), founded about 1095 and issued a rule in 1218. Houses were established in France, Spain, and Italy. The members devoted themselves to sufferers of "St. Anthony's Fire," which was probably the condition of ergotism. Hospitals were developed for the victims of this disease, who were lovingly cared for by the Brothers. The hallucinatory manifestations of ergotism have been vividly described in the literature. An interesting account of an outbreak of ergotism in 1951 in Pont Saint-Esprit in France is described by Fuller (1968) in his book *The Day of St. Anthony's Fire.*

The origin of the Beguine movement is uncertain, and the derivation of its name is obscure. It is usually credited to a priest of Liège, Lambert le Begue, who encouraged the settlement of *mulieres sanctae* around his church—among them the daughters of barons, knights, and nobles—in what has come to be regarded as the first beguinage. The Mulieres Sanctae were individual women who identified themselves with a monastery by donating a part of their substance (if they were rich) or voluntary service (if they were poor). They took no vows and lived in their own homes. Eventually these women gathered together into a communal life. They took vows of chastity and obedience for the time they were in residence but did not give up rights to property or possessions. They were free to marry and leave at any time. The Beguines of Flanders were one of the most prominent secular nursing orders. Later, many of these communities became Tertiaries of St. Francis or St. Dominic.

The organization was extremely simple. Two to four women lived together in small houses built in an enclosed precinct and grouped around a church or hospital. Such beguinages were picturesque in their simplicity. Those at Bruges (c. 1184) and Ghent (c. 1234) in Belgium are well known. Each community was self-contained and fixed its own rules, which were approved by the bishop of the diocese. Because there was great diversity in the Beguines, it is difficult to render an adequate description of their work. Their original objective seems to have been religious; they strived for perfection and reform of the Church and the saving of souls. Members ranged from the rich to the poor, the noble to the humble, and their work varied. Their dress varied according to location.

The Beguines supported themselves by teaching, spinning and other handicrafts, and care of the sick in hospitals. They started a visiting nursing service in the neighborhood homes, and fees were charged if the families were able to pay. Hospital work became one of their chief interests and led to the erection of their own hospitals, where they nursed. One of the most famous is the Hotel Dieu at Beaune, France, which was founded in 1443. These hospitals were also staffed by the Sisters of Matilda, an order established specifically for this purpose by the Beguines. During wars, famines, and epidemics, members of the order converted their cottages into hospitals; they also served as nurses on battlefields.

The Beguines were always popular with the people, but they met with resistance and suffered a certain amount of persecution from ecclesiastical authorities. Clerics could not tolerate their independence and striking innovations in community life. The Beguines were accused of heresy and in 1215 were forbidden by the Pope to found any more such groups. In spite of several periods of persecution, they flourished and expanded. By the end of the thirteenth century there were few communities without a Beguinage, and the order had spread to neighboring countries. It is estimated that there were some 200,000 Beguines by that time. Gradually a decrease in numbers and size of these organizations occurred for various reasons. The Beguines retain a corporate existence in Belgium today. According to one source, they constitute

> as historically interesting a community of women as anywhere be found. The freedom and independence of their original mode of existence, their self-supporting character, the irreproachable dignity and quiet, simple usefulness of their lives, continue unchanged. They have passed through vicissitudes and perils, but always safely.
>
> *Nutting and Dock, 1937, p. 271*

Other groups of women appeared somewhat later. The Sisterhood of the Common Life gathered about Gerhard Groot, who was an idealist and leader of thought. The Sisters, like the Beguines, took no binding vows but held no private property. They lived together in a conventional manner and were preeminently visiting nurses in the cities along the Rhine. Their habit was a simple gray dress, and they were self-supporting. The order of men, the Brothers of the Common Life, was also founded by Groot. The Brothers devoted themselves to the sick poor and taught children who were bedridden. They became known as the schoolmasters of the time. Thomas à Kempis lived and studied with this community.

Another interesting confraternity was the brotherhood of Misericordia, which was started about 1244 in Florence. Founded primarily as a volunteer ambulance society, it was composed of a group of religious laymen. The members functioned in many Italian cities and became known as the "Masked Brotherhood." This arose from the members' belief that their contributions would gain spiritual reward only if they prevented themselves from being recognized by others.

The order of the Alexian Brothers was formed in 1348 to assist with the care of the victims of the bubonic plague. This group of laymen also undertook the burial of the dead. St. Alexius, a fifth century Roman who nursed the sick in a hospital at Edessa, was chosen as their patron saint. This occurred in 1469, when the group organized under Augustinian rule. The sick continue to be cared for by this order. Several large general hospitals for men and boys, a rest home, and a home for elderly men are supported and serviced by its members. The Alexian Brothers also staff Memorial Hospital and Clinic at Boys Town, Nebraska. At one time the Alexian Brothers' Hospital School of Nursing in Chicago was the largest male nursing school in the United States.

Growth of Hospitals

During the late Middle Ages Pope Innocent III encouraged the development of hospitals in European cities. Church executives or influential citizens who visited with him were invited to study the model Santo Spirito Hospital and were encouraged to organize simi-

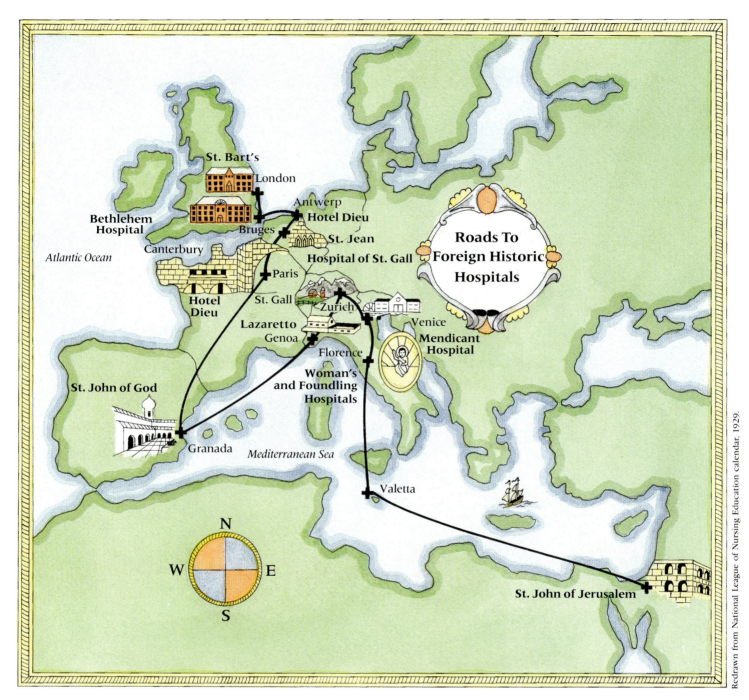

Map of the ROADS TO FOREIGN HISTORIC
HOSPITALS.

lar institutions in their own communities. This idea of city hospitals was met with support and approval, and in some cases hospitals passed amicably from ecclesiastical to secular control. The number of hospitals rapidly escalated, and the size of the institutions varied greatly. Several factors contributed to the demand for more hospitals: existing hospitals had been organized as orphanages, hospices for travelers and the sick, and almshouses; communicable disease was uncontrolled; urban life had been hastily developed; and crowded living conditions were contributing to the spread of disease.

In general, the hospitals were erected to care for the sick poor. The wards were very large; privacy was frequently provided by the use of cubicles. The structures were usually beautiful, having been constructed at a time when every public building was to be a work of art. The larger ones were similar in architectural form to the churches of the period.

171

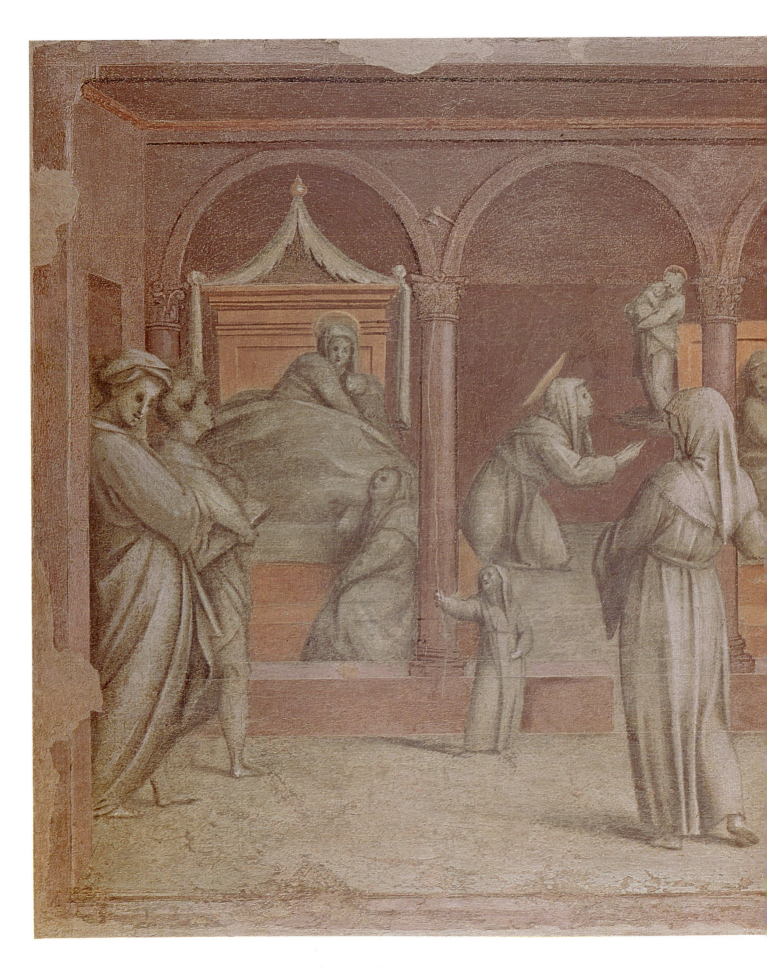

Pontormo, HOSPITAL SCENE, *early sixteenth century. Accademia, Florence, Italy. (SCALA/ Art Resource, NY).*

172

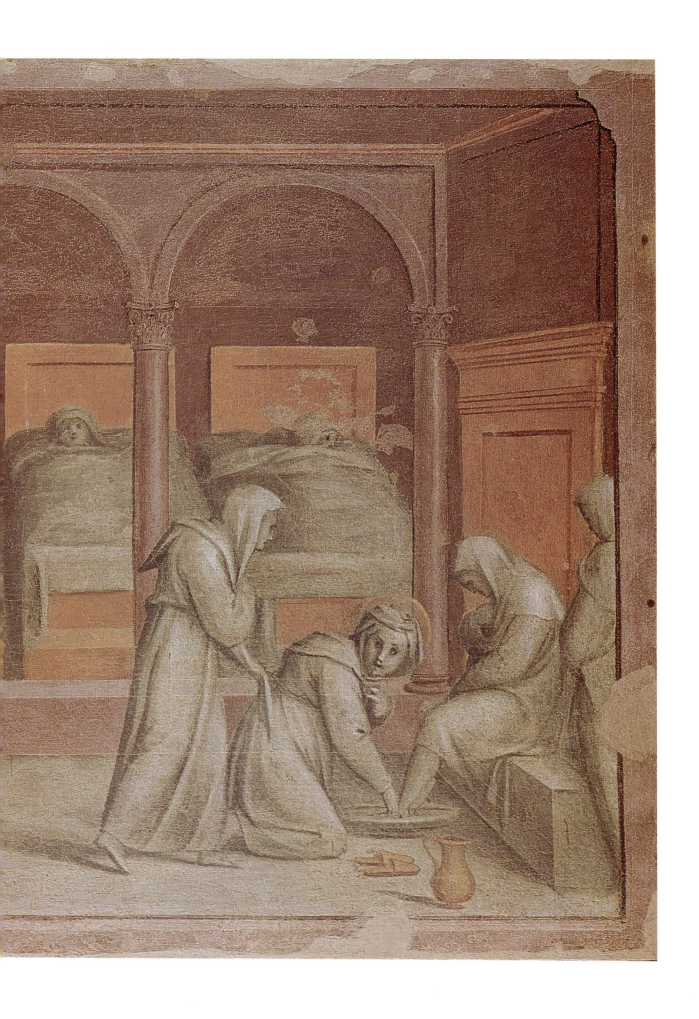

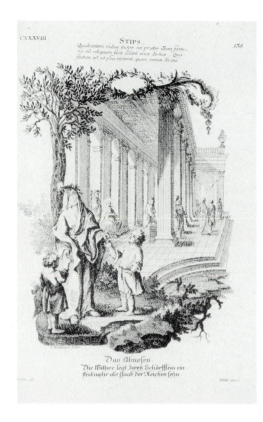

The depiction of ALMS in the 1758–1760 Hertel Edition of Cesare Ripa's ICONOLOGIA. From BAROQUE AND ROCOCO PICTORIAL IMAGERY, edited by Edward A. Maser, 1971 Dover Publications, New York.

Indeed, the appearance of a main hall or ward would have suggested an ecclesiastical interior to a modern observer. Straw pallets were replaced by wooden beds, and curtains or partitions supplied some privacy. Linen and woolen supplies became more ample, and a large place would have its own farms to provide food and its own wind or water mills to prepare "corn" (wheat) for the patients. Although the buildings were still cold and dark by modern standards, they were a great improvement over the bare and humble dwellings of the "dark ages."

Shryock, 1959, pp. 109–110

Management and hygienic practices varied from hospital to hospital; they were sometimes good and sometimes bad. The hospitals, which were usually well endowed, were built on carefully chosen sites. Medieval hospitals were a place to keep, not cure, the patients. The aspect of cure evolved slowly and did not become widespread until the late nineteenth century. Nursing care, which was largely custodial in nature, was provided twenty-four hours a day. It was done primarily by monks and nuns, although servants were used part of the time. It is difficult, however, to determine where the division of labor actually occurred. As centuries passed, there were not always enough nurses. Other changes began to occur: the sickbed began to hold more than one patient; patients were sometimes not only dirty but ill fed; the practice of using individuals of low character to augment inadequate nursing staffs became more common. At least a hint of a decline in nursing was present, a decline that would ultimately occur and persist for a long, dreadful time.

A custom of this period was to display paintings in the hospitals as diversional therapy for patients. St. John's Hospital at Bruges in Belgium offers an example of this practice. Established in 1118 by Augustinian monks and nuns as a hospice for travelers, its older buildings are preserved as a museum. Six paintings by the Flemish master Hans Memling are located in this hospital.

The first English hospital was doubtless that at York, built by Athelstane about 936. It was also a poorhouse and had a ward for

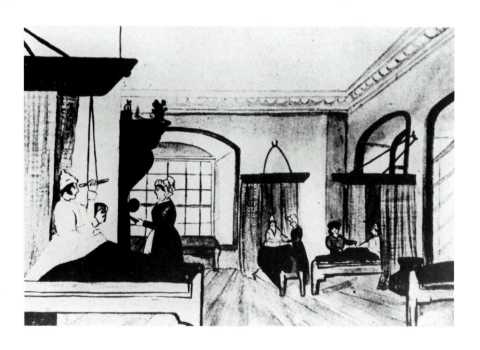

RAHERE'S WARD, *1832. From a contemporary drawing by a patient. St. Bartholomew's Hospital, London, England.*

174

lepers. St. Giles' Hospital was built by Queen Matilda in 1101 for the care of forty lepers. The Queen was also instrumental in the building of the Hospital of St. Katherine in London in 1148. Women of noble birth did the nursing in these hospitals; they did district nursing in the homes of the poor. The charter of these hospitals incorporated both types of nursing service.

St. Bartholomew's Hospital probably has the longest continuous

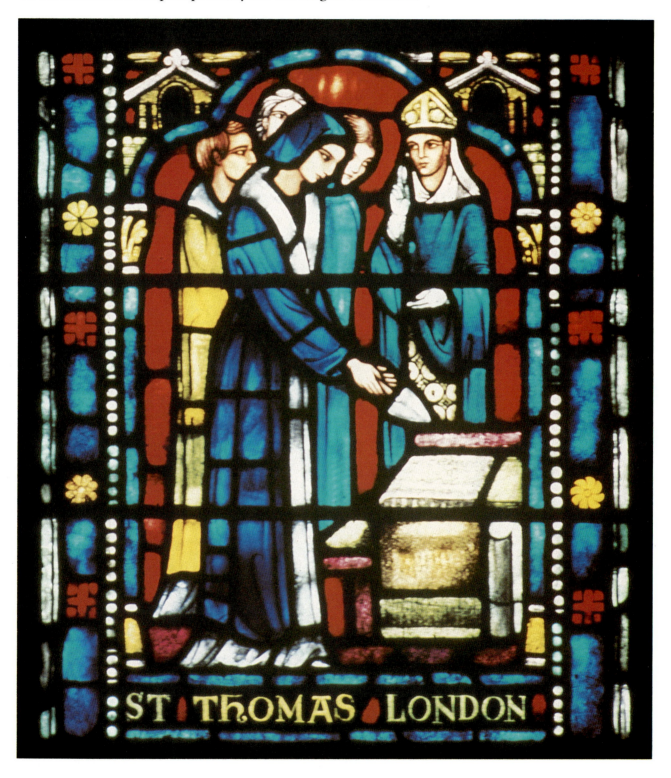

Designed by Reynolds, Francis, & Robnstock. ST. THOMAS' LONDON, *c. 1938. Stained glass. Panel from* THE NIGHTINGALE WINDOW, *Washington Cathedral, Washington, D.C. Courtesy of Morton Broffman.*

Florence Nightingale is shown laying the cornerstone of the hospital building.

record of service of any hospital in the British Empire. It was founded in 1123 by Rahere, who rose to fame as a jester to Henry I and then joined the Augustinian monks. Rahere became a convert after a pilgrimage to Rome, where he became critically ill. He promised to build a church and hospital in honor of St. Bartholomew if he recovered and reached England safely. During the Reformation the hospital was seized by Henry VIII. The pleas of the lord mayor and citizens of London resulted in a new charter for it to become a hospital once again. Originally a poorhouse and orphanage, St. Bartholomew's was exclusively a hospital by the thirteenth century.

St. Thomas' Hospital was founded in 1213 by Richard, Prior of Bermondsey. This institution was made famous in the nineteenth century, when the first school of nursing was established there by Florence Nightingale. Because of its strategic location in a densely populated area of London on the main route to Rome and other cities, St. Thomas' became a hospital for the sick, a refuge for the poor, and a hospice for travelers and pilgrims. Lepers were not admitted but sent to the nearby Lock Hospital (St. Thomas' Hospital paid their

William Hogarth, THE RAKE IN BEDLAM, *c. 1735. From the series entitled* THE RAKE'S PROGRESS. *British Museum, London, England.*

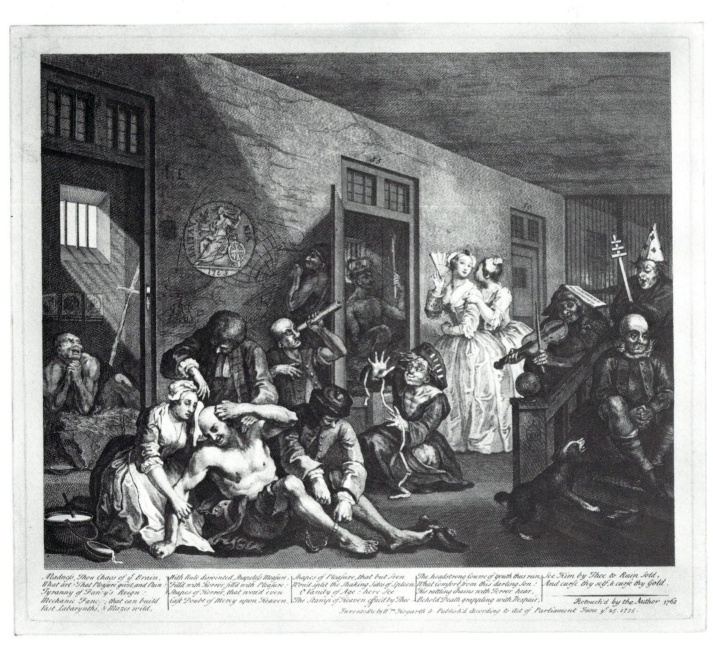

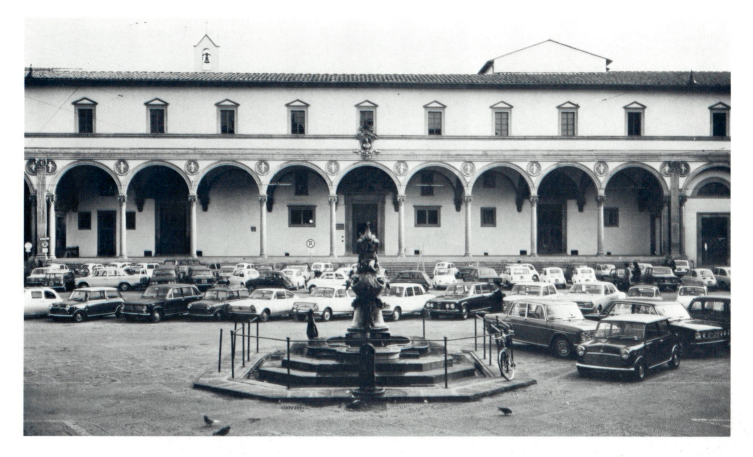

Filippo Brunelleschi, Ospedale degli Innocenti. Begun 1419; completed mid–fifteenth century. Piazza della SS. Annuziata, Florence, Italy. (Archivi Alinari, Florence).

bill). There was a "foule" ward for contagious diseases, a men's and a women's ward; children were also admitted. In addition, there was a lying-in ward for unmarried women, which had been donated by the famous Richard Whittington.

Bethlehem Hospital was the first English institution for the mentally ill. It was founded in 1247 by Simon FitzMary, sheriff of London, as a priory. Originally a hospice of St. Mary of Bethlehem, it was designated a hospital about 1330. During the fourteenth century it was mentioned as a lunatic asylum that rapidly became infamous for the brutal treatment of its inmates. It has been said that once patients responded to treatment they were sent out into the streets to beg for a living. They wore metal armbands to identify themselves as mental patients and were called "Tom o'Bedlams." Violent patients were chained in cells, and they became one of the tourist attractions of London in the eighteenth century. Admission fees provided a source of revenue for the hospital. The name of the hospital was gradually contracted into "Bedlam." This word is used today to describe a place where fools chatter.

Ospedale Santa Maria degli Innocenti was built in 1451 as a foundling asylum for abandoned children. Such children either died or became the property of the person who found them. Many times the children were picked up and sold for money, and they were constantly at the mercy of the slave-traders. This Hospital of the Innocents in Florence was built with funds from a guild of silk merchants. The structure itself embodied beautiful architecture. It was adorned with the famous medallions of Andrea della Robbia (1435–1525). A type of foster parent plan was initiated in which the parents promised to treat the orphans as their own children. Either the hospital or the foster parents taught the children a trade.

Andrea della Robbia's terracotta tondos
from the facade of Filippo Brunelleschi's
Ospedale degli Innocenti in Florence.
(Archivi Alinari, Florence).

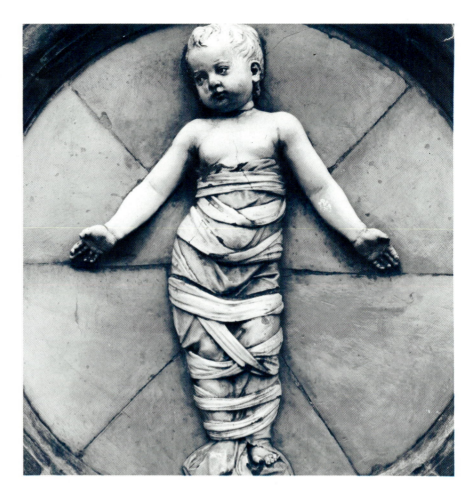

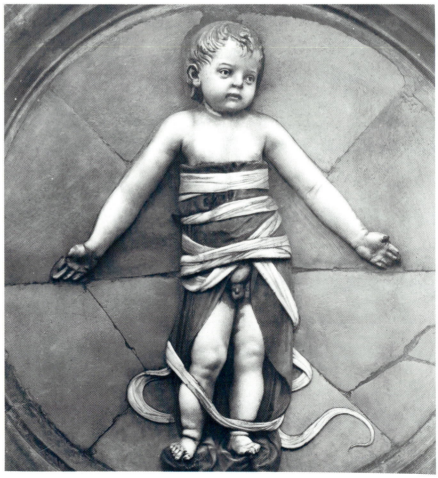

Medicine in the Late Middle Ages

As hospitals were built in the cities of Europe, the universities with their medical schools were also developing. The revival of a lay medical profession brought physicians into the hospitals during the later medieval period. The most reputable physicians were those who had attended universities and had received the degree of doctor of medicine. The beginning of a connection between physicians and hospitals occurred as physicians were called into the institution to see or follow a patient. The physician might even be paid a retainer fee if summoned on a regular basis.

> Medicine saw its darkest days in the early medieval period. During the later medieval period, two currents may be seen in medical practice. A vain speculation with little or no concern for obvious facts and search for truth is quite apparent; on the other hand, the foundation for scientific medicine was being laid through the rediscovery and translation of the old masters and through more frequent use of dissection of human bodies to study human anatomy and disease processes in human tissues. Prior to this time, the teaching of anatomy was based almost entirely on Galen. Most of Galen's observations were derived from animal dissections.
>
> *Frank, 1953, pp. 109–110*

There continued to be an enormous amount of faulty knowledge and superstition during this time. Undoubtedly the majority of it had been passed down from the ancient world and from tribal ancestors.

> Apothecaries prescribed such ridiculous remedies as crocodile dung or cheaper substitutes for the common people who could not afford such an exotic cure. Even the great surgeon, Pare, considered powdered mummy and unicorn's horn as a valuable remedy. In early modern times the potato was used as a medication before it was accepted as a staple food, coffee and tea were thought to prevent acidosis....
>
> *Sellew and Nuesse, 1946, p. 113*

The use of astrology and alchemy were accepted practices; physicians consulted the horoscopes of their patients as well as medical books to determine treatments. Humoral therapy was still trusted. The astrological signs were used to determine when to take medicine or when to be bled, since the humors were supposedly controlled by the planets. Various other techniques were developed and put into practice by physicians in this period. They included the use of extraordinary medicines such as the horn of the unicorn, a narcotic inhalation for anesthesia, the use of spices for drugs and leeches for bloodletting, and the examination of urine.

St. Hildegarde (1098?–1179), the "Sybil of the Rhine," was a leading medical authority during this time. She was born at Bockelheim of noble, wealthy, and religious parents. At the age of eight, she was sent to be educated at the Benedictine cloister at Disibodenberg. Hildegarde entered this monastery and eventually became its abbess at the age of thirty. Eventually she established another Benedictine cloister near Bingen on the Rhine.

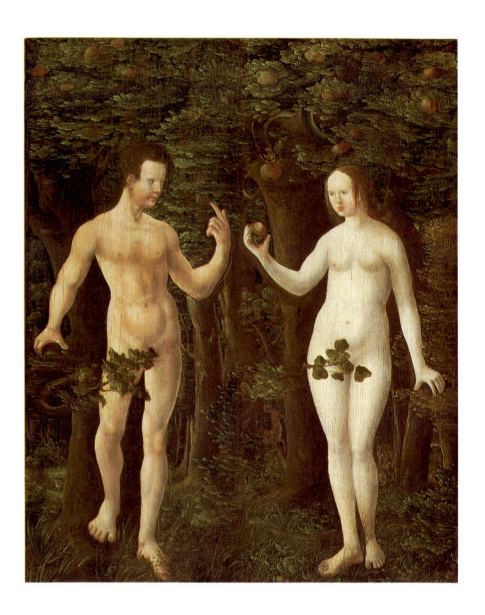

Workshop of Albrecht Altdorfer, ADAM AND EVE, *center panel of* THE FALL OF MAN, *c. 1525. Transferred from wood to hardboard, 38.2 × 15.6 cm. National Gallery of Art, Washington, D.C., Samuel H. Kress Collection 1952.*

During her life of eighty-one years, Hildegarde accomplished many things. Considered to be one of the greatest women of the twelfth century, she was a mystic, poet, prophetess, and physician. She ascribed her extraordinary intellectual powers to a kind of revelation granted to her frequently in a trancelike state. Hildegarde foretold such things as the downfall of the German Empire, the approach of the Reformation, and the disasters of the papacy (Nutting and Dock, 1937). She consistently communicated with kings and princes. Pilgrims frequently sought her advice and counsel; invalids came to her to be cured.

Hildegarde's knowledge embraced medical science, nursing, music, herb gardening, natural science, and spiritual and religious philosophy. She was a prolific writer on many subjects, including theology and physiology. Her greatest achievement, however, was her knowledge of medicine. Hildegarde was more conspicuous as a physician than as a nurse, although she combined the arts of both in her work. (No account of nursing work as such or mention of the care of the sick, however, is found in her biographies.) Whether she actually practiced medicine or nursing is unknown, yet her vast knowledge is certain (Eckenstein, 1896). Hildegarde wrote two medical books between 1151 and 1159, when she was nearly sixty years of

180

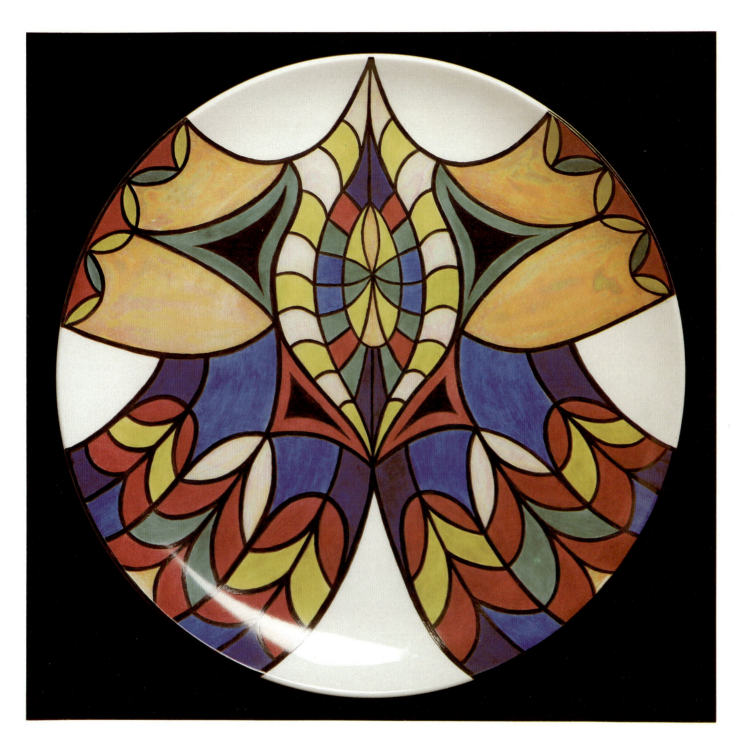

Judy Chicago, "Hildegarde of Bingen," plate from THE DINNER PARTY, *1979. China-painted porcelain, 35.6 cm diameter. Through the Flower, Benicia, California.*

age. One of these, *Liber Simplicis Medicinae,* which contained nine books, was edited in the sixteenth century under the title *Physica St. Hildegardis.* The other, *Liber Compositae Medicinae,* contained five books that dealt with the causes, symptoms, and cure of disease. Normal and abnormal psychology were also discussed. Hildegarde referred to anxieties, obsessions, idiocy, phobias, and mental illness and stated: "When headache, vapours, and giddiness attack a patient simultaneously they make him foolish and upset his reason. This makes many people think that he is possessed by an evil spirit, but that is not true" (Butler, vol. 9, 1934, p. 234). Another important work by Hildegarde was *Liber Operum Simplicis Hominis,* which was concerned with anatomical and physiological subjects. The range of subjects contained in these works is amazing. Hildegarde foretold

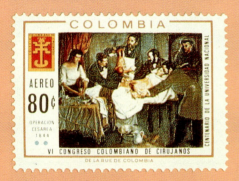

Colombia's 1967 eighty-cent air mail stamp was issued in observance of the Sixth Congress of Colombia Surgeons held in Bogota. The multicolor reproduction is of Grau's painting, THE FIRST CAESAREAN SECTION (1844), showing a nurse as a member of the surgical team. Courtesy of Howard B. Hurley.

autoinfection, recognized the brain as the regulator of all the vital processes, understood the influence of the nervous system, and discussed the vibration and pulsation of blood in the veins. Her mental distinction gave her a natural supremacy over her contemporaries.

Obstetrics. The care of the pregnant woman and the infant has always been a sensitive index of social progress. Contrary to popular opinion, childbearing has become more difficult as civilization has advanced. This has been particularly true among city populations. The rather simple outdoor life of primitive women and wives of serfs on feudal manors was substituted in the city by rather monotonous work that taxed one part of the body. In addition, city life was unhygienic in many ways. In those countries where rickets prevailed, a woman's pelvis was often deformed and Caesarean operations were thus necessary to save the mother and child. Often the mother died because medieval surgery was crude. Returning Crusaders spread syphilis, which became an important cause of infant, and sometimes maternal, fatality. Intermarriage occurred and often resulted in the union of a man and woman of different body structures. Thus a woman might give birth to a child too large for the size of her pelvis.

During the Middle Ages the *midwife,* not the physician, delivered infants. Only in difficult cases was a barber/surgeon asked to help with the delivery. The unborn child was sometimes killed and the body removed with crude instruments introduced through the vagina. Reputable physicians attended pregnant women only in rare instances, usually if the woman was of noble birth or was the king's mistress. In fact, the services of a physician in this area were not valued and strong prohibitions existed against their use. A Doctor Wertt of Hamburg was burned at the stake in 1522 for attending a delivery dressed as a woman.

Numerous paintings depict the practice of obstetrics by midwives. The delivery is portrayed in a variety of ways and different themes are depicted: guarding of the lying-in chamber from medical interference; presence of the midwife and the child nurse; different positions used for delivery, such as sitting or squatting; and types of appliances (obstetrical chair, V-shaped stool, beds) used.

Shortly after 1500 several events occurred that affected obstetrical care. The first book on obstetrics, *The Garden of Roses for Pregnant Women,* was written by Eucharius Roslin in 1513 at the request of the Duchess of Brunswick. The best-known practices of obstetrical care were reinforced; full of superstitions, this book sanctioned the crudest practices of midwives (Haggard, 1929). The *podalic version* was introduced in France by Ambroise Paré. This technique was used when a child was not in the proper position for a normal delivery; the surgeon's hand was inserted into the uterus and the child was grasped by the feet and turned. A school of midwifery was opened at the Hôtel Dieu in Paris in the sixteenth century. The Chamberlen brothers invented the obstetrical forceps in 1588. This instrument was kept a secret and passed on to the son of one of the brothers.

Epidemics and Plagues

In the fourteenth century, a catastrophic disease, Black Death, swept over the European continent and England four times. The worst occurrence was in 1348. Black Death is generally believed to have been a plague of the bubonic type, which results from the bite of an in-

182

fected parasite. Primarily a disease of rodents, particularly rats, it is transmitted to humans by parasites, such as fleas, that have fed on the diseased rodents. Direct contact with an infected person can also transmit the disease. Rats on vessels that were being used to transport supplies spread the disease over the greater part of Europe. The name *Black Death* came from the fact that dark hemorrhagic spots appeared under the skin of its victims. The outbreak of bubonic plague in the fourteenth century is considered to be one of the most devastating crises that ever occurred in human history. The sudden and unusual character of the disease brought terror to the people.

> The Black Death, which caused the unprecedented mortality of one-fourth of the population of the earth (over sixty millions of human beings), appeared in Europe about 1348, after devastating Asia and Africa. . . . Sweeping everything before it, this terrible plague brought panic and confusion in its train and broke down all restrictions of morality, decency and humanity. Parents, children and lifelong friends forsook one another, everyone striving to save only himself and to come off with a whole skin. Some took to vessels in the open sea only to find that the pestilence was hot upon them; some prayed and fasted in sanctuaries, others gave themselves up to unbridled indulgence, or. . . . fled the country to idle away their time in some safe retreat; others lapsed into sullen indifference and despair. The dead were hurled pell-mell into huge pits, hastily dug for the purpose, and putrefying bodies lay about everywhere in the houses and streets.
>
> *Garrison, 1913, pp. 127–128*

The sweating sickness began in England and spread over the continent about the same time. This virulent disease is thought to have been influenza. Large numbers of people died within a day or a few hours after the first symptoms appeared. The onset was accompanied by chills, fever, headaches, stupor, cardiac pain, vomiting, fatigue, and profuse sweat. Unfortunately, some of the care that was rendered probably hastened the patient's end. It was believed that the patient must sweat continuously for twenty-four hours. Therefore windows and doors were closed, stoves were lighted, and furs were piled on the ill. Attendants stayed with the patients, attempting to keep them awake so that they might retain their senses. Various techniques were used to accomplish this, such as whipping the body with branches or dropping vinegar into the eyes. It was remarked that the patient was "stewed to death" (Jamieson and Sewall, 1950).

Tremendous changes took place in the last centuries of the Middle Ages. The feudal system deteriorated. Cities and a middle class society developed. Luxury and misery, learning and ignorance existed side by side. The changing needs of society prompted the beginning of reforms.

*T*he transition from medieval times becomes quite evident toward the close of the fifteenth century. Among the momentous forces that again changed the existing social order were movements whose seeds were planted in preceding centuries and which came to fruition in this era. Those forces were the Renaissance, the Protestant Revolt or Reformation, nationalism, the discovery of a new world, oceanic commercial enterprise, and the diffusion of knowledge through the printed word. All of these forces influenced the healing arts in one way or another.

Sister Charles Marie Frank

NURSING IN TRANSITION

The Dark Period and the Dawn of Modern Times

The centuries that immediately followed the Crusades were marked by great social changes. These changes began as early as 1250, tended to accelerate about 1450, and by 1750 had become dominant as the modern characteristics in Western Europe (Shryock, 1959). Between the fall of Constantinople (1453) and the Battle of Waterloo (1815), a variety of revolutions served to expand man's idea of the universe and the meaning of human life. Yet these forces also threatened to destroy the social recovery that had been accomplished thus far. The economic, industrial, intellectual, political, and religious revolutions inevitably had far-reaching effects upon every aspect of life, including the treatment of the sick and the sick poor, the management of hospitals, and the status of nursing. These movements demonstrated the currents of popular feeling that increased tensions in most of Europe: the dominant Church with its large temporal power had become oppressive; the intellectuals were criticizing the doctrines of extreme ecclesiasticism; the laboring classes were bitter toward serfdom and oppression; and the religious were yearning for a return to a simpler faith with greater observance of ceremonials. The time was ripe for change.

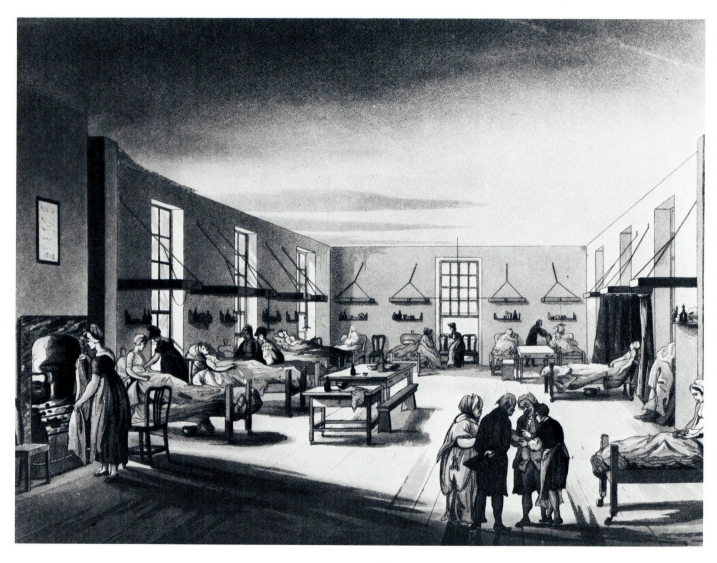

After Thomas Rowlandson, INTERIOR AT MIDDLESEX HOSPITAL, LONDON, *c. 1808. Etching and aquatint. National Library of Medicine, Bethesda, Maryland.*

■ RENAISSANCE AND REFORMATION

To the sixteenth century belong two great movements, the Renaissance and the Reformation. Each was a result of the spirit of revolutionary change and man's quest for new knowledge and beauty. Probably the same social forces that produced the intellectual movement known as the Renaissance brought a split within the Church that eventually divided Christianity into warring sects. Together, these movements ushered in the "modern era" in which society was aware of the new world of Columbus, the old world of the Near and Far East, the new laws of Newton, and the old learning of the Graeco-Roman ages. The scientific method of inquiry was initiated, and secularism became the modern spirit. All established institutions were affected during this transition period, which produced new institutions and also modified the old ones. Those having to do with the

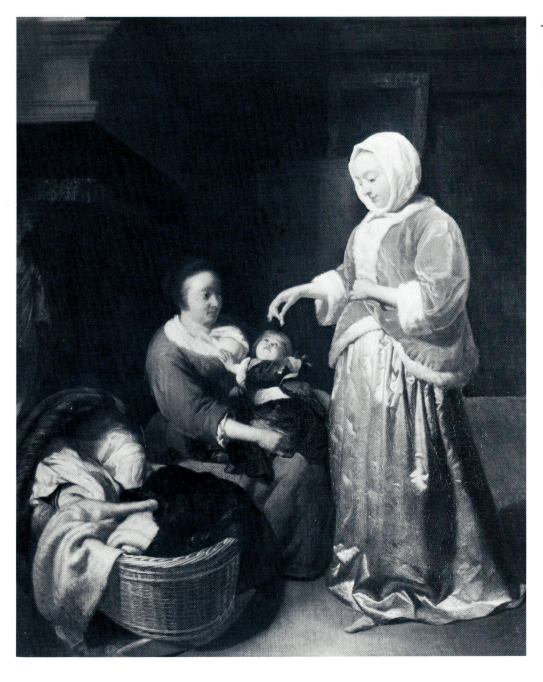

Joost van Geel, MOTHER WITH NURSE AND CHILD. *Wood. Museum Boymans-van Beuningen, Rotterdam, Netherlands.*

care of the sick were, perhaps, affected the most. Reforms promoted by the changing needs of the society began to occur, although in some instances they were slow in coming.

The Renaissance

The chaos of the Middle Ages subsided with the unparalleled phenomenon known as the Renaissance. This period in history was called a *rinascita,* or rebirth, by Giorgio Vasari (1511–1574), a Florentine artist and architect who believed that the major motivation for its evolution was a return to the cultures of ancient Rome and Greece. It was a period characterized by shifts in standards that were evident in literary and intellectual circles. Of primary importance was the decline in the power of the Church in temporal matters accompanied by a rise in intense secular interest in worldly affairs. The dominant spirit of the Renaissance was an interest in the things of the earth without reference to God.

> In the sixteenth century men rejected the Church but held on to their belief in Christ. In the seventeenth century the intellectuals rejected the divinity of Christ but retained their belief in the Deity.... In the eighteenth century, the Age of Enlightenment, the "philosophers" openly rejected God Himself and substituted Reason. In the nineteenth century religious indifferentism, materialism, general unbelief and atheism spread among the masses.
>
> *Devane, 1948, p. 55*

With this lost sense of relationship to God, the movement became characterized by both gullibility and skepticism, which led to a renewal of pagan superstitious practices and witchcraft. Yet outstanding Christian humanists emerged during this time, and renowned saints lived exemplary lives.

The Renaissance indeed has been viewed as both a blessing and a curse. It brought about a tremendous renewal of interest in learning in the areas of classical literature, humanism, and expressions of beauty. It was therefore also known as the period of Humanism or the Revival of Learning. This renewal of interest in the arts and the sciences had a positive influence on the medical advancement in the Renaissance period. The learning, however, engendered materialistic, secularistic, and individualistic tendencies in the people. The society divided into two classes, the intelligentsia, who lived luxurious lives, and the working classes, who were oppressed because of their lack of knowledge and worldly possessions. Intellectual superiority and moral laxity emerged and drastically affected the political and religious character of the European people.

The Renaissance began in Italy about 1400 and permeated Western Europe during the ensuing century. The new state of mind reflected itself in literature, painting, sculpture, and architecture. In addition, increasing wealth made it possible for art to penetrate the middle class. Painting, which had been limited to religious subjects and idealized themes from the Christian tradition, expanded to include the depiction of contemporary life. In Italian Renaissance

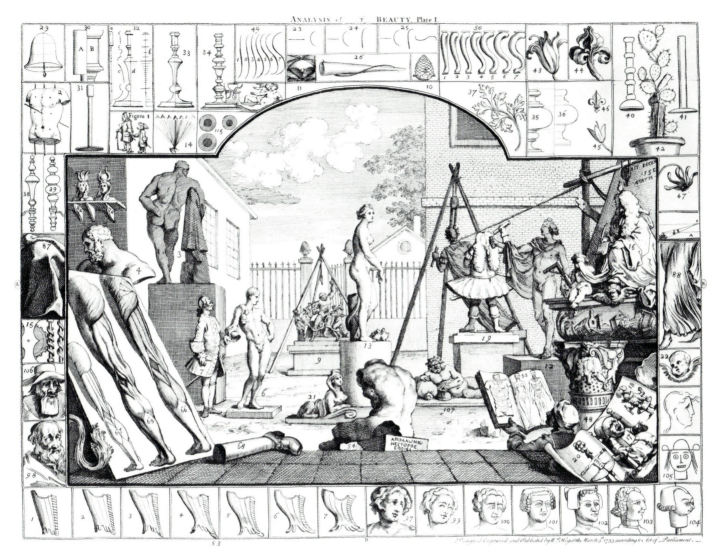

William Hogarth, ANALYSIS OF BEAUTY, *Plate I, c. 1753. Engraving, approx. 36.8 × 49.5 cm. British Museum, London, England.*

painting, however, religious subjects still predominated. Renaissance painting, noted for its human quality, was "realistic" and attempted to reproduce natural objects as they actually appeared. During this era prominent and innovative artists portrayed real people with increasing skill in perspective and color. Students from the school of Florentine art who left an indelible mark in this field included Leonardo da Vinci (1452–1519), Michelangelo (1475–1564), who painted frescoes in the Sistine Chapel, and Raphael (1483–1520). Titian (1477–1576) led a second group of students from the Venetian school. The Florentine school was noted for form and grace of line; the Venetian school, for its mastery of color.

Leonardo da Vinci was perhaps the most versatile of the artists of the Renaissance. His masterpiece, "The Last Supper," was painted on a wall of the refectory in a monastery at Milan. Da Vinci was the first artist to consider anatomy for reasons other than its practicality.

Leonardo himself made anatomical preparations from which he produced drawings, of which more than 750 are extant, representing the skeletal, muscular, nervous, and vascular systems. The illustrations were often supplemented with annotations of a physiological nature. Leonardo's scientific accuracy was greater than that of Vesalius, and his artistic beauty remains unchal-

189

lenged. His correct assessment of the curvature of the spine went otherwise undiscovered for more than a hundred years. He depicted the true position of the *fetus in utero* and first noted certain anatomical structures. The sketches were seen by only a few contemporaries and were not published until the end of the last century.

Petrucelli, 1978, p. 410

Leonardo painted marvelous variations in expressions on the faces of his subjects. Reactions of fear, frustration, pain, joy, and happiness appeared natural and lifelike.

The northern schools of painting, notably the Dutch and the Flemish, gave rise to artists such as Peter Paul Rubens (1577–1640), Anthony Van Dyck (1599–1641), and Rembrandt van Rijn (1606–1669). The Dutch masters tended to abandon religious themes and devote themselves to merchants, princes, or scenes from everyday life. They were interested in human dissection and left excellent examples of this, as in Rembrandt's classic *Lesson in Anatomy*.

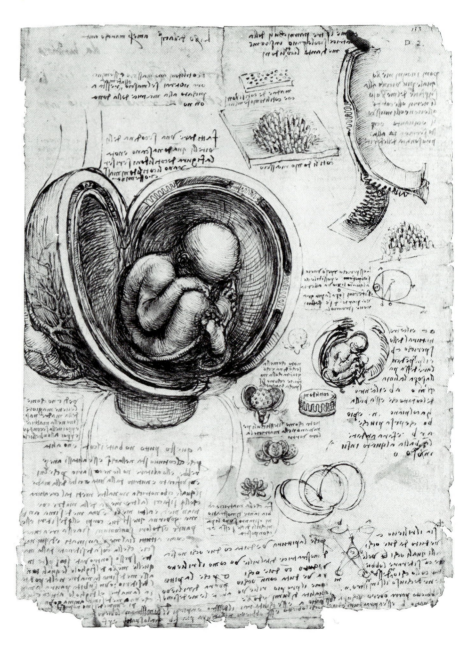

Leonardo da Vinci, EMBRYO IN THE WOMB, *c. 1510. Pen and ink. Royal Collection, Windsor Castle. Copyright reserved. Reproduced by gracious permission of Her Majesty Queen Elizabeth II.*

The Reformation

The Reformation (Protestant Revolt), which began in 1517, started as a reform and ended as a revolt. It was a religious movement that resulted in a division in Christianity. The Reformation was precipitated by two major factors: (1) the widespread abuses that had become a part of Church life and practice, such as the selling of indulgences and pardons, the veneration of relics, and the ignorance and depravity of the clergy, and (2) doctrinal difficulties. Essentially, a showdown occurred between the philosophy of St. Augustine, which dominated the early Church, and that of St. Thomas Aquinas, which gained preeminence in the thirteenth century. The more liberal doctrine of Aquinas permitted man free will to choose between good and evil and to achieve grace both through good works and faith. Reform had been advocated for many centuries by influential individuals from within and without the Church. Erasmus scoffed at the ridiculous abuses, and Thomas More prayed for internal revision. The Church, however, did not take action and thereby paved the way for drastic intervention. By the time Martin Luther (1483–1546) pinned his ninety-five theses to the castle church door at Wittenburg in 1517, many people were ready to oppose the established regime.

The rebellion against the Pope and the patriarchal rule of the Church was led by Martin Luther. Luther, once a German mendicant monk, became the leader of a group of dissatisfied people who broke away from the Catholic Church. These separatists were called *Protestants* ("those who protested"), a group that was to be comprised of many religious denominations. The followers of Luther were called Lutherans, and the Lutheran Church of today still adheres to his doctrine. The Lutherans rapidly declared both the independence of their congregations from the Pope and the right of each state to choose between the new Church and the old. Where there had been only one Europe, there was henceforth two. The Western world was divided into Catholics, who adhered to the teachings of Christ as dictated by the Church, and Protestants, who rejected the authority of this Church.

Within a few years northern Germany, Norway, Sweden, and Denmark were Lutheran. In addition, the success of Lutheranism encouraged other revolts against Catholic authority. During the next century many sects arose, such as Anabaptists, Mennonites, Quakers, Calvinists, Presbyterians, Puritans, and Anglicans. Each interpreted the doctrine in a slightly different way; each was certain of the absolute truth necessary for salvation. Although this division weakened Protestantism, it enhanced society by insisting upon each individual's right to think for himself. Some of these groups ultimately established churches that were as intolerant of opposition as was Catholicism.

Correction of abuses within the Church finally came with the Council of Trent, a general council of church authorities called at Trentino, Italy, in 1545. In order to identify means of removing causes of criticism and clarify the Church's position, this council continued its sessions for eighteen years, until 1563.

> The Council defined attacked points of Christian theology, established disciplinary measures for clergy, religious and laity, and prepared a catechism of Christian doctrine for parish use. The means taken to bring about the real reform are sometimes referred to as the Counter-Reformation.
>
> *Frank, 1953, p. 130*

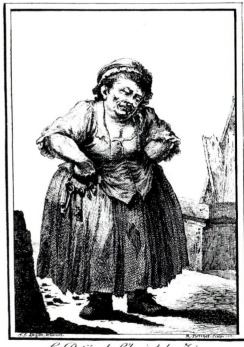

La Portière de L'hopital des Toicuses.

THE DOORKEEPER AT TOICUSES HOSPITAL.
From the PICTURE BOOK OF GRAPHICS ARTS 1500–1800, *volume 6. Compiled by Georg Hirth, published in Munich by Knorr & Hirr, 1882. British Library, London, England.*

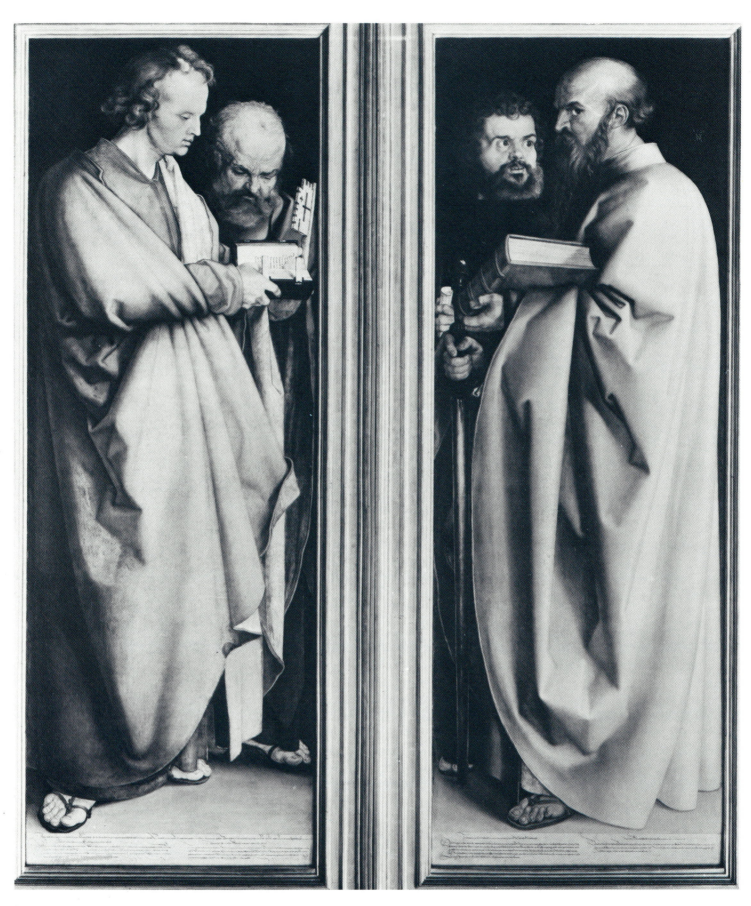

Albrecht Dürer, FOUR APOSTLES, *1526. Panel, approx. 214.6 × 76.2 cm (each). Alte Pinakothek, Munich, Federal Republic of Germany.*

The four apostles symbolize the four temperaments. From left to right, St. John represents the sanguine temperament; St. Peter, the phlegmatic; St. Mark, the choleric; and St. Paul, the melancholic.

However, efforts to reconcile Catholicism and Protestantism failed, and Europe drifted into a tragic struggle between the two groups. The result was an era of hatred, civil conflict, the development of multiple factions to foster individuality, and an international conflict known as the Thirty Years' War (1618–1648). People had also begun to depart for the New World, where they might ensure for themselves a true freedom in religion.

The Reformation had no direct effect on hospitals in Catholic countries, and some hospitals did indeed survive in Protestant countries. Yet the majority of hospitals operated by the Catholic religious orders were closed or controlled by the Protestants. Monks and nuns were driven out of the institutions in the Protestant countries, which caused a tremendous shortage of people to care for the sick and the poor. The plight of the unfortunates became unbearable as they were reduced to a state of disgraceful pauperism. (Under Catholicism the poor had been esteemed.) Hospitals became places of horror, since there was no qualified group to take the place of the nursing religious orders. The most serious consequences occurred in England, where Henry VIII suppressed all the religious orders and confiscated the property of some 600 charitable endowments. Women were recruited from all sources to fill the nursing ranks. Many of these women were assigned nursing duties in lieu of serving jail sentences. This "Dark Period of Nursing," between 1550 and 1850, saw nursing conditions at their very worst.

The seeming ambivalence of Protestant countries toward their sick and poor was the result of two conflicting influences: the desire to make money, to be rich and powerful, and the desire to be the chosen of God by doing works that would provide a state of "grace." Laws and customs discouraged the humane care of the downtrodden and the weak, yet tremendous efforts were made to raise money to open hospitals and provide the necessities of life. This dichotomy had the most serious effect on nursing.

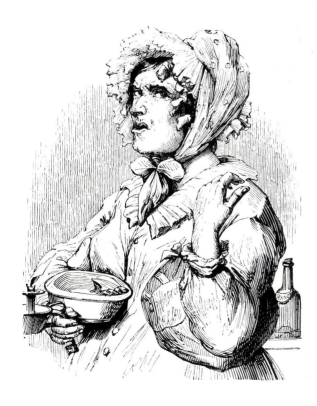

THE NURSE, *c. 1840. Cartoon illustrating the popular idea of the nurse of the day. The Mansell Collection, London, England.*

■ THE AGE OF REVOLUTIONS

The intellectual, political, industrial, and economic revolutions were strong motivators for changing the ideas and activities of man, as was the religious revolt. These movements—complex, varied, and interrelated—all were influences that brought about the Renaissance. It was a time of flux, and these factors were crucial to the development of new necessities and new circumstances in the life that had evolved. The modern world was being born, but it would experience severe labor pains and harsh growing pains.

The Political Revolution

The political life that was characterized by feudal institutions in medieval times gave way to the establishment of national states during the Renaissance. These national states developed in the part of Europe that had previously been unified under the Holy Roman Empire. Unity was achieved through monarchs who gradually overthrew feudal lords. Authority was centralized in the monarchy; a system of private ownership and private enterprise took shape. Individuals and nations sought power through the accumulation of wealth and the grasping of opportunity.

Other changes occurred as nationalism progressed. The language and customs of the capital were spread throughout the entire kingdom. The trend toward a national language had begun and fostered a growing pride in the land. Individuals in the literary field began to work in their own tongue instead of using Latin. This patriotism was also stirred by wars against other peoples, which were initiated by the ambition of kings. National competition developed and resulted in armed interventions. One great struggle followed another until the Seven Years' War (French and Indian War) in 1754, which earned first place for England. However, poverty and discontent followed the wars, and a series of revolutions erupted in an endeavor to create more democratic forms of government. The American Revolution (1775–1783), the French Revolution (1789–1795), and the Latin American Revolution (1800–1825) reflected a reaction against human inequality and an emphasis on individual rights. Finally, the Napoleonic wars began in 1797 and ended in 1815 with the Battle of Waterloo. This particular conflict buried dictatorship for a time.

The Economic Revolution

The physical world was explored by England, France, Spain, Portugal, and Holland over the space of three centuries (1450–1750). New lands were discovered. North and South America, New Zealand, and the ocean islands were seized from less civilized peoples and colonized. India, China, and Africa were rediscovered and forced into trade with Europe. Man's world was doubled in size and his dream of wealth expanded proportionately. Vast riches from trade with the Old and New Worlds poured into Europe. Particularly significant was the bullion carried from the Americas by Spain, which put more gold and silver into circulation in Western Europe than ever before. It is

194

estimated that the circulating gold and silver in 1500 was worth $2 million; by 1600 its worth had increased to $2 billion. A revolution in economic thought and practice was thus created. (Bullion could also have included precious stones.) A capitalistic economic system, sometimes referred to as *merchant capitalism,* began to take form.

Mercantilism developed in response to economic activity for national ends. It began to emerge as early as the fourteenth century and was dominant during the seventeenth and early eighteenth centuries. This system held that a nation's wealth was determined by the amount of precious metals in its treasury. Government regulated industry, agriculture, and labor. Furthermore, government controls would ensure the maintenance of a stable economy and an increase in the stockpile, particularly through a favorable balance of trade. The state would create laws to force an excess of exports over imports and reap the profit in bullion. Businessmen became the dominant class in their community and were led by merchant princes. (Shakespeare's title character in *Merchant of Venice* [1596] impressed men of England as the dynamic business leader.) Private enterprise, competition for markets, and expectations of gains were vital components of this system.

The Industrial Revolution

The industrial revolution began in England at approximately 1750 and drastically upset traditional life-styles. With the rise of the capitalist economic system, medieval craftsmen became dependent upon capitalists for wages. At first, craftsmen labored in their own homes, but by 1700 the factory system of production had gained popularity.

> The factory system is marked by the wage relationship between the employer and employees, by mass production, and by the tendency to enlarge steadily the size of the productive units. This system requires centralized direction and elaborate financial outlays....
>
> *Sellew and Nuesse, 1946, p. 143*

Unfortunately, a belief prevails that the industrial system was suddenly introduced during this time because of inventions in the textile industry. The real revolution, however, was underway before the occurrence of such inventions, which served to accelerate the process. Machinery did, however, standardize quality, and master craftsmen were forced to give up their crafts and lands and become laborers (factory hands) for rich men. All types of industries were affected and efficiency became the key to success. In addition, as the era of invention unfolded, the number of manufacturing cities grew.

The Intellectual Revolution

The intellectual or scientific revolution was precipitated by the discoveries of Copernicus (1473–1543), Galileo (1564–1642), and Newton (1642–1727). Their work demonstrated that the earth was not the center of the universe but revolved in accordance with universal laws over which man had no control. Experimentation, measurement, and instruments to improve sight or hearing became important aids to observation and the development of the new science, "experimental philosophy." The inductive method of thought was introduced as scholars began to observe facts and phenomena and determine solutions to the mysteries of life through a process of reasoning.

Numerous discoveries occurred in the physical sciences that seemed to revolutionize human thought. Nicholas Copernicus demonstrated that the earth turns on its axis and moves in an orbit around the sun. Johannes Kepler (1571–1630) further developed this theory. Isaac Newton discovered the law of gravitation. Simon Stevin (1548–1620) developed the use of decimals. John Napier (1550–1617) and Henry Briggs (1561–1630) promoted the use of logarithms. René Descartes (1596–1650) invented analytic geometry. A number of other individuals were also instrumental in advancing the physical sciences. These sixteenth century discoveries led to the invention of the telescope, microscope, thermometer, barometer, and pendulum clock.

The field of the biological sciences was also advancing and would become basic to the progress of medical science. The work of Andreas Vesalius (1514–1564), the founder of modern anatomy, was thought to be revolutionary. His findings were based upon investigation rather than speculation. William Harvey (1578–1657) described the circulation of the blood, proof of which was published in 1628 in his *Anatomical Dissertation Upon the Movement of the Heart.* Robert Hooke (1635–1703) described the cellular structure of plants. Anton van Leeuwenhoek (1632–1723), using the recently invented microscope, discovered protozoa and bacteria and described human spermatozoa.

Advances in technology interfaced with progress in the sciences. This was particularly evident with the greatest of the Renaissance inventions, the printing press. Letters could be stamped on paper by movable type, and after the year 1500 manuscripts were rapidly superseded by printed volumes. The first complete book printed in this manner was the famous Gutenberg Bible (1454). Books became cheaper and available to all educated men. Scientists were thus able to read one another's books, exchange ideas promptly, build on published works, and communicate findings.

■ NEW DIRECTIONS IN MEDICINE

The birth of the scientific method of inquiry profoundly influenced the development of medicine in the Renaissance period. Medical men, like other scientists, benefited by the development of experimentation. Indeed, the majority of scientists *were* physicians. Yet the line between science and magic remained blurred. Quacks and charlatans continued to appear and appeal to the poor and the ignorant, who depended on this type of "medicine man" and self-medication. This was necessary because physicians were the elite group during this period and they took care of only the upper classes.

The New Anatomy

The first movement in the advance of medical science was the growth of anatomical knowledge and its application to surgery. The Flemish anatomist Andreas Vesalius was undoubtedly the leader in this area. His work, which was based on human dissection, replaced crude medieval concepts and corrected over 200 mistakes in the works of Galen (Shryock, 1959). Vesalius's *De Humani Corporis Fabrica* (*The Fabric of the Human Body*) of 1543 illustrated both verbally and visually the dissected parts of the human body—the skeleton, muscles, vascular system, abdomen, and so forth. The findings of Vesalius were revolutionary and were not well received by his colleagues, who derided him and ignored his work. After Vesalius' death his students continued his work. They included Gabriele Fallopio (1523–1562), the discoverer of the fallopian tubes.

Ambroise Paré (1510–1590), a Parisian surgeon, transformed the practice of surgery by applying anatomical knowledge with the scientific method. He began his career as a barber's apprentice, became an assistant at the Hôtel Dieu, and finally was a surgeon in the army. He brought back the use of ligatures for bleeding vessels caused by gunshot wounds (his colleagues treated such wounds with boiling oil). Paré brought together the surgeons of the universities and the barber surgeons who were relied upon by the people. His practical genius included improvements in artificial limbs, trusses, hernia operations, and the glass eye.

Theophrastus Bombastus von Hohenheim (1493–1541), better known as Paracelsus, was one of the most unusual men in medical history. Paracelsus viewed the body as a sort of glorified chemical retort and initiated the chemical approach to physiology. He stressed that alchemists should stop attempting to make gold and start making medicines. Paracelsus particularly advocated the use of mercury, arsenic, lead, iron, sulfur, and antimony. He thus earned the title of Father of Pharmacology, in spite of the fact that he combined the use of chemicals with astrology. Paracelsus, an eccentric Swiss physician who had trained in Italy, consistently rebelled against authority. It is said that he publicly burned the books of Galen and other classical works. Paracelsus was one of the few surgeons of his time who renounced the accepted theory that pus was normal in the healing process. His was a daring approach to the field of medicine (Haggard, 1933).

The value of the new methods and the transition from anatomy to physiology was clearly illustrated by work done in the area of the heart and blood vessels.

> Galen had declared that the vascular system centered in the liver, and that blood ebbed and flowed through the body via a septum between one side of the heart and the other. But anatomists now found that no such septum existed and this cast doubt on the whole theory.
>
> *Shryock, 1959, p. 140*

William Harvey (1578–1657) solved the problem by demonstrating with animals the actual circulation of the blood with the heart acting as a central pump. These findings were published in his *Exercitatio*

Anatomica de Motu Cordis et Sanguinis in Animalibus (*On the Movement of the Heart and Blood in Animals*), one of the most important works in medicine and biology. Unfortunately, Harvey was ridiculed and became known to some as the "circulator." To others, he was known as the Father of Modern Medicine, since his most valuable contribution was the establishment of physiological experimentation.

The value of anatomical studies was demonstrated during the Renaissance. Wide-reaching effects of these studies occurred in medicine, particularly in the areas of surgery and physiology. In addition, they logically led to the acceleration of the field of pathology.

Three Centuries of Progress

The seventeenth century saw the beginnings of attempts to explain the mechanics of the human body. Jerome Fabricus (1537–1619) was the first embryologist. Athanasius Kircher (1602–1680), a Jesuit monk, used a microscope and connected microorganisms with contagion. Anton van Leeuwenhoek perfected the microscope and described bacteria and protozoa. The development of the clinical method was the contribution of Thomas Sydenham (1624–1689), who advocated the subjection of old theories to new scientific observation. His efforts to observe cases and to experiment with treatments led him to propose new methods of handling the sick. Sydenham provided detailed descriptions of prevalent diseases and influenced the trend of medicine by emphasizing fresh air to replace the stuffiness of the sick room. The autopsy was also found to be useful during this period.

The real importance of these discoveries was the provision of frameworks for thought about normal and deviant functioning of the human body. These innovations served to illustrate a specific trend in medical thought, the readiness of enlightened men to discard old ideas for new ones. Increasingly, medical and scientific names of renown began to emerge:

> Marcello Malpighi, the greatest of the microscopists and founder of the science of histology; Willis, de Graaf, Peyer, Brunner, Stensen, Glisson, Van Deventer, the father of modern midwifery; Priestley who isolated oxygen; Lavoisier who discovered the interchange of gases in the process of respiration; Pott, John Hunter, the surgical pathologist; Pringle, founder of modern military medicine. . . .
>
> *Frank, 1953, p. 132*

In addition, this century witnessed the changing of alchemy to chemistry by Robert Boyle (1627–1691). His knowledge of the nature of a pure substance overturned the ancient and long-revered theory that the four elements are earth, air, fire, and water. With this change the old humoral theory of health and illness was no longer relevant and a new theory was needed. One of the first new models was offered by René Descartes (1596–1650), whose *De Homine* was the original modern attempt at a physiology text.

It took the first fifty years of the eighteenth century for all of this new knowledge to be organized and digested. Advances continued to be made during this new century, but they were not as bold or as conspicuous as those of the previous one. They were nevertheless important in improving the standards of medical practice. Albrecht von Haller (1708–1777) systematized the new discoveries and made them available to practitioners. Giovanni Morgagni (1682–1741) correlated diseases of the organs with symptoms arising from impaired organic functioning. John Hunter (1728–1793) used his studies in

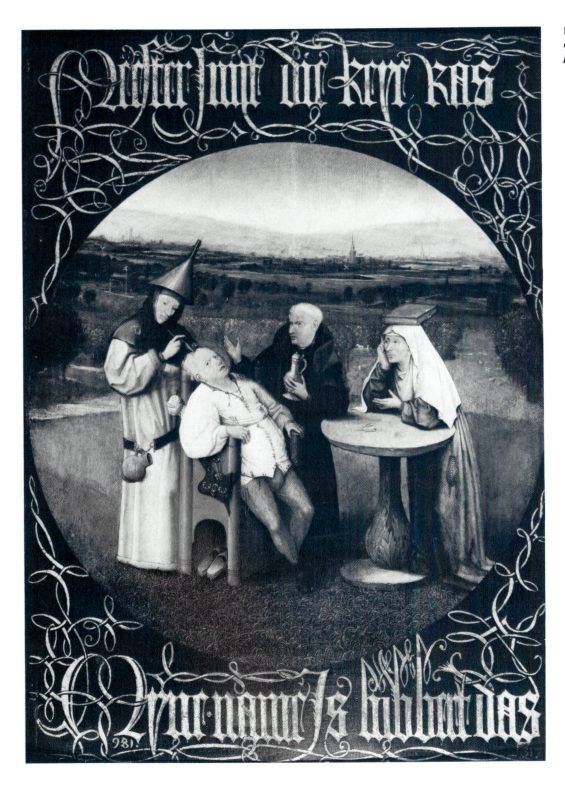

EXTRACTION OF THE STONE OF MADNESS. *Museo del Prado, Madrid, Spain.*

comparative anatomy in new operative procedures and developed a simple and safe operation for aneurysm.

In the eighteenth century smallpox was prevalent and took many lives. Edward Jenner (1749–1823), an Englishman, discovered a satisfactory method of vaccination against smallpox in 1798. This procedure, with certain modifications, is still used today. In spite of its proven efficiency and effectiveness, however, vaccination has been avoided by some people.

Psychiatry developed as a separate branch of medicine in the latter part of the eighteenth century. The mentally ill had received cruel and inhumane treatment in the sixteenth and seventeenth centuries. Vicious practices were associated with the idea that the mentally ill were "possessed" of a demon or even the Devil himself. Certain physicians protested that mental disease was a medical problem and that the mentally ill should be treated in a humane fashion. Vincenzo Chiarrigi (1759–1820) established sound treatment of the mentally ill in the hospital that he directed. A Quaker, William Tuke, introduced more understanding methods in a retreat (York Retreat, managed by the Society of Friends) that he had established. Philippe Pinel (1745–1826), a physician and director of two hospitals in Paris, was probably the most famous leader in this area. He abandoned the use of restraining chains and advocated acceptance of the mentally ill as human beings in need of medical assistance, nursing care, and social services.

During this same period instruments were invented for measurement and inspection of the body. A pulse watch was made by Sir John Flayer (1647–1734) in 1707. This watch ran for exactly one minute and then stopped. Leopold Auenbrugger (1722–1809) initiated the use of percussion. This technique had been unique to innkeepers, who tapped wine kegs to determine the remaining volume. René Théophile Laënnec (1781–1826) devised the stethoscope after listening to heart sounds through a tube of rolled-up paper tied with a string. This was followed by a cylinder made of light wood, about twelve inches long, that could be taken apart by unscrewing it into two pieces. (Dr. Cammann of New York developed the binaural stethoscope.)

Advances in medicine continued into the nineteenth century. One of the greatest contributions was the result of the work of Louis Pasteur (1822–1895). His discoveries laid the foundation for the science of bacteriology. The principles relating to attenuation of viruses, preventive vaccination against disease-producing organisms, treatment of rabies, and the discovery of the process of "pasteurization" were all significant works that enhanced the practice of medicine and the prevention of disease. Robert Koch (1843–1910), one of Pasteur's contemporaries, discovered the causes of cholera and tuberculosis. Joseph Lister (1827–1912) became one of the greatest men in the history of surgery. He introduced the use of antiseptics in operating rooms as a preventive measure against infection. During Lister's time "hospitalism" was accepted as an unavoidable evil in surgery. This name was applied to the infectious epidemics that stalked the hospital wards and took many lives. Anyone who was fortunate enough to recover from surgery often regained only partial health. Such morbidity and mortality were not acceptable to Lister, who scientifically studied its causes and perfected his techniques. Other very important discoveries were facilitated by the work of Pasteur.

In 1879, Neisser discovered the gonococcus; in 1880, Eberth described the typhoid bacillus; in 1882, Koch reported the discovery of the tubercle bacillus; in 1883, Klebs and Loeffler discovered the *Bacillus Diphtheriae* and Salvioli described the pneumonococcus that he found in thoracic exudates and tissues; in 1892, Welch and Nuttal first described Welch's bacillus (gas infection); and in 1897, Shiga discovered the dysentery bacillus.

In 1895, Röntgen discovered x-rays; in 1896, Marie and Pierre Curie isolated radium, and Widal introduced his agglutination test for diagnosing typhoid fever.

Frank, 1953, p. 213

By the middle of the nineteenth century other instruments of diagnosis came into being. The stethoscope, the mercury thermometer, and x-rays had become important adjuncts to the practice of medicine. The introduction of ether and chloroform as general anesthetics greatly aided the practice of surgery. The science of bacteriology had become the basis for modern medicine and surgery. Indeed, medicine had made revolutionary progress. Many individuals, only a few of whom have been mentioned here, had made significant contributions. A rapid series of discoveries had occurred over the three centuries, and these would forever change the direction of medicine.

PHILIPPE PINEL ORDERING THE CHAINS REMOVED FROM THE MENTALLY ILL, *c. 1793. World Health Organization, Geneva, Switzerland.*

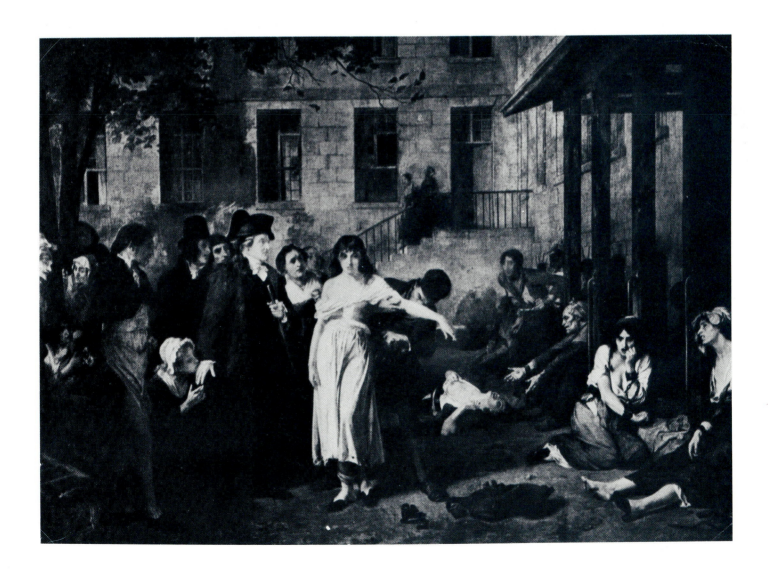

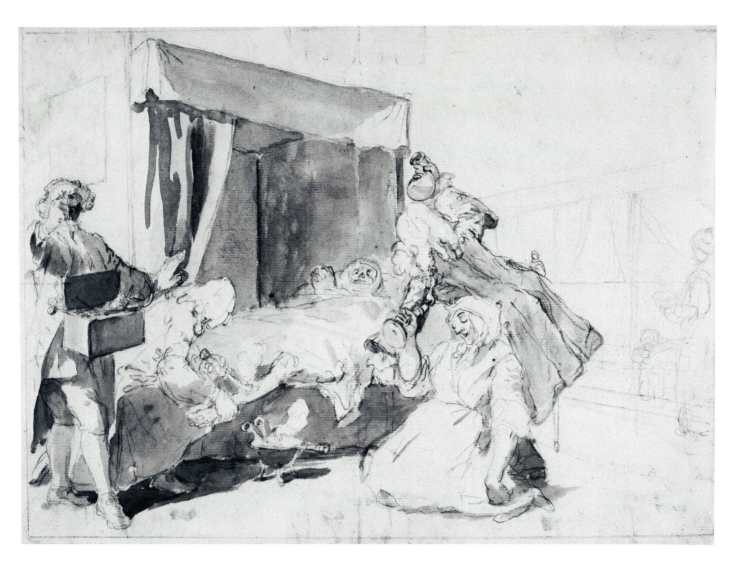

William Hogarth, AN OPERATION SCENE IN
A HOSPITAL, *mid–eighteenth century. Pencil
and grey wash over chalk. The Pierpont
Morgan Library, New York.*

Obstetrics and Infant Welfare

The serious problem of infant and maternal death rates in the eighteenth century was tackled in Europe and the British Isles. Since
exact statistics were not available, however, it is difficult to assess the
change with any accuracy. The maternal death rate had many causes,
including poor or no prenatal care, poor nutrition from ignorance
and poverty, infectious disease in early pregnancy, and the dreaded
hospital infection—puerperal fever. In some instances it was also
precipitated by delivery at the hands of ignorant and filthy midwives.

In the eighteenth century all but the wealthy used midwives for
the delivery in normal cases; surgeons were called in for difficult
cases. The destruction of the child and removal of its body, however,
were less frequently done by the surgeons because of Paré's introduction of the podalic version and the invention of the obstetrical
forceps by Peter Chamberlen. Yet surgeons tended to interfere with
the deliveries, either with instruments or manually, so that their
efforts to relieve mothers often brought death to both the mother
and the infant. In the latter part of the eighteenth century, particularly in England, physicians assumed the care of pregnant women.
They replaced surgeons in difficult cases and even in some normal
deliveries. The "consultant in midwifery," the predecessor of the

202

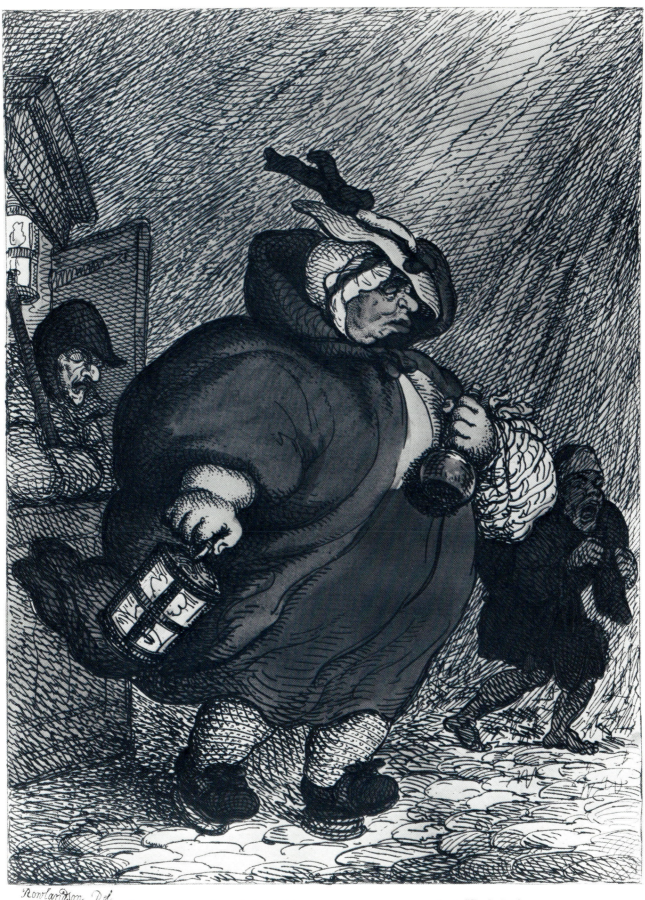

A MIDWIFE GOING TO A LABOUR

Thomas Rowlandson, A MIDWIFE GOING TO A LABOUR, 1811. British Museum, London, England.

obstetrician, became a specialist who was separate from both physicians and surgeons. Two other events occurred that assisted with the improved status of the mother: the addition of the study of obstetrics to the medical curriculum and the advent of lying-in hospitals. In the lying-in hospitals, however, improved maternal death rate was dependent on the conditions that existed in them. In some, where conditions were the worst, the rate fluctuated between ten and twenty percent of the mothers who delivered in the institutions.

As an answer to the problem of puerperal fever, William Hunter (1718–1783) proposed noninterference during delivery. During his time the number of cases of puerperal fever had increased to tragic proportions. Since the cause of the infection was unknown and the danger of contracting it was high, Hunter's solution seemed plausible. However, some of his followers became so adamant about noninterference that some patients were allowed to die who might have otherwise been saved.

Ignaz Philipp Semmelweis (1818–1865) also became concerned about the problem of puerperal fever. Born in Budapest, he received his doctor's degree and the degree of master of midwifery from the University of Vienna. Semmelweis was granted a position as assistant director of the obstetric clinic at the Lying-in Hospital in Vienna, where he was appalled by the high maternal mortality rate resulting from puerperal sepsis (childbed fever). He began to observe and analyze patient care and noticed a curious fact. He noted a difference between the maternal mortality rates of two clinics. The incidence of the fever and death was lower in the clinic where midwives practiced, but it was higher in the one where medical students practiced. Semmelweis determined that the spread of infection occurred because of the careless habits of the medical students, who went directly from the dissecting (autopsy) table to deliveries or to examinations of prenatal or postpartum patients. Therefore he demanded that the students wash their hands with soap and water, then wash them with chlorinated lime. As a result of this practice, there was a remarkable decrease in death rate, from 10 percent to a little over one percent. *The Cause, Concept, and Prophylaxis of Childbed Fever,* published in 1861, provided an account of this valuable research. Unfortunately, the work of Semmelweis was ridiculed and was not accepted by his colleagues. The criticism he suffered apparently led to his eventual mental illness. In 1865 he died from blood poisoning, a condition that he had fought to eliminate.

Oliver Wendell Holmes (1809–1894), a graduate of Harvard, also fought to eliminate childbed fever. Holmes, who abandoned the study of law for medicine, in 1829 wrote the essay, "The Contagiousness of Puerperal Fever," now considered a medical classic. This work was published five years before the research of Semmelweis became known and was bitterly attacked by the medical community. Like Semmelweis's theory, Holmes's idea regarding the cause of puerperal fever was correct. He republished the essay in 1855 with an introduction that criticized what he thought were unjust remarks. Gradually the cause of the disease as identified by both Holmes and Semmelweis was accepted.

The plight of the child in this time was vividly depicted by the extremely talented British painter and engraver William Hogarth (1697–1764). Hogarth criticized the social problems of his day, which were present in a world craving the pleasures of life. His pic-

GIN LANE.

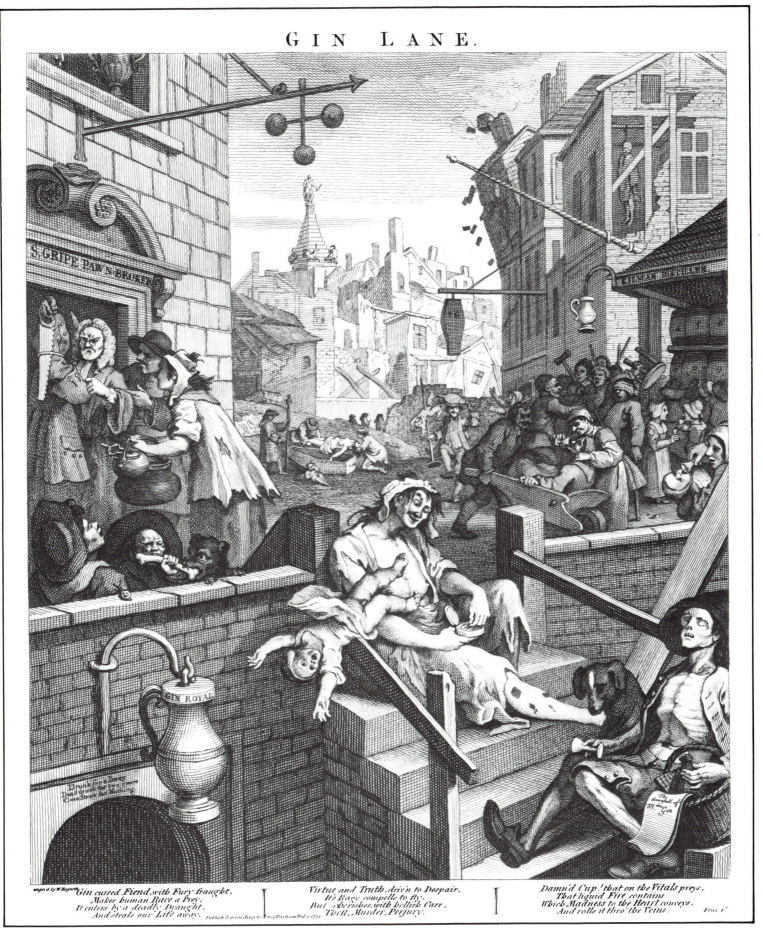

Gin cursed Fiend, with Fury fraught.
Makes human Race a Prey;
It enters by a deadly Draught,
And steals our Life away.

Virtue and Truth, driv'n to Despair.
It's Rage compells to fly.
But cherishes with hellish Care,
Theft, Murder, Perjury.

Damn'd Cup! that on the Vitals preys.
That liquid Fire contains
Which Madness to the Heart conveys.
And rolls it thro' the Veins.

William Hogarth, GIN LANE, c. 1750. Engraving. British Museum, London, England.

tures were stories of the frailties of human nature, usually displayed in a scene of horrible devastation. In the *Works of Charles Lamb,* a section entitled "On the Genius and Character of Hogarth" explains the extraordinary gift of this artist with the observation that most "pictures are looked at—his prints we read" (Lamb, vol. 1, 1818, p. 70).

The abandoned child had become a serious problem in the eighteenth century. There was public callousness and indifference to the practice of extensive infanticide. This attitude needed to be changed before strides could be made to reduce infant mortality. Evidence was also available that demonstrated infant death from neglect, cruelty, and illness.

> The exact statistics are not available, but in the early part of the century, the infant mortality rate for children under five years of age was 50 per cent. In London between 1730 and 1750, 75 per cent of all the babies christened were dead before the age of five. Of 10,272 infants admitted to the Dublin Foundling Hospital during 21 years (1775–1796) only 45 survived, a mortality of 99.6 per cent. Many famous foundling hospitals of the period had similar records. Even Queen Anne, who presumably received the best of care, lost 18 children in early infancy.
>
> *Dolan, Fitzpatrick, and Hermann, 1983, pp. 111–112*

The infant death rate was also caused by factors other than neglect and cruelty. These included *headmouldshot,* the overriding of the sutures of the cranium; *horseshoehead,* the separation of the sutures usually associated with congenital cranial defects; and *overlying,* the practice of nurses sleeping with infants. In addition, wet

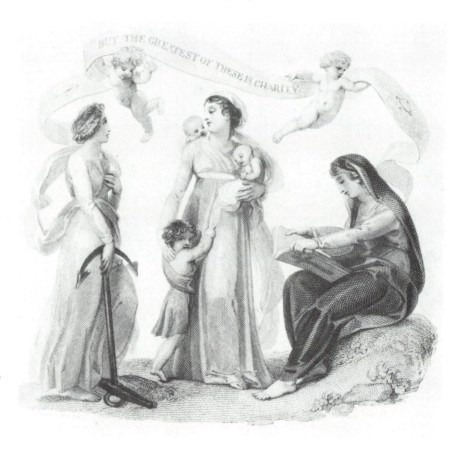

Designed by Thomas Stothard, R.A., HOSPITAL FOR THE MAINTENANCE AND EDUCATION OF EXPOSED AND DESERTED YOUNG CHILDREN, *1809. Engraving. British Museum, London, England.*

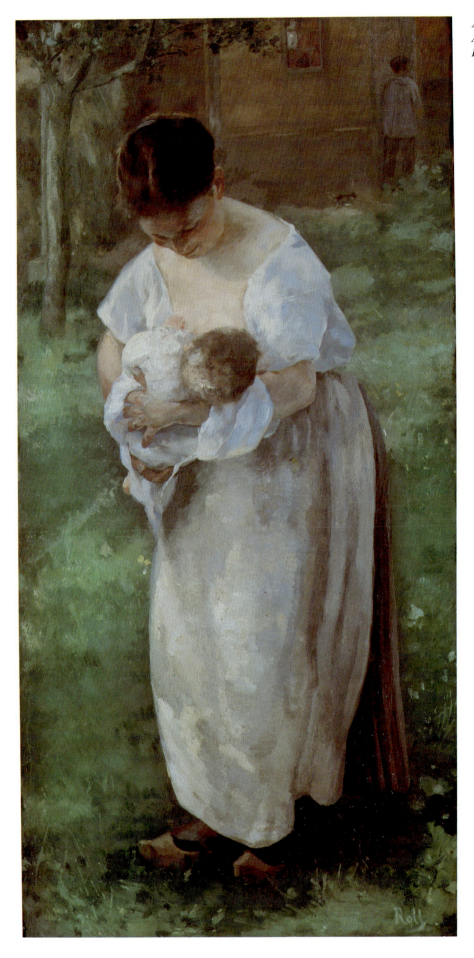

Alfred Roll, THE WET NURSE. *The Bridgeman Art Library Ltd./Musée des Beaux Arts, Lille, France.*

nurses were frequently hired and they sometimes transferred disease to the child. Just as there were nurses who infected their sucklings, there were also infants who infected their nurses (Robinson, 1946). Bottle feeding, too, was a potential contributor to infant death through the contraction of disease from contaminated milk and water. Another cause of infant death was the common occurrence of "dropping," the practice of abandoning the infant on doorsteps of wealthy homes or simply leaving them to freeze or starve in the street. Finally, infanticide continued into the nineteenth century.

As in most complex social movements, it is difficult to establish all the reasons for improvement in the infant death rate. However, this improvement was in no small part a result of the efforts of several

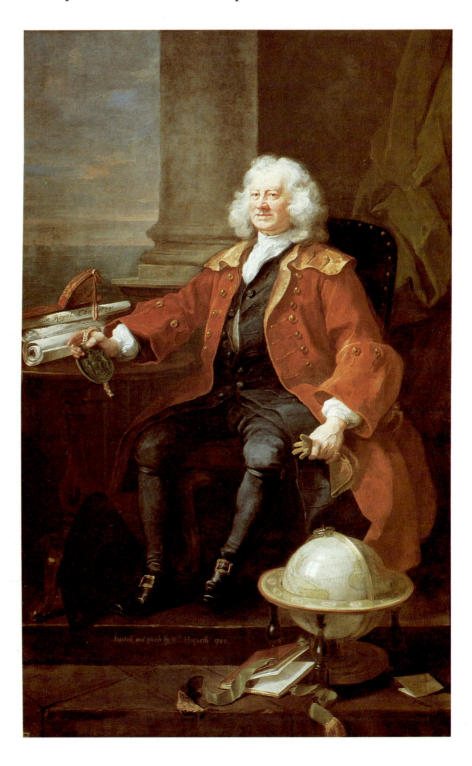

William Hogarth, CAPTAIN CORAM, *1740. Canvas. Thomas Coram Foundation for Children, London, England.*

individuals who wished to alleviate the high infant mortality. Among these were Thomas Coram (1668–1751) of England, who labored to establish the Hospital for Foundlings in London (1738); Jonas Hanway (1712–1786), who was involved with the parish workhouse movement in England and persuaded Parliament to enact laws for relief of infants of the poor; George Armstrong (?–1781), one of the first English pediatricians, who was a staunch advocate of infant welfare and the prime leader in the dispensary movement that culminated in the establishment of the Dispensary for the Infant Poor on April 24, 1769. Perhaps the most significant development was a work titled "An Essay upon Nursing and Management of Children," which appeared in London in 1750. It was written by William Cadogan (1711–1797), who became a physician to the Foundling Hospital after receiving master of arts, bachelor of medicine, and doctor of medicine degrees at Oxford. Cadogan was the first to write a simple, understandable book of instructions addressed to mothers about the care and feeding of infants and young children. Some might consider him the Doctor Spock of the era! A now familiar passage dealt with Cadogan's plea for maternal feeding:

> There would be no fear of offending the husband's ears with the noise of the squalling brat. The child was it nurs'd in this way would be always quiet, in good humour, ever playing laughing or sleeping. In my opinion a man of sense cannot have a prettier rattle (for rattles he must have of one kind or another) than such a young child. I am quite at a loss to account for the general practice of sending infants out of doors to be suckled or dry-nursed by another woman, who had not so much understanding, nor can have so much affection for it as the parents: and how it comes to pass that people of good sense and easy circumstances will not give themselves the pains to watch over the health and welfare of their children: but are so careless as to give them up to the common methods, without considering how near

Designed by Thomas Stothard, R.A., THE WORK OF CHARITY SCHOOLS, CHILDREN RESCUED FROM WANT AND MISERY, TO BE CLAD AND EDUCATED, *c. 1790. Engraving. British Museum, London, England.*

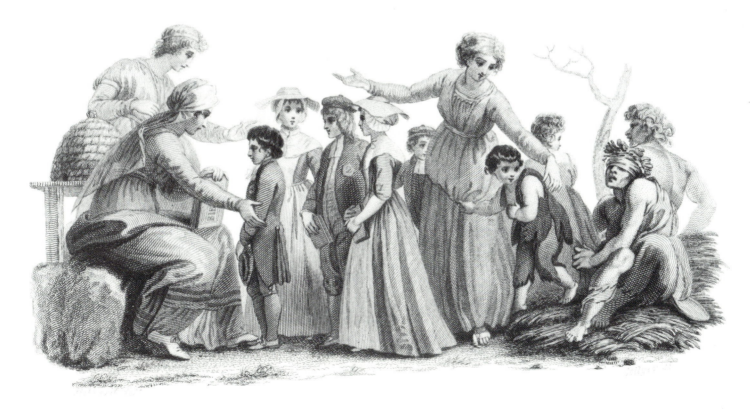

it is to an equal chance that they are destroyed by them. The ancient custom of exposing them to wild beasts or drowning them would certainly be a much quicker and more humane way of despatching them.

Quoted in Robinson, 1946, p. 83

Cadogan was an apostle of maternal breast feeding; no other woman's milk was good enough for the child. He also stressed daily baths for infants, loose clothing, and frequent changes of clothing.

Disease Epidemics

Epidemics continued to ravage Europe from the sixteenth through the nineteenth centuries. Devastating outbreaks of typhus and bubonic plague occurred and reduced the masses of the population to a pitiful state. These plagues were particularly ravaging because of the social decay that had resulted from urban industrialism. The epidemics of this early modern period forced physicians to accept a realistic view of medicine. Advances in medical knowledge and sanitation were frequently offset by the health hazards that existed in the large cities.

Jean-Honoré Fragonard, THE VISIT TO THE NURSERY, before 1784. Canvas, approx. 73.7 × 92.1 cm. National Gallery of Art, Washington, D.C., Samuel H. Kress Collection 1946.

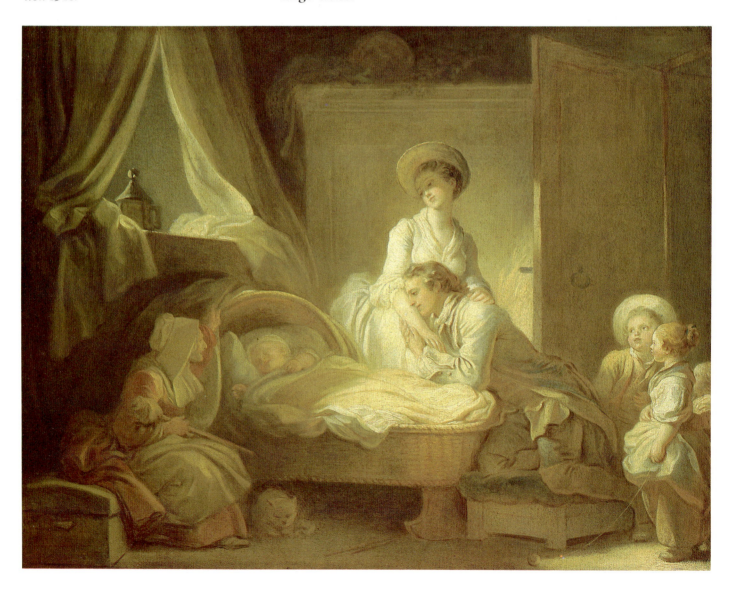

It is clear that health conditions were probably no better or worse than those that had existed in previous centuries. Yet urban living conditions facilitated the precipitation of diseases: sanitation was poor, sanitary facilities were lacking, sewage disposal was inadequate, cities were filthy, public health laws were lacking, water supplies were impure, and dirt and congestion inevitably brought pests such as rats, lice, and bedbugs, which carried infection. Congestion had increased, but its implications for health had been ignored. Epidemics of typhus were evidently spread to the European nations through foreign trade. Dark rooms served to increase the rate of tuberculosis. Since the value of fresh air was not understood, doors and windows were closed when someone was ill. Windows in hospitals and homes were frequently blocked up or bricked over for economical reasons.

Approximately one third of the population of London died in the plagues that swept England in 1603 and 1625. Other diseases were equally destructive: typhus caused a large proportion of deaths in the eighteenth century; smallpox was responsible for the death or disfigurement of one out of every ten people in Europe. Conditions resulting from smallpox were even worse in new settlements, where immigrants carried the infection to natives. At one point Cotton Mather wrote that nine of ten, "nay 99 out of 100," of the Indians perished from smallpox. Cholera epidemics occurred frequently and with the greatest severity in the slum areas. During the nineteenth century major outbreaks of this disease occurred in 1832, 1849, and 1866.

The home of the person who contracted plague was boarded up, and the well members of the family became prisoners of the house and the disease. The imprisonment usually lasted at least a month after all trace of the disease had disappeared. The plague physician wore an elaborate dress—a long red or black leather gown, leather gauntlets, a mask with glass-covered openings for the eyes, and a long beak filled with fumigants and antiseptics. He carried a container of sweet-smelling spices, a meagre attempt to thwart the stench in the air. Fires were burned continuously in the streets to help purify the air. The dead were buried at night, usually with great precautions.

The spread of syphilis became so far-reaching that it could truly be called one of the great plagues. Although it was differentiated from epidemic diseases by the close of the fifteenth century, it was thought to be spread in the same manner, through proximity to an infected person. At first the sexual nature of this disease was unknown and no social stigma existed. Social attitudes changed very rapidly, however, as people became aware that syphilis was transferred through sexual relations. Secrecy was common among those who had contracted the disease and led to the foregoing of treatment and the spread of the disease through marriage. At this time barber surgeons treated syphilitic sores with salves that contained mercury; this treatment was extremely painful.

Urban life, trade, and industrialism contributed to the overwhelming health hazards that existed during these centuries. The situation was confounded by the lack of an adequate means of social control. Reforms were desparately needed. Eventually the organization of physicians, hospitals, and public health activities arose from the alterations brought about by the industrial revolution.

■ HOSPITALS AND REFORMERS

The Reformation brought about the widespread movement toward suppression of monasteries that was led by Martin Luther and Henry VIII. The immediate result of monastic dissolution was that established hospitals and inns were taken away from the public, who had been dependent on them for many years. This was followed by a period of rapid deterioration in the care of the sick and the poor. A decline in the quality of public service, particularly for the sick, thus occurred and created a long period of stagnation and decay. As wars were waged for religious opinion, the sick and the poor were being neglected. The unselfish devotion of the religious orders was no longer available in Protestant countries, where these orders had been oppressed. In this age of callousness and brutality, neither officials nor physicians took any particular interest in elevating nursing or in improving the conditions of hospitals.

Hospital Decay

After the Protestant Revolt, charitable activities were usually divided along religious lines or delegated to secular authorities. The religious struggles had no direct effect on hospitals in Catholic lands such as Spain and Italy. Many small institutions, however, were closed in Protestant countries when the nursing orders were suppressed, and this led to either the necessity for modifications in the large city establishments or the development of city hospitals. Severe utility replaced the beauty that previously had been associated with institutions for the sick.

> The hospitals of cities were like prisons, with bare, undecorated walls and little dark rooms, small windows where no sun could enter, and dismal wards where fifty or one hundred patients were crowded together, deprived of all comforts and even of necessaries. In the municipal and state institutions of this period the beautiful gardens, roomy halls, and springs of water of the old cloister hospital of the Middle Ages were not heard of, still less the comforts of their friendly interiors.
>
> *Nutting and Dock, 1937, p. 500*

Unsanitary conditions that prevailed in these hospitals led to outbreaks of epidemics. Diseases were seldom segregated. "It was not uncommon for the sick to be thrown into beds already occupied by several bedfellows—the dead or the delirious, side by side, perhaps, with those who still lived and retained their reason" (Jamieson and Sewall, 1950, pp. 268–269). Beds were so close together that cleaning was almost impossible. Consequently, all types of rubbish remained under them. Bed baths were not attempted; bleeding and purging were the usual treatments for all conditions. Mismanagement, inadequate staffing, and exploitation were common occurrences within these facilities. Men who were civil appointees assumed leadership and withheld authority from the women (matrons), who were placed in charge of the secular help doing the "nursing" of the day. Control of nursing was thereby lost by women. This was truly a period of the most complete and general masculine supremacy in the

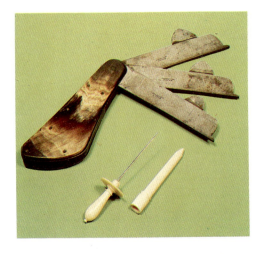

BLEEDING KNIFE AND LANCING PIN, *c. 1790.*
The Bridgeman Art Library Ltd./Private Collection.

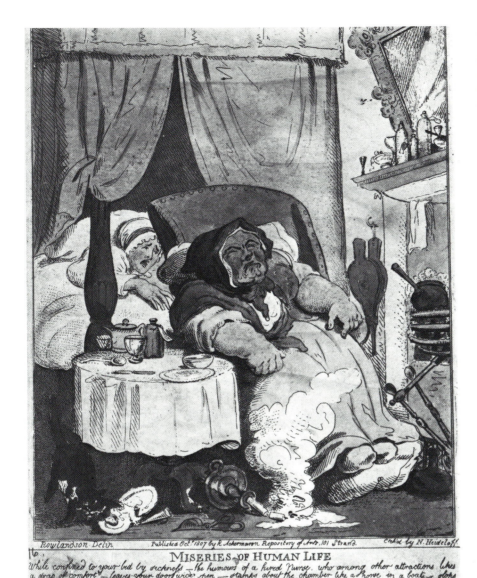

After Thomas Rowlandson, WHILE CONFINED TO YOUR BED BY A SICKNESS: THE HUMOURS OF A HIRED NURSE, *c. 1807. Hand colored etching. From Rowlandson's* MISERIES OF HUMAN LIFE. *National Library of Medicine, Bethesda, Maryland.*

history of nursing. Women were without a voice in both hospital management and nursing organization. In addition, the typical nurses were usually the dregs of society, those individuals who were immoral, drunken, and illiterate. The actual squalor of the times is evident in a portion of the regulations (1789) of the Royal Hospital at Haslar, which were hung in the wards:

III. That no dirt, bones, or rags, be thrown out of any window, or down the bogs, but carried to the places appointed for that purpose; nor are any clothes of the patients, or others, to be hung out of any of the windows of the house.

IV. That no foul linen, whether sheets or shirts, be kept in the cabins, or wards, but sent immediately to the matron, in order to its being carried to the wash-house; and the nurses are to obey the orders of the matron in punctually shifting the bed and body linen of the patients, *viz.* their sheets once a fortnight, their shirts once in four days, their nightcaps, drawers, and stockings once a week, or oftener if found necessary.

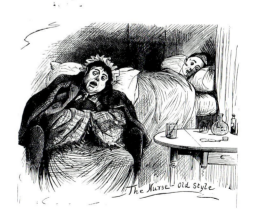

THE NURSE OLD STYLE, *c. 1879. Cartoon illustrating the drunken nurse dozing at the bedside of an alarmed patient. The Mansell Collection, London, England.*

213

V. That no nurse or other person do wash in the water closets. . . .

VIII. That no nurse do admit any patients, on any pretense whatsoever, into her cabin, nor suffer any person to remain in it at night, not even her husband or child.

IX. That any person concealing the escape of any patient from her ward, or that has not made due report, at the agent's office, of her having missed such patient, be discharged the hospital, upon proof thereof.

X. That all nurses who disobey the matron's orders, get drunk, neglect their patients, quarrel or fight with any other nurses, or quarrel with the men, or do not prudently or cautiously reveal, to the superior officers of the house, all irregularities committed by the patients in their wards (such as drinking, smoking tobacco in the wards, quarrelling, destroying the medicines, or stores, feigning complaints and neglecting their cure) be immediately discharged the service of the house, and a note made against their names, on the books of the hospital, that they may never more be employed.

Howard, 1791, pp. 180–182

The English Scene

The most serious consequences in health care occurred in England. It must be remembered, however, that an inward and religious revolution had taken place in England, especially in London, long before Henry VIII legalized its outward and visible form. Many people were ready for the break with Rome, the divorce between Henry and Catherine, and the suppression of the monasteries. This sovereign used the Protestant Revolt to free himself from papal authority with the excuse of the Church's refusal to sanction his divorce. An ulterior motive was based in the fact that monastic properties represented one fifth of his kingdom. Henry VIII suppressed all orders and confiscated the property of over 600 charitable endowments. Many of these had been devoted to beggars, orphans, the elderly, and the poor as well as to those who were acutely ill. Eventually the civil government was forced to take over the general public relief, and this culminated in a "Poor Law" system developed during the reign of Elizabeth.

All the London hospitals were closed in two waves, the smaller ones in 1538 and the larger ones (income over £200 per annum) in 1540. The fate of the larger English hospitals was particularly important, since they essentially limited their work to the care of the sick. Decisions about their outcome ultimately affected the future of both medicine and nursing. The effect was immediate because "England alone among European countries possessed no hospital system" (Evans and Howard, 1930, p. 69). It was not long before the citizens begged that hospitals be given to the city to be financed and run by civil authorities. In 1547 the city of London petitioned Henry VIII's son, Edward VI, who reigned from 1547 to 1553, for permission to take over the largest hospitals—St. Bartholomew's, St. Thomas's, Bridewell, Bethlehem, and Christ's.

The city arranged to govern these hospitals through a "court" of governors, undertook to add to their endowments, maintained them through private subscription and "rates" (taxes), and assigned to each a specific responsibility for the solution of one social problem. St. Bartholomew's and St. Thomas's hospitals were to care for the sick poor; Bridewell, the unemployed; Bethlehem, the insane; and Christ's, the orphans. With the passage of time the individual functions changed. St. Bartholomew's and St. Thomas's hospitals progressed toward the cure aspect of the general hospital as opposed to the medieval custody function. Bridewell became a workhouse and a house of correction. Bethlehem became known as "Bedlam," since knowledge regarding the treatment of the insane was lacking. Christ's Hospital became one of the leading schools of England. Such was the beginning of the civilian control of hospitals and the advent of lay nursing in England. Care of the sick in these institutions gradually deteriorated for about 300 years, since England possessed no nursing class. Other Protestant countries followed trends similar to those in England with reorganization of city hospitals.

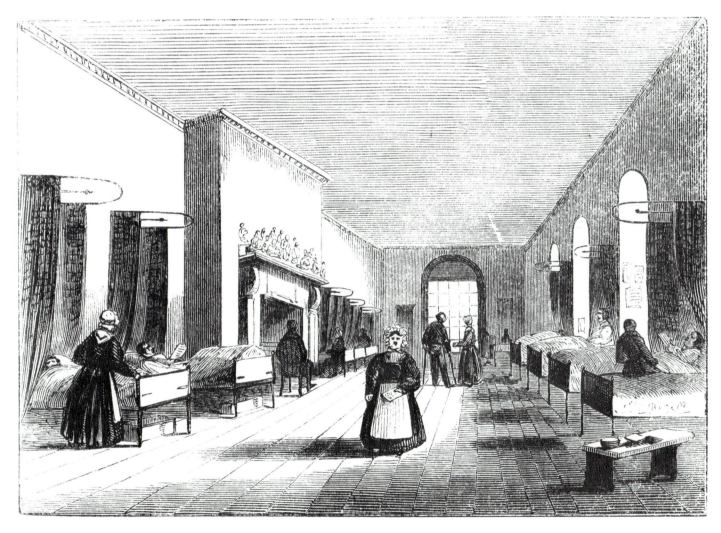

W.A. Delamotte, RAHERE'S WARD, *1844. Drawing. St. Bartholomew's Hospital, London, England.*

This picture has unfortunately been labeled a "Gamp" type nurse simply because she wears the usual dress of her class at that period. The Dickens character Sairey Gamp was a monthly nurse who attended the sick in their homes and whilst hospitals, by no means excluding this one, undoubtedly had many nurses who were uncaring gin-swillers, it is recorded that the Sister of Rahere Ward at the time of this picture was: "stout, ruddy, positive and very watchful . . . she could report correctly the progress of a case; and from her wages she saved all she could and left it in legacy to the hospital." St. Bartholomew's Hospital, London, England.

215

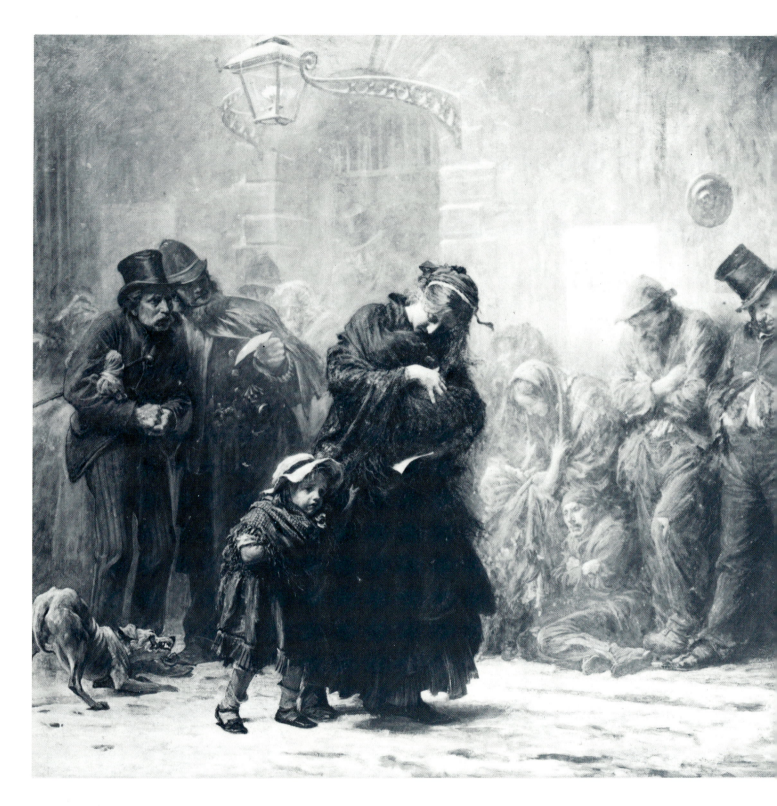

Religious Nursing Orders

The sixteenth century also saw renewed activity in nursing within the Church itself. Various religious orders devoted to this cause originated in this period. More than 100 female orders were founded specifically to do nursing. In fact, orders multiplied so rapidly and some had so little permanence that information about them is unavailable. Most prominent among these was an order of men, the Brothers of St. John of God, or the Brothers of Mercy. The name was derived from the inscription on their almsboxes: "Brothers, do good"

216

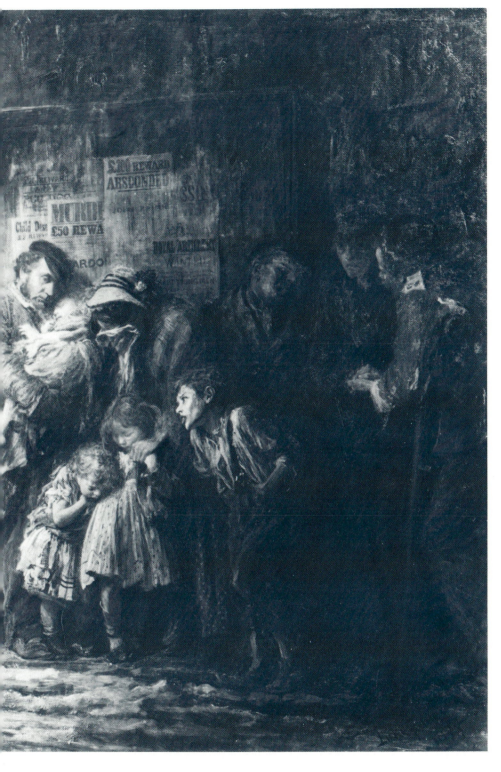

Samuel Luke Fildes, APPLICANTS FOR ADMIS-
SION TO A CASUAL WARD, *1874. Canvas.
Royal Holloway College, London, England.*

("Fate bene, fratelli"). This order was founded in Spain in 1538 by a
Portuguese, Jean Ciudad (1495–1550), known as John of God (Juan
di Dios). After spending 18 years as a soldier, he vowed to devote his
life to God if he recovered from a wound received in battle. In 1540
John opened a hospital in Granada and invited a group of friends to
assist with the nursing care. At first these Brothers were laymen, not
monks, and they worked without a rule until 1570. They were mendicants who devoted themselves to nursing, hospital work, the distribution of medicines, the tender care of the mentally ill, abandoned
children, and the visitation of the sick at home. Those in need were

cared for in a very loving and special way. Homeless vagrants, the crippled, and even derelicts received devoted nursing service. It is said that St. John himself carried on his back the deformed who were unable to walk or crawl to the hospital. The Brothers of St. John eventually opened hospitals at Madrid, Cordova, Toledo, Naples, and Paris. This order spread over a large part of the civilized world within 50 years of its founding. Its members were probably the best known nursing Brothers (baumherzigen Bruder) in Catholic Germany by the eighteenth century. Paintings of Juan di Dios frequently show wards of a hospital in the background.

Another notable nursing order of men, the Nursing Order of Ministers of the Sick, was founded by St. Camillus De Lellis (1550–1614). This Italian order did hospital work and specially cared for those stricken with the plague in Rome in 1590. Conflicting information exists regarding the early life of St. Camillus. What is important, however, is that a series of illnesses that necessitated his hospitalization stirred him to devote himself to the care of the sick. The members of his order, popularly known as the Camillian Fathers and

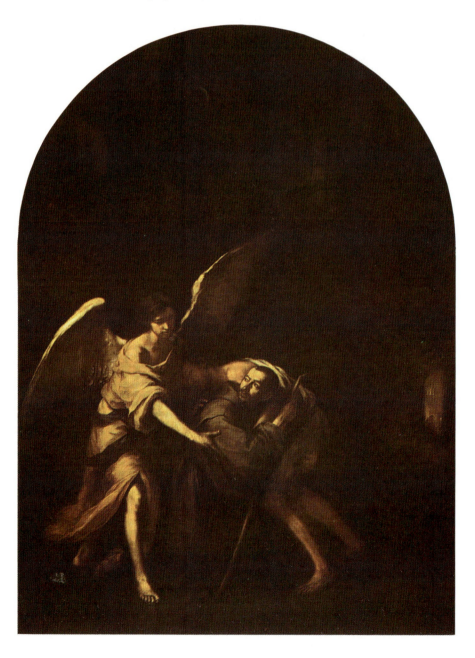

Bartolomé Esteban Murillo, ST. JOHN OF GOD CARRYING THE SICK TO THE HOSPITAL, *c. 1670. Canvas. Hospital de la Caridad, Sevilla, Spain.*

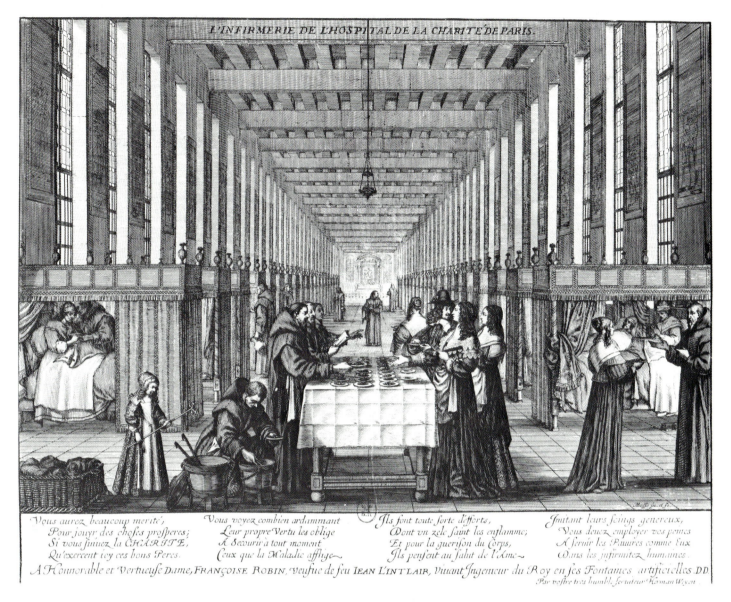

L'INFIRMERIE DE L'HOSPITAL DE LA CHARITE DE PARIS.

Vous aurez beaucoup merité,
Pour jouyr des choses prosperes;
Si vous suiuez la CHARITE,
Qu'exercent icy ces bons Peres.

Vous voyez combien ardammant
Leur propre Vertu les oblige
A Secourir a tout moment
Ceux que la Maladie afflige

Ils font toute sorte d'efforts,
Dont vn zele saint les enflamme;
Et pour la guerison du Corps,
Ils pensent au salut de l'Ame

Imitant leurs soings genereux,
Vous deuez employer vos peines
A seruir les Pauures comme Eux
Dans les infirmitez humaines.

A Honnorable et Vertueuse Dame, FRANÇOISE ROBIN, Veufue de feu IEAN L'INTLAIR, Viuant Ingenieur du Roy en ses Fontaines artificielles. DD.
Par vostre tres humbl. seruateur Herman Weyen.

Brothers, took the three regular vows plus a fourth, a pledge to the work of nursing. They wore a red cross on their cassocks.

Perhaps the most interesting of these later organizations and one that has maintained importance until the present day is the Sisters of Charity founded by St. Vincent de Paul (1576–1660). This order developed at a time when destitution and disease from continual wars were overcoming France. Political unrest was also very great. St. Vincent offered solutions to these problems that were both revolutionary and visionary. He was a quiet, unassuming French Catholic priest (Franciscan) whose experiences in his earlier life prepared him to assist with the sufferings of humanity. Of particular note was his capture by Barbary pirates and his sale as a slave to the Turks. St. Vincent described this experience in a personal letter:

> This is how they set about disposing of us. After having stripped us naked, they bestowed on each of us a pair of breeches, a linen doublet and a cap, and marched us through the streets of Tunis, whither they had come in order to sell us. After having perambulated the town five or six times with chains round our necks, we were taken back to the boat for the dealers to come and see who could eat and who could not, by way

Abraham Bosse, ANNE OF AUSTRIA VISITING THE INFIRMARY OF THE CHARITY HOSPITAL IN PARIS, *c. 1635. Etching, 22.2 × 32.1 cm. Philadelphia Museum of Art: SmithKline Beckman Corporation Fund.*

of proving that our wounds were not mortal. When this was over they led us into the marketplace, where the dealers came and inspected us precisely as one does when one is buying a horse or an ox, opening our mouths to examine our teeth, feeling our sides, probing our wounds, making us walk, trot and run, carrying burdens the while, then setting us to wrestle in order to judge of our respective strength, and indulging in hundreds of other brutal proceedings.

Quoted in Robinson, 1946, p. 63

Eventually, St. Vincent was able to return to Paris, where he was appalled at the conditions of the poor and the sick poor in such a large town. He began to assist the Brothers of St. John of God with the care of patients in the Charité Hospital in Paris. His interests soon, however, reached out into provincial communities, and in 1617 he moved to the country parish of Châtillon-en-Bresse. Here St. Vincent was asked to appeal on behalf of a destitute family, and he became distressed at the indiscriminate relief that was called forth. The family was inundated by well-meaning individuals. This event vividly demonstrated charity's waste from lack of control. It proved to be the motivating force for St. Vincent's institution of a society of ladies called the Confrérie de la Charité (Dames de Charité), whose members visited the sick in their homes to render both nursing care and spiritual consolation. This was the first society for organized aid in which a service was offered to as many people as possible, with a

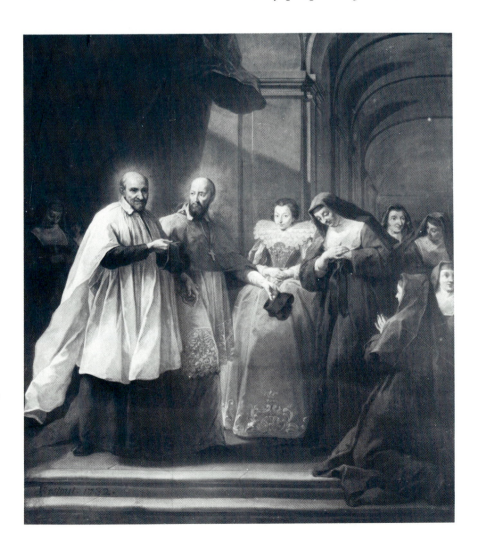

Jean Restout II, ST. VINCENT DE PAUL APPOINTED AS ALMONER TO THE SISTERS OF THE VISITATION, *c. 1729. Church of Saint-Marguerite, Paris, France. (Photographie Bulloz)*

St. Vincent was instrumental in reforms for the poor and hospital reforms. Groups of men and women who formed under his counsel constituted the first societies for organized charity.

220

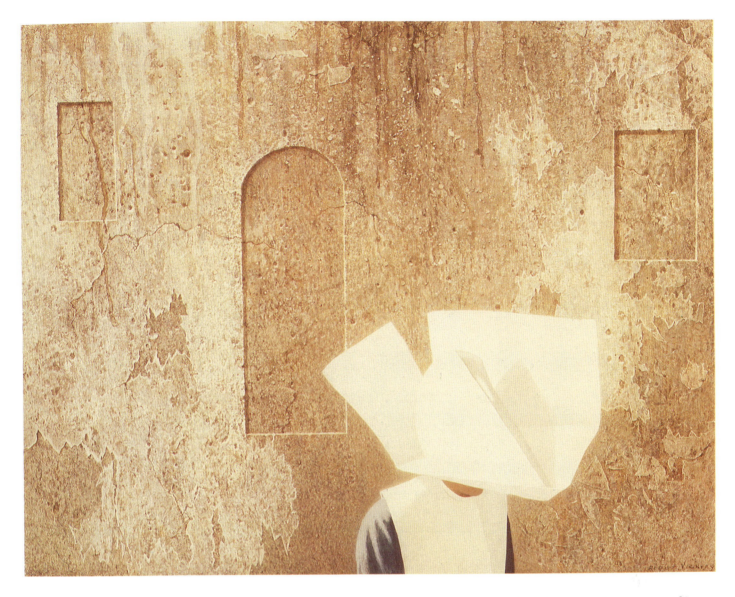

Robert Vickrey, SISTER OF CHARITY, 1965. Tempera. I.B.M. Corporation with concurrence of ACA Gallery, New York.

The Sisters of Charity were organized by St. Vincent de Paul and were perhaps the most widespread and best loved of all nursing orders. They took charge of hospitals, the poor, asylums, and parish work. They became widely known as visiting nurses, since they also cared for the poor and the sick in their homes.

minimum of duplication. The membership of eleven women took no vows or made any kind of promises. From this simple beginning, associations arose in numerous towns and villages. At first, all the branches were composed of women, but later a branch for men was founded at Folleville. The extension of services into homes in the centuries that followed St. Vincent became a regular feature of the work of certain communities. Sympathy for the poor was combined with a genius for organized reform and led to a system of social service, a method to help people help themselves.

Mlle. Le Gras (1591–1660) became the first supervisor of these community nurses. St. Louise de Marillac, as she was later known, was a woman of noble birth and a widow when she became associated with the work of St. Vincent. In 1629 and 1631 she was sent on a tour of the provincial associations to investigate their work and assist them with improvements in their care. A secular nursing order called Les Filles de Charité, or the Sisters of Charity, was founded in 1633, and St. Louise became its superior. The Filles were initially under no written rule but merely followed a few regulations that had been drawn up by Mlle. Le Gras. Young single girls were recruited; they were required to be intelligent, refined, and sincerely interested in

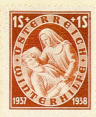

A semi-postal emission from Austria in 1937 consisted of four denominations each with a surcharge for charitable purposes. Included were stamps depicting nurse and infant, nursing of the aged and the illustrated value showing a Sister of Mercy with patient. Courtesy of Howard B. Hurley.

Nicaragua's 1963 issue of a three-stamp set marked the 300th anniversary (in 1960) of the deaths of St. Vincent de Paul and St. Luisa de Marillac. Known as "the nurse of the poor," St. Luisa de Marillac was founder of the Sisters of Charity of St. Vincent de Paul. This nurse was canonized in 1934. Courtesy of Howard B. Hurley.

the sick poor. An educational program was established to include experience in the hospital, home visits, and care of the sick. Such was the modest and humble beginning of the now famous Sisters of Charity. (They, perhaps, should be called Daughters of Charity, since St. Vincent always referred to them as "Filles.")

On March 25, 1634, approximately one year after this community was formed, St. Louise formally took a vow to devote herself to this life. She thus became the first Sister of Charity of St. Vincent de Paul. In the year 1642, the first four Sisters took vows that were, and still are, only annual. This order was a tremendous innovation because it was active yet uncloistered. (The Church insisted that consecrated virgins be cloistered.) St. Vincent was adamant in this regard and expressed his ideal quite eloquently:

> Their convent must be the houses of the sick; their cell the chamber of suffering; their chapel the parish church; their cloister the streets of the city or the wards of hospitals; in place of the rule which binds nuns to the one enclosure, there must be the general vow of obedience; the grating through which they speak to others must be the fear of God; the veil which shuts out the world must be holy modesty.
>
> *Nutting and Dock, 1937, p. 436*

The Sisters' spiritual training was in the hands of St. Vincent, who provided a weekly lecture conference. These talks were written down by St. Louise, and about 160 have been preserved. "They are a model of simplicity and clearness and remain the earliest as well as one of the best series of addresses on nursing ethics" (Seymer, 1932, p. 54). The organizational pattern of this order was composed of the following:

- ☐ A selected group, with set regulations restricting acceptance.
- ☐ A common home with experienced supervision.
- ☐ A system of instruction.
- ☐ A probation of two months followed by a training period of five years.
- ☐ Protection by the use of uniform dress of a type which would distinguish them from the people about them, and at the same time be secular.
- ☐ Annual renewal of vows, or freedom to leave for marriage or change of occupation.

Jamieson and Sewall, 1950, p. 323

The dress of the Sisters of Charity did indeed become distinctive—a gray-blue gown and apron of rough woolen cloth, a stiff white collar, and a white spreading headdress called a cornette. In 1809 the Sisters were introduced into America by Mother Elizabeth Seton (1774–1821), the first American-born person to be canonized. A community was established at Emmitsburg, Maryland, after the rule of the Motherhouse in France had been obtained. It was not until 1815 that Mother Mary Aikenhead organized a community in Dublin.

The work of the society was ever expanding into new fields. One important role was the development of special skills in caring for abandoned children. With the encouragement of St. Vincent, the

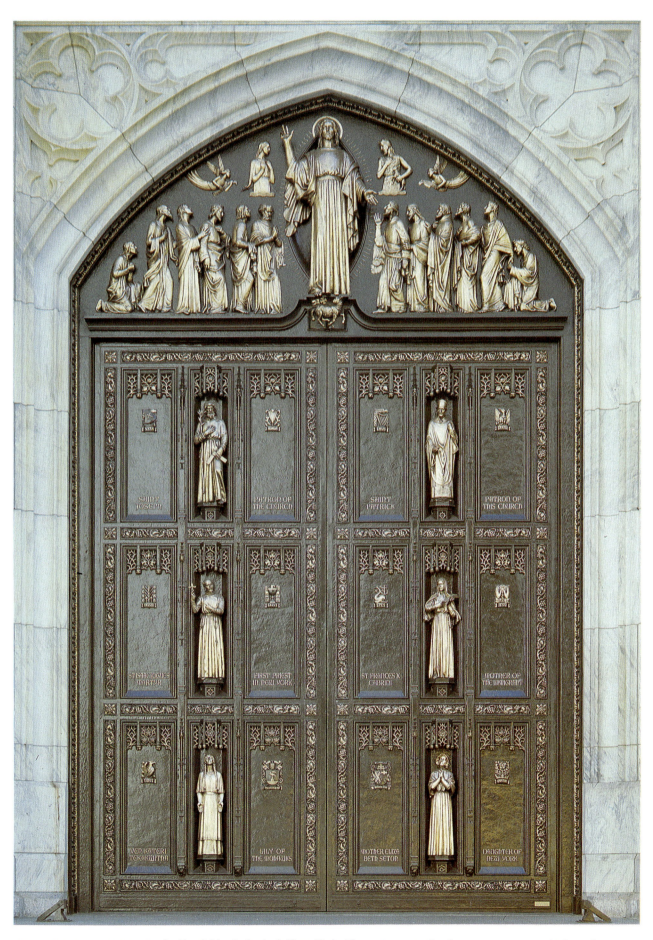

THE GREAT BRONZE DOORS. *St. Patrick's Cathedral, New York. The statues on the doors are: top row, St. Joseph and St. Patrick; middle row, St. Isaac Jogues and St. Frances X. Cabrini; lower row, Venerable Kateri Tekakwitha and St. Elizabeth Ann Seton.*

223

ST. VINCENT DE PAUL BEING SHOWN THREE SMALL CHILDREN, *eighteenth century. From a painting in the old Paris Foundling Asylum. Musée de l'Assistance Publique, Paris, France.*

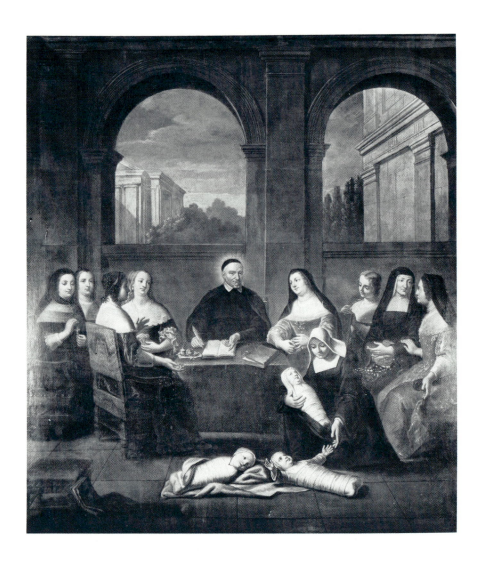

women went into action to save these doomed children. They wandered the dark streets and gathered the babies who had been thrown away. Unwanted infants were frequently brought to the Hospice des Enfants Trouvés et Orphelins, established by Vincent's disciples, where the Sisters of Charity served as nurses. This organized relief for the foundlings of Paris led to the portrayal of St. Vincent with orphans in his arms, wrapped in his cloak. The Sisters also took charge of hospitals, foundling asylums, and homes for the insane, and they engaged in general parish work. They taught in schools, gave heroic service during many wars, and offered care to lepers. The modern principles of visiting nursing and social service were sown during this time.

Humanitarian Efforts

The existence of actual deterioration in hospitals during this time is beyond dispute. A period of stagnation had set in, and little or no progress in the art of nursing was made, particularly in Protestant countries. There is evidence of the squalor of the hospitals and the inferiority of the attendants within them. The era of reform, however, was about to come. A number of humane individuals were stirred by the painful social conditions of the eighteenth century and began to labor for change. Of those reformers who lived before the nineteenth century, one of the best known was John Howard (1727–1789). Howard, an English philanthropist, spent his life and fortune examining and reporting on the conditions of prisons, dungeons, pest-houses, hospitals, and asylums. His series of investigations was probably the most powerful factor in the improvement of public institutions in this era. Howard's writings depicted the story of the degradation of often forgotten human beings. Although prisons and lazarettos were his chief concern, he left graphic notes of what he observed in hospitals. His reports on hospitals were the most authentic of the time and emphasized the necessity for fresh air and cleanliness. Howard's only praise was extended to the Sisters of Charity and the Beguines. His accounts were varied, sometimes limited to a few sentences and other times consisting of long commentaries, as in the case of the Knights of St. John's Hospital at Malta:

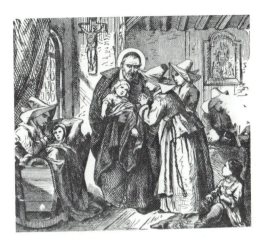

ST. VINCENT DE PAUL, *nineteenth century. Engraving. The Bettmann Archive, New York.*

> One ward is for patients dangerously sick or dying; another for patients of the middle rank of life; and the third for the lower and poorer sort of patients. In this last ward (which is the largest) there are four rows of beds; in the others, only two. They were all so dirty and offensive as to create the necessity of perfuming them; and yet I observed that the physician, in going his rounds, was obliged to keep his handkerchief to his face. . . .
>
> From the kitchen (which is darker and more offensive than even the lower hall, to which it adjoins) the broth, rice soup and vermicelli are brought in dirty kettles first to the upper hall, and there poured into three silver bowls, out of which the patients are served. . . .
>
> The number of patients in the hospital during the time I was in Malta (March 28th to April 19, 1786) was from five hundred and ten to five hundred and thirty-two. These were served by the most dirty, ragged, unfeeling and unhuman persons I ever saw. I once found eight or nine of them highly entertained with a delirious *dying* patient. The governor told me that they had only twenty-two servants, and that many of them were debtors or criminals, who had fled thither for refuge.
>
> *Howard, 1791, pp. 58–60*

The writings of John Howard were serious and had their effect. However, they penetrated society very slowly, and for another generation or two shameful conditions continued in both hospitals and nursing. Through Howard's efforts vast prison reforms ultimately occurred and conditions were vastly improved.

Interest in reform grew steadily, and the movement brought about many changes that influenced health care and nursing. Humanitarian leaders emerged and dwelt upon a sense of social responsibility for the welfare of others. One of these was the notable social reformer, Elizabeth Gurney Fry (1780–1845), who was closely identified with practical reforms and the revival of nursing. Elizabeth Gurney was a deeply religious Quaker who married Joseph Fry and settled in London. She was beautiful, a gifted speaker, and the mother of eleven children. She, too, gave conspicuous service in prison reform based on principles similar to those of John Howard. She visited Newgate Prison in 1813 and was appalled by the conditions and treatment of the incarcerated prisoners. Murderers, sex offenders, thieves, the mentally ill and retarded were all housed together in

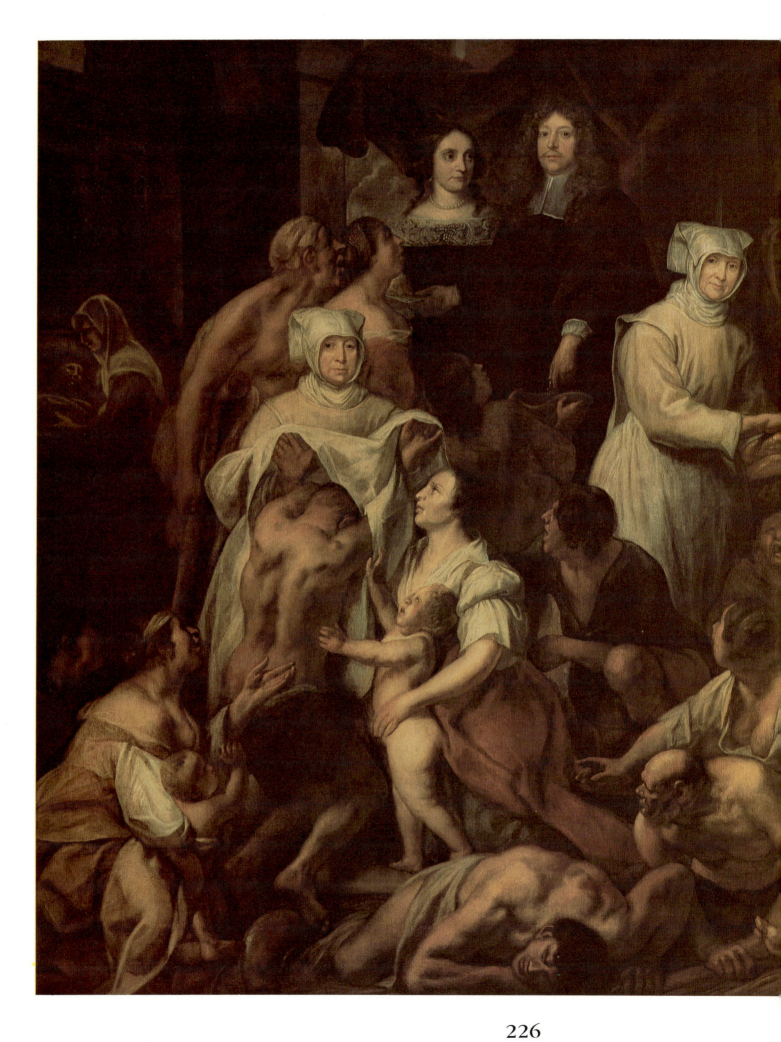

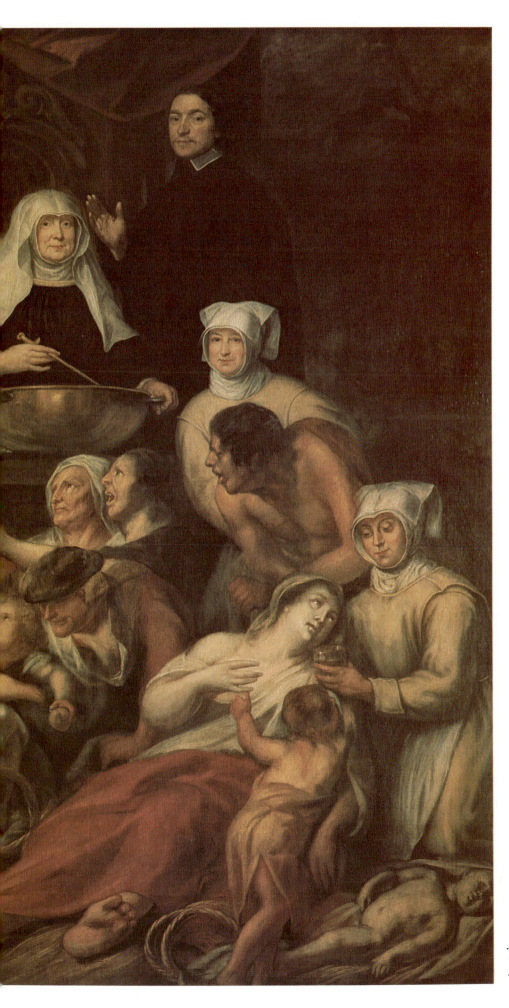

Jacob Jordeans, THE SISTERS OF CHARITY
OF ANTWERP, *c. 1635. Koninklijk Museum
Schone Kunsten, Antwerp, Belgium.*

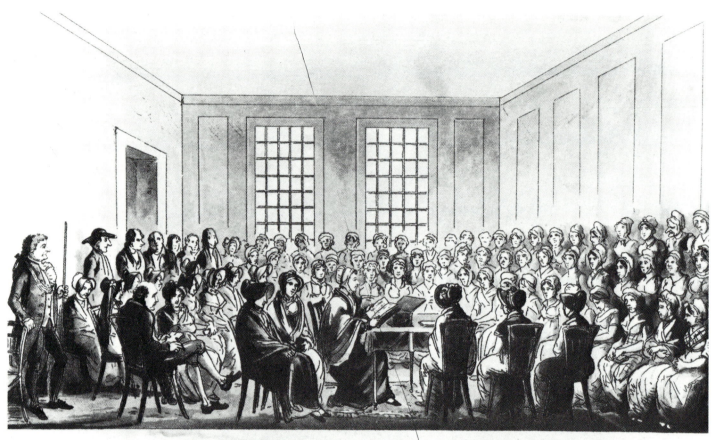

"AN HOUR IN NEWGATE" *Exhibiting M.rs FRY and her friends, as published by the* QUAKERS.

dark, damp, and poorly ventilated living quarters. Even children were inmates of this prison; they accompanied their parents if there were no relatives who could or would care for them. Such children were thus raised in an environment where there was a scant supply of food and little or no adequate clothing. Although the exterior of Newgate was beautiful, conditions within the walls were deplorable, as a description of the women's quarters illustrates:

> They occupied two long rooms, where they slept in three tiers, some on the floor and two tiers of hammocks over one another.... When I first entered, the foulness of the air was almost insupportable; and everything that is base and depraved was so strongly depicted on the faces of the women who stood crowded before me with looks of effrontery, boldness and wantonness of expression that for a while my soul was greatly dismayed.
>
> *Whitney, 1936, p. 193*

> The infirmary was not much better: On going up, I was astonished beyond description at the mass of woe and misery I beheld. I found many very sick, lying on the bare floor or on some old straw, having very scanty covering over them, though it was quite cold; and there were several children born in the prison among them, almost naked.
>
> *Whitney, 1936, p. 184*

In *David Copperfield* Charles Dickens vividly portrayed Newgate using humorous, pointed descriptions of the existing evils. Few who read his story realized that it was one of personal experience.

Dickens' father had been locked up in debtors' prison, where the entire family had resided until a fortunate legacy set them free. This novel brought the conditions of the English gaols to the attention of groups that may have ignored the reports of Mrs. Fry.

In 1817 Elizabeth Fry established an association for improving the lot of women prisoners in Newgate Prison. She began a program of instruction for the children, arranged for sewing rooms for the women, found books for those who wanted to read, and was instrumental in developing a prison shop where materials produced in the prison could be sold outside (income from the sales would go to the workers). In 1818 she visited other prisons in the British Isles and became known for her investigations of prison conditions and her attempts to arouse public opinion.

Mrs. Fry, who became widely known as a philanthropist, eventually founded a society for visiting nursing that had its origin in her prison work. This group of ardent workers was called the Society of Protestant Sisters of Charity (1840). They were not, however, affiliated with any church and later were known as the Institute of Nursing Sisters. The members were prepared for private nursing only, to nurse the sick of all classes in their homes. These women received no classroom or theoretical instruction; for several hours a day for a few months' period, they visited Guy's Hospital in London, where they obtained a minimum of practical experience. A similar organization was founded among the Quakers in Philadelphia at a later date.

Elizabeth Fry kept in close contact with other leaders of humane thought. Among these was Amalie Sieveking (1794–1859) of

ELIZABETH FRY READING TO THE PRISONERS IN NEWGATE PRISON, 1823, *nineteenth century. From an engraving after Jerry Barratt. Religious Society of Friends, London, England.*

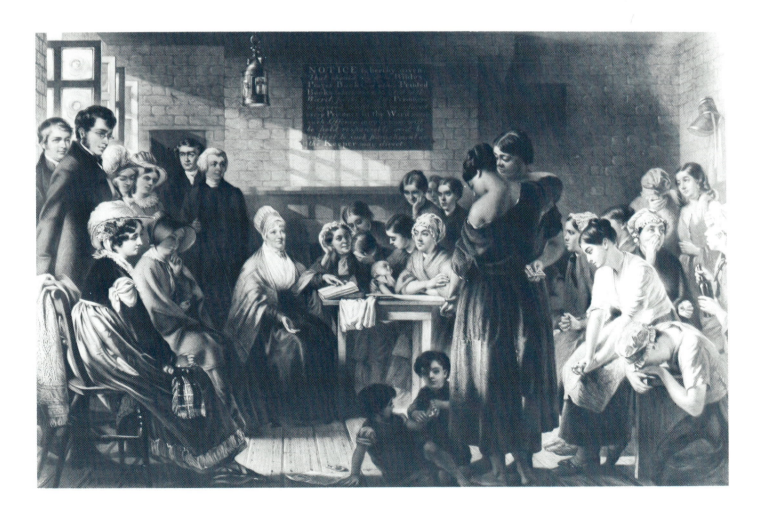

Hamburg, Germany, a well-known author who was prominent in the "women's movement." Amalie wished to develop a Protestant counterpart of the Sisters of Charity but was not successful. She therefore formed a group of volunteers, the Friends of the Poor, who visited the poor and the sick and gave nursing care in homes. Both men and women were originally included in this organization, and the women were called "nurses" rather than "deaconesses." Amalie was also interested in the establishment of better housing for low-income groups, distribution of food, finding employment for the disabled, and other types of social service for the poor. She enlisted the aid of women who were interested in a larger sphere of women's work outside the home. From this time, social work and nursing thus became closely connected to feminist movements.

More than a century later, the efforts of Dorothea Lynde Dix (1802–1887) on behalf of the insane in the United States were comparable to the work of Howard and Fry. She focused on two distinct problems: the care of the criminal and the care of the mentally ill. Dorothea Dix found that many of the prisoners were actually mentally ill and their treatment was negligible. Her efforts, begun at the age of thirty-nine, eventually earned her the title of "The John Howard of America." Her constructive work in surveying the needs of the mental patients and prisoners in Massachusetts led to the establishment of more than thirty psychiatric hospitals in the United States. One of these, Butler Hospital, was founded in Rhode Island with the backing of a wealthy and influential gentleman named Cyrus Butler.

The accomplishments of Dorothea Dix were many, including the construction of the first state psychiatric hospital in Trenton, New

Francisco Goya. THE MADHOUSE, *c. 1812–19. Canvas. Real Academia de Bellas Artes de San Fernando, Madrid, Spain.*

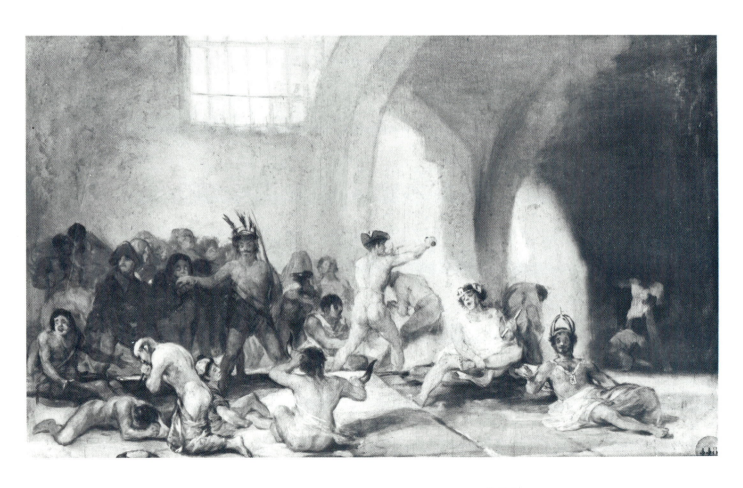

230

Jersey; the elevation of standards of care for the mentally ill in the United States and Canada; and the systematic and careful recording of observations to be presented to the legislature to elicit support for humane treatment of the mentally ill. Miss Dix had personally observed the incredible practices associated with these patients: some were confined in cages, closets, and cellars; other patients were chained and naked; and some were beaten into submission with rods or other implements. Her crusades continued for approximately twenty years and resulted in a system of mental hospitals under government control. Legal commitment based on medical diagnosis, abolition of restraints, and expertness of supervision provided the backbone of these institutions.

Dorothea Dix was the pioneer crusader for the mentally ill in the United States. Before her endeavors, few people realized that the mentally ill needed humane treatment or that they were classified by law as comparable to criminals. Frequently the mentally ill were used as entertainment for the public, who paid a fee to witness their antics. In some locations they were kept in almshouses or jails. The most unfortunate aspect of this situation was that mental illness was thought to be incurable. Consequently, incentives for reform were lacking, and efforts toward change were not understood. It thus took a persistent individual such as Miss Dix to initiate a movement to correct an unpardonable situation.

■ SOCIAL REFORMS AND NURSING

The great revival of learning left the care of the sick untouched and unimproved. This was probably because of the prevailing thought that nursing was a religious rather than an intellectual occupation. Therefore scientific improvement was not considered necessary. Yet the religious motive was lacking in the lay persons who were employed to care for the sick after the Reformation had occurred. Intelligent persons could not be persuaded to undertake nursing in the offensive municipal hospitals. Nursing slipped back into its ancient position of menial work, and the disagreeable features of nursing assumed prominence.

The latter half of the period between 1500 and 1860 AD saw nursing conditions at their worst. The "Dark Period of Nursing" had indeed arrived. In general, the lay attendants or nurses were illiterate, rough, and inconsiderate, oftentimes immoral, alcoholic. When a woman could no longer earn a living from gambling or vice, she might become a nurse. Nurses were drawn from among discharged patients, prisoners, and the lowest strata of society. They scrubbed, washed, cleaned, worked long hours (sometimes 24 to 48 hours at a stretch) and essentially led a life of drudgery. Roaches, other insects, and vermin plagued the nurses in the hospitals of this period. Pay for nurses was poor and was frequently supplemented in any way possible. The nurses expected and took bribes whenever they could be obtained. This deplorable status of nurses and nursing continued throughout this period. There was little organization associated with nursing and certainly no social standing. No one would enter nursing who could possibly earn a living in some other way. As nurses, even the Sisters of the religious orders came to a complete standstill professionally because of a persistent sequence of restrictions from the middle of the sixteenth century (Nutting and Dock, 1937).

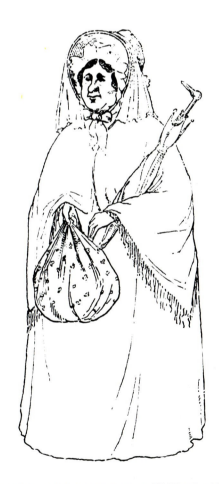

"SAIREY GAMP," A NURSE OF SIXTY YEARS AGO, *c. 1907. Illustration from the Wellcome Trustee's* PROFESSIONAL NURSES DIARY. *Wellcome Museum for the History of Medicine, London, England.*

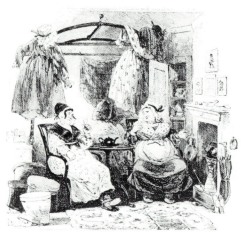

MRS. GAMP PROPOSES A TOAST. *From Charles Dickens'* MARTIN CHUZZLEWIT. *The Bettmann Archive, New York.*

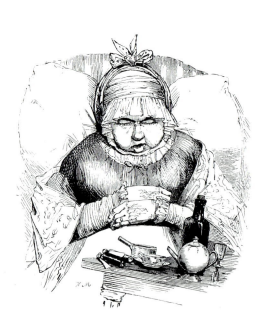

THE MONTHLY NURSE, *c. 1840. This illustration appeared around 1840 with the following passage from* TRISTRAM SHANDY: *"From the very moment the mistress of the house is brought to bed every female in it, from my lady's gentlewoman down to the cinderwench, becomes an inch taller for it." The Mansell Collection, London, England.*

The search into the social evils of the eighteenth century included an examination of nursing. Hogarth's cartoons and Charles Dickens' later descriptions of nurses were effective caricatures. In *Martin Chuzzlewit* (1844) Dickens depicted nursing conditions through the immortal characters of Sairey Gamp and Betsy Prig. Mrs. Gamp represented the hired attendant for the sick, the private duty nurse; Mrs. Prig portrayed the hospital nurse. Sairey Gamp was, in reality, not a fictitious character but an actual nurse Dickens' friend had hired for a member of his family. Both of these women cheated their employers, tricked their patients and stole their rations and possessions. They demanded that the patients pay for extra little services, and they were deliberately cruel to the sick who were at their mercy. In a later preface to the novel (November 1849), Dickens remarked:

> Mrs. Sarah Gamp is a representation of the hired attendant on the poor in sickness. The Hospitals of London are, in many respects, noble institutions; in others, very defective. I think it not the least among the instances of their mismanagement, that Mrs. Betsy Prig is a fair specimen of Hospital Nurse; and that the Hospitals, with their means and funds, should have left it to private humanity and enterprise, in the year Eighteen Hundred and Forty-nine, to enter on an attempt to improve that class of persons.
>
> *Dickens, 1910, p. xxviii*

Mrs. Gamp's first appearance in the novel occurred when she was summoned by Mr. Pecksniff to prepare the body of Anthony Chuzzlewit for burial:

> She was a fat old woman, this Mrs. Gamp, with a husky voice, and a moist eye, which she had a remarkable power of turning up and showing the white of it. Having very little neck, it cost her some trouble to look over herself, if one may say so, to those to whom she talked. She wore a very rusty black gown, rather the worse for snuff, and a shawl and bonnet to correspond. . . . The face of Mrs. Gamp—the nose in particular—was somewhat red and swollen, and it was difficult to enjoy her society without becoming conscious of a smell of spirits. Like most persons who have attained to great eminence in their profession, she took to hers very kindly; insomuch, that setting aside her natural predilections as a woman, she went to a lying-in or a laying-out with equal zest and relish.
>
> *Dickens, 1910, pp. 312–313*

Leigh Hunt, a contemporary of Dickens, also gave his version of the midwife specialist, which Sairey also professed to be. (Mrs. Gamp considered herself a monthly nurse, or, as her signboard boldly stated, "midwife.")

> Her greatest pleasure in life is, when lady and baby are both gone to sleep, the fire bright, the kettle boiling, and her corns quiescent. She then first takes a pinch of snuff, by way of pungent anticipation of bliss, or as a sort of concentrated essence of satisfaction; then a glass of spirits—then puts the water in the teapot—takes another glass of spirits (the last having been a small one, and the coming tea affording a "counteraction")—

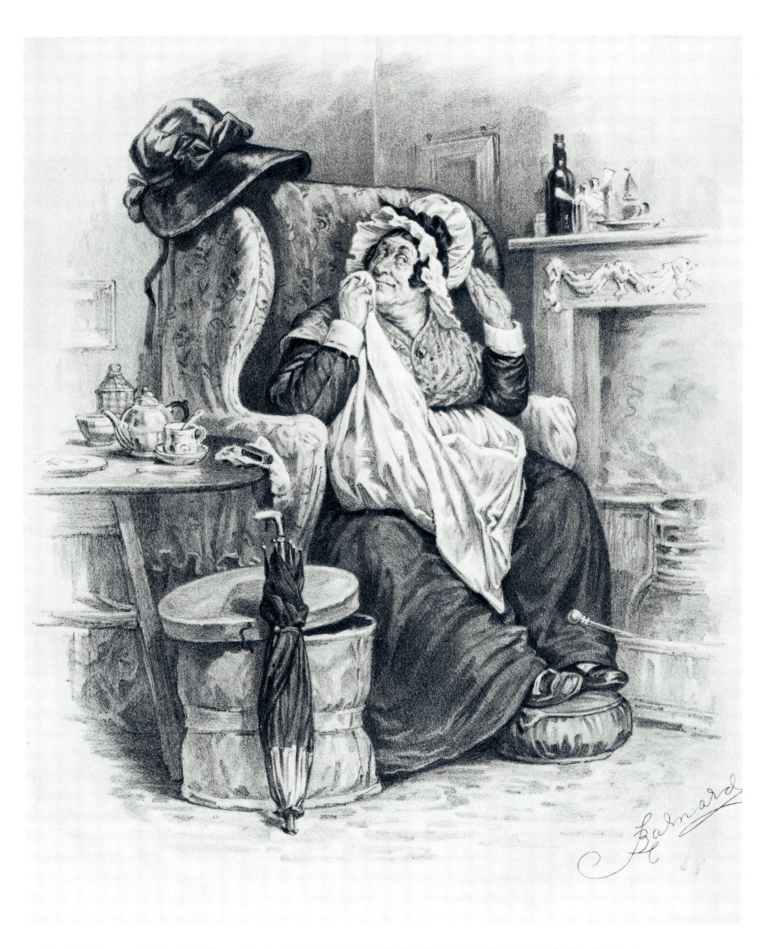

Frederick Barnard, MRS. GAMP. *From Charles Dickens'* MARTIN CHUZZLEWIT *first published in 1844. The Bettmann Archive, New York.*

233

then smoothes down her apron, adjusts herself in her arm-chair, pours out the first cup of tea, and sits for a minute or two staring at the fire, with the solid complacence of an owl—perhaps not without something of his smore, between sneeze and snuffbox.

Hunt, 1889

Help was needed for the prevailing nursing situation, and public interest in its improvement began to be demonstrated among various groups. Doctors, clergy, and philanthropic citizens advocated the establishment of nursing systems of a different character. Some favored a system under religious auspices, others a secular plan involving paid nurses. This public concern resulted in the beginning of significant changes that directed steady reform in nursing.

The Birth of Modern Nursing

One of the most important factors in the regeneration of nursing was the Deaconess Institute at Kaiserswerth, Germany, established in 1836 by Pastor Theodor Fliedner (1800–1864). The deaconess orders, which had existed at the time of Christ, were revived by the Protestant churches during the nineteenth century. This movement was sparked by the recognition of the need for the services of women. In a number of instances women were prompted by religious motives to perform social services and the care of the sick became their chief duty. Kaiserswerth became the most significant organization of Protestant deaconesses for nursing service; it is credited with creating the first modern order of deaconesses.

THE DEACONESS INSTITUTE AT KAISERSWERTH, *c. 1848. Engraving. The Bettmann Archive, New York.*

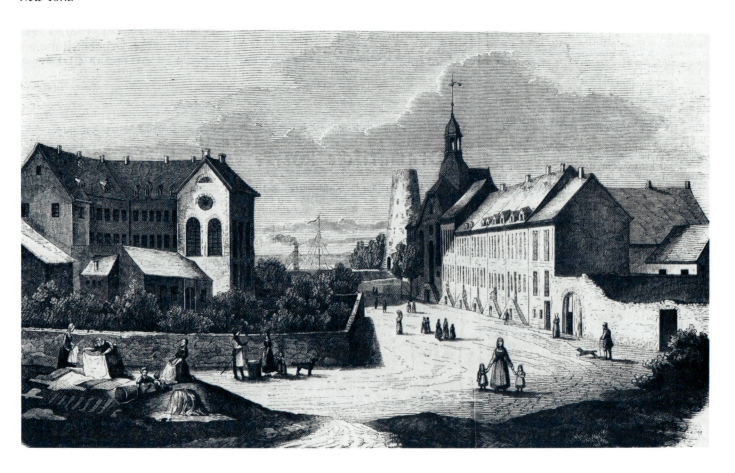

This institute was started on a modest scale, yet made an indelible impression on the whole of nursing that was to follow. It indirectly influenced individuals such as Florence Nightingale, who stayed there for a brief time. Pastor Fliedner, who had been appointed to the parish of Kaiserswerth in 1822, began his social work by founding a German Prison Association (Rheinisch-Westfälischer Gefängnisverein) in 1826. The first of its kind in Germany, it was inspired by the work already done in prison reforms in England and Holland. Fliedner had traveled abroad to raise money for his struggling parish and observed these changes firsthand. He met Elizabeth Fry and was impressed with her work at Newgate Prison. He inspected hospitals, almshouses, and prisons in Holland, where he observed the work of deaconesses. He married Friederike Münster (1800–1842) in 1828, and their joint activities in prison reform led to the start of a small refuge for discharged prisoners in 1833. This asylum, as it was called, was the first of many units that formed the institute.

The Fliedners next turned their attention to the care of the sick and opened a small hospital with a training school for deaconesses. This hospital was started in a house and the first deaconess, Gertrude Reichardt, the daughter of a physician, was admitted in 1836. By the end of the first year, six other women joined her for training. These deaconesses took no vows but simply promised to work for Christ. Although they received no salary, they were taken care of for life, an arrangement known as the *motherhouse system*. It was an offspring of the monastic system and offered security, since the deaconesses were provided with a permanent home and protection. They were sent out to district, hospital, and private duty assignments or to distant mission fields. Their dress was a plain blue cotton gown with a white apron and a large turned-down collar. A white muslin cap with a frill around the face was tied under the chin with a large white bow. Long black cloaks and black bonnets over their caps were worn outdoors.

The movement of the institute expanded rapidly and "by 1840 the work at the Kaiserswerth hospital had grown so much that two other adjoining houses were bought; by 1842 the total bed capacity was over two hundred, and the institute itself, now too small to house all the Deaconesses, had to be rebuilt" (Seymer, 1932, p. 63). The training of the deaconesses was designed to prepare them for both teaching and nursing. The program in nursing included a rotation in hospital clinical services (experience on wards for men, women, and children as well as on those for communicable disease, convalescents, and sick deaconnesses), instruction in visiting nursing, theoretical and bedside instruction in the care of the sick, instruction in religious doctrine and ethics, and enough pharmacy to pass the state examinations for pharmacists. This program of study took three years. An interesting principle was enforced in that the nurses were required to follow the physician's orders exactly and that the physician alone was responsible for the outcome.

It is interesting to see how much of their system and detail our modern training schools have inherited from the Motherhouse — the probationary system, and the school for preparatory training; the letters from clergyman and physician as to character and health; the allowance of pocket-money; the grading of work, from easy to difficult; the chain of responsibility; the grading of pupils from probationer to head nurse, with the superintendent at the head; the class-work and lectures; and every principle of discipline, etiquette, and ethics. The combination of a semi-military form of professional discipline with social equality, found in the Motherhouse, gave the pattern to the early American schools even more than did the English schools, whose system of class distinctions was never established in America.

Nutting and Dock, vol. 2, 1907, p. 40

A framework of organization evolved at Kaiserswerth that incorporated many facets of service. These were divided into four areas: nursing, relief of the poor, the care of children, and work among the unfortunate women who were prisoners and "Magdalens." The institute became so well known that many individuals came to study its methods. Friederike, the ambitious and energetic cofounder of Kaiserswerth, died in 1842. After her death, Pastor Fliedner married Caroline Bertheau (1811–1892), who had acted for three years as superintendent of the female surgical department of the Hamburg Hospital. Her nursing experience proved to be extremely valuable to the continuation of the work at the institute. The Kaiserswerth influence spread far beyond the German boundaries. In 1849 Fliedner escorted four deaconesses to Pittsburgh, Pennsylvania, where they were to assume responsibility for the Pittsburgh Infirmary (currently

THE CHILDREN'S HALL IN THE DEACONESS INSTITUTE AT KAISERSWERTH, *c. 1850. Engraving. The Bettmann Archive, New York.*

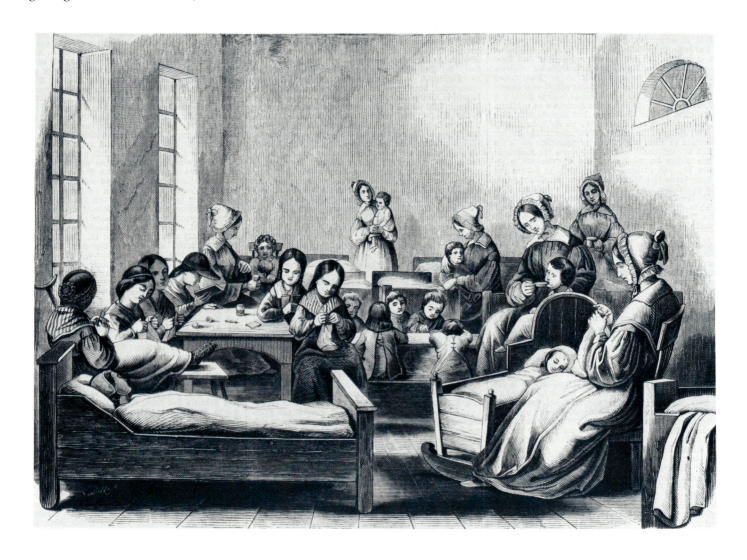

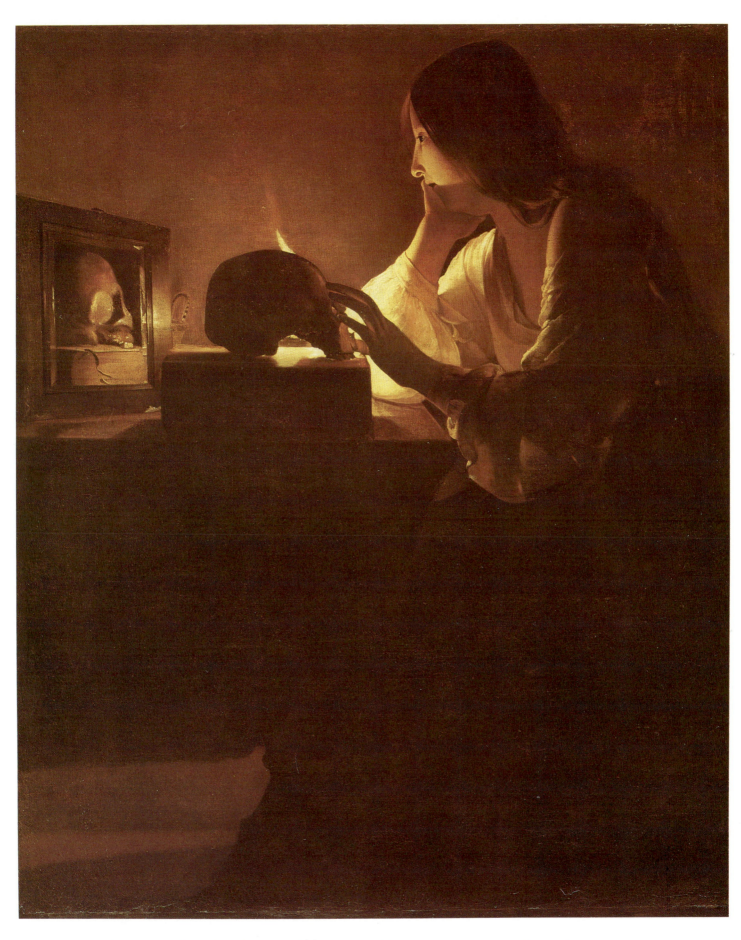

Georges de La Tour, THE REPENTANT MAGDALEN, *c. 1640. Canvas, 113 × 92.7 cm. National Gallery of Art, Washington, D.C., Ailsa Mellon Bruce Fund 1974.*

Passavant Hospital); other branches were founded in Jerusalem, Smyrna, Constantinople, Beirut, and Alexandria. Graduates of the program went to all corners of the globe to assist with the care of the sick and the needy. These beginnings set the stage for the founding of a new system of nursing by Florence Nightingale, whose reforms drastically changed the care of the sick throughout the world.

The Nightingale Revolution

> Miss Nightingale introduced sanitary science through female nursing in military hospitals by reducing the death rate of the British Army from 42 to 2 per cent (1854–55); protested against the corridor system of hospitals and fought for pavilions (1856); printed her extensive octavo on the health of the army (1858); issued the anonymous blue book on military sanitation in which she demonstrated the frightful but preventable mortality of the recent war (1859); showed the relationship of sanitary science to medical institutions (*Notes on Hospitals,* 1859); wrote the authoritative text of modern nursing (*Notes on Nursing,* 1859); established the Army Medical School at Fort Pitt, Chatham, and chose its faculty (1860); and founded the first training school for nurses (St. Thomas's Hospital, 1860). Florence Nightingale epitomized her lifework when she wrote in a private note: "I stand at the altar of the murdered men, and, while I live, I fight their cause." Florence Nightingale was the greatest war nurse in history.
>
> *Robinson, 1946, p. 129*

It is doubtful whether any woman's story has been repeated oftener than that of Florence Nightingale. Yet existing accounts fall short in efforts to document totally her place in the sphere of social progress. Unquestionably, she was a significant individual in nursing's history and has been identified as the pioneer and founder of modern nursing as well as a reformer of hospitals. Florence Nightingale pursued a mission of service to humanity throughout her lifetime. Her achievements are especially impressive when viewed against the background of social restraints on women in Victorian England. Some still question which of her numerous contributions are the greatest. Certainly her efforts to reform the military health care system in Britain and her development of a solid nursing program built on sound professional standards are at the top of the list. Other of her endeavors are less well known, including her work in the area of statistical analysis. However, a recent article about Nightingale by Bernard Cohen identified her as "a pioneer in the use of social statistics and in their graphical representation" (Cohen, 1984, p. 128).

There is indeed controversy among biographers regarding the "true essence" of Florence Nightingale. For the most part, she is portrayed as a saint. Yet she has long been recognized to have had faults by some of the principal authors: Cook (1913) noted that she was hard on her friends and intolerant of other points of view; Strachey (1918) saw her as an eagle rather than a swan; Goldsmith (1937) depicted her with frankness; Woodham-Smith (1951) did not emphasize her faults but did not ignore them and considered her to be not only a saint but a woman of the world. A recent author, however, F.B. Smith (1982) dismisses the earlier biographers as hagiographers

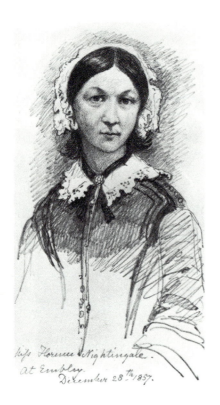

G. Scharf, FLORENCE NIGHTINGALE AT EMBLEY, *1857. Pencil drawing. National Portrait Gallery, London, England.*

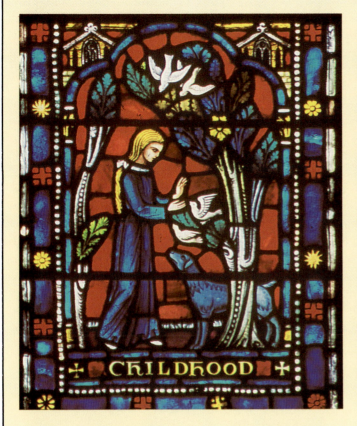

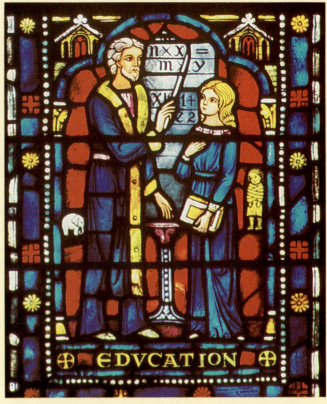

Designed by Reynolds, Francis, & Rohnstock. CHILDHOOD,
c. 1938. Stained glass. Panel from THE NIGHTINGALE
WINDOW, *Washington Cathedral, Washington, D.C. Courtesy
of Morton Broffman.*

*As a child, Florence Nightingale nursed wounded birds and
animals. She is shown feeding the birds while her favorite
dog looks up eagerly.*

Designed by Reynolds, Francis, & Rohnstock. EDUCATION,
c. 1938. Stained glass. Panel from THE NIGHTINGALE
WINDOW, *Washington Cathedral, Washington, D.C. Courtesy
of Morton Broffman.*

*William Nightingale is shown teaching his daughter,
Florence.*

who were blinded by the belief that those who do good deeds must
be good themselves. It would seem that his purpose is to specifically
malign Miss Nightingale, to expose her as a fraud. Yet whatever is the
truth regarding her personal side certainly does not detract from
her many accomplishments. She was a "rarely versatile genius who
starred in many roles and played them all with distinction" (Stewart,
1939, p. 208).

Florence Nightingale (1820–1910) was born in Florence, Italy,
on May 12, 1820 to wealthy English parents who resided at Embley
Park, Hampshire, in the summer and at Lea Hurst, Derbyshire, in the
winter. The birth occurred during one of her parents' travels on the
Continent, and they named the child for the city of her birth. Florence was raised in England with her elder sister Parthenope and received a thorough education. By the time she was seventeen she had
mastered several ancient and modern languages, was well read in
literature, philosophy, religion, history, political economy, and science, and had mastered higher mathematics. She was probably better
educated than most men of her time. At a very early age she expressed a desire to enter nursing; her parents objected because of the
hospital conditions of the day. Not surprisingly, they hoped that she
would give up her unusual ambition, marry, continue in the social
circles to which she was accustomed, and have children.

The details of Florence Nightingale's life at home, her education, her friends, and her travels are too extensive to relate in this book, but they have been amply dealt with in several biographies. This background is, however, important to an understanding of the driving force in her life, her struggle for independence and freedom to pursue a career in nursing. A series of events transpired during the sixteen years it took Miss Nightingale to overcome family obstacles, some of which were particularly significant in her quest to become a nurse. She systematically studied various institutions she visited while engaging in continental travel. Perhaps the crucial period of her career began with a visit to friends in Rome (1847), where she entered into a lifelong friendship with Mr. and Mrs. Sidney Herbert. Sir Sidney was to have the greatest influence on her life, since it was through him that she later went to the Crimea and with him that she formed "the little war office." On this particular journey she also became familiar with the nursing of Roman Catholic sisterhoods. Her travels took her to Egypt, Greece, and eventually Germany, where she spent a fortnight at Kaiserswerth. Later in 1847 she enrolled in the program for nursing at Kaiserswerth and finished the three-month program. She spoke of this institute as her "spiritual home,"

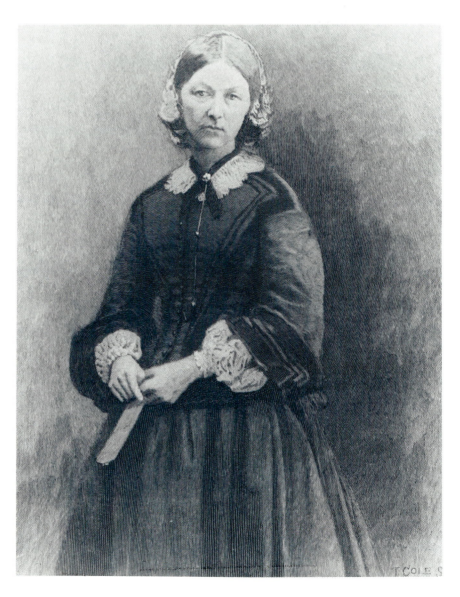

T. Cole, FLORENCE NIGHTINGALE, *c. 1850. Wood engraving. National Library of Medicine, Bethesda, Maryland.*

240

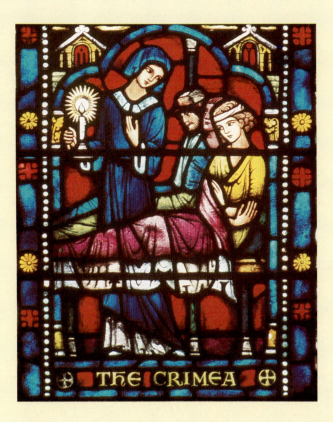

Designed by Reynolds, Francis, & Rohnstock. THE CRIMEA, *c. 1938. Stained glass. Panel from* THE NIGHTINGALE WINDOW, *Washington Cathedral, Washington, D.C. Courtesy of Morton Broffman.*

The great work for which Nightingale is best remembered is symbolized by the well-known subject, "The Lady of the Lamp."

although she would not admit that she had "trained" there. In her opinion the hospital work of the deaconesses was not on a level with the rest (Cook, 1913). In 1853 Miss Nightingale studied in Paris under the Sisters of Charity at the Maison de la Providence. Returning to London, she assumed an administrative position as superintendent of the Establishment for Gentlewomen During Illness. She remained for a year and succeeded in creating a model institution by the standards of the day. However, she was disappointed that she was unable to initiate a formal training school for nurses. As she began to plan and prepare for the superintendent's position at King's College Hospital, British and French troops invaded the Crimea in support of Turkey's dispute with Russia. This event precipitated an unexpected opportunity for achievement.

The hour and the woman.   In his biography of Florence Nightingale, Cook (1913) used the chapter heading "The Hour and the Woman" to express the period of Miss Nightingale's life during the time of the Crimean War. No other phrase could better describe the union that occurred between the national need and the woman who was most fit to meet it. Soon after the outbreak of the Crimean War, England rang with the stories of the base at Scutari. With the British Army was the first war correspondent, William Howard Russell of *The Times* (London), who quickly dispatched vivid reports of conditions of soldiers and the utter inadequacy of their care in October of 1854.

It is with feelings of surprise and anger that the public will learn that no sufficient preparations have been made for the proper care of the wounded. Not only are there not sufficient surgeons . . . not only are there no dressers and nurses . . . there is not even linen to make bandages . . . it is found that the commonest appliances of a workhouse sick-ward are wanting, and that the men must die through the medical staff of the British army having forgotten that old rags are necessary for the dressing of wounds. . . . The manner in which the sick and wounded are treated is worthy only of the savages of Dahomey. . . . Here the French are greatly our superiors. Their medical arrangements are extremely good, their surgeons more numerous, and they have also the help of the Sisters of Charity, who have accompanied the expedition in incredible numbers. These devoted women are excellent nurses.

Woodham-Smith, 1951, p. 85

An appalling picture of the army's inefficiency was thus presented to the public; it illustrated the high death rate from wounds, infections, cholera, and lack of adequate care. The country was seething with rage, and a letter in *The Times* demanded angrily, "Why have we no Sisters of Charity?"

Sir Sidney Herbert, by then the Secretary of War, decided to defy precedent and for the first time in English history send a contingent of female nurses to military hospitals. He knew of one woman capable of bringing order out of the chaos and immediately wrote his remarkable letter (October 15, 1854) to Florence Nightingale requesting her services. It contained a plea to supervise the military hospitals in Turkey:

There is but one person in England that I know of who would be capable of organising and superintending such a scheme. . . . The selection of the rank and file of nurses will be very difficult: no one knows it better than yourself. The difficulty of finding women equal to a task, after all, full of horrors, and requiring, besides knowledge and goodwill, great energy and great courage, will be great. . . . My question simply is, Would you listen to the request to go and superintend the whole thing? You would of course have plenary authority over all the nurses, and I think I could secure you the fullest assistance and co-operation from the medical staff, and you would also have an unlimited power of drawing on the Government for whatever you thought requisite for the success of your mission . . . but I must not conceal from you that I think upon your decision will depend the ultimate success or failure of the plan. Your own personal qualities, your knowledge and your power of administration, and among greater things your rank and position in Society give you advantages in such a work which no other person possesses.

Woodham-Smith, 1951, pp. 87–89

Florence Nightingale was appointed superintendent of the Female Nursing Establishment of the English General Hospitals in Turkey. She left for the base hospital at Scutari on October 21, 1854, accompanied by thirty-eight nurses (she realized that several were unfit but time was of the essence). They included ten Roman Catholic Sisters from Bermondsey, eight Anglican Sisters from the Sel-

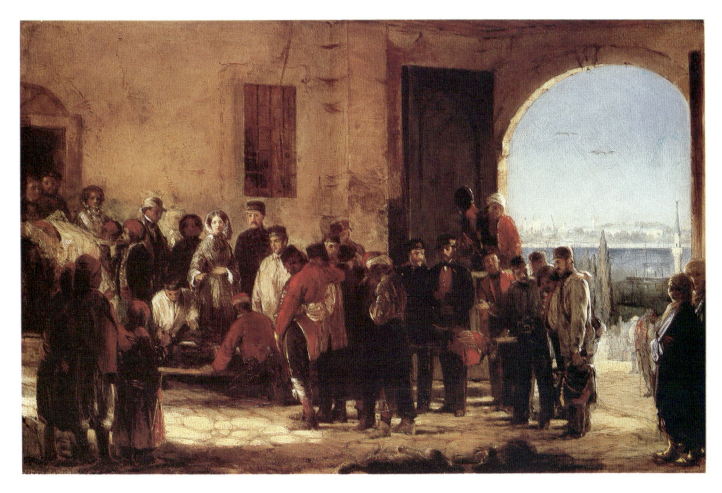

Jerry Barratt, FLORENCE NIGHTINGALE RECEIVING THE WOUNDED AT SCUTARI, *late nineteenth century. Canvas. National Portrait Gallery, London, England.*

Ionite order, six nurses from St. John's House, and fourteen from various hospitals. The vast Barrack Hospital, which resembled a hollow square with a tower at each corner, was crowded with four miles of beds. It was designed to accommodate 1700 patients, but between 3000 and 4000 were packed into it. Candles sticking in empty beer bottles lit up endless scenes of human agony. An open sewer that attracted rats and vermin was immediately under the building. There was no water, no soap, no towels, few utensils of any sort, no knives or forks, and putrid food. It took four hours to serve a meal that for all practical purposes was not edible. Men lay practically naked or in ragged uniforms clotted with blood. When available, canvas sheets were used; these were so coarse that the wounded men begged to be left in their blankets. Essential surgical and medical supplies were lacking, and there was no dietary or laundry equipment of any kind. The death rate was 42.7 percent.

Miss Nightingale demonstrated her skill as an administrator. She was, however, hampered by military authorities who resisted every change that she suggested. They resented the fact that her authority was independent of the armed services, that she was a civilian, and that she was a woman. In addition, she had to reckon with the unreliability of many on her nursing staff. Yet none of her difficulties with doctors was as wearing as those with her nurses. In the midst of appalling horror, this type of situation occurred:

> I came out, Ma'am, prepared to submit to everything, to be put
> on in every way. But there are some things, Ma'am, one can't

243

submit to. There is the Caps, Ma'am, that suits one face and some that suits another. And if I'd known, Ma'am, about the caps, great as was my desire to come out to nurse at Scutari, I wouldn't have come, Ma'am.

Woodham-Smith, 1951, p. 119

Overcoming these obstacles and obtaining the obvious necessities, Miss Nightingale transformed a place of horror into a haven where patients could truly convalesce. She set up five diet kitchens, a laundry, coffee houses that provided music and recreation (canteens), reading rooms, and organized classes. In the evening, after the other nurses had retired, she made solitary rounds. She stopped to observe the condition of the sickest patients. These rounds were made with her famous lamp or lantern, which had a wind shield that prevented the candle within it (placed in a candlestick) from being extinguished. Longfellow immortalized this "Lady with a Lamp" in his poem of 1857, "Santa Filomena." The greatest measure of Miss Nightingale's success was the overall drop in the mortality rate—to 2.2 percent—that occurred within six months' time.

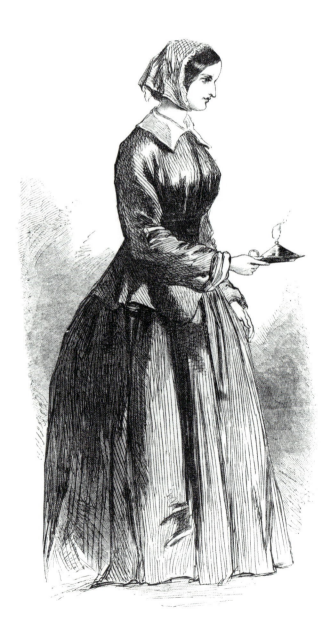

FLORENCE NIGHTINGALE. *Wood engraving.* HARPER'S WEEKLY, *June 6, 1857. National Library of Medicine, Bethesda, Maryland.*

When the conditions at the Barrack Hospital were reasonably satisfactory, Miss Nightingale went across the Black Sea to the Crimea, where two British hospitals were located near the seaport of Balaclava. On horseback or in a carriage the army had given her, she covered the distances between them. She visited the front and the hospitals but contracted "Crimean Fever" and nearly died. The English soldiers wept at the news of her illness and all of England waited patiently for her recovery. The strain from the illness and the nursing care she had provided undermined her health to the point that she was never able again to work with her former vigor. For the rest of her life she remained a semi-invalid. Miss Nightingale returned to England in July 1856, four months after the end of the war. A testimonial was presented to her by the English public in the form of fifty thousand pounds. This sum was obtained by compulsory subscription from the soldiers of the Crimea and donations from the public. It was deposited into the Nightingale Fund, which later was used for a training school for nurses.

Two figures emerged from the Crimea as heroic, the soldier and the nurse. In each case a transformation in public estimation took place, and in each case the transformation was due to Miss Nightingale. Never again was the British soldier to be ranked as a drunken brute, the scum of the earth. He was now a symbol of courage, loyalty, and endurance, not a disgrace but a source of pride. . . . Never again would the picture of a nurse be a tipsy,

MISS NIGHTINGALE'S CARRIAGE AT THE SEAT OF WAR. *Illustration from the* ILLUSTRATED LONDON NEWS, *August 30, 1856. National Army Museum, London, England.*

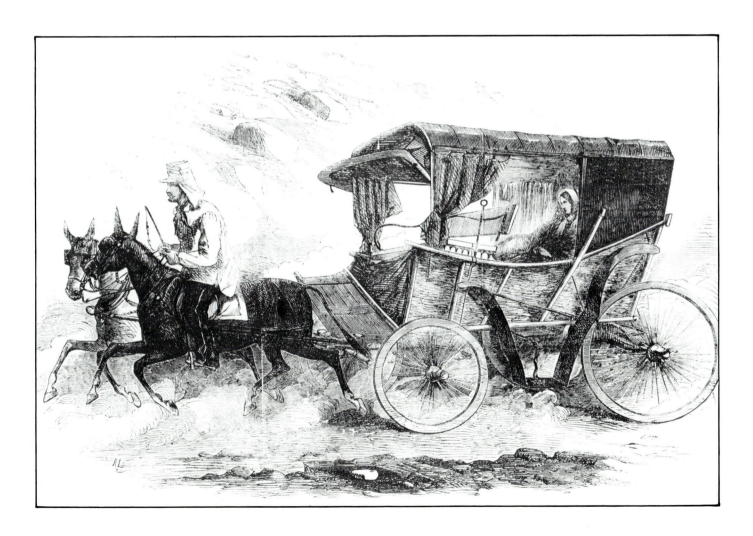

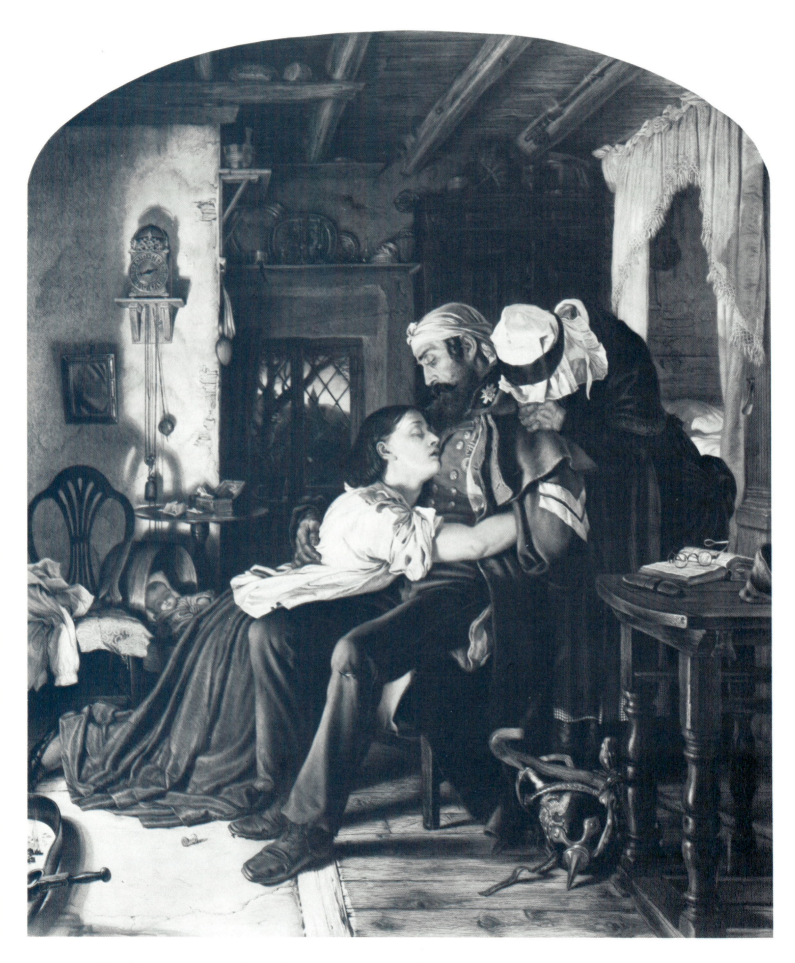

HOME! RETURN FROM THE CRIMEA, *nineteenth century. Engraving. Victoria and Albert Museum, London, England.*

promiscuous harridan. Miss Nightingale had stamped the profession of nurse with her own image . . . in the midst of the muddle and the filth, the agony and the defeats, she had brought about a revolution.

Woodham-Smith, 1951, p. 179

Before departing from the Crimean theater, Florence Nightingale made a pledge to the dead soldiers to fight for their cause. She insisted on a formal investigation of military health care, which led to the establishment of a Royal Commission on the Health of the Army in 1857. Miss Nightingale published her own views in an 800-page book titled *Notes on Matters Affecting the Health, Efficiency and Hospital Administration of the British Army,* which included a section of statistics accompanied by diagrams. She called the diagrams "coxcombs" because of their vivid colors; these polar-area charts depicted the statistic being represented in proportion to the area of a wedge in a circular diagram. These statistics were Miss Nightingale's most compelling argument for the improvement of medical care in military and civilian hospitals. After five years of hard fighting for reforms, her efforts were realized. Army hospitals and barracks were

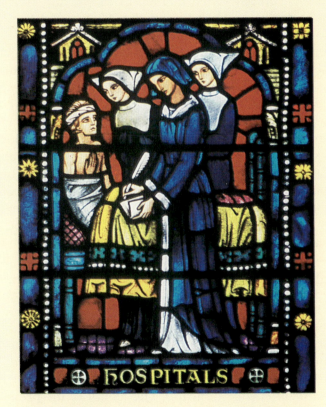

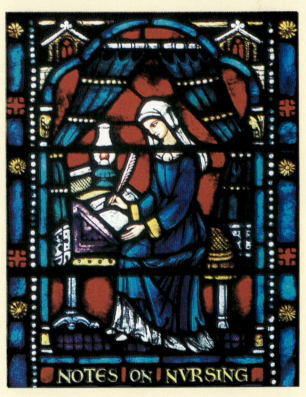

Designed by Reynolds, Francis, & Rohnstock. HOSPITALS, *c. 1938. Stained glass. Panel from* THE NIGHTINGALE WINDOW, *Washington Cathedral, Washington, D.C. Courtesy of Morton Broffman.*

Florence Nightingale visited hospitals at home and abroad. Here she takes notes at the bedside of a patient in the hospital of St. Vincent de Paul in Paris.

Designed by Reynolds, Francis, & Rohnstock. NOTES ON NURSING, *c. 1938. Stained glass. Panel from* THE NIGHTINGALE WINDOW, *Washington Cathedral, Washington, D.C. Courtesy of Morton Broffman.*

Miss Nightingale is shown writing NOTES ON NURSING, *the work that provided an enormous motivation for the study of nursing.*

reconstructed on a sanitary basis, a sanitary code for the Army was developed, a military medical college was established, recreational clubs were founded, and the Army's procedures for gathering medical statistics were reorganized.

Florence Nightingale exercised a somewhat similar influence over British administration in India. Vast irrigation projects and economic reforms were enacted by the government on the strength of two of her reports, *Observations on the Sanitary State of the Army in India* (1863) and *Life or Death in India?* (1873). This revolution in the military hospitals was carried over into civilian hospitals. The work was aided by *Notes on Hospitals* (1859), an exhaustive study on hospital planning and administration. Miss Nightingale also drew up a standard nomenclature on diseases and devised a Model Hospital Statistical Form that was approved at the International Congress of Statistics, held in London in the summer of 1860. As a recognized authority, she was frequently consulted about the plans for new hospitals in England, Australia, the United States, and Canada. Plans for the Johns Hopkins Hospital in Baltimore were taken to England for her criticism.

The Nightingale school.

Florence Nightingale developed the first organized program of training for nurses. The Nightingale Training School for Nurses opened in 1860 as an entirely independent educational institution financed by the Nightingale Fund. A council of distinguished persons had been appointed to administer the fund and negotiate the establishment of the school. The members investigated the existing London hospitals and chose St. Thomas's Hospital, where the resident medical officer, R.G. Whitfield, was sympathetic and the matron, Mrs. Wardroper, had made her mark by exhibiting an upright character, an unremitting devotion to her task, and success in reforming hospital abuses. An overwhelming majority of London physicians opposed the project. Out of 100 physicians queried, only four favored the school. Strong opposition came from within St. Thomas's itself through John Flint South, a senior consulting surgeon. South vehemently opposed the school and published a pamphlet, *Facts Relating to Hospital Nurses* (1857), in which he asserted: "As regards the nurses or ward-maids, these are in much the same position as housemaids, and require little teaching beyond that of poultice-making." Miss Nightingale's ill health prevented her from taking charge of the program, but she acted as a chief adviser for many years.

The aims of the Nightingale school were to train hospital nurses; to instruct nurses in the training of others; and to train district nurses for the sick poor. Consequently, students went into homes as well as into hospitals to care for and teach patients and families about the preservation and maintenance of health. The length of the program was one year, after which the nurses were drafted on the staff of a hospital for two years' further experience. A distinction was made between ordinary probationers and "lady nurses," which reflected the British class consciousness. The former were drawn from relatively uneducated levels, and their expenses were paid by the Nightingale Fund; the latter were gentlewomen who paid their own way (tuition fees) and were expected to become future matrons. The graduates of this program were destined to become nursing leaders on an interna-

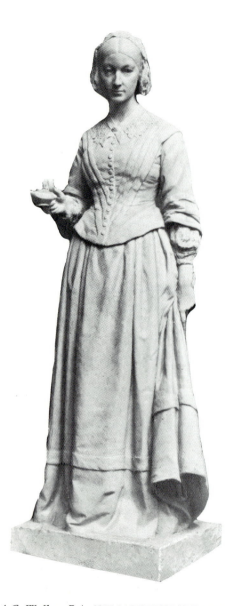

A.G. Walker, R.A., THE LADY WITH THE LAMP. *Stone. Crimean Memorial, London, England. By permission of the Royal College of Nursing of the United Kingdom.*

tional scale. As soon as they were available, they were in demand by other hospitals.

The Nightingale school was extremely important to nursing. It served as a model for other schools, sent graduates to foreign lands, and raised nursing from degradation and disgrace to the rank of a respectable occupation for women. The opening of the school was the opening of a new way of life for women. Gone forever, at least in England, was the reign of Sairey Gamp and Betsy Prig.

A small book of seventy-seven pages written by Florence Nightingale, *Notes on Nursing* (1859), held special interest for nurses. It was used as a text in the Nightingale school as well as in many schools founded by the nurses who studied there. In 1860 the book was rewritten, enlarged, and translated into Italian, German, and French. Concern over the meagre number of available copies prompted a reprinting in 1946. The fundamental principles that were set forth in this book remain as true today as when they were written. Their scope is described in the preface:

> The following notes are by no means intended as a rule of thought by which nurses can teach themselves to nurse, still less as a manual to teach nurses to nurse. They are meant simply to give hints for thought to women who have personal charge of the health of others.
>
> *Nightingale, 1859, p. iii*

After the founding of the school, fifty years remained, for Miss Nightingale survived until the age of ninety. This half century was spent in constant and fruitful activity. She died in August 1910 and was buried in the family plot at East Wellow, near Romney, in Hampshire. A small cross with her initials and dates marks the site of the grave. The family refused burial in Westminster Abbey in respect of Miss Nightingale's wishes. There are numerous monuments to her in various places in the world: in London, Derby, Milbank, Florence, Calcutta, and in St. Paul's Cathedral, St. Thomas's Hospital, the Royal Infirmary, and the Episcopal Cathedral in Washington, D.C. In this last structure is the famous and beautiful stained glass "Nightingale Window," composed of six panels that depict the events in the life of Miss Nightingale.

One need not review all the "causes" to which Florence Nightingale gave of herself in order to appreciate her role as a creative social force. She was a living memorial to a new type of thought that would forever influence the direction of nursing.

> The definite dividing-line between the old nursing and the new, is the demarcation between pre-Nightingale nursing and Nightingale nursing. In the sense that Hippocrates (460–370 BC) was the father of medicine, Florence Nightingale (1820–1910) was the founder of nursing: systematized medicine is thus an ancient art, while organized nursing is a recent art. Miss Nightingale hewed a new profession out of centuries of ignorance and superstition. The greatness and the goodness of Florence Nightingale combined to emancipate woman from the curse of not finding her work: Florence Nightingale gave to woman the blessed work of the trained nurse of the human race.
>
> *Robinson, 1946, p. 129*

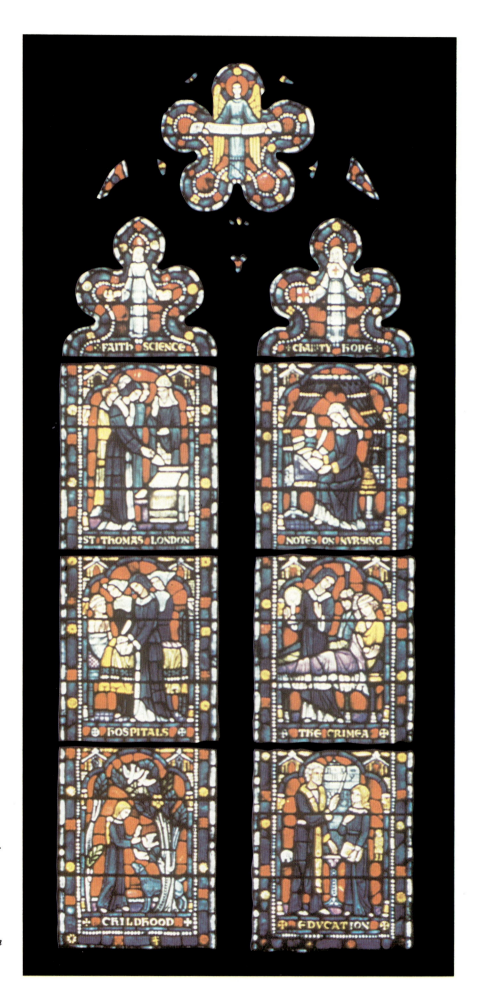

Designed by Reynolds, Francis, & Rohnstock.
THE NIGHTINGALE WINDOW, *c. 1938. Stained glass. Washington Cathedral, Washington, D.C.*

The window was dedicated in 1938 and portrays the theme of "The Glorification of Nursing." The six medallions are wrought in richly glowing colors and depict six phases of Miss Nightingale's life.

The Birth of the Red Cross

A further stimulus for nursing reform culminated in the development of the international Red Cross organization. Its founder was J. Henri Dunant, an investment banker from Geneva, Switzerland. A humanitarian, Dunant had journeyed to Italy to secure a meeting with Napoleon III of France, but found himself at Solferino, where he was a witness to the horrors of the bloodiest battle of the war between France and Austria. He was depressed by the lack of medical services; only two physicians were attending to some 6000 wounded men. Dunant enlisted local people to give whatever aid and nursing care was possible. He subsequently appealed to various European governments to set up an international organization that would provide volunteer nursing aid on battlefields.

Dunant repeatedly referred to Florence Nightingale and her work in the Crimea as the inspiration behind his crucial trip to Italy. Her work had also fortified his belief in the feasibility of such an organization. In 1862 he published the famous *Recollections of Solferino* (Un Souvenir de Solferino), which contained the idea for the birth of the Red Cross. He first presented his plan to the Society of Public Utility in Geneva (1863). After five years of hard work, Henri Dunant observed the gathering of a national congress at Geneva to consider the ways and means of accruing volunteers to serve in the event of another war. On August 22, 1864, twelve governments signed what is now known as the Treaty of Geneva. It contained principles to govern and protect those wounded in war, the supplies needed for their care, and the personnel attending the wounded

BATTLE OF SOLFERINA, JUNE 24, 1859, *which gave cause to the foundation of the Red Cross by Jean Henri Dunant. The Bettmann Archive, New York.*

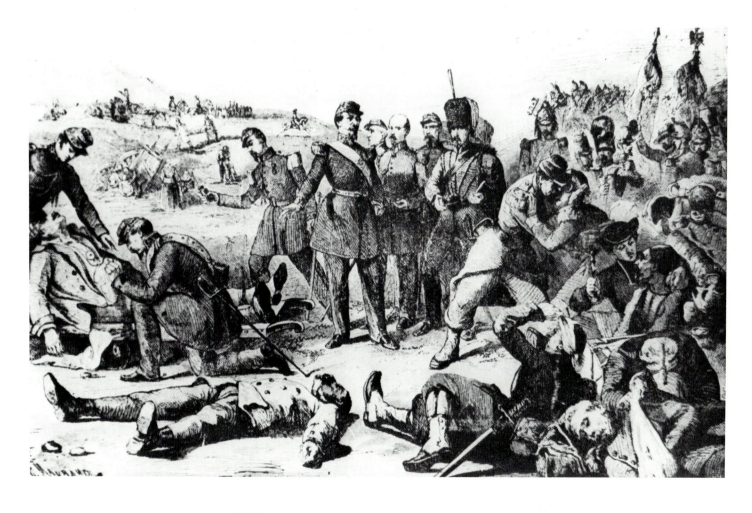

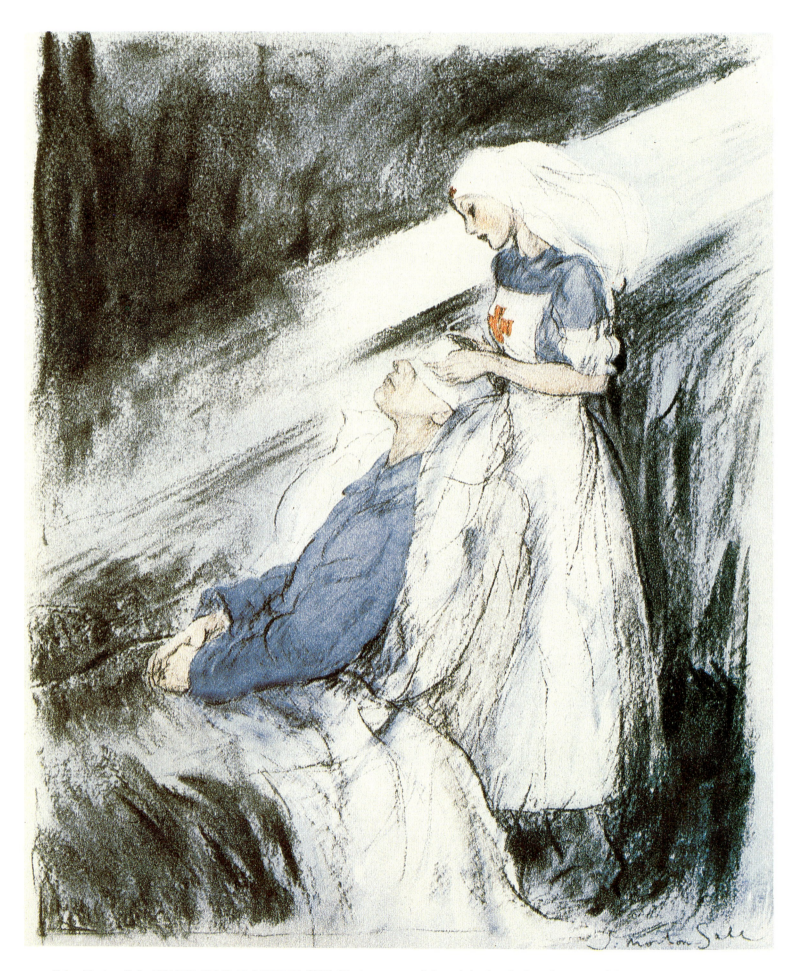

John Morton-Sale, THE RED CROSS OF COMFORT, *1939. Photogravure of the original painting. Courtesy of the Artist.*

through the use of a single determined emblem. The design chosen for the common flag of the organization was that of the flag of Switzerland with its colors reversed—a red cross on a white background. (The Red Cross societies of Moslem nations use a red crescent on a white background for their flag. Iran has a red lion and sun, which for many years has been the Persian national symbol.) Each government agreed to honor Red Cross nurses as noncombatants and to respect their hospitals and other facilities. In addition, societies in neutral countries would be permitted to render humanitarian services to either side.

National Red Cross societies were built up in many countries, and some older groups that had carried on relief work in the earlier wars of the nineteenth century became affiliated with it. The Geneva treaty was signed by England in 1870. The United States refrained from confirming it until 1882, only after Clara Barton, with rugged determination, paved the way for Congress to ratify it.

*I*n the early nineteenth century, the status of
nursing in the United States was not unlike that
in England prior to the influence of Florence Nightingale. Large city hospitals were in existence and
nurses were haphazardly trained in the hospital.
There were few trained nurses and no formal training programs. The Civil War, much like the Crimean
War in the case of England, brought the need for
skilled nurses to the attention of government agencies, and brought about the first major reforms in
nursing in this country. In the latter half of the
century, the growing sense of social responsibility for health, the improved status of women
in society, and the influence of the Nightingale
concept, all contributed to the development of nursing education and improved nursing practice. The
United States produced many women who greatly
influenced nursing during the same period
that Florence Nightingale made her
reforms, and later.

Gloria M. Grippando

254

THE DEVELOPMENT
OF NURSING
IN AMERICA

The social movements that had characterized several centuries in Europe had their American counterparts. The time of the Reformation, which had split European nations into Catholic and Protestant, was also a period of great discoveries and early emigration to America. Groups from the Old World migrated to various regions of the New World, bringing their customs with them. These customs included those related to the care of the sick. The earliest evidence of nursing, however, in the Western hemisphere was among the preliterate peoples who inhabited North, Central, and South America. Even before the Jesuit Fathers of France had pioneered in medicine and the Catholic Sisters had established mission hospitals, the Indians of the Americas had practiced crude methods of medical and surgical treatment. They had their own folk and magic medicine and could care for their sick without knowledge of medical science. The newcomers were often impressed by the native "medicine men," who served in the role of doctors, and herbwomen (the latter assumed the functions of nurses). According to Nutting and Dock (vol. 2, 1907), the Aztecs and the Incas had built their hospitals and taken care of their sick in the very dawn of history. In *Native Races of the Pacific States of North America,* Bancroft states that in all of the larger cities of ancient Mexico there were endowed hospitals attended by physicians, surgeons, and nurses and that the Mexicans had studied and practiced medicine from ancient times; women physicians were common and obstetricians were women. Shryock, however, makes the statement that "even the civilized Indians of Mexico and of Peru had developed nothing in the way of such institutions ... of hospitals and nurses there was no evidence" (Shryock, 1959, p. 170).

Although discoveries had been made in the New World before the time of Columbus, no lasting colonies had been established. A northwest passage to India was being sought by navigators and sailors. Thus Columbus named the natives he encountered in the Western world *Indians,* since he thought they were on a land that was part of India. As new lands were discovered, they were generally bestowed on the sovereigns who had financed the expeditions. It was hoped by specific governments that the expeditions would lead to the attainment of wealth and trade from the new lands. Ultimately, kingdoms would be extended and empires created. Columbus, Vespucci, Balboa, Hudson, Cartier, Drake, and others were supported in their endeavors by their homelands. Other factors compelled individuals to journey far from their native lands: freedom from religious persecution and a desire by missionaries to convert the so-called heathens to Christianity.

■ SETTLEMENTS OF THE NEW WORLD

The settlements of the New World were closely tied to the mother countries of Spain, France, and England. The new territories or colonies were thought to exist for the advantage of the homeland, and trade with them was organized from that perspective. Adventurers who were fascinated by tales of the strange new lands and the fabulous wealth that supposedly existed there left their homelands to explore and conquer. Many of the colonists also included members of religious orders who became the teachers, nurses, and physicians of the new lands.

Need for additional provision for care of the sick was created when the first boatload of adventurers started out from Europe. Crude conditions of travel led to deadly outbreaks of scurvy, as well as of disease contracted before leaving the homeland. On his second trip, Columbus was careful to bring a physician. Explorers, conquerors, and conquered—all were exposed to infections for which they had no immunity. Unfortunately, it was almost simultaneous with this need that the period of depression in European nursing was being induced by the Renaissance and the Protestant Revolt—a depression to be prolonged by revolutions to establish religious freedom and the civil rights of man. A great era of discovery opened up and facilitated the spread of disease, at a time when opportunities for its control were becoming fewer and less adequate than ever.

Jamieson and Sewall, 1950, p. 279

The problems of medical care and nursing were met in different ways by the different colonists and were usually dependent upon the customs of the homelands. Spain was best prepared because Protestantism had not weakened her Church. Religious orders of the Catholic Church accompanied the Spaniards to America. In addition to protecting the public health, they explored and converted pagans to Christianity. Nursing was clearly a function of the religious, which included devoted service and the salvation of souls. As hospitals were erected, they were also controlled by the religious, who supported the institutions through gifts they had received. France also used the Dominicans, Franciscans, and Jesuits and later the nursing orders, but England had no comparable support. Organization was lacking and individuals were given the responsibility for medicine and nursing. Eventually, in those colonies settled by Protestant countries, nursing was done by persons hired at low wages or supplied by inmates of houses of correction.

Spanish America

Spain rapidly established colonies from Mexico to Peru during the 1500s. These colonies became a large and energetic realm nearly 100 years before the first permanent settlements of other Europeans were established. In some areas native peoples were able to mingle their culture with that of the conquerors. In others, particularly in the chief centers such as Lima and Mexico City, Spanish civilization followed the pattern of the homeland. The University of Mexico and the University of Lima were founded in 1551, and the various departments of theology, arts, rhetoric, grammar, Scripture, canon law, civil law, and medicine were present. Here the medical science of the Renaissance was cultivated and the first medical schools appeared: the first at the University of Mexico in 1578, the second affiliated with the University of Lima prior to 1600.

In 1519 Hernando Cortez conquered what we now call Mexico. His conquest brought into Spanish possession the great wealth of the Aztecs, Toltecs, Mayas, and Incas. The well-meaning reigning chief of the Aztecs, Montezuma, had received Cortez into his palace. Montezuma had been taught to believe in a white god, appearing in the form of Cortez. Montezuma was met, however, with cruelty. He was imprisoned and his capital of Tenochtitlan was seized. The Aztecs had risen to a high degree of culture; their temples and pyramids are thought to predate those of Egypt. They had acquired large amounts of gold, silver, and precious stones, which were seized and shipped back to Spain. The Indians were cruelly treated and in some cases nearly decimated. Where they proved to be unfit for work in the mines, Negro slavery was introduced. Missionaries protested the inhumane treatment of the natives and slaves and tried to improve their situation.

The medicine of the Aztecs was highly developed. The Aztecs had hospices for the care of the sick, used minerals as drugs (they had knowledge of 3000 plants) and soporifics to deaden pain, and had midwives for prenatal and postpartum instruction as well as for assistance at deliveries (Frank, 1953). The god of medicine was Tzapotlatean. So skilled were the Aztec surgeons and physicians that Cortez asked the Spanish government to refrain from sending medical men from Spain; he preferred the Indians because he believed they were superior. The Incas were not as advanced. They used purging, bloodletting, trephining, amputation, and potions made from a single herb. The Incas believed that the cure for a particular disease would be found in the area in which the disease was prominent; therefore quinine from the cinchona tree was found in the malaria-infested jungles.

The devoted missionaries followed the conquerors and established a church in every Indian and Spanish town. Missions were founded along the outposts of Spanish claims. These extended from California to Texas, and to Paraguay and Chile. They were also founded in Spanish Florida. Junipero Serra, a Franciscan friar, was responsible for this extensive project, which eventually reached as far north as the Mission San Francisco. These missions were government supported and operated schools and manual training centers.

Beautiful churches, buildings, bridges, roads, and aqueducts were built under Spanish rule. Gratitude to God for success found

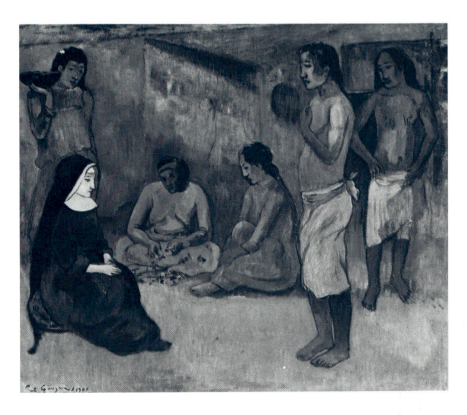

Paul Gauguin, SISTER OF CHARITY, *1902. Canvas, 64.8 × 76.2 cm. Courtesy of the Marion Koogler McNay Art Museum, San Antonio, Texas, Bequest of Marion Koogler McNay.*

258

expression in the development of charitable institutions, frequently in the form of hospitals. Approximately thirty hospitals were erected between 1524 and 1802, and the majority of them were staffed by religious men and women. The first hospital on the American continent was built in the Tenochtitlan capital (later renamed Mexico City) by Cortez in 1524. According to legend, this hospital was built on the site where Cortez first met Montezuma. It was originally named the Hospital of the Immaculate Conception (Hospital de Nuestra Senora O Limpia Concepcion); it is now called the Hospital of Jesus of Nazareth (Hospital de Jesus Nazareno). This building is a reflection of the beauty and spaciousness of Spanish hospital architecture under Moslem influence. Cortez donated funds for the completion of the hospital and also built a convent and a seminary. In his will he left an endowment for the hospital to thank God for his successes and to expiate his sins. This institution was to care for rich and poor alike. In 1528 the hospital of Santa Fe (Holy Faith) was built in what is now New Mexico. In Lima several institutions were built, including almshouses, hospitals, and lazarettos for those afflicted with contagious diseases. Hospital care, however, was reserved for the sick poor, and most of the nursing was done by the Sisters of Charity of St. Vincent de Paul.

The French in America

The first permanent settlement of the French was established in 1605 at Port Royal in Nova Scotia. The Canadian area of North America had been visited earlier: Norwegians had landed there about 1000 AD; John Cabot, a Venetian under King Henry VII, sighted land near the Gulf of the St. Lawrence; Frenchmen arrived in the area early in the sixteenth century. In 1534 Jacques Cartier, under Francis I, sailed for the North American continent. He returned to France after finding neither gold nor a northwest passage to the Orient. When Cartier returned a year later, he sailed into the St. Lawrence River, where he found established Indian villages. According to Frank (1953), Cartier questioned the natives about the name of the country. Thinking that he was referring to the village, they answered "Kanata," which meant "the place where we live." Therefore Cartier called the land Canada, its present-day name. This land has also been referred to as "New France."

Cartier was followed to Canada by explorers, Franciscan Friars, Jesuits, Dominicans, and other settlers. The French priests soon summoned help from the motherland for religious women to teach the children and care for the sick. The first woman to nurse in this new land, however, was Maria Hubou (the name of her second husband). She was the wife of the surgeon-apothecary Louis Hébart, whom Samuel de Champlain, the famous explorer, brought with him in 1617 (Gibbon and Mathewson, 1947). The Jesuits published reports of the need for aid in the *Jesuit Relations.* They sought to establish schools for Indian children, build hospitals for the sick, and make general improvements in all social conditions. The Europeans had transmitted measles, smallpox, and tuberculosis to the natives, who blamed the white man for the destruction of their race. The priests found it almost impossible to combat the diseases with the prevailing conditions of the land. They were thwarted in their at-

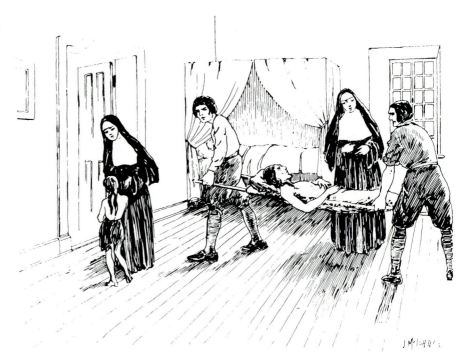

tempts by dirt, cold, crowded living conditions, lice, and the savagery of the natives.

Great interest arose in the men and women of France through Jesuit publications and reports. Duchess d'Aiguillon, a niece of Cardinal Richelieu, was moved into action. She signed a contract in 1637 with the Augustinian Hospitallers of Dieppe for their services as hospital Sisters and sent workmen to lay the foundations for the first hospital in New France. The Hôtel Dieu at Quebec opened in 1639 and was staffed by three Sisters of the Order of St. Augustine (Augustinian Sisters) upon their arrival on August 1, 1639. These Augustinian nuns belonged to a cloistered order and had been prepared to care for the sick. They wore a white woolen dress with a black leather belt and black veil. All three were from good French families: Marie Guenet de St. Ignace; Anne Lecointre de St. Bernard; and Marie Forestier de St. Bonaventure de Jésus. They encountered many hardships, and within eight months one of the Sisters had died.

> The Hospital Nuns arrived at Kebec on the first day of August of last year (1639). Scarcely had they disembarked before they found themselves overwhelmed with patients. The hall of the Hospital being too small, it was necessary to erect some cabins, fashioned like those of the savages, in their garden. Not having furniture for so many people, they had to cut in two or three pieces part of the blankets and sheets they had brought for these poor sick people. In a word, instead of taking a little rest and refreshing themselves after the great discomforts they had suffered upon the sea, they found themselves so burdened and occupied that we had fear of losing them and their hospital at its very birth. The sick came from all directions. . . . their stench was so insupportable, the heat so great, the fresh food so scarce and so poor. . . . In brief, from the first of August until the month of May, more than one hundred patients entered the hospital, and more than two hundred poor savages found relief there.
>
> *Kenton, 1925, pp. 169–170*

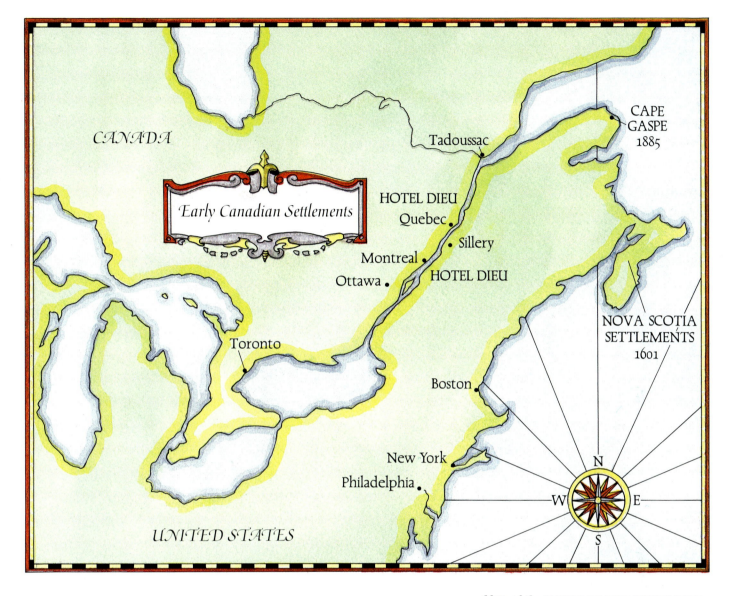

Map of the EARLY CANADIAN SETTLEMENTS.

The hospital in Quebec had a facility similar to an outpatient department that was used for the treatment of Indians who were not sick enough to be hospitalized. Indian women were trained by the Sisters to assist with the care of the sick, but their duties were chiefly domestic, such as cooking, cleaning, and preparing supplies. During the period from 1640 to 1644, the Augustinians went to Sillery, the Jesuit mission not far from Quebec, to care for the natives, but they returned when the Iroquois became hostile.

The Ursuline Sisters accompanied the Augustinians on the voyage from France. They were an order of teaching nuns enlisted by Madame de la Peltrie, who had undertaken the establishment of a mission school for the Indians. However, they were soon schooled in the care of the sick in order that they might assist during the epidemics. Smallpox broke out in the school, and the Ursuline dwelling was rapidly turned into housing for the infected. In this emergency hospital many Indians died until the disease finally ran itself out. This short-term instruction in the care of the sick could be regarded as the earliest training and supervision of nurses in America. As soon as it was feasible, the Ursuline Sisters returned to the work for which they had initially been prepared.

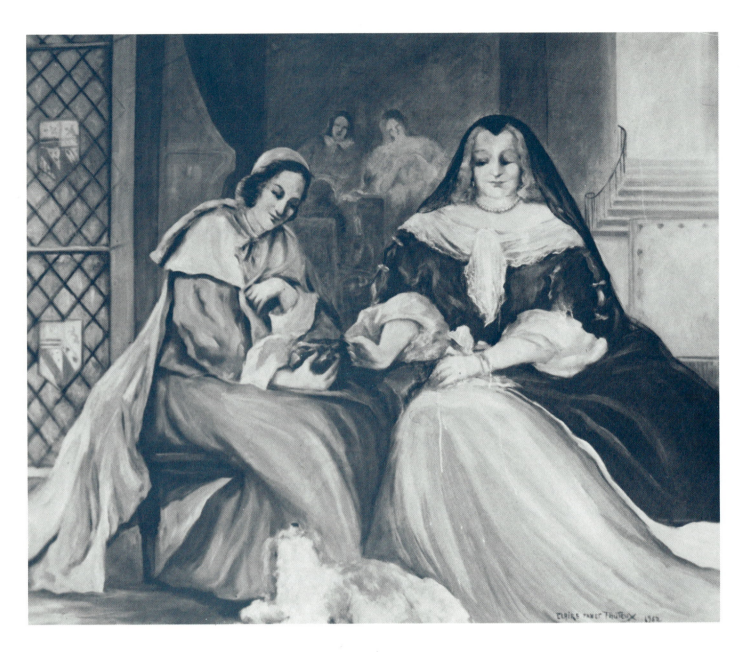

Claire Fauteux, JEANNE MANCE. *Courtesy of the Hôtel Dieu, Archives des Religieuses Hospitalières de Saint-Joseph, Montréal, Canada.*

A second settlement was founded about 200 miles farther up the St. Lawrence. Included in the original plans for "Montreal" were a school and a hospital, with the latter deemed to be an immediate necessity. The establishment of this hospital is the story of Jeanne Mance (1606–1673), a romantic figure in Canadian nursing and considered to be the founder of the Hôtel Dieu of Montreal as well as the co-founder of Montreal itself (Gibbon and Mathewson, 1947). She was the daughter of wealthy French parents and had been educated at an Ursuline convent. From her earliest childhood, Jeanne Mance had demonstrated a religious inclination. She received instruction in nursing care while assisting the Ladies of Charity in 1638 during a severe epidemic. Upon her arrival in Canada, she was also permitted to enter the Augustinian cloister at Quebec, where she waited for completion of the construction of the fort at Ville Marie, the future Montreal. Here Jeanne Mance was provided an excellent opportunity to learn more about nursing and the administration of a hospital. She arrived in Montreal on May 17, 1642, under the financial sponsorship of the wealthy philanthropist, Madame de Bullion, who wanted her to erect a hospital there.

The inhabitants of the settlement lived in peace for about a year. The floods and then the warring Iroquois followed. More than half of the settlers met death at the hands of the Iroquois. In a tiny cottage hospital inside the fort, Jeanne Mance tended to men wounded by arrows. She compounded her own medicines, treated chilblains and frostbite, practiced bloodletting, and cared for the Iroquois Indians as well as the colonists. By October 1644 a larger hospital had been established in a building sixty by twenty-four feet; it was divided into two wards, servants' quarters, a kitchen, and a room for Mlle. Mance. The hospital was surrounded by a palisade and protected by a moat because of the ever-threatening Iroquois. For almost fifteen years Jeanne Mance did all of the nursing here with the help of a few assistants. She earned the reputation of being the "first lay nurse of Canada" and of North America as well.

Jeanne Mance returned to France in 1657 to seek financial support and recuit personnel. Three hospital nuns from the Society of St. Joseph de la Flèche (Hospitallers of St. Joseph) returned to Montreal to staff the Hôtel Dieu with Jeanne Mance as the administrator, a position she held until her death in 1673. The Sisters suffered from a variety of misfortunes during the first century of the hospital's ex-

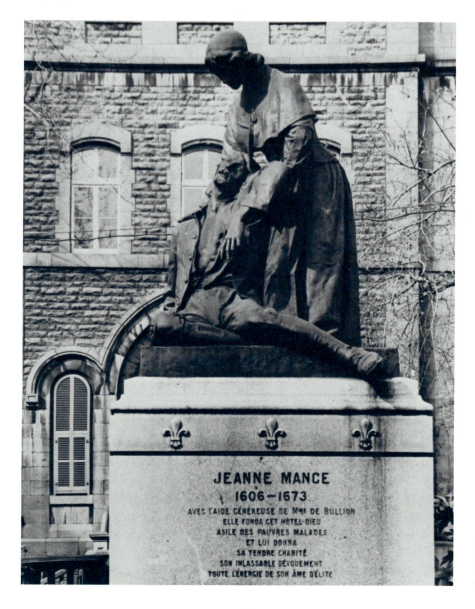

JEANNE MANCE
1606—1673
AVEC L'AIDE GÉNÉREUSE DE Mᵐᵉ DE BULLION
ELLE FONDA CET HÔTEL-DIEU
ASILE DES PAUVRES MALADES
ET LUI DONNA
SA TENDRE CHARITÉ
SON INLASSABLE DÉVOUEMENT
TOUTE L'ÉNERGIE DE SON ÂME D'ÉLITE

Philip Hebert, JEANNE MANCE. *Courtesy of the Hôtel Dieu, Archives des Religieuses Hospitalières de Saint-Joseph, Montréal, Canada.*

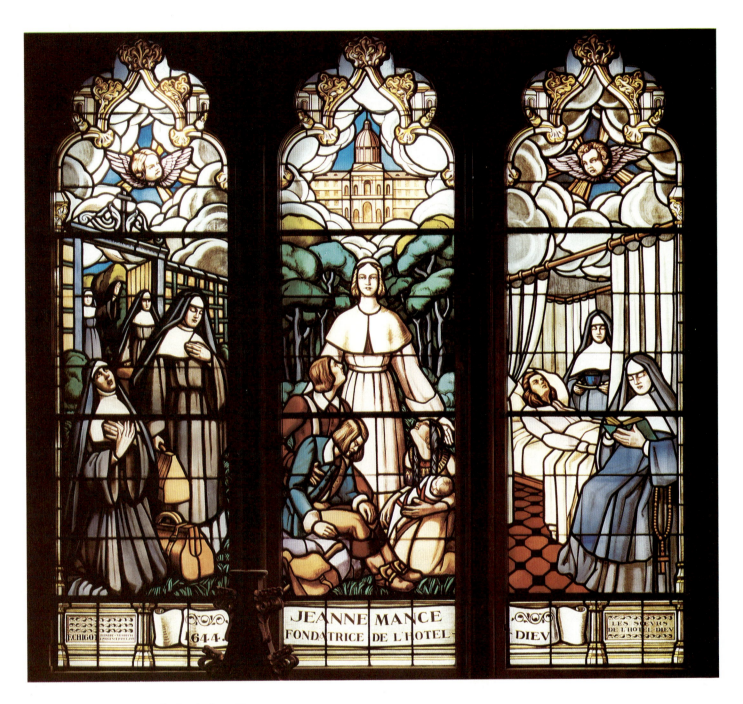

JEANNE MANCE WINDOW. *Stained glass. The Notre-Dame Basilica, Montréal, Canada.*

Jeanne Mance, one of the most romantic figures in the history of Canadian nursing, is depicted surrounded by patients in the central panel. In the left panel, the first three sisters, Hospitallers of St. Joseph, leave France in 1659. The right panel shows them caring for patients in Montréal.

istence—Indian attacks, severe poverty, fire, earthquake, and famine. They persevered and eventually experienced considerable prosperity and recognition for their good work. The next century saw all French developments at Montreal and Quebec pass into English control as a result of the Seven Years' War.

A number of other hospitals and orders were organized in Canada. One of particular note was the order of Grey Nuns established by Madame Marguerite Marie d'Youville in 1739. The members were not cloistered and were thus able to carry their work into the homes of the needy. The Grey Nuns were Canada's first district nurses. However, they were misunderstood because people were not comfortable with nuns walking freely on the streets.

Early nursing in Canada did not particularly affect the development of nursing in the country that later would become the United States. The French settlements of New Orleans and those farther up the Mississippi River, however, had an influence on American nursing. This territory was called Louisiana in honor of France's king. It, too, was ravaged by epidemic diseases, particularly yellow fever and smallpox. All of the scourges of a seaport area were encountered. New Orleans needed teachers and nurses. An almshouse had been built there and housed criminals, indigents, the mentally ill, and the sick poor. This inspired Jean Louis, a French sailor, to leave 12,000 livres upon his death to "Serve in perpetuity to the founding of a hospital for the care of the sick of the City of New Orleans . . . and to secure the necessary things to succor the sick" (Henrietta, 1939, p. 249). Ursuline Sisters arrived from France in 1727 to nurse in the new hospital. The hospital, which was legally named L'Hôpital des Pauvres de la Charité, developed slowly and went through several name changes. It eventually became the great and famous Charity Hospital of New Orleans. The Ursuline Sisters were very active throughout Louisiana. They opened numerous hospitals and performed many heroic deeds that reached a peak with the nursing done during the Battle of New Orleans. In later years they restricted themselves to teaching, and their work was carried on by the Daughters of Charity.

The English Colonies

Europeans emigrated to the English colonies for a variety of reasons, including freedom from religious oppression, a spirit of adventure, and the chance to start again. It is said that approximately a quarter of a million came as indentured servants. They committed themselves to work for a number of years to pay for their passage. Many of them came from the gaols and debtors' prisons, seeking an opportunity to begin a new and rewarding life.

England laid claim to that portion of the Atlantic coast that was between the claims of Spain and France. Colonization was a private affair in that the English government granted permission to an individual or a chartered company to establish a colony. Royalties were paid to the Crown; profits and losses were assumed by the proprietors. The first permanent English settlement in America was made in Jamestown in 1607 by the London Company. The area was named "Virginia," after the virgin queen, Elizabeth. The colony faced many hardships and suffered Indian massacres, illness, starvation, and a heavy mortality. Medical care was lacking and little of what could be called nursing was available. The first three years in the new colony was a period of human devastation. All but sixty of the original 500 settlers died from malnutrition or dietary insufficiency. A shipload of women arrived in Jamestown in 1619 to be auctioned off as wives. During that same year the first slaves were brought from Africa.

A succession of colonies followed Jamestown. A group of Separatists, who were later known as Pilgrims, sailed on the *Mayflower* and landed at New Plymouth in 1620. This group was augmented by the Puritans, who were being persecuted in England. (The Plymouth Company was later incorporated as the Massachusetts Bay Company, which became identical with the Massachusetts colony.) In 1626 the Dutch East India Company established a colony called "New Netherlands," which was located in what is now Staten Island, Manhattan, and Delaware. The principal town, called "New Amsterdam," was lo-

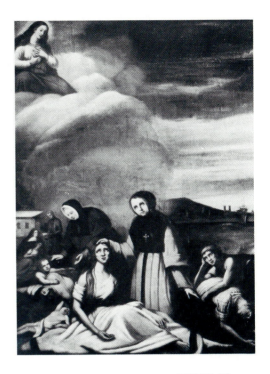

Theophile Hamel, GREY NUNS, SISTERS OF PROVIDENCE AND HÔTEL DIEU SISTERS CARING FOR THE IRISH IMMIGRANTS. *Chapelle Notre-Dame-de-Bonsecours, Montréal, Canada. By permission from Claude Labrecque, Chaplain of Notre-Dame-de-Bonsecours.*

This painting is in honor of the nuns and priests who died caring for the Irish immigrants arriving in Montréal suffering from the fatal epidemic of pest in 1847.

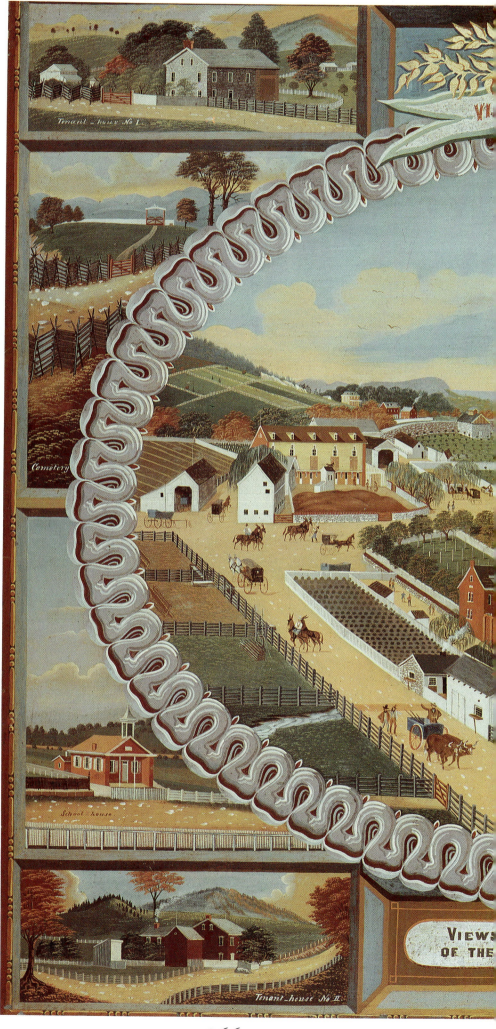

Charles C. Hofmann, THE BERKS COUNTY ALMSHOUSE, *1878. Metal, approx. 81.3 × 99.1 cm. National Gallery of Art, Washington, D.C., Gift of Edgar William and Bernice Chrysler Garbisch 1953.*

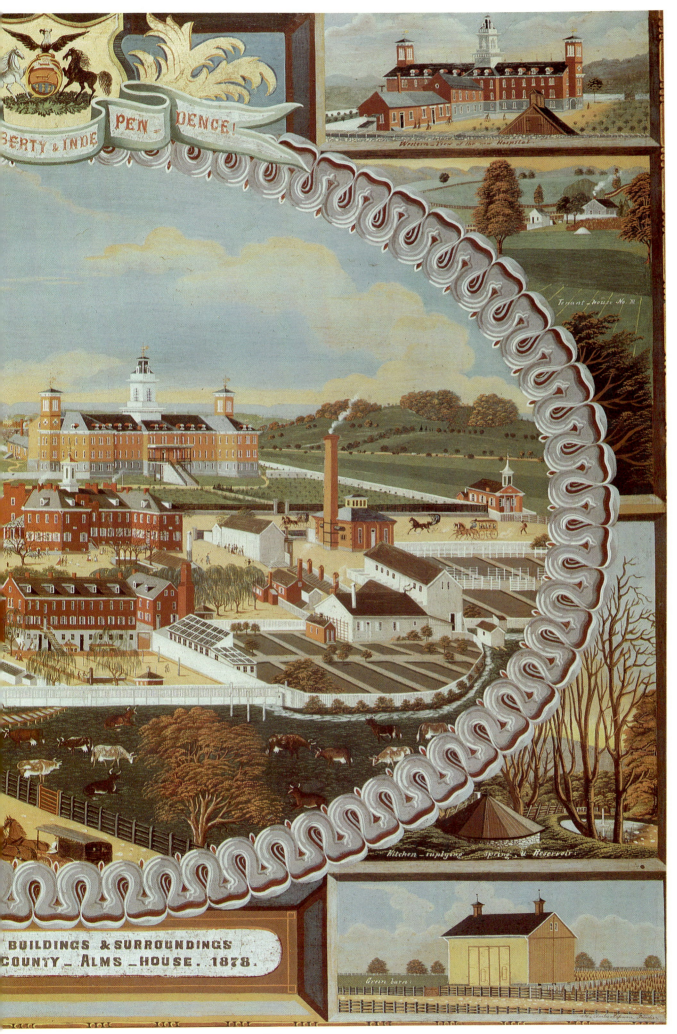

Western View of the new Hospital.

Tenant House No. III.

Kitchen supplying Spring & Reservoir.

Green barn.

BUILDINGS & SURROUNDINGS
COUNTY ALMS HOUSE. 1878.

cated on Manhattan. Maryland was founded as a refuge for English Catholics in 1633 by Lord Baltimore, Cecil Calvert, a group of Jesuits, and 300 carefully selected colonists. Connecticut and Rhode Island were founded as a result of grievances among members of the Massachusetts colony. Pennsylvania was given to William Penn by Charles II in payment of a debt to Penn's father. This Quaker colony was noted for tolerance and religious freedom. English colonization became a reality as other equally important settlements developed. There was, however, little similarity and unity among them. Each colony was self-governed, and there was no central power to coordinate them. They remained isolated and even antagonistic toward one another for almost a century and a half. Their differences were particularly caused by religious beliefs, although varying temperaments and the prevalence of bigotry played a role.

The Pilgrim Fathers brought a stern philosophy with them to the New World, and it was not conducive to the development of institutions for the care of the sick. They took it for granted that welfare work was a function of private charity or the state. It was assumed that families would look after their own unfortunates and therefore public refuge was unnecessary. Early treatments of diseases consisted largely of prayer intermingled with much superstitious medical practice. Samuel Fuller, a deacon, acted as a physician in New England for thirteen years after his arrival on the *Mayflower*. Physicians did not need a degree; the educated men among the colonists (clergymen, governors, or schoolteachers) were thought to be well equipped

Winslow Homer, NEW YORK CHARITIES– ST. BARNABUS HOUSE, 304 MULBERRY STREET. *Engraving, approx. 22.9 × 33.7 cm.* HARPER'S WEEKLY, *April 18, 1874.*

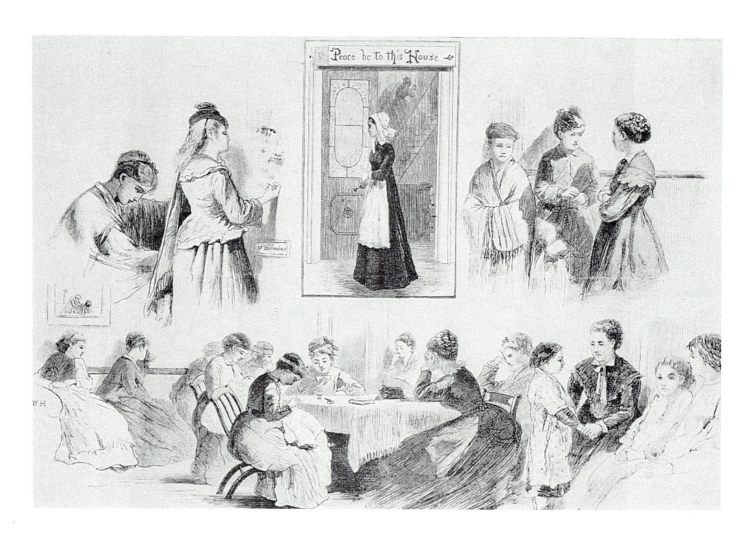

enough to handle the role of a physician. Ignorant quacks were in abundance. Indian folklore soon became incorporated into the overall scheme.

> Obviously this clerical and lay medicine would have to be very primitive. It was a peculiar mixture of religious medicine, folk-medicine, and scientific principle. One invoked the word of God, let blood, or prescribed drugs, to the best of one's understanding. We must not forget that at this period European medicine, even when practiced by physicians, was effective only in exceptional cases.
>
> *Sigerist, 1934, p. 37*

The English settlers lacked the organized service of the convent or the mission, the experience of nuns and priests. Consequently, hospitals developed slowly in the original thirteen colonies. Social welfare was considered to be the responsibility of the individual, the family, or the neighborhood. Relatives or friends supplied nursing care when needed. Otherwise, nursing fell to those persons who were inclined to do it. When the settlements reached a certain size, however, some sort of public refuge had to be provided. The colonists followed the pattern of the homeland and ultimately organized institutions for the sick and the poor. This was not done out of Christian charity as much as for social convenience. The poorhouse and the hospital were placed under one roof, and the conditions were similar to those found by Elizabeth Fry in Britain.

Dean Cornwell, OSLER AT OLD BLOCKLEY. *Canvas. Courtesy of Wyeth Laboratories, Philadelphia, Pennsylvania.*

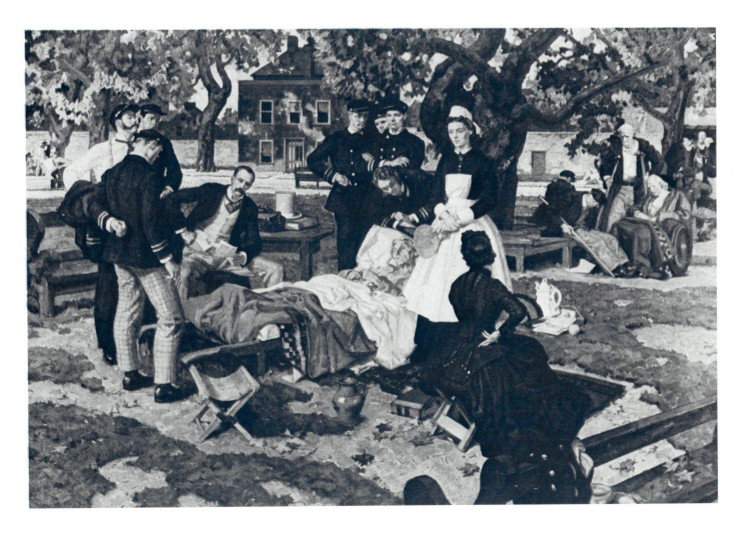

■ HOSPITAL DEVELOPMENT
   IN AMERICA

The growth of hospitals in colonial America was slow. In the 150 years prior to the American Revolution (1776–1784), approximately five hospitals were founded outside of Canada. The earliest were not hospitals in the true sense of the word. They were usually almshouses that included infirmaries where the sick poor were attended by inmates. Regarded by some as the first hospitals in the English colonies, they later evolved into separate municipal hospitals.

Several hospitals claim to have been the first established in America. This discrepancy is directly related to the definition of *hospital* and the specific focus of the institution. As indicated above, many of these early hospitals were developed as poorhouses; the care of the sick was incidental. However, the earliest hospital on record was established in New Amsterdam by the Dutch West India Company in 1658. Located on Manhattan Island, it served to care for sick soldiers and slaves coming into port as cargo on company ships.

The Philadelphia Almshouse, which was erected in 1731, cared for the sick, the indigent, the insane, the infirm, prisoners, and orphans. In 1919 the hospital was separated from the almshouse. From 1835 to 1902 it was called Philadelphia Hospital. In 1902 the name was changed to the Philadelphia General Hospital. Servants, criminals, and paupers cared for the sick. This institution is usually designated as the "oldest hospital in continuous service" and was affectionately known as "Old Blockley." It offered the typical picture of the almshouse of the late eighteenth and early nineteenth centuries. The treatment of the insane was particularly disheartening. The female lunatics were under the supervision of a male keeper who was assisted by two male paupers. These men slept among the insane and entirely managed the violent cases, even bathing and dressing the women. "Some of the patients, even in their madness, shrunk from this rude handling and raved with the increased fury at their indecent exposure. Revolting to decency as this practice was, it was not without difficulty, and only by degrees, abandoned" (Nutting and Dock, vol. 2, 1907, p. 333). In addition, it was the custom to permit the public to visit these insane wards to stare, laugh, and jeer at the inmates.

The nursing in this institution was as crude and indifferent as anything that had taken place in London. During a cholera outbreak in 1832, for example, the attendants were found to be continuously intoxicated. In their drunken state, they fought over the beds of the sick or lay in a stupor beside dead bodies. The situation was improved only with the introduction of the Sisters of Charity of Emmitsburg, who undertook the task of reform. This transpired after investigations in 1793 and 1832, which brought the shocking conditions to light. Unfortunately, after the Sisters departed, unsatisfactory conditions returned and remained for a long time. Finally, Alice Fisher, a Nightingale nurse, arrived in 1884 and proceeded to upgrade the quality of nursing care.

Bellevue Hospital had its beginnings in the small hospital established by the West India Company in 1658. It was sold in 1680 and a better building was provided. In 1736 another new building was added to serve as a "Publick Workhouse and House of Correction of New York." This building became the immediate predecessor of

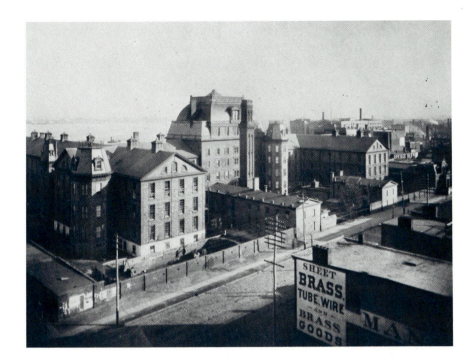

BELLEVUE HOSPITAL, *New York City, c. 1885.*
Courtesy of the New-York Historical Society,
New York.

Bellevue and stood where New York's city hall presently stands. It was rebuilt and enlarged several times. Buildings changed according to societal needs, and the city eventually assumed a share of the expense of charity. In time, the present Bellevue Hospital was concentrated on the bank of the East River. The building was originally (1794) used as a pesthouse to serve victims of yellow fever and for several years was used only when yellow fever broke out in the city. In 1811 more ground around the hospital was bought, and a new almshouse was built and dedicated on July 29, 1811. Officially opened in 1816, this institution contained the almshouse, a penitentiary, wards for the sick and the insane, and rooms for the resident physician, warden, and attendants. The sick were cared for by paupers or prisoners, political graft flourished, and epidemics were frequent. For many years Bellevue was a "house of horrors."

> Hospitals were as a rule in a disgraceful state of degradation.
> They were dirty and ill ventilated, they reeked with infection,
> so that patients who came in suffering from one disease, or from
> a wound, caught another disease or some virulent infection.
> The death rate was fearfully high, sometimes actually more than
> 50 per cent. In the days before Lister, hospital surgery was
> extremely discouraging. The only nurses that could be obtained
> for hospitals were women who did the menial work besides
> caring for the patients.
>
> *Walsh, 1929*

A committee was designated in 1837 to investigate the deplorable state of the hospital. According to Carlisle (1893), the prevailing conditions cited by the committee included filth, no ventilation, overcrowded wards, no clothing or supplies, patients with high fever lying naked in bed, putrefaction, and vermin. In addition, it was stated that the resident physician—with his students, the matron, and the nurses—had left the building. As a result, the pesthouse, the prison, and later the psychiatric wards were removed to Blackwell's Island. A new era began with the creation of a medical board in 1847. The

271

almshouse and hospital, however, remained together until 1848, when Bellevue began its ensuing career as a hospital.

Bellevue was probably the first institution to establish an ambulance service (1869). Provisions were made for emergency treatment:

> Beneath the driver's seat was a box containing a quart flask of brandy, two tourniquets, a half-dozen bandages, a half-dozen small sponges, some splint material, pieces of old blankets for padding, strips of various lengths with buckles, and a two-ounce vial of persulphate of iron.
>
> *Kane, 1934, p. 332*

Charity Hospital of New Orleans was founded with funds left by a sailor, Jean Louis, in 1737. This money, designated to be used for the establishment of a hospital for the care of the sick, included funds to purchase equipment. It served as both a hospital and an asylum for the poor. Several catastrophes occurred, and the hospital was rebuilt in 1832. The Sisters of Charity were placed in control of the institution in 1834.

In 1751 the first institution deserving of the name *hospital* was founded in Philadelphia through the efforts of Dr. Thomas Bond and other Philadelphia physicians. This group proposed that a general hospital be established there and worked to obtain contributions. With the assistance of Benjamin Franklin, they were able to secure funds from the Province (State) of Pennsylvania and from private donors. The Pennsylvania Hospital became the first hospital in the United States that was designed solely for the curative care of the sick. The insane, too, were placed in the category of those who were ill and needed treatment. After careful selection, servant-nurses were employed. The seal of this institution is that of the Good Samaritan: "Take care of him and I will repay thee." The hospital's medical library was the best in the area for a long time. The most renowned physician of colonial times, Dr. Benjamin Rush (1745–1813), served the mentally ill in Pennsylvania Hospital. His most famous work, "Medical Inquiries and Observations Upon Diseases of the Mind," was published in 1812 and contained a foresighted approach to care. A separate department for the mentally ill was developed in 1841, and

SICK WOMAN IN WARD OVERRUN BY RATS IN BELLEVUE HOSPITAL. *Engraving from* HARPER'S WEEKLY, *1860. Museum of the City of New York, New York.*

This illustration appeared with the following, "We give herewith a picture of the beds in Bellevue Hospital in this city, in one of which the newborn child of Mary Connor was eaten by rats on Monday morning, April 23 . . . the building's swarming with rats, as many as 40 having been found in the bathtub one evening, and Mary Connor herself mentions that in her agony, she felt them running over her body."

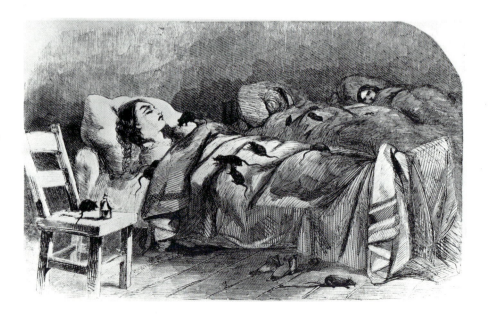

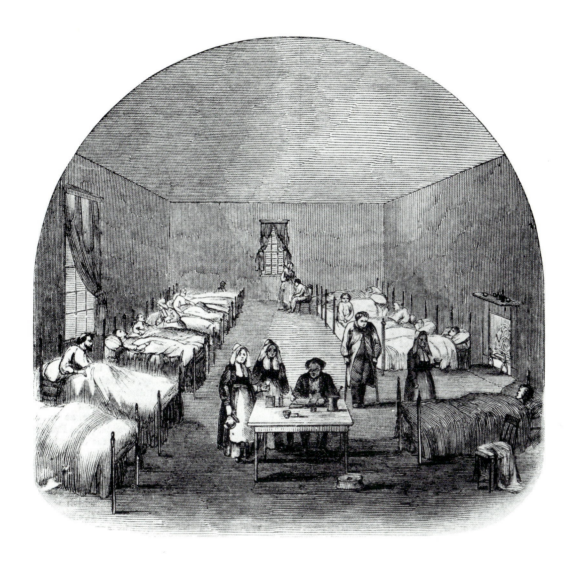

THE WARD, *New Orleans 1859. The Bettmann Archive, New York.*

it was referred to as "Kirkbride," after Dr. Thomas Kirkbride, who was in charge of the service for forty-two years. Before this time, lunatics had been caged in the basement of the general hospital.

The New York Hospital received its charter in 1771. According to Nutting and Dock (1907), however, it did not receive patients until January 1791. The original building burned to the ground. The hospital was used by British and Hessian soldiers as a barrack, and it suffered the disorganizations of war. It was backed by the most prominent and cultured citizens, and its attendants were probably superior to those of Bellevue and Blockley. The care offered to patients was also better than that given in the almshouses. Dr. Valentine Seaman gave the nurses a series of lectures that focused on anatomy, physiology, maternal nursing, and the care of children. The latter lectures were published in *The Midwife's Monitor and Mother's Mirror* in 1800. Dr. Seaman regarded midwives as indispensable; he believed that they should be thoroughly and carefully taught. He did not seem to make a clear differentiation between midwivery and nursing.

Other hospitals that still carry on public service, along with several dispensaries, originated prior to 1860. In 1786 the Quakers established the Philadelphia Dispensary to care for the sick in their homes. It was independent of any hospital, and finances were taken care of through appeals to public sympathy. The concept that large numbers of people needing treatment were not sick enough to be hospitalized was a relatively new one. As a result of this idea, the

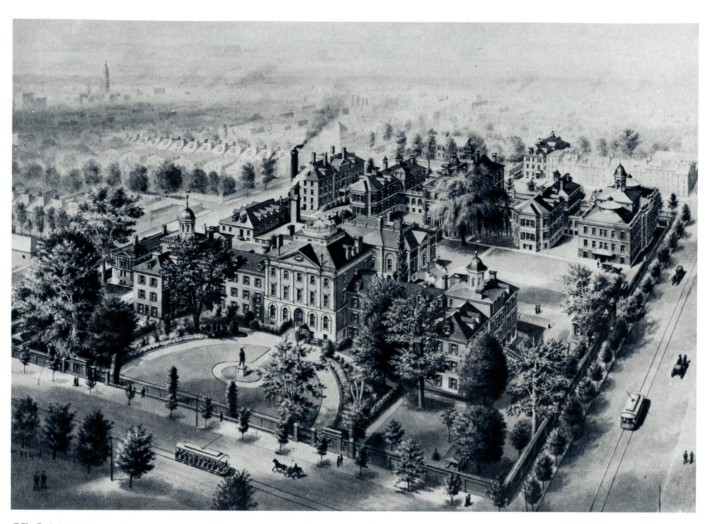

P.T. Goist, VIEW OF PENNSYLVANIA HOSPITAL IN THE EARLY TWENTIETH CENTURY. *Engraving. Courtesy of Pennsylvania Hospital, Philadelphia.*

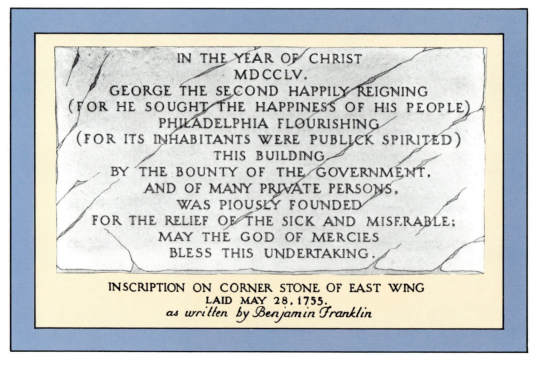

IN THE YEAR OF CHRIST
MDCCLV.
GEORGE THE SECOND HAPPILY REIGNING
(FOR HE SOUGHT THE HAPPINESS OF HIS PEOPLE)
PHILADELPHIA FLOURISHING
(FOR ITS INHABITANTS WERE PUBLICK SPIRITED)
THIS BUILDING
BY THE BOUNTY OF THE GOVERNMENT,
AND OF MANY PRIVATE PERSONS,
WAS PIOUSLY FOUNDED
FOR THE RELIEF OF THE SICK AND MISERABLE;
MAY THE GOD OF MERCIES
BLESS THIS UNDERTAKING.

INSCRIPTION ON CORNER STONE OF EAST WING
LAID MAY 28, 1755.
as written by Benjamin Franklin

CORNERSTONE OF PENNSYLVANIA HOSPITAL, *1755, with an inscription written by Benjamin Franklin. Courtesy of Pennsylvania Hospital, Philadelphia.*

274

expense of hospital care became unnecessary. Medical, surgical, and obstetrical services were offered under the supervision of Dr. Joseph Warrington. Physicians treated individuals without charge and made home visits when necessary. The dispensary was a success and the idea spread to other cities. The New York Dispensary was opened in 1791; the Boston Dispensary, in 1796. The latter had the first dental, lung, and evening pay clinic for working people in the nation; in addition, it housed the first food clinic in the world. Unfortunately, the dispensaries sank into neglect and almost obscurity when public and professional interest turned to hospitals. Services dwindled until a first-aid service and the issuance of free medicines were the only remaining functions.

■ MEDICINE IN THE COLONIES

Medicine could offer little help against rampant disease and sickness in colonial America. Medieval methods were used in diagnosis, and treatments generally were not scientifically based. Emetics, purgatives, and bleeding continued to be the chief methods employed in the care of the sick. Brandy and whiskey became favorite remedies for febrile illnesses and continued to be so for a number of years. By the middle of the nineteenth century, however, the contributions to scientific knowledge made by Pasteur, Lister, Koch, and others began the modern era of medicine and surgery. The science of bacteriology provided the foundation. The introduction of ether and chloroform as general anesthetics facilitated surgical practice. These advances altered the course of medical history to the point that concepts of illness, treatments, and hygienic practices at the end of the century bore little resemblance to what they had been in the beginning. "Looking back, one may say that medicine was groping in the dark

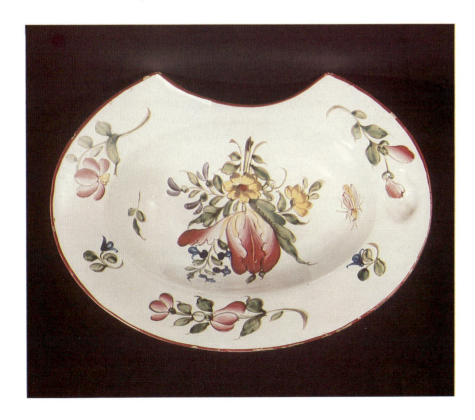

BLEEDING BOWL, *c. 1760. Strasburg porcelain. The Bridgeman Art Library Ltd./Private Collection.*

275

but was seeking light with growing anticipation. New concepts as well as further knowledge were essential if light was to be found" (Shryock, 1959, p. 195).

Serious health problems were brought to the New World with the migrants who left Europe. Scarlet fever, diphtheria, influenza, typhoid, typhus, tuberculosis, yellow fever, and other infectious diseases produced epidemics that were a constant nightmare. Scurvy and pellagra were the prevalent nutritional diseases and indicated a lack of proper food, particularly among the poorer classes. One in five individuals was afflicted with smallpox, which proved to be a formidable and dreaded disease. Fear became so great that experiments with inoculation were undertaken. Nearly all physicians opposed it, but the prominent clergy supported it. The opposition was apparently because of the risk factor involved with inoculation (occasionally deaths followed). The process of inoculation represented the beginnings of preventive medicine or, more specifically, immunology. A modified form called vaccination replaced the use of smallpox inoculation. Developed and reported in 1798 by Edward Jenner, it employed the use of the cowpox "virus," which proved to be safer and equally effective.

The true nature of disease remained an enigma. In addition, few persons understood how the prevailing practices used with disease and illness worked. They were ignorant of the action within the body that brought about the observed effects. In many instances it was enough just to know that it worked. "Learned men" gave advice on care of the sick and surgical care. Many laymen thus functioned as physicians without ever receiving a formal medical degree. Colonial physicians were generally poorly educated. According to some sources, the title of "doctor" was not even used in the colonies before 1769. It was an age of few doctors and profiteering quacks.

> Of medicine the Puritans knew little and practiced less. They swallowed doses of weird and repelling concoctions, wore charms and amulets, found comfort and relief in internal and external remedies that could have had no possible influence upon the cause of the trouble, and when all else failed they fell back upon the mercy and will of God. Surgery was a matter of tooth-pulling and bone-setting, and though post-mortems were performed, we have no knowledge of the skill of the practitioner. The healing art, as well as nursing and midwifery, was frequently in the hands of women. . . . The men who practiced physic were generally homebred, making the greater part of their living at farming or agriculture. Some were ministers as well as physicians. . . . There were a number of regularly trained doctors—though not a physician had more than a smattering of medicine.
>
> *Andrews, vol. 6, p. 82*

Men who could afford the expense went to Europe to study in the medical schools of Edinburgh or Vienna. Otherwise, the young student of medicine was apprenticed to a practicing physician, to whom he paid a fee (usually $100) as well as rendering services about the house and stables. He was permitted to observe his master treat patients and upon completing the duration of the apprenticeship would receive the textbooks and instruments essential for his practice. Observation, reading, and practice comprised the learning techniques. The average time spent in this process was approximately 144 weeks or close to three years. The preceptors ultimately became a powerful force that prevented progress in medical education and care.

As the colonies continued to develop, the issue of medical education increased in importance. Yet the medical departments did not find a place in colleges or universities until Harvard, the first American university (founded in 1636) was over one hundred years old. They were then organized rapidly and included the College of Philadelphia in 1765 (later a part of the University of Pennsylvania); King's College in 1767; Harvard in 1783; and Dartmouth in 1798. Other programs developed in the next century and included those established at Yale in 1810 and Johns Hopkins University in 1893.

> When the nineteenth century dawned, America had only four small medical schools to supply physicians for its burgeoning population, compelling most doctors to acquire their training by apprenticeship. In 1807 the University of Maryland Medical School was organized by a small group of Baltimore physicians as a private venture, and in succeeding years dozens of these proprietary medical schools came into existence. Three or four physicians would apply for a state charter, rent or buy a building, and begin advertising for students. The school year ordinarily lasted from eight to fourteen weeks, and the course work consisted exclusively of listening to lectures. Many proprietary schools granted degrees after one academic year, although they usually required the student to have served a one- or two-year apprenticeship prior to admission. Since these schools were dependent upon student fees for income, few applicants were ever turned down and even fewer failed to graduate.
>
> *Lyons, 1978, p. 534*

Approximately 400 medical schools were established before 1860, and many of them graduated poorly educated physicians. The quality of instruction was poor, libraries were inadequate, there were no laboratories, and dissection opportunities were limited. Unfortunately, little had been done to regulate these programs. The formation of the American Medical Association in 1847 finally led to the reform and advancement of medicine. This organization advocated the improvement of medical education, the establishment of a code of ethics, and the promotion of public health measures. The advent of this association moved American medicine toward professionalization. The A.M.A. created a permanent committee on education in 1904, and it became the A.M.A. Council on Medical Education in 1906. This council persuaded the Carnegie Foundation for the Advancement of Teaching to evaluate medical schools according to the ability of their graduates to pass licensing board examinations. Abraham Flexner was employed by the foundation to survey the field. His report, the Flexner Report (1910), was a damning indictment of medical education and brought foundation money to the higher quality schools; the weaker schools were forced out of business. The council, in turn, classified the schools on an A, B, C basis, which played a primary role in the standardization of medical education.

The remarkable progress that was finally achieved in the scientific basis of patient care was illustrated by Thomas Eakins (1844–1916). This American artist left two paintings that vividly present a "before" and "after" look of the medical scene. The same amphithe-

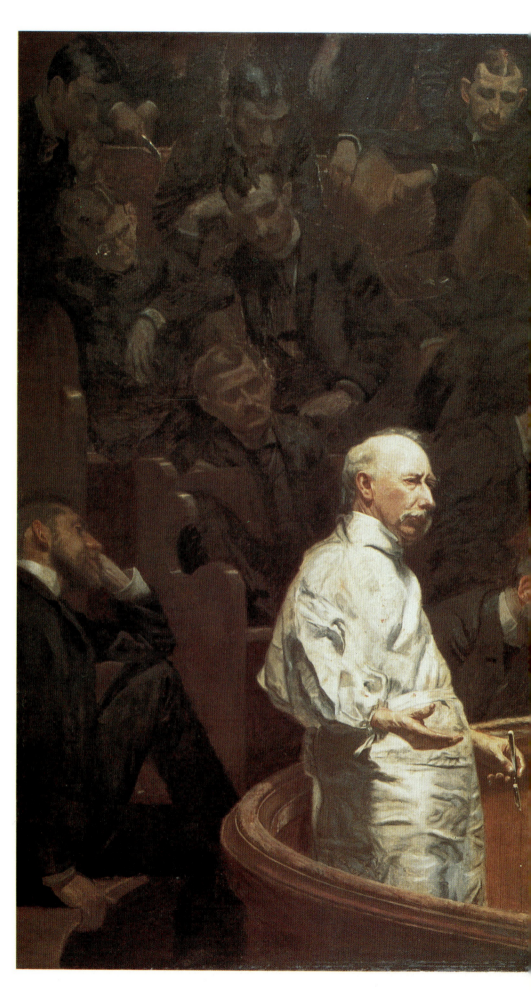

Thomas Eakins, THE AGNEW CLINIC, *1898. Canvas, 331.5 × 179.1 cm. University of Pennsylvania, School of Medicine, Philadelphia.*

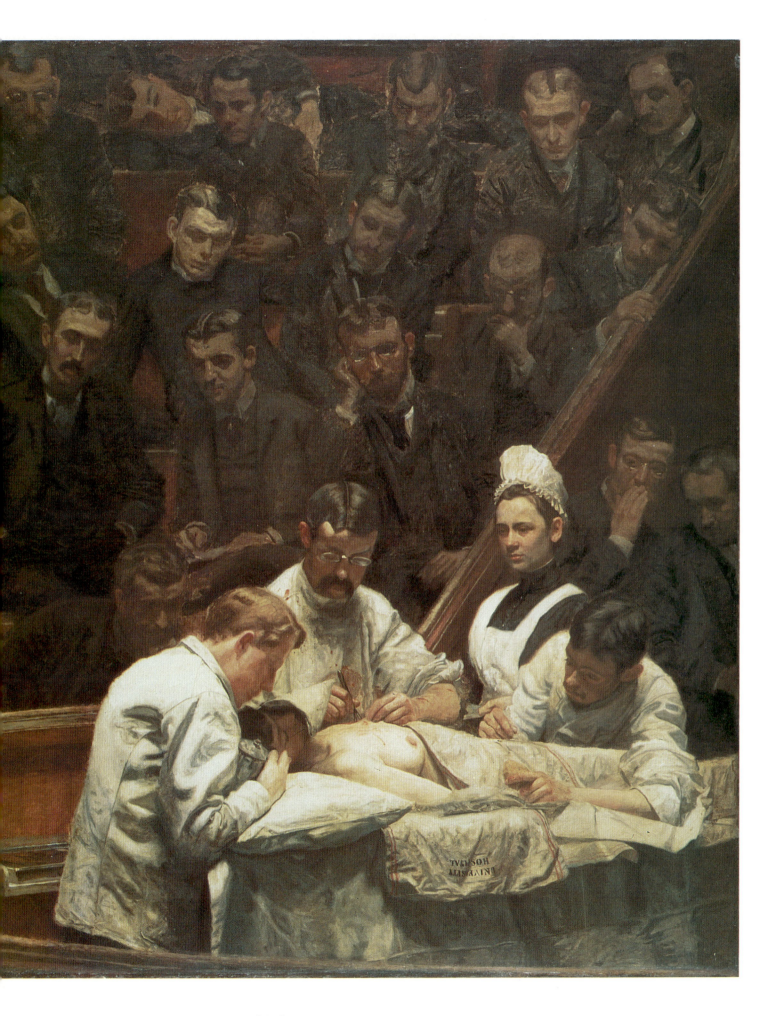

279

ater was used for the setting of each painting. The *Gross Clinic* (1875) depicts grand rounds in which Dr. Gross explains the surgical operation being performed to medical students. It appears that he is totally unaware of the patient and oblivious to the horror of the patient's mother, who sits to his right. The *Agnew Clinic* (1898) depicts a distinct change. The surgeons wear gowns, the patient is covered, ether is being used, and a nurse (nursing schools had finally opened) has joined the operating team. The needed reforms had begun to occur.

■ RELIGIOUS NURSING ORDERS IN AMERICA

Many priests and nuns came to America with the French and Spanish settlers and supplied at least a minimum of nursing care to the Catholic communities. The Augustinian Nuns, Ursuline Nuns, and Sisters of Charity are most often mentioned in the history of nursing service in the hospitals of North and South America. Religious orders of women also contributed greatly to nursing care during the Civil War. Their organization and motivation provided a distinct advantage over the so-called lay nurses of the day. The members of these orders had some education and had been carefully instructed. Those recruited to these orders were usually refined, intelligent women with a sincere interest in the care of the sick.

Among the earliest religious communities that took part in the care of the sick in hospitals and homes in the United States was the Sisters of Charity of Emmitsburg, Maryland. This order was founded by Mother Seton (1774–1813) in 1809. Elizabeth Ann Bayley Seton became the first native-born American to be canonized for her charitable works. Her original community was known as The Sisters of Charity of Saint Joseph, but in 1850 the members united with the

QUARTERS AND CHAPEL OF THE DAUGHTERS OF CHARITY AT LINCOLN HOSPITAL IN WASHINGTON, D.C., *c. 1860. National Library of Medicine, Bethesda, Maryland.*

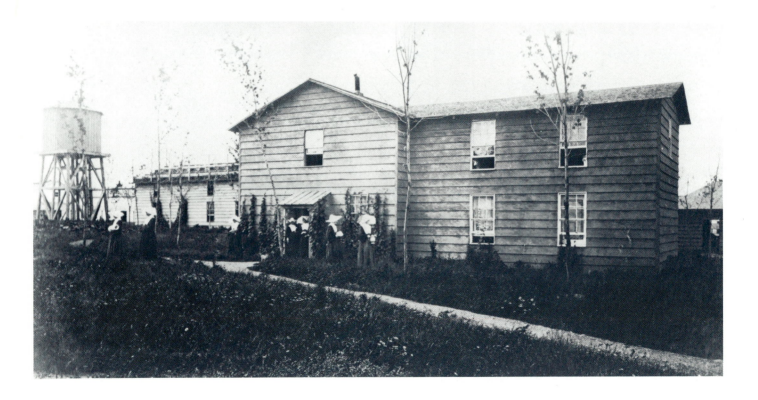

worldwide community of the Sisters of Charity of St. Vincent de Paul. A habit of blue with a large linen headdress ("cornette") was chosen at this time in lieu of the original dress of the community. (The founding group wore a habit that resembled Mrs. Seton's widow's dress.) Different branches eventually bore the name of Sisters of Charity: the Sisters of Charity of New York (Black Cap Sisters of Charity); the Sisters of Charity of Greensburg, Pennsylvania, of New Jersey, of Cincinnati, Ohio, and of Halifax, Nova Scotia; and the Sisters of Charity of Nazareth, Kentucky. The latter community was founded by Mother Catherine Spalding; its members used horses for travel to the homes of patients. These orders were also called by other names: Gray Sisters, Gray Nuns, or Daughters of Charity. Opportunities were provided in nursing education, the delivery of nursing service, and parochial education.

Elizabeth Seton was the daughter of Dr. Richard Bayley, an eminent American physician who was the first professor of anatomy at King's College (now Columbia University). She married William Seton, a banker, in 1794. Upon her husband's early death, she was left with five children and no financial support. Her conversion to Catholicism alienated friends who otherwise might have assisted her. Elizabeth Seton and other society matrons established the Widow's Society in New York to raise money for poor widows, to visit them in

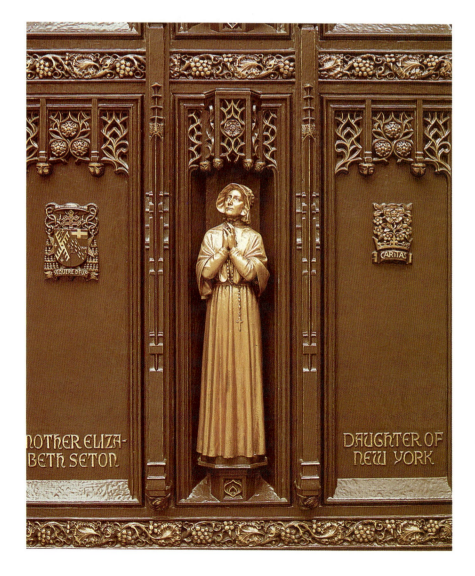

"St. Elizabeth Ann Seton," detail from THE GREAT BRONZE DOORS. St. Patrick's Cathedral, New York.

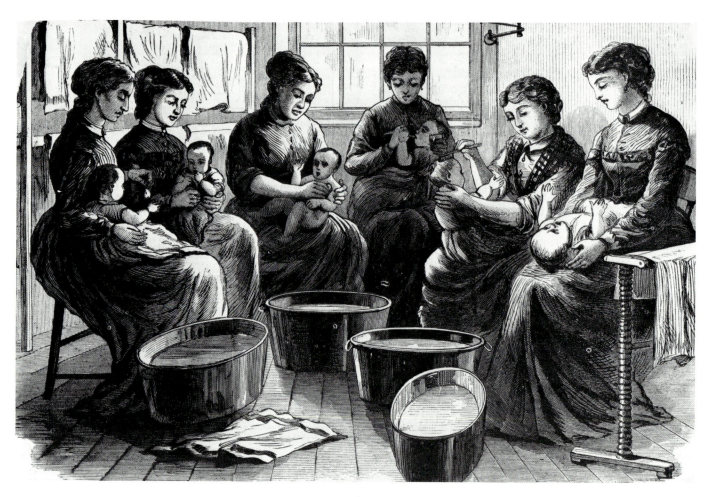

FOUNDLING HOSPITAL OF SISTERS OF CHARITY,
"WASHING THE BABIES", *1869. Engraving. The
Bettmann Archive, New York.*

their homes, and to nurse and comfort them. She turned to teaching and opened a school for girls in Baltimore. This event was the beginning of parochial education in the United States. A piece of land in Emmitsburg was chosen for the school, and it was not long before other young women joined her and became Sisters in this teaching order.

These Sisters of Charity became well known for their remarkable work in hospital nursing and nursing during epidemics. They were asked to manage a number of hospitals, including the Marine Hospital in Baltimore, the Mullanphy Hospital in St. Louis, "Old Blockley" in Philadelphia, and the Charity Hospital of New Orleans. Nursing thus became an important branch of their work. The members were also instrumental in founding several hospitals and mental and foundling asylums.

Demands for nursing care by the religious orders increased as the settlements of the new country progressed. The various Catholic nursing orders responded rapidly and developed extensive networks throughout the country. The Sisters of Mercy, the Sisters of the Holy Cross, the Irish Sisters of Mercy (who came to America in 1843), the Dominicans, the Sisters of the Poor of St. Francis, and other communities worked in hospitals, homes, and in all types of settings. The majority of them also nursed under fire on the battlefields. They founded hospitals everywhere and provided the highest standards of nursing of the times. Many of the first hospitals in America were named Mercy Hospitals, such as those in Pittsburgh, Chicago, and San Francisco. They were the better hospitals that were available at the time of the Civil War.

282

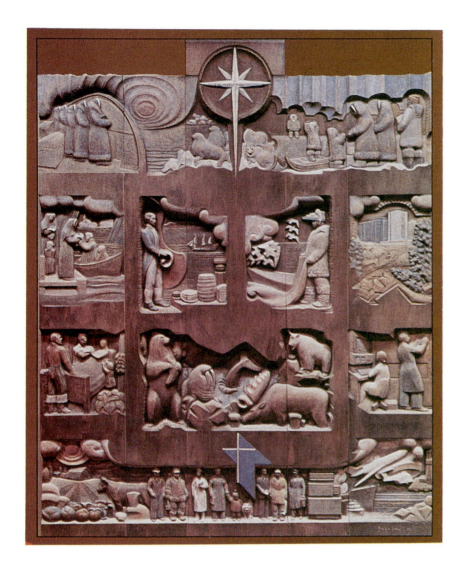

Sisterhoods of the Protestant Church also contributed to the nursing effort in America. The Episcopal Sisterhood of the Holy Communion was founded in New York in 1845 by Pastor Muhlenberg at what is currently St. Luke's Hospital. The work of the English Lutheran Church began with four deaconesses who were brought to Passavant's Hospital in Pittsburgh by Pastor Fliedner in 1849. In Baltimore there was a branch of the English All Saints Sisters. The English Sisterhood of St. Margaret's (Episcopal) was brought to Boston about 1869, the beginning of its forty some years of service to the Children's Hospital of that city. Many deaconess hospitals were established, particularly in the Midwest. Protestant religious nursing groups also gave nursing care to the sick and the wounded during the time of the Civil War.

■ THE REVOLUTIONARY WAR

Colonial wars were fought from 1607 until the Revolution. These wars involved Indians, emigrants, loyalists, patriots, and colonist against colonist. The desire for independence grew stronger and stronger as the colonists became more self-sufficient. Yet until 1774 they considered themselves Britons. In that year Patrick Henry made

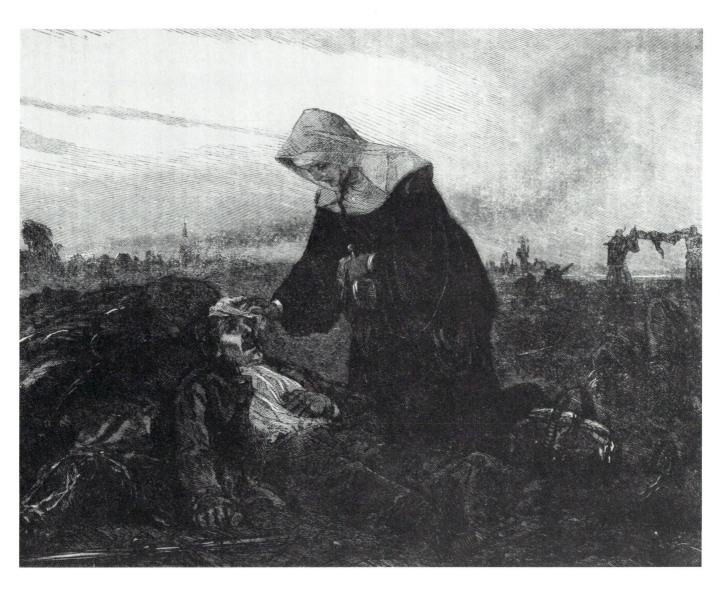

AFTER THE BATTLE, *1881. Engraving. The*
Bettmann Archive, New York.

his famous statement: "The distinctions between Virginians, Pennsylvanians, New Yorkers, and New Englanders are no more. I am not a Virginian but an American." The inevitable conflict between the British Crown and the colonies terminated in the Revolutionary War.

The American Revolution involved all the English colonies along the Atlantic coast. The colonies were, however, ill prepared for the burdens, the expense, and the organization necessary to wage war on their own. The hastily mobilized army had no medical corps, no Red Cross, and no trained nurses (Jamieson and Sewall, 1950). The nuns of the Catholic Church placed themselves and their hospitals at the disposal of the military authorities, since they were the only organized groups with some knowledge of nursing. Goodnow quotes a colonial writer who vividly depicted this state of affairs:

At the start of the war the tale of the medical department was a sorry one. There was practically no organization nor discipline. Surgical instruments were few. Drugs were few and bad; opium and quinine were scarce and ether was then unknown. Trained nurses and scientific nursing did not exist. Blundering assistants called "mates" were the only help the surgeons had.

Goodnow, 1942, p. 182

284

Several private homes in Cambridge were made into hospitals after the Battle of Bunker Hill, and Dr. John Warren was placed in charge. These are regarded as the first military hospitals. Other hospitals were established in Boston, where the nurses were mostly men. Women made no attempt at organized nursing, although meagre records indicate that a few women were actually employed as nurses to care for the soldiers. According to a congressional resolution of July 17, 1775, there would be one nurse to every ten patients in the personnel for military hospitals (Hahn, 1927). These women were to be paid one fifteenth of a dollar per day, the equivalent of two dollars per month (Stimson, 1925).

The government authorities were not indifferent to the condition of the military hospitals; however, they were involved with the general burdens of a revolution. Finally, in 1777 General Washington ordered that women be obtained to nurse the soldiers. Many women were subsequently employed, but they did little more than cook and serve meals. Often women followed their husbands to the battlefield and nursed them under the greatest of obstacles. Little surgery was performed because there were no aneshetics; the main type of surgery was amputation. There were frequent epidemics from scarlet fever, dysentery, and smallpox. Food rations were meagre, and shoes and clothing rapidly wore out. An interesting commentary about the aftermath of the war was rendered by Robinson:

> War, with its sudden collections of sick, wounded, and maimed, stimulates the progress of medicine: "The War of the Revolution was the making of medicine in this country." In the change from colonial to national medicine, the casualty was woman: woman was not ignored, she was expelled. The female practitioner, denied the opportunity and instruction of the new time, ceased to exist. Trained male obstetricians, invading the lying-in chamber, thrust out the immemorial midwife. As later expressed by a Boston physician (1820): "It was one of the first and happiest fruits of improved medical education in America, that females were excluded from practice; and this has only been effected by the united and persevering efforts of some of the most distinguished individuals of the profession." In the male monopoly of medicine, there was no room for the trained nurse: any grandmother, any destitute old woman who could be hired, was requisitioned as nurse, and none other was desired.
>
> *Robinson, 1946, p. 139*

■ NURSING IN THE CIVIL WAR (1861–1865)

At the outbreak of the Civil War, the Union had no army nurse corps, ambulance service, field hospital service, or organized medical corps. There was still no group of trained nurses in the country, but after the first battles the need for nurses became imperative. Many religious orders volunteered and offered their services. They provided nursing care in their own hospitals, in army hospitals, and on the battlefield. Approximately 600 Sisters from twelve orders participated during this critical period in history. They were given permission by President Abraham Lincoln to purchase any supplies needed for their

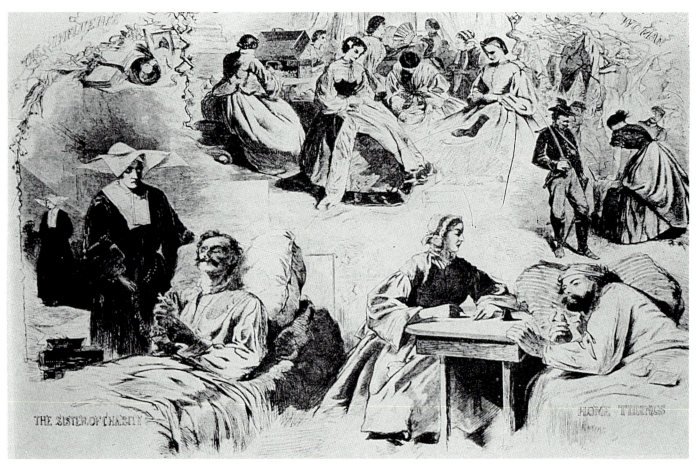

Winslow Homer, OUR WOMEN AND THE WAR. *Engraving, approx. 34.3 × 52.1 cm.* HARPER'S WEEKLY, *September 6, 1862.*

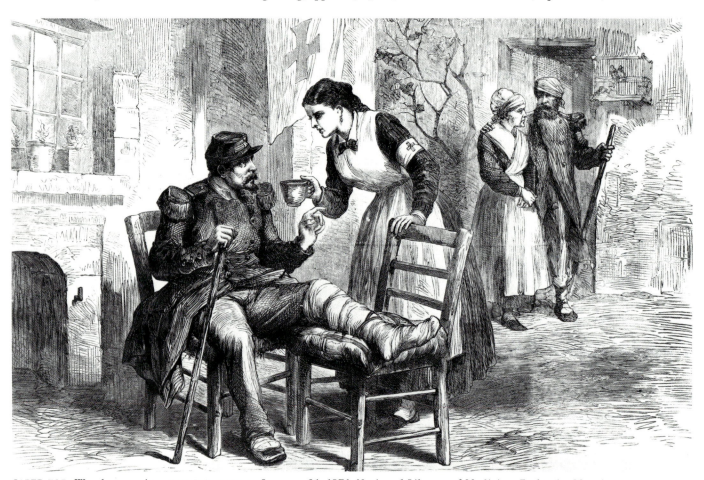

CARED FOR. *Wood engraving.* HARPER'S WEEKLY, *January 21, 1871. National Library of Medicine, Bethesda, Maryland.*

work. Lincoln knew that most "good nursing" was being done by these religious sisterhoods, that they had helped in epidemics, that they were already organized and were accustomed to discipline and obedience to authority. He, therefore, supported their efforts to the fullest. There were not, however, enough Sisters to care for the large number of sick and wounded. Hundreds of other women and men simply appeared in the camps and offered their services. With and without experience, they assisted with nursing care in whatever way they were able. The majority were volunteers, although some received compensation. It is estimated that between 2000 and 10,000 women or more were engaged in nursing and hospital administration during the Civil War. (The large range is a result of the variance in citations in reference materials.) The most famous of these were Dorothea Lynde Dix, Clara Barton, Louisa May Alcott, Mary Ann "Mother" Bickerdyke, and Walt Whitman.

The total number of men lost either from battle injuries or from disease during the American Civil War was 618,000, 360,000 of whom were Union soldiers and 258,000 Confederates. Many of these died on the battlefield. Those with less serious wounds faced inadequate sanitary conditions and a generally awkward and unorganized medical corps. Septicemia, erysipelas, gangrene, and tetanus were common complications among the wounded. Almost any type of building became a military hospital; base hospitals were located in hotels, churches, warehouses, schools, farmhouses, and other public buildings. In addition, structures were hastily erected or tents were pitched. Even the Capitol was used, with 400 soldiers nursed in the

ELEVEN VIGNETTES OF SCENES IN THE U.S. ARMY'S CITIZENS VOLUNTEER HOSPITAL, *c. 1860. Lithograph. National Library of Medicine, Bethesda, Maryland.*

These scenes depict the Army's Citizens Volunteer Hospital in Philadelphia during the Civil War where volunteer nurses served in the wards.

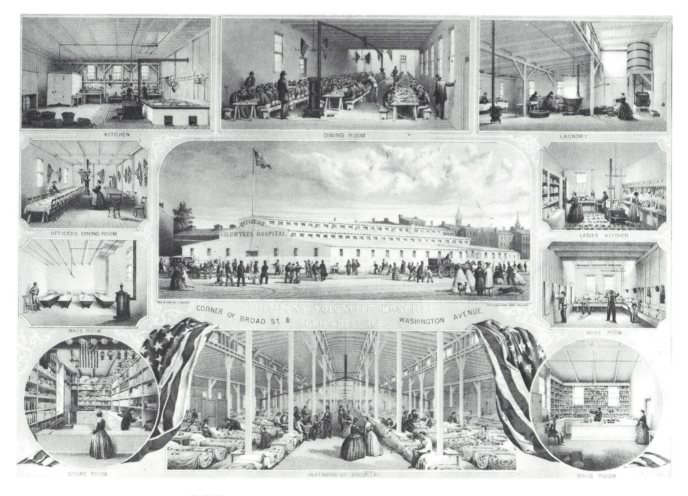

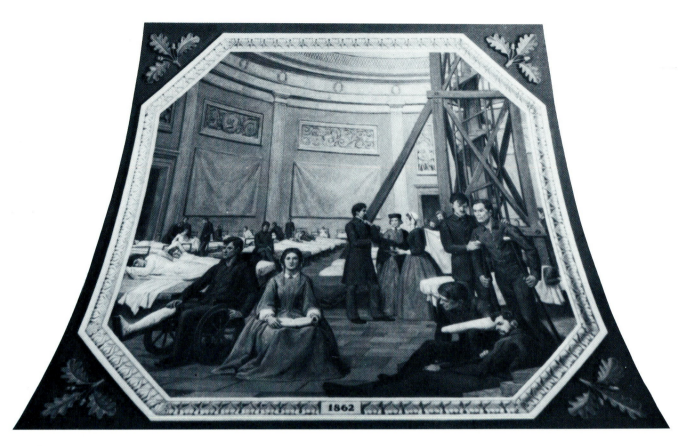

Allyn Cox, ROTUNDA AS A HOSPITAL DURING THE CIVIL WAR, 1862, *corridor, House Wing. Library of Congress, Washington, D.C.*

Senate and House and 300 in the Rotunda. Ward masters and orderlies were available in many of the hospitals to do as much nursing as possible. Women nurses gave medicines, tended to the diets, and dressed wounds.

The sick and injured were originally removed from the battlefield in hand litters. Later a medical transport service was organized with horse-drawn covered wagons used as ambulances. These springless wagons often inflicted much pain on the wounded as they bumped for hours over badly kept roads. Hospital trains were furnished by the railroads. Vessels along the Eastern seaboard and the Mississippi water route were used to evacuate patients and as "floating hospitals." The first Navy hospital ship, the steamer *Red Rover,* was put into service. Captured from the Confederates, this steamer was converted into a floating hospital and then added to the Federal fleet of ships. The Catholic Sisters of Mercy volunteered to do the nursing on board and can be considered the first Navy nurses. A description of the *Red Rover* was provided in a letter to Flag Officer A.H. Foote:

> I wish that you could see our hospital boat, the *Red Rover,* with all her comforts for the sick and disabled seamen. She is decided to be the most complete thing of her kind that ever floated, and is in every way a decided success. The Western Sanitary Commission gave us, in cost of articles, $3,500. The icebox of the steamer holds 300 tons. She has bathrooms, laundry, elevator for the sick from the lower to the upper deck, operating room, nine different water closets, gauze blinds to the windows to keep the cinders and smoke from annoying the sick, two separate kitchens for sick and well, a regular corps of nurses, and two water closets on every deck.

Roddis, 1935, p. 92

288

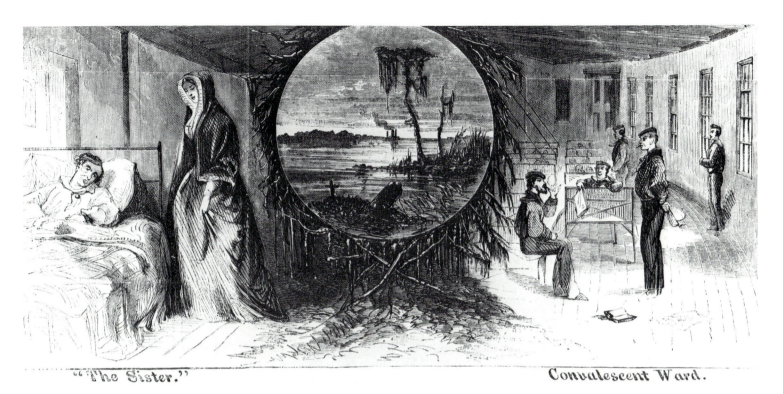

"The Sister."   Convalescent Ward.

THE SISTER AND CONVALESCENT WARD ON THE NAVAL HOSPITAL SHIP "RED ROVER." *Wood engraving.* HARPER'S WEEKLY, *May 9, 1863. National Library of Medicine, Bethesda, Maryland.*

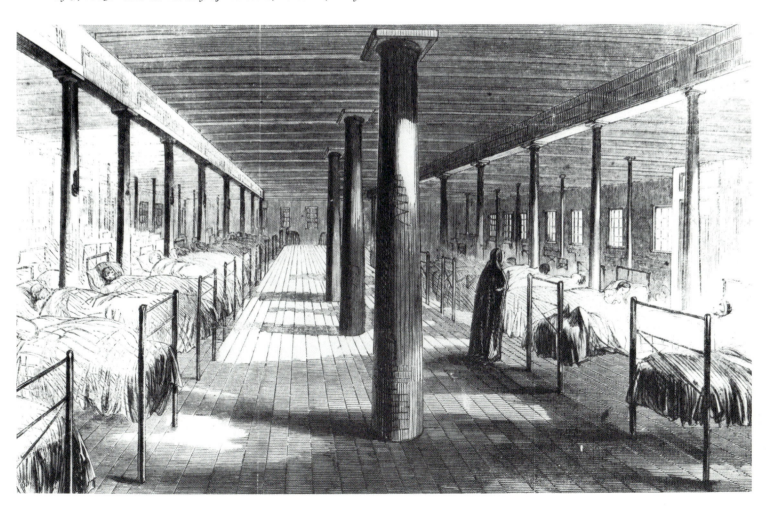

Theodore R. Davis, THE WARD. *Drawing. From* HARPER'S WEEKLY, *1863. Naval Audiovisual Center, Washington, D.C. Scene from one of the wards on the "Red Rover" Hospital Ship during the Civil War.*

289

United States Sanitary Commission

Within a month after Lincoln's initial request for soldiers, Dr. Elizabeth Blackwell, America's first woman physician, organized the Women's Central Association for Relief in New York City. Miss Louisa Lee Schuyler was elected president. Through the efforts of this group and similar ones, the Rev. Dr. Henry W. Bellows and four physicians were persuaded to go to Washington to plead for the establishment of a sanitary commission. This commission would act as advisor to the medical department of the Army and would investigate the health conditions of the Union Army. After both governmental and military opposition was overcome, the United States Sanitary Commission was established by order of President Lincoln on June 3, 1861. Its aim was stated as "a simple desire and resolute determination to secure for the men who have enlisted in this war, that care which it is the duty of the nation to give them" (Boardman, 1915, p. 53). A sum of $5 million in cash and $15 million worth of supplies was raised. This organization has been called the forerunner of the American Red Cross.

The Women's Central Association for Relief became a branch of the Sanitary Commission. Where branches did not exist, it stimulated the formation of new ones. It coordinated all the relief organizations throughout the country and sent nurses to areas where they were needed most. Preparatory programs were planned for the nurses at

Thomas Nast, HEROES AND HEROINES OF THE WAR, *nineteenth century. Engraving. Chicago Historical Society, Illinois. Represented in this print are the many diverse activities of the United States Sanitary Commission which provided nurses both on and off the battlefield, as well as helping to make supplies and raise money to support health care.*

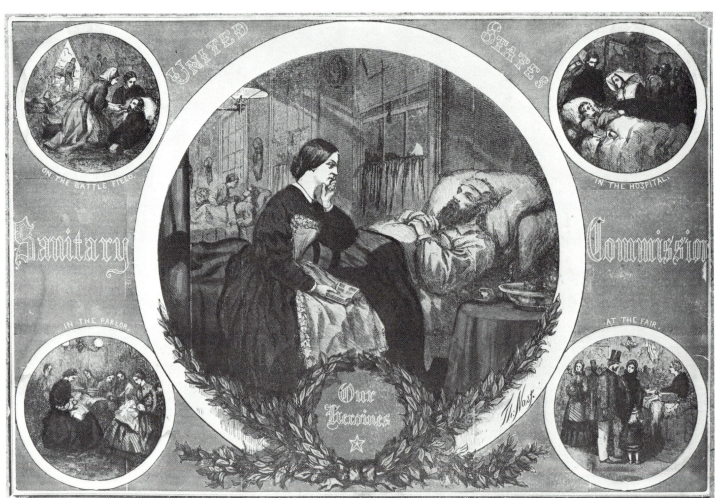

HEROES AND HEROINES OF THE WAR.

290

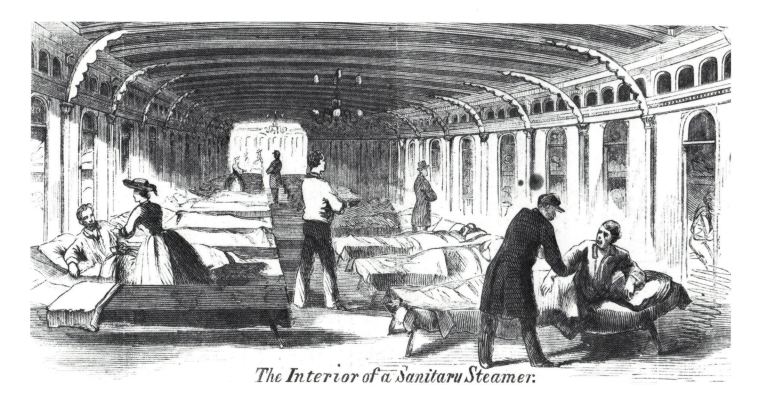

The Interior of a Sanitary Steamer:

New York Hospital, Bellevue Hospital, and several Boston hospitals. The nurses received one month's observation and work experience. The Western Sanitary Commission was distinct from the Eastern one but cooperated with it. It operated hospital steamers on the Ohio and Mississippi rivers in addition to a hospital train. The Confederacy had no such organization, but a number of women's groups rendered valuable service to the cause of the war.

The Sanitary Commission wished to secure the most healthy conditions in the military camps, hospitals, and on transports. It first inspected the Army camps in the vicinity of Washington and found these to be lacking in a variety of areas, including sanitation and hygiene, rations, and space. The report revealed that fifteen percent of the Northern regiment physicians were poorly qualified or totally incompetent. Soon after, the Northern forces suffered defeat at the

THE INTERIOR OF A SANITARY STEAMER.
Engraving. From HARPER'S WEEKLY, *1862. Naval Audiovisual Center, Washington, D.C.*

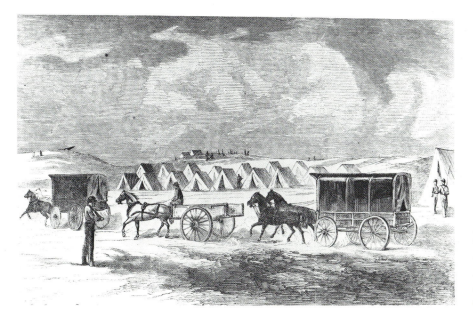

AMBULANCE TRAIN RETURNING FROM THE TRENCHES WITH WOUNDED DURING THE CAMPAIGN AT CHARLESTON HARBOR. *Engraving.* HARPER'S WEEKLY, *September 12, 1863. National Library of Medicine, Bethesda, Maryland.*

Battle of Bull Run, and an inquiry showed that the defeat lay in those conditions identified by the commission. In general, the soldiers had entered battle in an unfit condition.

After the first battles of the war, the wounded had practically no care. "Common soldiers, untrained, lazy, and indifferent or brutal, were cooks and nurses for the war hospitals, the largest of which had 40 beds. There were no medicines, no stores, nor ambulances. The camps were dirty and unsanitary." When they (the Sanitary Commission) first offered supplies and service, the Government Medical Bureau looked upon the proposal with suspicion; but its dire need soon forced it to accept. The Commission collected and distributed supplies of all sorts, planned camps and attended to their sanitation, tended the wounded on the field and in hospitals; in short, undertook a large share of the health work for the army. It provided such things as green vegetables, given by the farmers for the soldiers, thus preventing scurvy, the great army scourge.

Goodnow, 1942, pp. 190–191

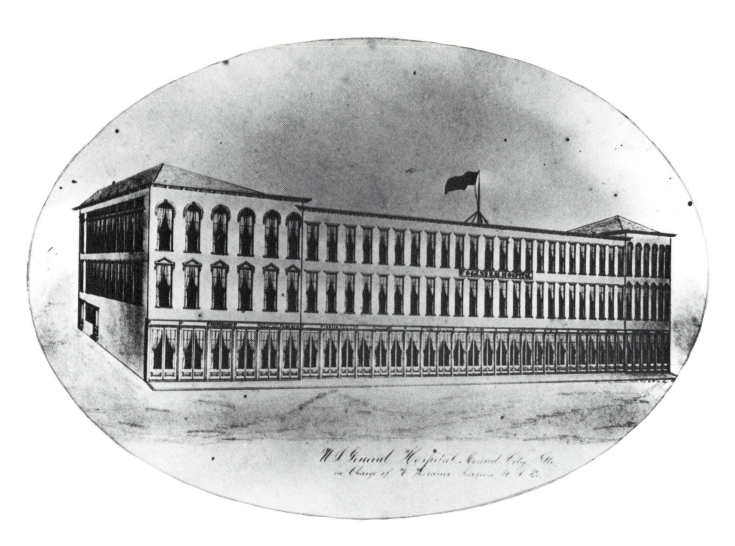

William Groth, U.S. GENERAL HOSPITAL DURING THE CIVIL WAR, *Mound City, Illinois. Naval Audiovisual Center, Washington, D.C. This hospital served as the staffing base for the USS "Red Rover."*

Dorothea Lynde Dix

On June 10, 1861, Dorothea Lynde Dix was appointed Superintendent of the Female Nurses of the Union Army by the secretary of war. This action provided for a corps of volunteer women nurses to be organized under her direction. Miss Dix was given the power to organize hospitals for the care of all wounded and sick soldiers, to appoint nurses, and to oversee and regulate specially donated supplies for distribution to the troops. Miss Dix was past the age of sixty when she received her appointment. She was not granted military rank, nor were the members of her corps. Although she did not have preparation in nursing, she possessed the necessary organizational skills from her previous humanitarian efforts in the area of mental health. Circular no. 7 of the surgeon general's office in the War Department read:

> In order to give greater utility to the acts of Miss Dorothy L. Dix as superintendent of women nurses in general hospitals, and to make the employment of such nurses conform more closely to existing laws . . . Miss Dix has been entrusted by the War Department with the duty of selecting women nurses and assigning them to general or permanent military hospitals. Women nurses

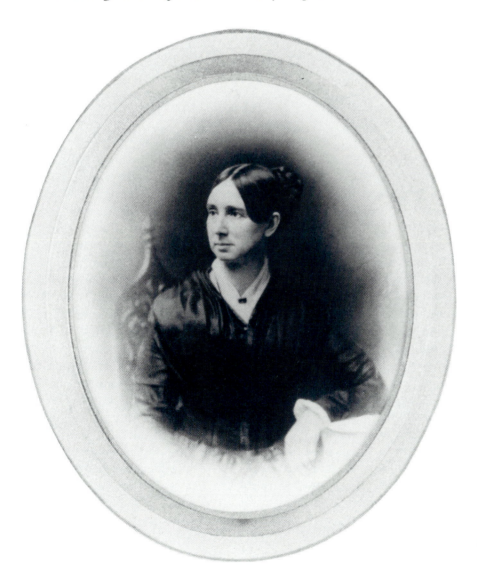

Portrait of DOROTHEA DIX. *National Library of Medicine, Bethesda, Maryland.*

293

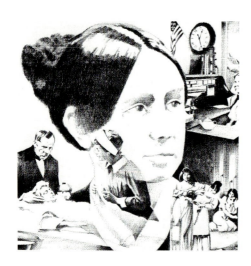

George Bestels, DOROTHEA DIX, *1893.*
Courtesy of the Upjohn Company,
Kalamazoo, Michigan.

are not to be employed in such hospitals without her sanction and approval except in case of urgent need. . . . Women wishing employment as nurses must apply to Miss Dix or to her authorised agents. Army regulations allow one nurse to every ten patients (beds).

Miss Dix's requirements for candidates were specified in circular no. 8, dated July 14, 1862. No candidate for a nurse position would be considered unless she was between the ages of 35 and 50. Matronly and plain-looking persons of experience, of superior education, and of serious disposition were to have preference. Habits of neatness, order, sobriety, and industry were prerequisites. All applicants were required to submit certificates of qualification and good character from at least two persons of trust who would testify to morality, integrity, and capacity for the care of the sick. Obedience to rules and conformity to special regulations were required and enforced. Dress was to be plain (colors of brown, gray, or black) and without ornaments. Those women who were accepted were to serve for at least a six-month period or for the duration of the war. Their compensation was to be forty cents a day and subsistence. Many women who were unable to meet the requirements ignored them and nursed during the war without official recognition or compensation. At the close of hostilities the office of the superintendent was abolished, and Dorothea Dix returned to her civilian life of reformative work in public institutions.

Clara Barton

During the Civil War, Clara Barton (1821–1912) became known as the "little lone lady in black silk." Nearly all war nurses were under the supervision of Miss Dix; the relief workers were associated with relief or aid societies, the Sanitary Commission, or religious organizations. Miss Barton, however, could not take orders or share authority and relied on her own initiative. She independently operated a large-scale war relief operation in which she arranged for huge quantities of supplies to be furnished to the Army and the hospitals. She also personally nursed in federal hospitals and with the armies on the battlefield and cared for the wounded of the Confederate armies. Her impartiality was expressed in the nursing care she extended to both whites and blacks, Northerners and Southerners. She frequently used her own resources to furnish such necessities as medical supplies, proper clothing, food, and bedding. On more than one occasion, bullets made holes in her dress and the men she was nursing were shot in her arms. Miss Barton eventually became one of the most prominent figures among the lay nurses of the Civil War. Her work embodied the ideals now characteristic of the Red Cross and became the foundation for her later success in the development of the American Red Cross (1881).

Clara Barton (Clarissa Harlowe) was born in North Oxford, Massachusetts. A former New England school teacher, she was appointed to a clerkship in the Patent Office in Washington, D.C., in 1854. This may have been the first time a woman held a government position. Miss Barton was, however, dismissed from this position be-

CHRISTIAN Herald

AND SIGNS OF OUR TIMES

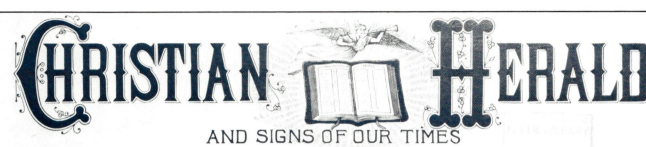

OFFICES: BIBLE HOUSE NEW YORK.

COPYRIGHT 1898, BY LOUIS KLOPSCH.

VOLUME 21.—NUMBER 10.

Rev. T. De Witt Talmage, D.D., Editor.

NEW YORK, MARCH 9, 1898.

PRICE FIVE CENTS.

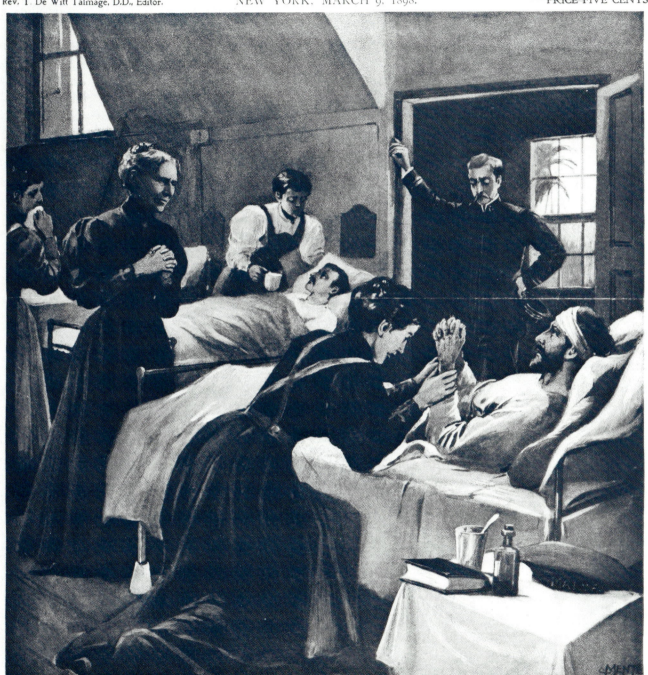

"I AM WITH THE WOUNDED."—Clara Barton's Cable Message from Havana to "The Christian Herald."

"I am with the wounded," flashed along the wire
  From the isle of Cuba, swept with sword and fire.
    Angel sweet of mercy, may your cross of red
      Cheer the wounded living; bless the wounded dead.

"I am with the starving," let the message run
  From the stricken island, when this task is done;
    Food and money plenty wait at your command.
      Give in generous measure; fill each outstretched hand.

"I am with the happy," this we long to hear
  From the isle of Cuba, trembling now in fear.
    May the great disaster touch the hearts of men,
      And, in God's great mercy, bring back peace again.

—JAMES CLARENCE HARVEY.

"I AM WITH THE WOUNDED." *Clara Barton's cable message from Havana from the cover of the* CHRISTIAN HERALD, *March 9, 1898. The Christian Herald Association, Chappaqua, New York.*

cause of her outspoken opinions on slavery. She seemed to have a flair for being the first to arrive on a scene and the first to leave when others appeared. She was already in Washington giving aid to the Sixth Massachusetts Regiment when Dorothea Dix arrived. When peace was finally made, Clara Barton conducted a prolonged search at her own expense for 80,000 missing men of the Army. She also delivered 300 lectures about the battlefields of the Civil War and established the first national cemetery on the Andersonville grounds. Miss Barton was overcome by nervous prostration, a condition that had surfaced earlier, and was directed by physicians to go to Europe, where she remained for four years. A month after arriving in Europe, she learned about the International Red Cross.

Clara Barton served with the Red Cross in 1870 during the Franco-Prussian War. On the battlefields and in the ravaged cities of France, she repeated her American Civil War performance. She also observed the systematic organization and remarkable effectiveness of the Red Cross and promised that America would join. She was subsequently decorated with the Iron Cross by the Kaiser. After a four-year absence, Miss Barton returned to the United States and began her crusade for the establishment of the American Red Cross. A Red Cross Committee was finally formed in 1881, but it took until 1882 for the U.S. Government to ratify the Geneva Convention and give the committee official standing. Clara Barton became its first president and held this office until 1904. Her home in Glen Echo, Mary-

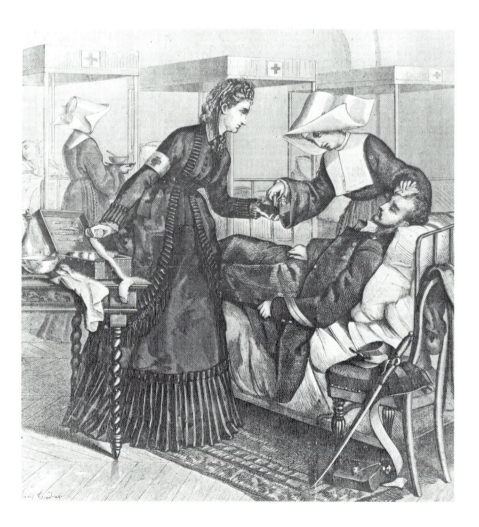

TWO NURSING NUNS AND A RED CROSS NURSE TEND CASUALTIES DURING THE FRANCO-PRUSSIAN WAR. *Wood engraving. From* LA MODE ILLUSTRÊE, *c. 1870. National Library of Medicine, Bethesda, Maryland.*

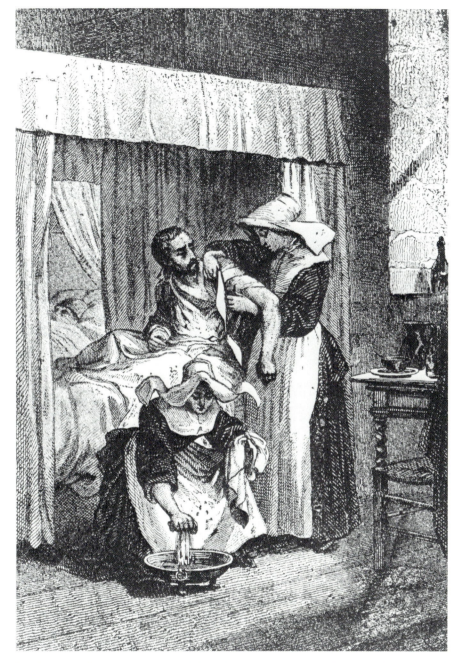

TWO NURSING NUNS CLEAN THE WOUND AND
BANDAGE THE ARM OF A SOLDIER, AN INCI-
DENT OF THE FRANCO-PRUSSIAN WAR, C. 1870.
Wood engraving. From Casimir Tollet's LES
EDIFICES HOSPITALIERS, *1892. National
Library of Medicine, Bethesda, Maryland.*

land, served as the national headquarters. According to the official charter, the Red Cross was dedicated

> to continue and carry on a system of national and international relief in time of peace and to apply the same in mitigating the sufferings caused by pestilence, famine, fire, floods, and other national calamities, and to devise and carry measure for preventing the same.

Assistance was first given in the United States during a yellow fever epidemic in Florida in 1888 and during the Johnstown flood of 1889. In 1909 the American Red Cross was reorganized under Jane Delano. At that time plans were made for a Red Cross Nursing Service to be staffed by a reserve corps of graduate nurses with specified qualifications. This pool of nurses acted as a supplement to the regular Army and Navy nurses as the occasion warranted.

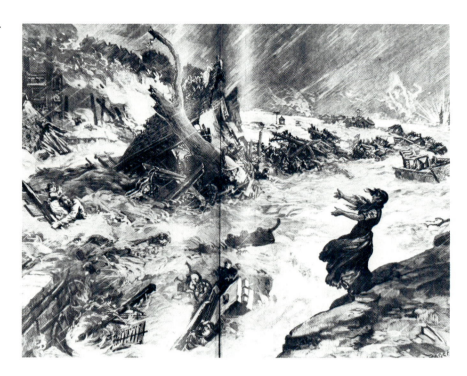

Volunteer Nurses

A large number of lay men and women volunteered as nurses during the Civil War. Many of them emerged as leaders and greatly influenced nursing during this period. All of them gave devoted service to the soldiers in time of need. They brought hope to the abandoned and gave faith to those who despaired. They nursed the sick and the wounded and comforted the dying. Most were amateurs, but their efforts had a positive effect on the troops.

> The Civil War is America's greatest tragedy, whose wounds have not healed with the balm of a century, yet it is a tragedy brightened by noble names in the North and in the South. America will lose a precious heritage if ever it permits these names to be forgotten. New ways and new names claim our attention, crowding out the old. From time to time, green leaves should be entwined with the sear laurels of the nurses of the Civil War.
>
> *Robinson, 1946, p. 207*

Mother Bickerdyke (Mary Ann Ball, 1817–1901) belonged to this saga of America. Her blanket-shawl, calico dress, and Shaker bonnet were indicative of her pioneer ways, which have passed with a period of American history. She was given the name *Mother* by the soldiers, as an affectionate term that expressed their gratitude. Mother Bickerdyke had been a widow from Galesburg, Illinois, with a moderate education and two small sons when she answered the call to help with the war effort. Her minister, Henry Ward Beecher, had issued a plea for some women of his congregation to proceed to government hospitals and battlefields to care for the sick and the wounded. She had taken a short course in homeopathy from Dr. Samuel Hahnemann and received a degree of Doctor of Botanic Medicine (Baker, 1952).

Mother Bickerdyke served under fire in nineteen battles from

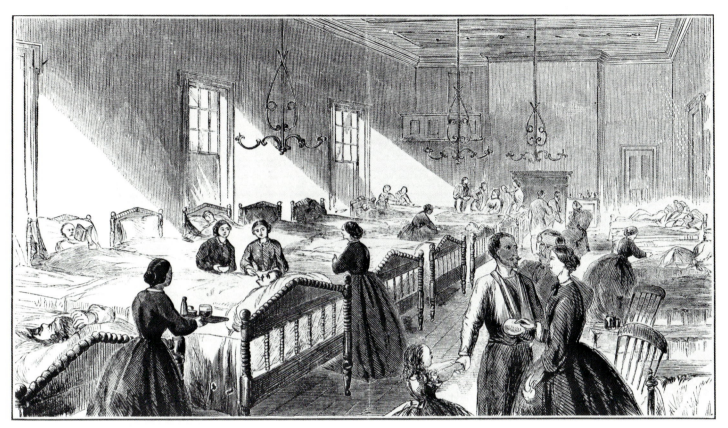

THE SOLDIERS' QUARTERS AT GEORGETOWN, D.C., DURING THE WAR 1861–1865. *From* LESLIE'S WEEKLY, *July 6, 1861. Culver Pictures, New York. Volunteer nurses attended the sick and the wounded at the U.S. General Hospital at Georgetown during the Civil War.*

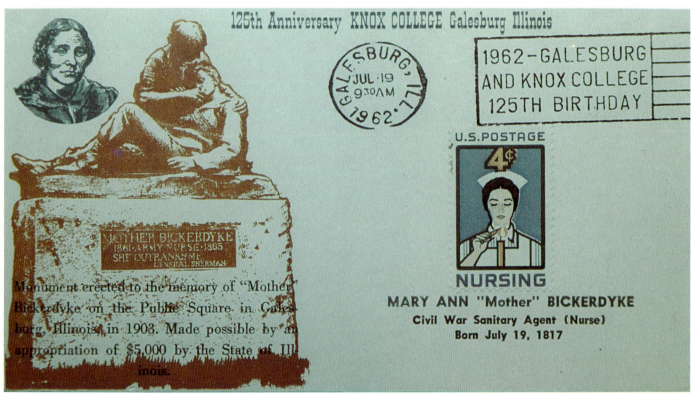

At the start of the Civil War she answered the call as a nurse. To the sick, wounded, and dying soldiers Mary Ann Bickerdyke was known as "Mother." She was one of the most capable and beloved women who ministered to the soldier casualties of that war. An Army surgeon said of her, "a large woman, strong as a man, muscles of iron, nerves of steel, sensitive but self-reliant, seeking all for others, nothing for herself." Knox College, Galesburg, Illinois, remembered her on its 125th anniversary with this commemorative cover in 1962, which is franked with the U.S. 1961 four-cent stamp honoring nursing. Courtesy of Howard B. Hurley.

299

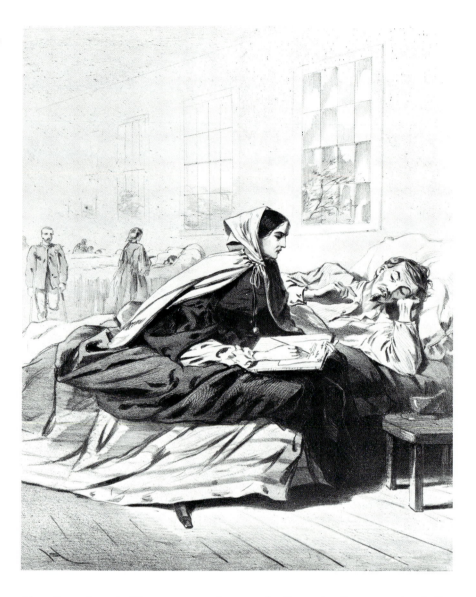

Fort Donelson in Tennessee to Savannah, Georgia. She organized diet
kitchens, laundries, and an ambulance service. She supervised the
nursing staff and distributed supplies. At night she often walked
through the abandoned battlefields, afraid that someone who was still
alive would be left. She became known as one of the greatest nurse
heroines of the Civil War, and numerous tales were told about her
exploits.

> Looking from his tent at midnight, an officer observed a faint
> light flitting hither and thither on the abandoned battlefield, and,
> after puzzling over it for some time, sent his servant to ascertain
> the cause. It was Mother Bickerdyke, with a lantern. Stooping
> down (among the dead) and turning their cold faces towards her,
> she scrutinized them searchingly, uneasy lest some might be left
> to die uncared for. She could not rest while she thought any
> were overlooked who were yet living.
>
> *Baker, 1952, p. 11*

Mary Ann Bickerdyke was indeed the soldier's friend. She fought
particularly hard for the rights and comforts of the common soldier.
Her accomplishments were recognized by the government at the
launching of the hospital ship, the SS *Mary A. Bickerdyke* in 1943 at
Richmond, California.

300

Louisa May Alcott (1832–1888) longed for a wider field of activity than that permitted a New England minister's daughter. She was a prominent advocate of women's rights, and at times this got in the way of her ambitions. Miss Alcott is best known for her books, *Little Women* and *Little Men,* and her poems and short stories were published in the *Atlantic Monthly.* This American novelist and writer of children's books served as a nurse at the Union Hospital at Georgetown (Washington, D.C.) for six weeks in 1862 to 1863 (Austin, 1957). This improvised hospital accommodated approximately 300 patients who were in various stages of injury and disease. Miss Alcott was placed in charge of a forty-bed ward, where she performed a variety of functions in her role of nurse. She dressed wounds, read novels to soldiers, wrote letters, made night rounds, and gave medicines. Her daily schedule was rather hectic, as portayed in her journal:

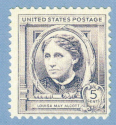

Louisa May Alcott is known primarily as an American author and writer of children's books, most notably LITTLE WOMEN. *Less well known is her service as a Civil War nurse. Born in Germantown, Pennsylvania, in 1832, she was remembered in the U.S. Famous Americans series of stamps issued in 1940. Courtesy of Howard B. Hurley.*

> Up at six, dress by gaslight, run through my ward and throw up the windows, though the men grumble and shiver. But the air is bad enough to breed a pestilence, and as no notice is taken of our frequent appeals for better ventilation, I must do what I can . . . for a more perfect pestilence box than this house I never saw—cold, damp, dirty, full of vile odors from wounds, kitchens, washrooms, stables. Till noon I trot, trot, trot, giving out rations, cutting up food for helpless "boys," washing faces, teaching my attendants how beds are made or floors are swept, dressing wounds, dusting tables, sewing bandages, keeping my tray tidy, rushing up and down after pillows, bed linens, sponges, and directions until it seems as if I would joyfully pay down all I possess for fifteen minutes' rest. At twelve comes dinner for the patients and afterward there is letter writing for them or reading aloud. Supper at five sets everyone running that can run . . . evening amusements . . . then, for such as need them, the final doses for the night.
>
> *Cheney, 1889, pp. 143–144*

Miss Alcott described the work done by the volunteer nurses in Civil War hospitals in letters that were published in 1863 in a book entitled *Hospital Sketches.* This is considered to be her first famous work.

Another writer, Walt Whitman (1819–1892), left a record of the care of the sick during the Civil War. This was done in a collection of poems, *Drum-Taps,* and in a diary, *Specimen Days and Collect,* which described his experiences as a hospital nurse in Washington. Walt Whitman was described by the Danish scholar Frederick Schyberg as a "natural and inevitable product of the tendencies, the struggles, the crises of America in 1860." Accounts of his ministrations to the wounded and his varied responses to the war were dispersed in dozens of notebooks, newspaper dispatches, letters, and other types of published and unpublished works. These were compiled, edited, and then published for the first time in *Walt Whitman's Civil War* in 1960.

Whitman was self-educated and learned the printer's trade in his boyhood. He subsequently worked at various jobs and was the editor of different newspapers. In 1862 he left his odd jobs to visit the Civil War front. Upon his return to Washington, he spent the rest of the war period as a volunteer nurse and companion to wounded soldiers.

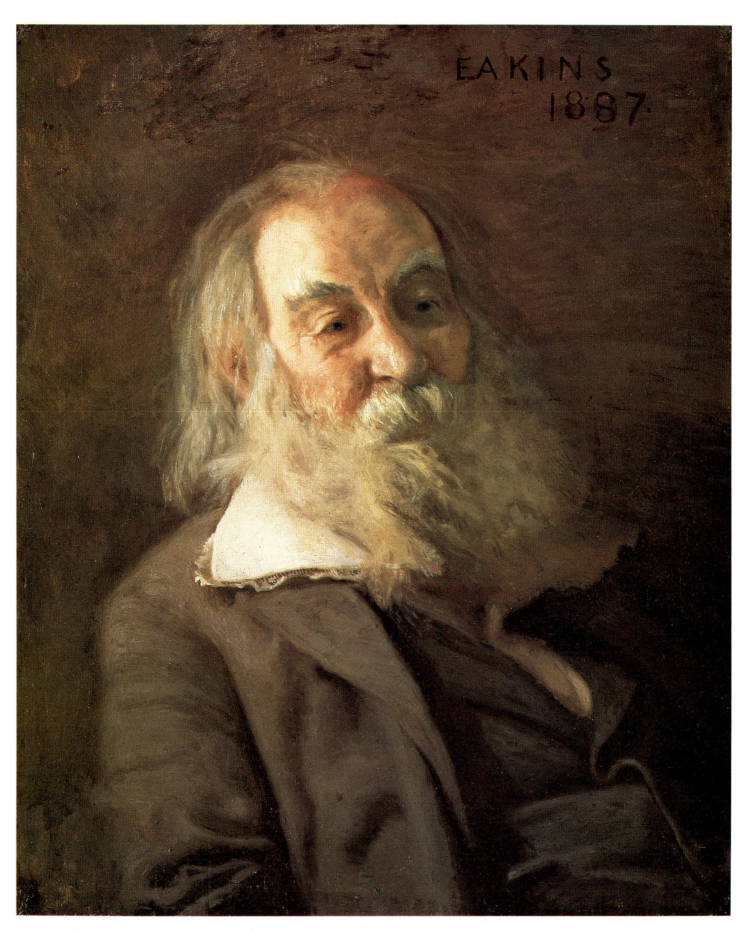

Thomas Eakins, WALT WHITMAN, *1887. Canvas. Courtesy of the Pennsylvania Academy of the Fine Arts, Philadelphia, General Fund Purchase.*

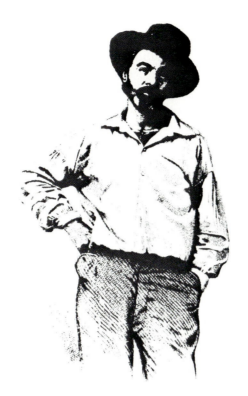

Portrait of WALT WHITMAN. *From* SELECTIONS FROM LEAVES OF GRASS BY WALT WHITMAN, *introduction by Walter Lowenfels, 1961 Crown Publishers Inc., New York.*

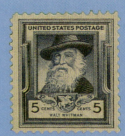

During the Civil War Walt Whitman worked as a volunteer hospital nurse in Washington, D.C., where he penned poetry about the conflict and wrote two of his most famous poems about President Abraham Lincoln, WHEN LILACS LAST IN THE DOORYARD BLOOM'D *and* O CAPTAIN! MY CAPTAIN! *The United States stamp in his honor as a Famous American was issued in February 1940 at Camden, New Jersey. Courtesy of Howard B. Hurley.*

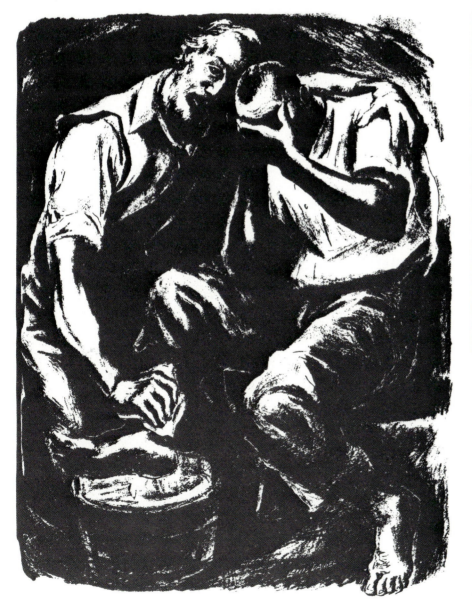

L. Daniel, WALT WHITMAN AS NURSE. *From* SELECTIONS FROM LEAVES OF GRASS BY WALT WHITMAN, *introduction by Walter Lowenfels, 1961 Crown Publishers Inc., New York.*

He did this while earning a modest living as a government clerk, a position from which he was fired in 1865 because of official disapproval of the sexual terminology in *Leaves of Grass*. Whitman spent his final years of life (1873–1892) as an invalid in Camden, New Jersey. Of all his Civil War poetry, Whitman's perceptions of the sufferings of the men and his efforts on their behalf are best described in "The Wound-Dresser":

Bearing the bandages, water and sponge,
Straight and swift to my wounded I go,
Where they lie on the ground after the battle brought in,
Where their priceless blood reddens the grass, the ground,
Or to the rows of the hospital tent, or under the roof's hospital,
To the long rows of cots up and down each side I return,
To each and all one after another I draw near, not one do I miss,
An attendant follows holding a tray, he carries a refuse pail,
Soon to be fill'd with clotted rags and blood, emptied, and fill'd
    again.

I onward go, I stop,
With hinged knees and steady hand to dress wounds,
I am firm with each, the pangs are sharp yet unavoidable,
One turns to me his appealing eyes—poor boy! I never knew
    you,
Yet I think I could not refuse this moment to die for you,
  if that would save you.

On, on I go, (open doors of time! open hospital doors!)
The crush'd head I dress, (poor crazed hand tear not the bandage
    away,)
The neck of the cavalry-man with the bullet through and through
    I examine,
Hard the breathing rattles, quite glazed already the eye, yet life
    struggles hard,
(Come sweet death! be persuaded O beautiful death!
In mercy come quickly.)

From the stump of the arm, the amputated hand,
I undo the clotted lint, remove the slough,
wash off the matter and blood,
Back on his pillow the soldier bends with
curv'd neck and side falling head,
His eyes are closed, his face is pale, he
dares not look on the bloody stump,
And has not yet look'd on it.

Whitman, 1961, pp. 44–45

Walt Whitman did not approve of women nursing in military hospitals. Even with his liberal views, he did not believe that it was a proper activity for respectable women. Yet many of the women who served as nurses in the Civil War were women from socially prestigious families who possessed strong political beliefs and educational backgrounds. Among them were the Woolsey sisters, Margaret Breckinridge, Harriet Foote Hawley, Ella Louise Wolcott, and Louisa Lee Schuyler.

The women of the Confederacy also gave heroic service during the Civil War. Religious Sisters and lay women volunteered to function as nurses. They opened their homes to sick and wounded sol-

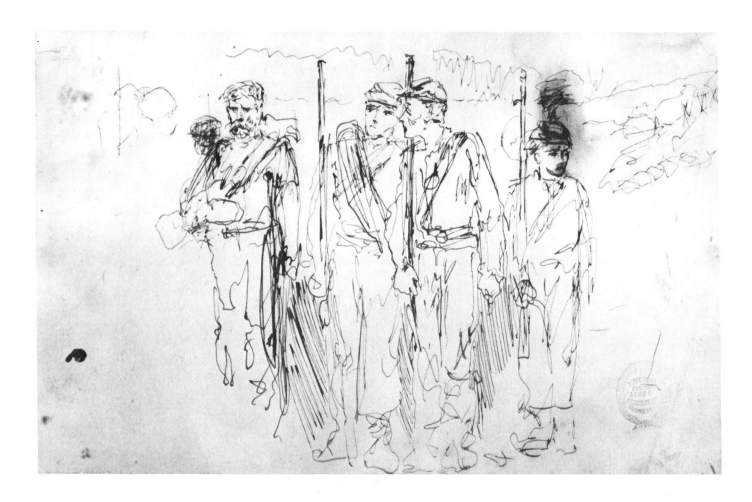

diers to be used as hospitals and convalescent centers. Some, as in the North, followed their husbands to war and to the battlefield, where they assisted in every way possible. The list included Kate Cumming, Ella King Newsom, Annie Johns, Betsy Sullivan, and a host of others. However, one individual in particular stands out. The Confederate Army did not appoint a director of nursing, but President Jefferson Davis granted the rank of captain to Miss Sally Louisa Tompkins

Winslow Homer, THE WALKING WOUNDED, *1861–62. Pen and ink on paper, approx. 18.8 × 12.5 cm. Courtesy of Cooper-Hewitt Museum, The Smithsonian Institution's National Museum of Design, New York, Gift of Charles Savage Homer.*

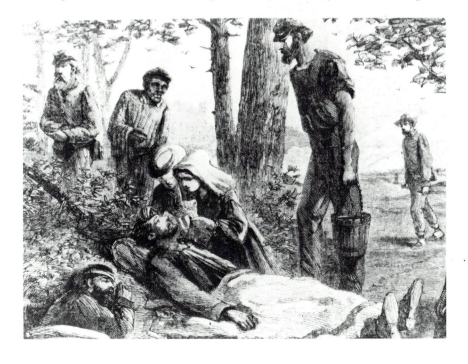

NURSES BEHIND THE LINES DURING THE CIVIL WAR, *c. 1860. Wood engraving. National Library of Medicine, Bethesda, Maryland.*

305

(1833–1916). She was the only woman to hold a commission in the Army of the Confederacy. Miss Tompkins was the daughter of a wealthy Virginian and had been active in the charitable works of her church. She established a private hospital in Richmond and maintained it entirely at her own expense. Miss Tompkins needed the rank in order to requisition supplies, but she refused to accept compensation for her work. The most serious and critical cases were brought to her independent institution because of its reputation. Yet the mortality was low, only 73 deaths out of 1333 patients.

Black women also made significant contributions to Civil War nursing. Some were volunteers; others were employed under the general orders of the War Department at a salary of ten dollars per month. There is, however, a paucity of published works relating to the specific and general contributions of Blacks in nursing, which makes it difficult to render a fair and comprehensive portrayal of their work. Several of them very competently cared for wounded soldiers in the Union Army. Harriet Tubman (1820–1913) was called the "Moses of her people" (Bradford, 1961) and is credited with making nineteen trips to the South to assist over 300 slaves in their quest for freedom (Miller, 1968). She was an abolitionist who became active with the Underground Railroad movement after her own es-

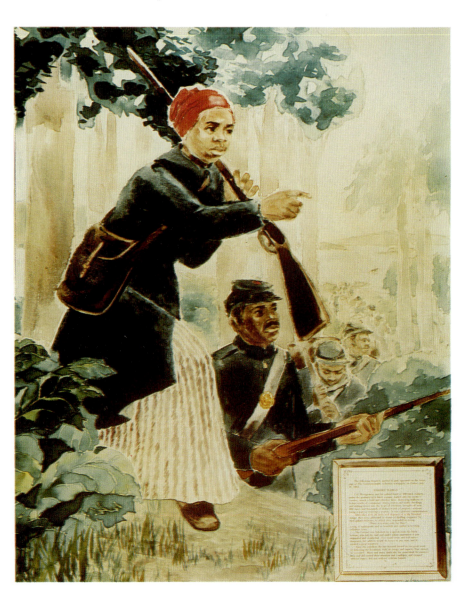

Joan Maynard, HARRIET TUBMAN, *1977.*
Defense Audiovisual Agency, Washington,
D.C.

306

cape to the North. At the onset of the Civil War, Harriet Tubman turned her energies to the care of those who needed her ministrations. She was a highly respected, fearless, and courageous individual who served the sick and suffering of her own race. According to Bradford (1961), Mrs. Tubman held the position of "nurse or matron" at the Colored Hospital in Fort Monroe, Virginia.

Sojourner Truth could be regarded as an early feminist. She was an ardent supporter of the women's movement and actively participated in the cause. She, too, competently assisted with the care of wounded soldiers for the Union Army. Susie King was the wife of Sergeant Edward King of the 33rd W.S. Colored Infantry. She was a

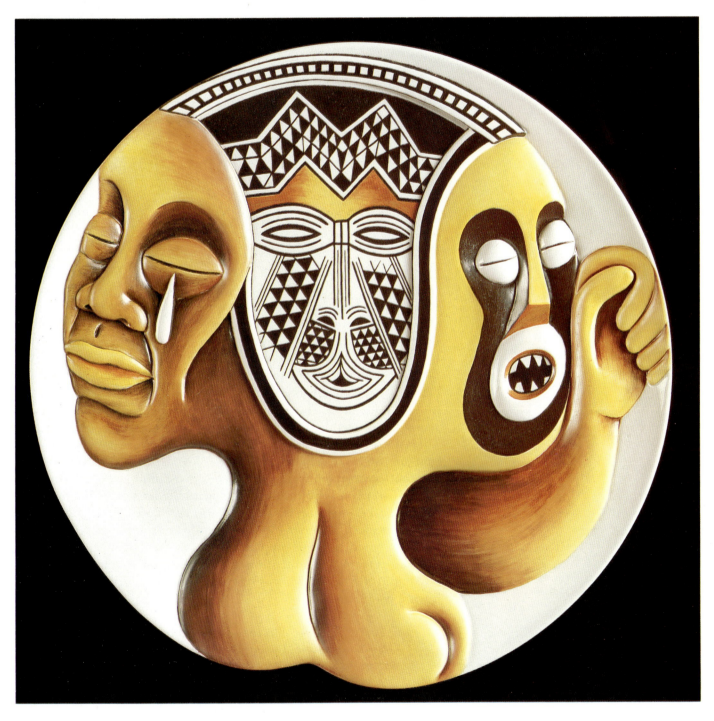

Judy Chicago, "Sojourner Truth," plate from THE DINNER PARTY, *1979. China-painted porcelain, 35.6 cm diameter. Through the Flower, Benicia, California.*

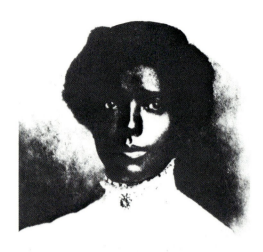

SOJOURNER TRUTH, *a nurse in the Civil War. Courtesy of W.B. Saunders Company, Philadelphia, Pennsylvania.*

volunteer nurse during the Civil War for over four years. Miss King was welcomed and respected by both physicians and soldiers and frequently accompanied Clara Barton on her rounds (Elmore, 1976). Her care went beyond the physical aspects; she read letters to the soldiers, offered comfort in whatever way possible, and even began to teach some of the soldiers to read and write.

Large numbers of men and women served as nurses in a variety of capacities during the Civil War. They were volunteers, members of the Army, persons from religious nursing orders, members of relief societies, or independent individuals who took it upon themselves to assist with the care for the sick and the wounded. These nurses represented all levels of society and constituted a myriad of intelligence, diplomacy, daring, and experience. Overall, they demonstrated a courageous spirit.

> The ordeal of the Civil War matured America; by that time America had made many contributions of first rank in medicine and surgery, but not a single contribution to nursing.... A century elapsed from the date of the Boston Tea Party (1773) to the opening of America's first Nightingale school for nurses (1873), and many believed that, of the two experiments, the latter was the more daring.
>
> *Robinson, 1946, pp. 145–146*

■ THE EVOLUTION OF SCHOOLS OF NURSING

The experiences of the Civil War emphasized the inadequate preparation of the majority of nurses who participated. Public interest in nursing was thus aroused, and awareness of the need to develop training programs for nurses increased. This movement was assisted by the large number of women from socially prominent families who had served. Their involvement and support lent a certain measure of respectability to the image of nursing. Two specific documents clearly indicated this rising interest in the potential development of nursing education. The first was written by a group of physicians; the second appeared as an editorial in a prominent women's magazine.

At the New Orleans meeting of the American Medical Association in 1869, Dr. Samuel D. Gross (1805–1884), chairman of the Committee on the Training of Nurses, presented a report. This committee had been appointed to investigate the best possible method to organize and manage institutions for the training of nurses. The strange neglect of nursing in the United States was identified and the need for good nursing emphasized. Early American efforts toward hospital reform were mentioned, and the vast extent of volunteer nursing in the Civil War was stressed. The committee made the following proposals:

I. That every large and well-organised hospital should have a school for the training of nurses, not only for the supply of its own necessities, but for private families; the teaching to be furnished by its own medical staff, assisted by the resident physicians.

II. That, while it is not at all essential to combine religious exercises with nursing, it is believed that such a union would be eminently conducive to the welfare of the sick in all public institutions, and the committee therefore earnestly recommend the establishment of nurses' homes, to be placed under the immediate supervision and direction of Deaconesses or lady superintendents.

III. That, in order to give thorough scope and efficiency to this scheme, district schools should be formed and placed under the guardianship of the county medical societies of every State and Territory in the Union, the members of which should make it their business to impart instruction in the art and science of nursing.

Proceedings of the American Medical Association,
1869, pp. 339, 351

Further suggestions related to the importance of forming societies of nurses, the qualities necessary for the nurse to possess, and the sending of copies of the report to medical societies all over the country. It is particularly interesting that in November of that same year Rudolf Virchow presented similar recommendations to a women's association in Berlin, Germany.

FIFTY YEARS, 1838 TO 1888. *Supplement to the* NURSING RECORD, *December 20, 1888. Courtesy of Croom Helm Ltd. Publishers, Kent, England.*

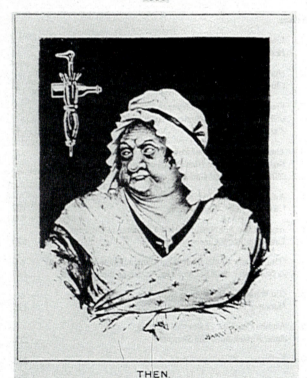

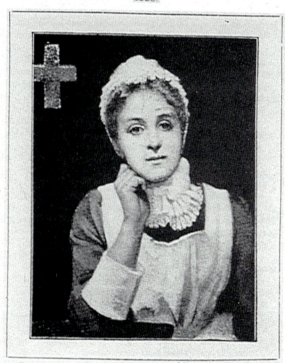

309

The *Godey's Lady's Book and Magazine,* popular in the late nineteenth century, strongly influenced women's fashions and manners. It had been founded by Louis A. Godey, who appointed Mrs. Sarah J. Hale as editor in 1837. Mrs. Hale's interest in the education of nurses was illustrated by an editorial, entitled "Lady Nurses," that appeared in the February 1871 issue:

> Much has been lately said of the benefits that would follow if the calling of sick nurse were elevated to a profession which an educated lady might adopt without a sense of degradation, either on her own part or in the estimation of others....
>
> There can be no doubt that the duties of sick nurse, to be properly performed, require an education and training little, if at all, inferior to those possessed by members of the medical profession. To leave these duties to untaught and ill-trained persons is as great a mistake as it was to allow the office of surgeon to be held by one whose proper calling was that of a mechanic of the humblest class. The manner in which a reform may be effected is easily pointed out. Every medical college should have a course of study and training especially adapted for ladies who desire to qualify themelves for the profession of nurse; and those who had gone through the course, and passed the requisite examination, should receive a degree and a diploma, which would at once establish their position in society. The "graduate nurse" would in general estimation be as much above the ordinary nurse of the present day as the professional surgeon of our times is above the barber-surgeon of the last century.
>
> *Hale, 1871, pp. 188–189*

The need for nurses was great. According to Hale, however, this need also involved a well-planned educational program that would generate "professional nurses." Her advice was not followed, and "training schools" for nurses eventually were established and proliferated.

A TRAINED NURSE, *a cartoon from the Rush Medical College yearbook,* PULSE, *1895. Rush-Presbyterian-St. Luke's Medical Center, Chicago, Illinois.*

This cartoon had the same historical validity as the other jokes under the title "Medical Terms Illustrated" in this yearbook. The word "trained" comes from the name of the nursing schools. In those days every nursing school was called a "training school."

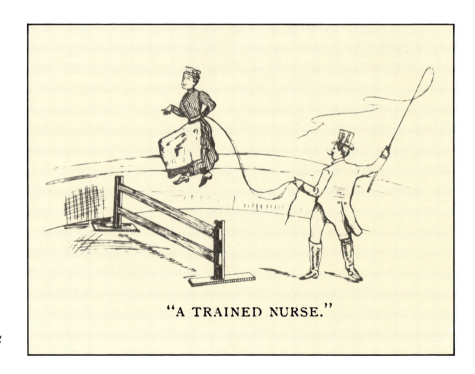

"A TRAINED NURSE."

First Instruction for Nurses

Until the inception of the first formal training schools for nurses, individuals who were involved with the care of the sick and midwives received intermittent lectures from physicians in the Eastern cities of the United States. This was in no way, however, an organized course of instruction. Most information was gleaned simply by doing nursing, such as it was. The only organized preparation available was offered in Catholic sisterhoods, and it was restricted to members of the order.

It is difficult to determine who should receive the distinction of having the first trained nurses in America. There were a number of individuals whose foresight led them to appreciate the need for training nurses. These pioneers attempted to rectify the situation. Dr. Valentine Seaman, a medical chief at the New York Hospital, is usually credited with initiating the first system of instruction for nurses on the North American continent. Below his portrait in the original hospital building is an inscription that praises his achievement: "In 1798 he organized in the New York Hospital the first regular training school for nurses, from which other schools have since been established and extended their blessings throughout the Community" (Nutting and Dock, vol. 2, 1907, p. 339). Dr. Seaman's lectures were described earlier in this unit.

Almost a generation later, the next attempt was made to train

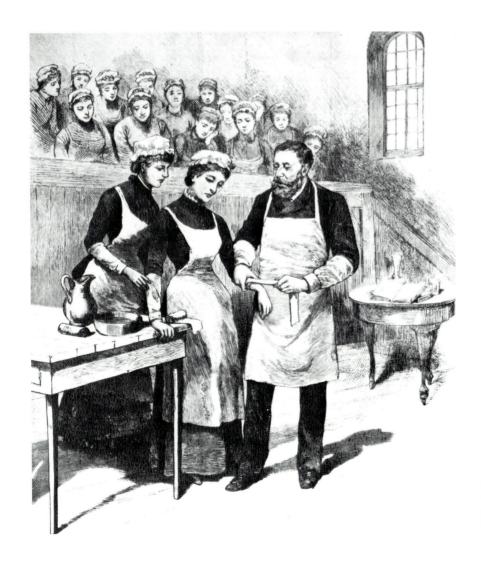

LECTURE ON BANDAGING AT THE BLOCKLEY TRAINING SCHOOL FOR NURSES IN PHILADELPHIA, *1886. The Bettmann Archive, New York.*

311

women for obstetrical nursing. This movement was initiated by Dr. Joseph Warrington of the Philadelphia Dispensary. As a result of his efforts, a society was formed on March 5, 1839. The basic purpose of the Nurse Society of Philadelphia was to provide an organization of women who would supply a maternity service in homes. Under the Quaker influence, a combined Home and School were opened in 1850; in time, service was extended to include medical and surgical patients. The women followed a plan of instruction that included lectures given by Dr. Warrington, demonstrations, and practice on a manikin. They received certificates and were eligible for calls after satisfactorily serving six cases. Accepted candidates, who were referred to as "probationers," had been thoroughly screened. The constitution of the society stated:

> Whereas, in our widely extended and densely populated city a large number of poor females are subject to great suffering and risk of life, during and shortly after the period of parturition, for want of competent nurses to guard them and their helpless offspring . . . the undersigned, impressed with the importance of

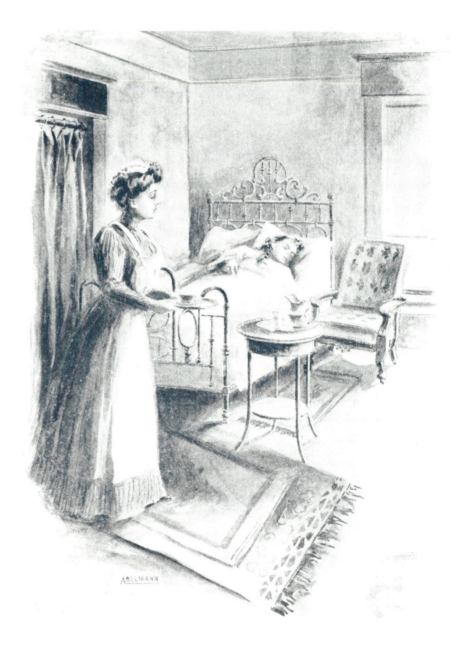

THE HOME NURSE. *The Bettmann Archive, New York.*

this subject, do associate for the purpose of providing, sustaining, and causing to be instructed as far as possible, pious and prudent women for this purpose, and do adopt the following regulations:

I. The Association shall be called the Nurse Society of Philadelphia.
II. The Board of Managers shall consist of twelve females, who are, or have been, heads of families.

Nutting and Dock, vol. 2, 1907, pp. 341–342

Early reports refer to this structure as the "First Nurse Training School founded in America" and the "First School in America established to Train Women as Nurses." In 1897 the plan of instruction was extended to one year.

Woman's Hospital of Philadelphia opened a training school in 1861. However, it progressed slowly until 1872, when it received an endowment. (This institution can be called the first endowed school of nursing in America.) This school was organized and conducted by two women physicians, Ann Preston and Emmelin Horton Cleveland. It was unique in the sense that it had been planned specifically with

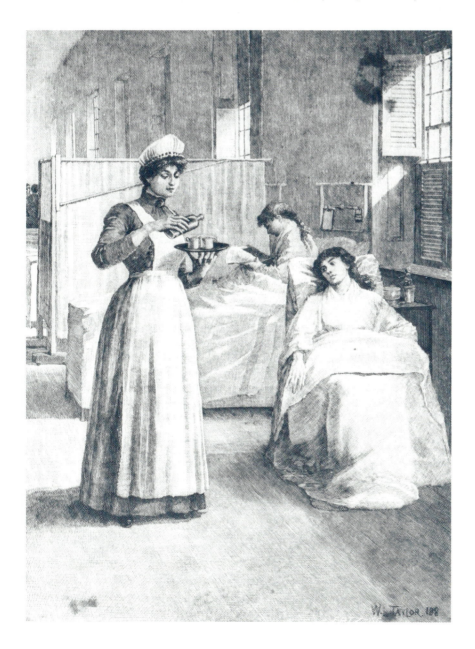

W.L. Taylor, NURSE ADMINISTERING MEDICINE TO AILING GIRL. *Woodcut. The Bettmann Archive, New York.*

the education of student nurses, rather than the care of patients, as its primary objective. In 1863 Dr. Preston wrote a pamphlet, *Nursing the Sick and the Training of Nurses*, which described the ideal nurse as having "the patience of hope [and] the faith of love. The good nurse is an artist!" The course of instruction lasted six months and covered content in surgery, medicine, obstetrics, poultice and plaster preparation, dietetic principles and methods of cooking.

Similar developments were transpiring in Boston. As early as 1860, the *New England Hospital for Women and Children* had attempted the teaching of nurses. This institution, staffed by women physicians, took the first step toward the development of a school of nursing with the arrival of Dr. Marie Zakrzewska in 1859. Upon her advice, the hospital charter issued in 1863 included a nursing school. The first bylaws were adopted on June 5, 1863, and declared the objectives of the institution to be:

> I. To provide for women medical aid by competent physicians of their own sex.
> II. To assist educated women in the practical study of medicine.
> III. To train nurses for the care of the sick.

Students were required to attend the entire six months' course, which included practice at the bedside of the patient. The first month was a probationary period. Few women applied, and only six were trained over the next two years. In 1872 the hospital moved to new quarters at Roxbury, Massachusetts, and admitted a class of five students to its newly formed training school. The specific plan of the school has been described in the following way:

> Young women of suitable requirements and character will be admitted to the Hospital as school nurses, for one year. This year will be divided into four periods; three months will be given respectively to the practical study of nursing in the Medical, Surgical, and Maternity Wards, and night nursing. Here the pupil will aid the head nurse in all the care and work of the wards under the direction of the Attending and Resident Physicians and Medical Students.
>
> In order to enable women entirely dependent upon their work for support to obtain a thorough training, the nurses will be paid for their work from one to four dollars per week after the first fortnight, according to the actual value of their service to the Hospital.
>
> A course of lectures will be given to nurses at the Hospital by the physicians connected with the Institution beginning January 21. . . . Certificates will be given to such nurses as have satisfactorily passed a year in practical training in the Hospital.
>
> *Munson, 1948, p. 552*

This school was under the direction of Dr. Susan Dimock. The students worked from 5:30 AM until 9:00 PM and slept in rooms near the ward in order that they might be immediately available if necessary. Their uniform consisted of a simple calico dress and felt slippers. Dr. Zakrzewska taught the simple details of nursing. There were no head nurses and no superintendent. The growth of the school continued, and in 1882 the course was extended to sixteen months. By this time the school had two head nurses and a superintendent of

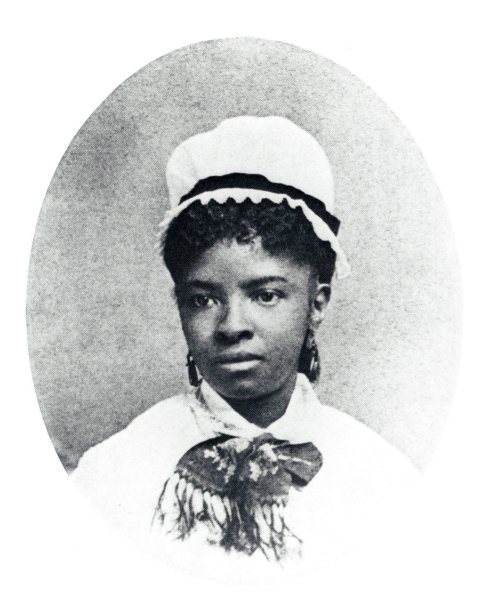

Portrait of MARY MAHONEY. *Schomburg Center for Research in Black Culture, The New York Public Library, New York.*

FIRST CONVENTION OF THE NATIONAL ASSOCIATION OF COLORED GRADUATE NURSES. *Schomburg Center for Research in Black Culture, The New York Public Library, New York.*

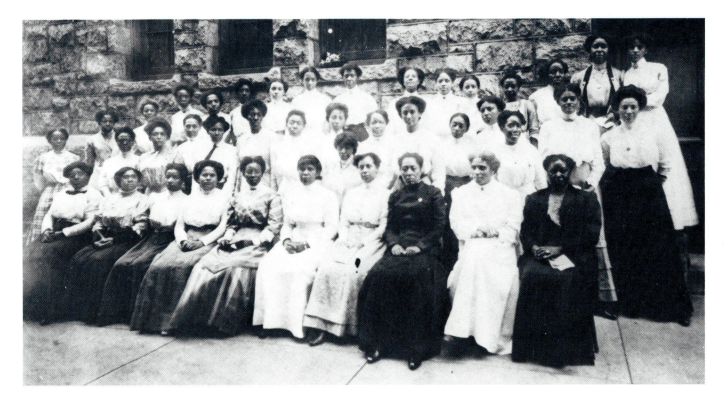

the training school. The program was lengthened to two years in 1893 and finally in 1901 to three years.

One student graduated at the end of the first year, on October 1, 1873. Melinda Ann (Linda) Richards (1841–1930) received her certificate and became known as the "first trained nurse in the United States" or "America's first trained nurse." She was overwhelmed with job offers upon her graduation but finally decided to accept the position of night superintendent at Bellevue Hospital. A variety of experiences awaited her there, some of which were particularly appalling. During her stay at Bellevue, Miss Richards made three significant contributions: she insisted on light at night (the gas had been turned so low that a lighted candle was necessary, but only two candles per week were allowed each ward); she instituted written case histories instead of verbal reports; and she exposed the mortality from puerperal fever, which thus led to the removal of mothers to Blackwell's Island (Robinson, 1946). After a year, Miss Richards went to the Boston Training School (Massachusetts General Hospital) as its superintendent. There she gave actual patient care as well as performing the required administrative duties.

Linda Richards went to England in 1877 to study nursing methods and became acquainted with Miss Nightingale. She went to Japan as a missionary and nurse, remained there for five years (1885–1890), and organized the earliest training school in the islands of the Orient. Miss Richards eventually returned to her alma mater and became the superintendent of the New England Hospital for Women and Children. Her later efforts, in collaboration with Edward Cowles, were directed toward the nursing of the insane. It is to her credit that for more than half a century she was an avid and active supporter of adequate education for nurses.

Mary Eliza Mahoney (1845–1926) completed the sixteen-month course of training at the New England Hospital for Women and Children on August 1, 1879. She is thus considered to be America's first Black professional nurse, the first Black nurse to graduate from a school of nursing. Miss Mahoney gave the welcoming address in 1909 at the first convention of the National Association of Colored Graduate Nurses. Throughout her life she primarily engaged in private duty nursing and worked for the acceptance of Blacks in nursing. After her death, the National Association of Colored Graduate Nurses established an award in her honor that was presented for the first time in 1936. The Mary Mahoney Medal is presented at the American Nurses' Association convention to an individual who has been instrumental in promoting equal opportunities to minority persons in nursing.

Separate schools for educating Black nurses eventually arose. They became a necessity in order that Blacks, who were banned from many schools, could receive training in nursing. The first of these was established at Spelman Seminary in Atlanta, Georgia, in 1886. Two similar institutions began in 1891, Hampton Institute in Virginia and Provident Hospital in Chicago. A school of nursing was also started at Tuskegee Institute in Alabama in 1892; it, however, was developed primarily to provide service rather than education. These schools experienced difficulties similar to those of the early white schools, but also suffered from societal prejudice toward Blacks.

Work was also begun in Canada to provide training for nurses. At about 1864 the community of St. Catharine's, Ontario, started a hospital with a little house, one nurse, a steward, and ideas for the

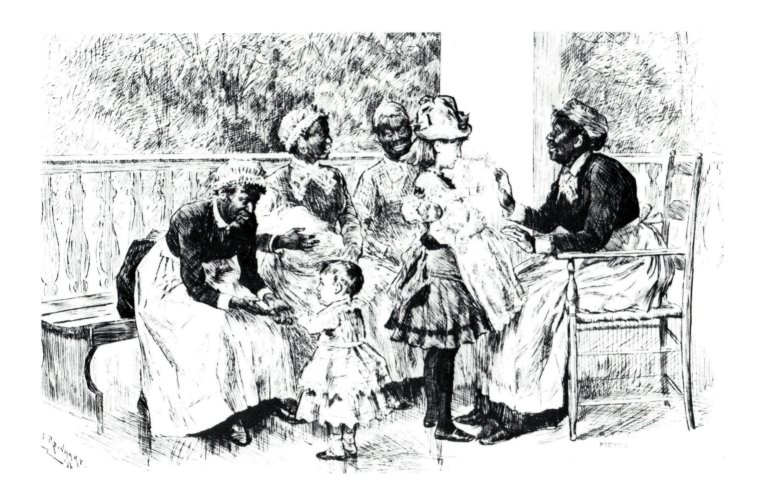

teaching of nurses. Under the direction of Dr. Theophilus Mack, a physician at the hospital and president of the board, the hospital grew steadily and definite teaching for nurses emerged in 1873. He was certain that the prejudice of many sick people against going into public hospitals would be overcome by a profession of trained lay nurses. At Dr. Mack's direction, a Miss Money was sent to England to bring back two trained nurses and five or six probationers. A system of training was in effect by 1874. The hospital was named St. Catharine's General and Marine Hospital. The nurses were required to stay for three years. For the first six months they were probationers without pay. They then received a stipend, board, and uniforms. The first annual report, dated July 1, 1875, illustrated the value of trained nurses:

J. Reinhart, COLORED NURSES, *1866. Schomburg Center for Research in Black Culture, The New York Public Library, New York.*

> The vocation of nursing goes hand in hand with that of the physician and surgeon, and they are absolutely indispensable one to the other. Incompetency on the part of a nurse renders negatory the best efforts of the doctor in the most critical moments, and has frequently resulted in loss of life. All the most brilliant achievements of modern surgery are dependent, to a great extent, upon careful and intelligent nursing, and the obstetrician knows only too well how fearful may be the consequences of ignorance and negligence on the part of attendants in the chamber of accouchement. The skilled nurse, by minutely watching the temperature, conditions of skin, pulse, respiration, and the various functions of all the organs, and reporting faithfully to the attending physician, must increase the chances of recovery two-fold.
>
> *Gibbon and Mathewson, 1947, p. 145*

317

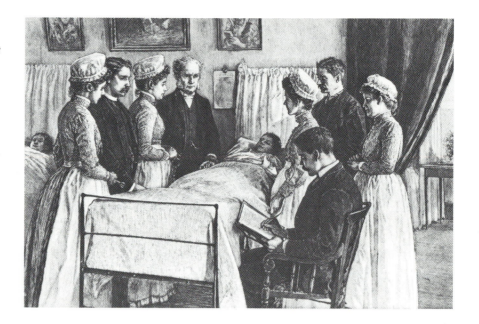

A CRITICAL CASE—A BEDSIDE CONSULTATION FOR THE BENEFIT OF STUDENTS AND NURSES AT BELLEVUE HOSPITAL, *1890. Engraving. The Bettmann Archive, New York.*

The Nightingale Plan in American Schools

Improvement in the care of the sick in both hospitals and homes rested with the development of a system of training nurses. The time was finally ripe for the organization of schools of nursing. Following the Civil War, interest in nursing education was high and culminated in the almost simultaneous appearance of three important schools. In 1873 the famous trio of schools that encouraged the steady progress of nursing evolved: Bellevue Training School in New York City on May 1, the Connecticut Training School in New Haven on October 1, and the Boston Training School (later the Massachusetts General Hospital Training School for Nurses) on November 1. These schools were initially based on the Nightingale model, but they were soon forced to deviate and follow a somewhat different path. The alterations that occurred greatly influenced the direction of nursing in America.

The earliest schools were created independently of hospitals by committees or boards that had the power to develop the schools. They were soon absorbed, however, into the hospitals to which they were attached because of a lack of endowment. This factor proved to be the greatest weakness in the system, since many hospitals soon discovered that schools could be created to serve their needs and a valuable source of almost free labor could be obtained.

In the absence of public or private support, the schools from the time of their inception faced financial problems of major proportions. An agreement by the school to give nursing service for the hospitals providing clinical experience was the primary means of overcoming this difficulty. This type of apprenticeship agreement was the factor promoting hospitals to establish schools on their own initiative. Having a school of nursing became accepted as the most popular and least expensive means of providing nursing care. The hospital was the master and the student nurse was the apprentice, with the latter giving free labor to the former in return for informal training in the traditional manner.

Ashley, 1976, p. 9

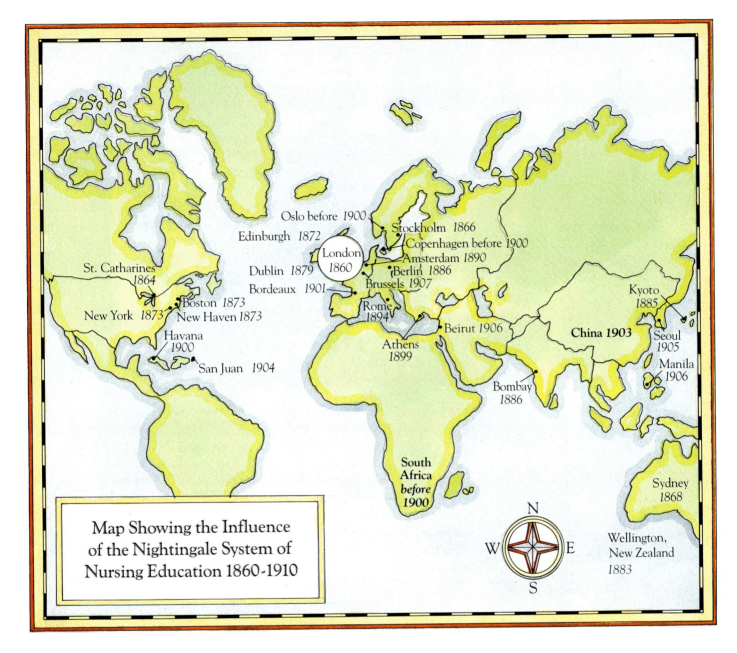

Map Showing the Influence
of the Nightingale System of
Nursing Education 1860-1910

Oslo before *1900*
Edinburgh *1872*
Stockholm *1866*
Copenhagen before *1900*
London *1860*
Amsterdam *1890*
Dublin *1879*
Berlin *1886*
Bordeaux *1901*
Brussels *1907*
Rome *1894*
Kyoto *1885*
China *1903*
Seoul *1905*
Beirut *1906*
Manila *1906*
Athens *1899*
Bombay *1886*
St. Catharines *1864*
New York *1873*
Boston *1873*
New Haven *1873*
Havana *1900*
San Juan *1904*
South Africa before *1900*
Sydney *1868*
Wellington, New Zealand *1883*

N
W E
S

Nursing care became the major product dispensed by hospitals. The real function of the school of nursing became *not education,* but *service.* In addition, no policy for control of the numbers of nursing schools or the standards for admission and graduation was established or accepted. Consequently, a proliferation of nursing schools occurred. The first decade of the twentieth century demonstrated a period of phenomenal growth, with the establishment of close to 700 new schools. All school functions were ultimately placed under the control and general direction of hospital authorities.

Bellevue Hospital Training School. Women involved in the reform movement following the Civil War turned their endeavors toward the improvement of hospitals. Miss Louisa Lee Schuyler and other women who had been prominent during the war effort and the U.S. Sanitary Commission founded the New York State Charities Aid Association in 1872. This voluntary body was concerned with the care of paupers, orphans, and the sick. One of its committees, with Mrs. Joseph Hobson as its chair, inspected Bellevue Hospi-

Map showing the INFLUENCE OF THE NIGHT-INGALE SYSTEM OF NURSING EDUCATION BETWEEN 1860–1910. *The dates indicate the approximate year of the first school of nursing in each country.*

319

tal and found it in a deplorable state of affairs. The nursing care was given primarily by women who were ex-convicts; fees were collected from the patients for the inadequate services they received; drunkenness and foul language were prominent; supplies such as soap, linens, and dishes were unavailable; conditions were particularly bad at night, when three night watchmen made periodic rounds of the wards. On the basis of the shocking report that was presented to the association, it was determined that the improvement of nursing was one of the essential ingredients for hospital reform.

A resolution passed in April 1872 and addressed to the Commissioners of Charity begged this group to consider a plan for establishing a training school for nurses. The commissioners, in turn, referred the plan to the medical board, which remained silent on the subject for a time. However, Dr. Gill Wylie of the hospital staff voluntarily visited England to study schools established under Florence Nightingale. Although he was unable to personally confer with Miss Nightingale, he received a letter from her upon his return home. This letter offered support and encouragement along with valuable information regarding the mechanics of a nursing school. In addition, it reiterated Miss Nightingale's position that the nurse and the physician have different aspects of service and render different kinds of care. Finally, opposition was overcome, although somewhat reluctantly, and the commissioners agreed to the use of six wards in Bellevue for the training of nurses. Funds were raised and a house was rented for the nurses' home. The purpose of the program was "to train nurses for the care of the sick in order that women shall find a school for their education and the public shall reap the advantage of skilled and educated labor" (Dock, 1901, p. 90). Sister Helen Bowden of the Sisterhood of All Saints was selected to direct the program. She was familiar with the Nightingale system and equated the conditions in Bellevue to those in the English workhouses. Therefore Sister Helen Bowden adopted a system that was very similar to that of St. Thomas's School. The Nightingale system became known in America as the "Bellevue System," since it was introduced in that institution.

The Bellevue Hospital Training School for Nurses was founded in May 1873, and five students enrolled in the first class. The program was one year in length, but the students were required to remain a second year in service. The students received only occasional lectures; the majority of time was spent in practical work through which they gained experience. They received ten dollars per month after completing a probationary period of one month. Initially, the students wore no uniforms, but after the first year the training school committee decided that a standard uniform should be adopted. (No nurse in America had ever worn a uniform.) This created a stir among the nurses, who were reluctant to wear uniforms. The committee very astutely granted Euphemia Van Rensselaer—one of the students with a distinctive family name, social position, and personal beauty—a two-day leave of absence from Bellevue. She returned in a uniform, apron, and cap that had been made especially for her. Her tailored uniform consisted of a long blue seersucker dress with white apron, collar and cuffs, and a white cap. Within a week every nurse was wearing the uniform, which eventually became the mark of a Bellevue nurse. A pin designed by Tiffany and Company in 1880 also distinguished the graduates of Bellevue.

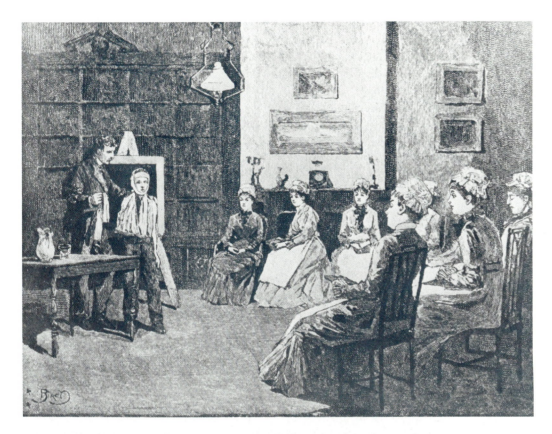

A LESSON IN BANDAGING, *The parlor in the Bellevue Hospital Nurses' Home in 1882. Wood engraving. From* CENTURY MAGAZINE, *November 1882, in "A New Profession for Women." National Library of Medicine, Bethesda, Maryland.*

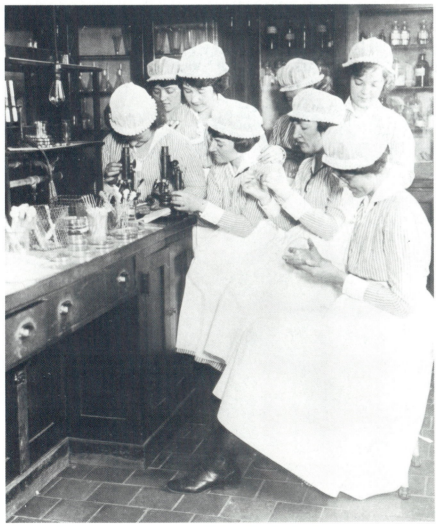

NURSES' TRAINING, *c. 1900. White Caps of Bellevue Hospital, New York, during instruction in a bacteriological lab. The Bettmann Archive, New York.*

The Bellevue school flourished and became one of the leading nursing schools in the country. In October 1874, Linda Richards became the night superintendent. A *Manual of Nursing* was published in 1876. Many brilliant leaders emerged from this program, including Isabel Hampton Robb, Lavinia Lloyd Dock, Mary Agnes Snively (a Canadian who fostered the progress of the training school at the Toronto General Hospital and the Canadian Nursing Association), and Jane A. Delano.

Connecticut Training School. The Connecticut Training School in New Haven was established through the efforts of Georgeanna Woolsey Bacon, her husband, Dr. Francis Bacon, and a wealthy philanthropist, Charles Thompson. Mrs. Bacon and her two sisters had served as nurses in the Civil War and remained actively involved in nursing. The training school, established as an organization separate from the hospital, opened in October 1873 with four students. It was controlled by a board of directors who contracted an exchange with the hospital whereby nursing service would be provided for educational services. Physicians supported the school from the very beginning. Miss Bayard, who had been trained at the Women's Hospital of Philadelphia, became the head of the school and it grew rapidly. By the end of the second year of operation, the first graduates were sent out to private families. By the fourth year the school was able to furnish superintendents of nursing to other hospi-

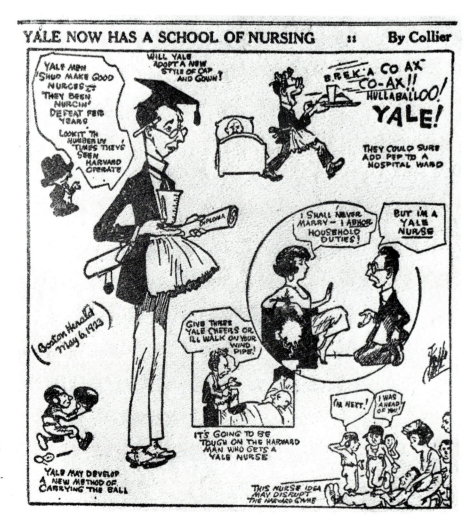

A napkin by Collier entitled YALE NOW HAS A SCHOOL OF NURSING, *c. 1940. Mugar Memorial Library, Boston University, Massachusetts. By permission from the* BOSTON HERALD AMERICAN.

tals. The school remained independent until 1906, when the hospital assumed control.

In 1879 the *New Haven Manual of Nursing,* created by a committee of both nurses and doctors, was published by the Connecticut Training School. It was a comprehensive text that found widespread acceptance among the nursing schools in the country. The school was one of the first to obtain a university affiliation (1924, Yale University) and an endowment of $1 million from the Rockefeller Foundation. The Yale School of Nursing was the first in the world that was established as a separate university department with an independent budget and its own dean, Annie W. Goodrich.

Boston Training School.

The Massachusetts General Hospital of Boston was the last of the three institutions to open a school for nurses. The idea was initiated by the Woman's Educational Association, which called a meeting to consider the subject. A training school committee was established to decide upon a plan, to ask for cooperation of the physicians, to raise funds, and to seek permission from the trustees of Massachusetts General to develop a school in connection with that hospital. The school of nursing began operation as the Boston Training School and opened its doors in November 1873 with a superintendent, two head nurses, and six pupils to take charge of two wards. Mrs. Billings, who had experience as a hospital nurse in the Civil War, was the first superintendent.

From the very beginning, the medical staff had not favored or supported the school. Unfortunately, under the new arrangement the wards did not run smoothly, and the school was identified as the source of the difficulties. The training school committee was given another year's trial only after assuring the trustees that a graduate nurse would be placed in charge of the school; at the end of that time, a decision would be made to either close or continue the school. Linda Richards was placed in charge, an event that marked a steady march of progress and success for the floundering program. She reorganized the school, conducted classes, and personally cared for patients. Because of the high quality of her nursing, Miss Richards

Harry Fenn, THE MASSACHUSETTS GENERAL HOSPITAL IN BOSTON. *Drawing. The Bettmann Archive, New York.*

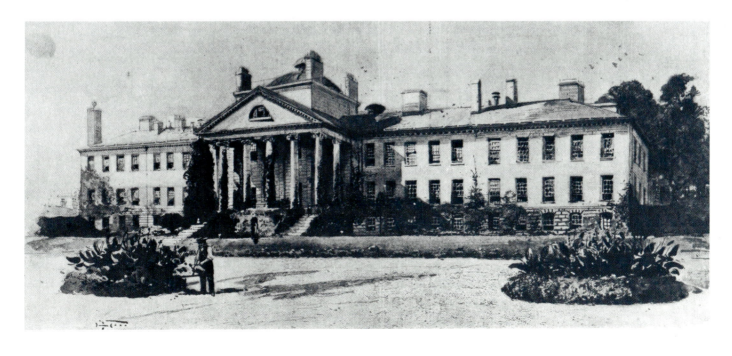

proved to be an excellent example for students to follow. The training committee administered the school until 1896, when control reverted to Massachusetts General Hospital because of financial problems.

These early schools soon proved their value, and by 1879 there were eleven training schools in the United States. By the turn of the century there were no less than 432 schools, and most of these had expanded their programs to two or three years. The standards, however, varied greatly among the schools. Active renovation in hospitals and the creation of new ones occurred between 1873 and 1895. One of these was Johns Hopkins Hospital (Baltimore), whose training school opened in 1889 under Isabel Adams Hampton (Robb). The function of the hospitals slowly changed from refuges of the destitute to institutions for the care of the sick and injured. The value of trained nurses had finally been proven, and this resulted in a growing demand for trained nurses.

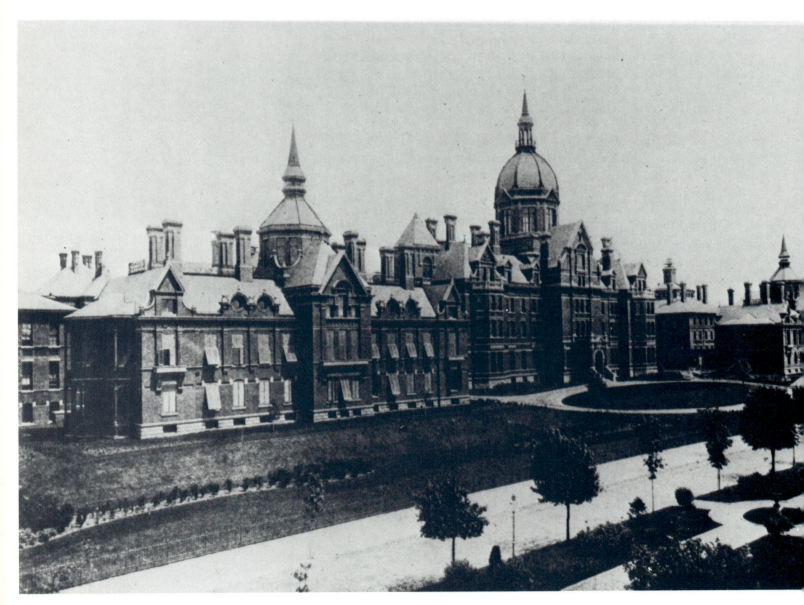

VIEW OF JOHNS HOPKINS HOSPITAL, *1889. Special Collections, Milbank Memorial Library, Teachers College, Columbia University, New York.*

324

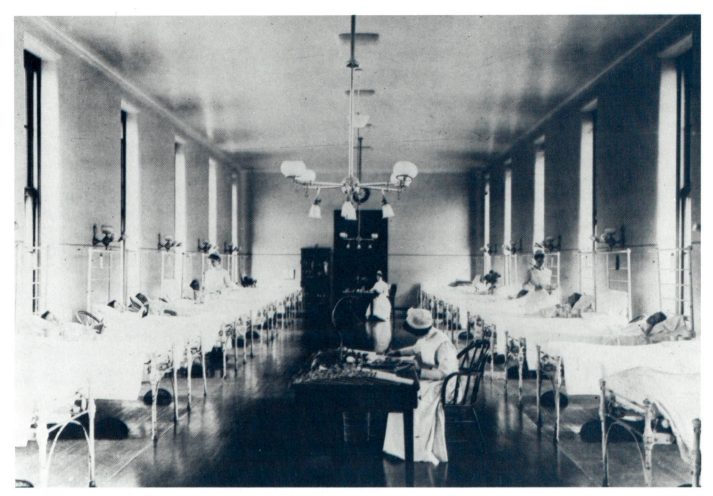

VIEW OF A WARD AT JOHNS HOPKINS HOSPITAL, *turn of the century. Special Collections, Milbank Memorial Library, Teachers College, Columbia University, New York.*

■ CANADIAN SCHOOLS

Canada had one of the earliest schools patterned after the Nightingale schools, the one located at the General and Marine Hospital in St. Catharine's (1874). The bylaws for nurses were laid down in the regulations for the training school (later called the Mack Training School) and were influenced by the Nightingale principles. The first of these bylaws stated:

> The nurses in the daily discharge of their duties must observe the strictest secrecy, and carefully avoid "gossip," their demeanour should be kind and respectful on all occasions, and when on duty at private houses, they are expected, in addition to taking the complete charge of their patients, to avoid giving unnecessary trouble, to wait upon themselves, and to pay the closest attention to the preparation of aliments for the sick, as well as to cheerfully assist in many matters not strictly within their duty—to faithfully carry out the physician's directions, and in the event of emergencies, to report any instance when the execution of his orders have been exceeded or omitted. To evince no bias to any favourite medical practitioner. To attend scrupulously to the special duties to the patient with the gentleness and exactitude taught by their superiors, and never to interfere with or criticize the treatment.
>
> *Gibbon and Mathewson, 1947, pp. 144–145*

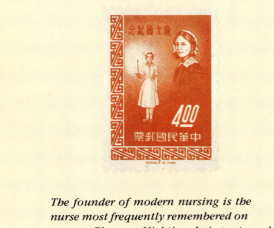

The founder of modern nursing is the nurse most frequently remembered on stamps. Florence Nightingale is portrayed by the Republic of China with a student nurse holding her candle. This 1964 stamp was issued to observe Nurses' Day, May 12. Courtesy of Howard B. Hurley.

Excerpts from "The First Annual Report of The St. Catharine Training School and Nurses' Home," dated July 1, 1875, are particularly enlightening:

> Every possible opportunity is seized to impart instruction of a practical nature in the art of nursing, while teaching will be given in chemistry, sanitary science, popular physiology and anatomy, hygiene and all such branches of the healing art as a nurse ought to be familiarized with.... The vocation of nursing goes hand in hand with that of the physician and surgeon, and they are absolutely indispensable one to the other.... By observing the known principles of hygiene, she will co-operate intelligently with him, also in placing the sufferer from disease in the best relation to the ground he is above, the surrounding heat, light, air, aliments he is sustained by, and the liquids he drinks. She will, likewise, by the proper precautions well recognized in hygiene, avert the evils of contagion or infection, and the spread of disease by noxious miasma.... Finally, she will inspire confidence, allay terror, soothe anxiety, and often quiet the mental state while taking care of the physical, and prevent injurious interference from officious by-standers.
>
> *Gibbon and Mathewson, 1947, p. 145*

The second Canadian hospital to consider the idea of a training school for nurses was Montreal General (1821). In 1875 the hospital board sought the assistance of Florence Nightingale in establishing a school. Five nurses were sent from St. Thomas's Hospital, but they were appalled by the environment and eventually resigned; one of the original five died of typhoid fever. The conditions in the Montreal General Hospital were much like those of Bellevue. Filth was the primary feature, with armies of rats scurrying about the wards and sometimes attacking patients. Other attempts were made to start the school, but they also proved unsuccessful. Finally, Nora Gertrude Livingstone, a graduate of the New York Hospital, succeeded in establishing a school in 1890. Under her direction the nursing school had its real beginning.

The history of the Toronto General Hospital was similar to that of Montreal General. From 1877, attempts were made to establish a training school, but it was not until 1884 that the real fame of the school began. At this time Mary Agnes Snively, a graduate of Bellevue Hospital, became the superintendent. She reorganized the school and developed a modern plan of work and study. During her tenure the school became well known throughout the nursing world as embodying the highest ideals in nursing. Miss Snively remained until 1910 and greatly elevated the standards of the Toronto school.

Other schools soon followed in Canada: the Children's Hospital at Toronto in 1886; the Winnipeg General (1887), which claims to have been the first hospital in Western Canada to start a training school for nurses; St. Boniface General in Winnipeg (1890); the Royal Jubilee at Victoria (1890); Victoria General in Halifax (1892); and the Royal Victoria at Montreal (1894). Miss Snively reported that by June 1909 there were seventy schools for nurses; of these, ten offered a two-year course, three had a program of two and one half years; and fifty-seven required a three-year course (Gibbon and Mathewson, 1947). The introduction of training schools for nurses became almost automatic for progressive Canadian hospitals after 1890. Trained nurses began to emerge in Canada almost simultaneously with those in the United States.

■ NURSING IN THE SPANISH-AMERICAN WAR

The war with Spain provided American nurses with their first experience in army nursing. Unfortunately, the Spanish-American War also graphically illustrated American deficiencies, such as the lack of a Red Cross nursing service, the need for an army nurse corps, and the lack of emergency reserves. The U.S. Army Medical Department was made up of approximately 983 members, but it had very little prestige. Certainly, the number of members was not adequate to care for the 28,000 members of the Regular Army. American battle casualties were small during this war, but hastily constructed army camps were devastated by typhoid fever, malaria, dysentery, and food poisoning. Epidemic diseases caused ten times more deaths than did bullets. Nurses were desperately needed. The Nurses' Associated Alumnae of the United States and Canada (renamed the American Nurses' Association in 1911) offered assistance, but the Army rejected it. The primary objection to the organization was that it had been in existence for a relatively short time and was not recognized as the spokesman for nurses. The offer had also come one day too late. The Daughters of the American Revolution had already volunteered, and Anita Newcomb McGee (1864–1940), their vice-president and a physician with no previous administrative experience, had been appointed in charge of the Army Nursing Service. Dr. McGee was given the position of acting assistant surgeon in the United States Army.

Congress authorized the employment of female nurses on a contract basis, which provided thirty dollars per month plus room and meals. The contract, however, did not provide for personal care if the nurses became ill. Dr. McGee preferred graduate nurses with proper endorsements from their own schools and suggested that all applicants be examined and cleared through the D.A.R. Some 8000 volunteer nurses were placed under contract and in essence represented the beginning of the current Army Nursing Corps. Nearly 1600 graduate nurses served; Catholic orders also served in large numbers, particularly the Daughters of Charity. The first nurses were appointed in May 1898, and they were stationed in Army hospitals in the United States, Puerto Rico, Cuba, Hawaii, and the Philippine Islands. In addition, they served on the hospital ship, the USS *Relief.* This ship carried supplies of medicines and dressings and enough equipment to outfit a 750-bed hospital for six months. Six women nurses were aboard when it left Tampa harbor.

The Army hospitals had been tended by hospital corpsmen who lacked training and experience. These men were recruits who were often the dregs of the units and were totally unqualified to care for the sick. They were guilty of unsanitary practices, such as using the same bucket for food and excrement, which helped spread disease throughout the camps. Consequently, conditions of the worst type met the nurses when they arrived. The nurses often worked day and night with inadequate supplies and shelter. They eventually won respect and recognition, not only from the servicemen but also from

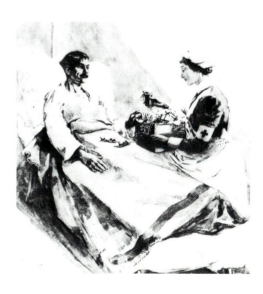

W.A. Rogers, A MESSAGE FROM HOME. *A hospital scene during the Spanish-American War. The Bettmann Archive, New York.*

327

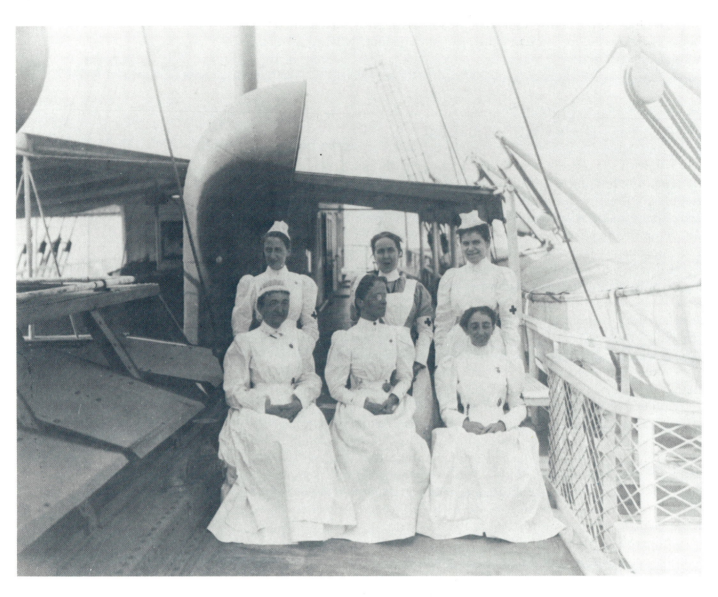

NURSES ON DECK OF THE HOSPITAL SHIP
"RELIEF" NEAR CUBA. *The Red Cross During
the Spanish-American War, c. 1898. National
Library of Medicine, Bethesda, Maryland.*

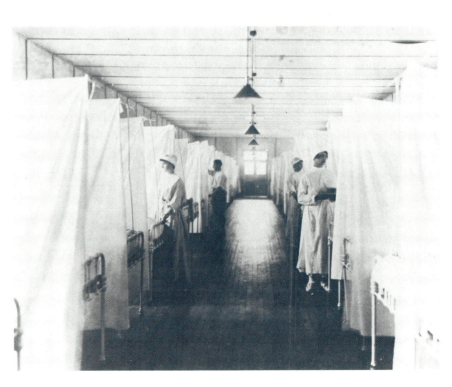

NURSES ON SCREENED BED WARD AT WALTER
REED HOSPITAL IN WASHINGTON, D.C.
*National Library of Medicine, Bethesda,
Maryland.*

the surgeons, who initially had been prejudiced against them. Thirteen nurses died while rendering nursing care during this war.

The Army was continually exposed to typhoid and yellow fever during the Spanish-American conflict. Therefore research was begun to investigate the cause and spread of typhoid fever. A committee headed by Major Walter Reed determined that flies and unclean practices were the obvious sources of the illness. Yellow fever had also been particularly virulent and the cause of many fatalities. A team of physicians, including Dr. James Carroll, Dr. Aristides Agramonte, Dr. Jesse W. Lazear, and Major Walter Reed, was sent to Cuba by the U.S. Government to find some method of control for this problem. Major Walter Reed and Dr. Agramonte consulted with Dr. Carlos Finlay, a physician in Havana, regarding his theory (of nineteen years) that yellow fever was caused by a common house mosquito. They then proceeded to conduct experiments requiring that human volunteers be bitten by mosquitos under controlled conditions so that reactions could be studied. The first volunteers were physicians; some survived, others died. These experiments proved that the mosquito now called *Aedes aegypti* was the yellow fever carrier and led the way to conquest of the disease.

Dean Cornwell, CONQUERORS OF YELLOW FEVER. *Courtesy of Wyeth Laboratories, Philadelphia, Pennsylvania. Drs. Jesse Lazear, James Carroll, Carlos Finlay, and Major Walter Reed investigating the mosquito-borne disease in Cuba following the Spanish-American War, August 27, 1900.*

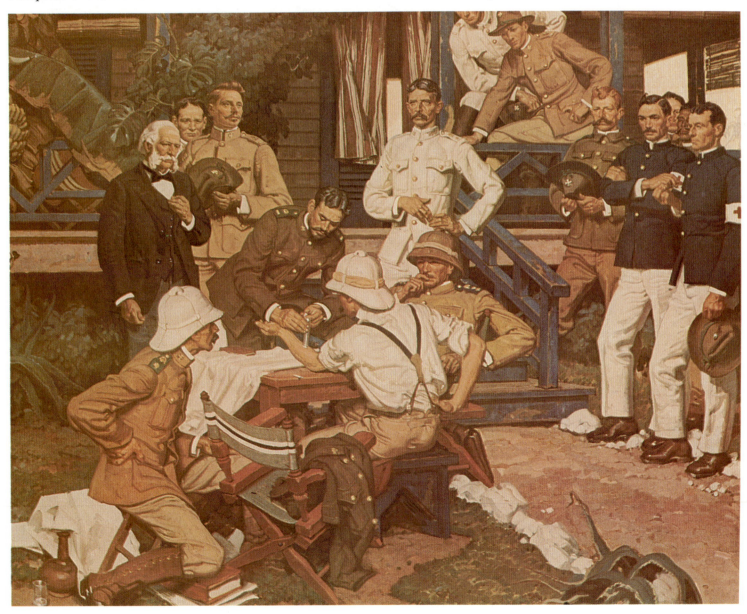

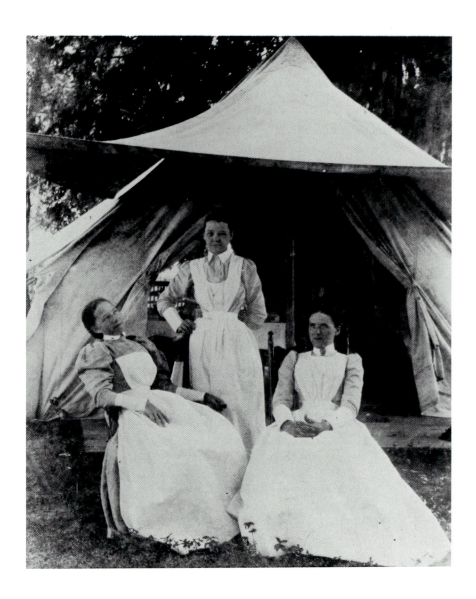

The last person to be used for the yellow fever experiment was
a nurse who gave her life. She was remembered by the medical
officer in charge of the hospital where her death occurred:

> On many occasions during the Spanish-American War the nurses
> showed heroism and devotion to duty equal to that of any
> soldier or sailor in battle. The majority of those with me at Las
> Animos Hospital, Havana, had not had yellow fever, yet they all
> unflinchingly nursed the malignant cases of that disease, staying
> by those who died, to the very last, trying to alleviate the suffer-
> ing and save life, their clothing, hands, and sometimes their faces
> smeared with blood and black vomit. One of those Las Animos
> [sic] nurses, Miss Clara Maass, gave up her young life from a high
> sense of duty. She thought she would be more useful in Cuba as
> a nurse after having had yellow fever, and requested to be bitten
> by infected mosquitos in order to contract the disease and be-
> come immune. I tried to dissuade her from the step, telling her
> that her life was too valuable to be exposed to such great risk. . . .
> Nevertheless, she insisted, and the fatal mosquitos were applied
> to her arm. Three or four days later, she developed a malignant,
> hemorrhagic case of yellow fever, from which she died in about
> a week.
>
> *Quoted in Frank, 1953, p. 259*

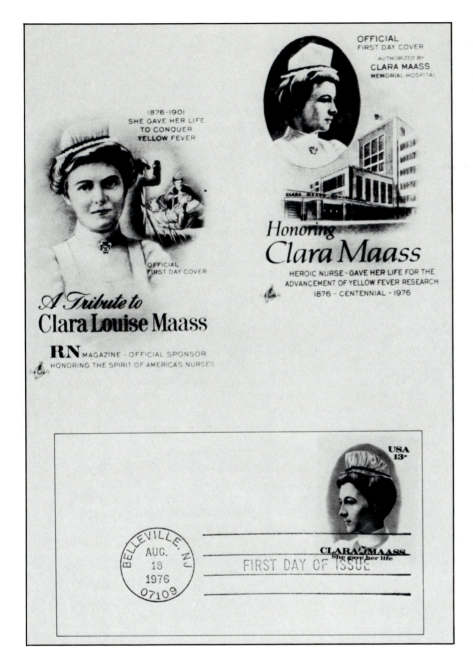

The official first day covers honoring nurse Clara Louise Maass, which were sponsored by RN MAGAZINE *and the Clara Maass Memorial Hospital to celebrate the 100th anniversary of her birth. Courtesy of Howard B. Hurley.*

Clara Louise Maass (1876–1901) graduated from the Christina Trefz Training School for Nurses of the Newark German Hospital in 1895. This hospital has since been renamed the Clara Maass Memorial Hospital. Miss Maass was one of the first five students to graduate from the two-year program. She remained on the staff and three years later became a head nurse. She volunteered to become a contract nurse with the U.S. Army during the Spanish-American War and served in Florida, Georgia, Cuba, and the Philippines. After her term of service was complete, Clara Louise Maass volunteered in response to Major William C. Gorgas's call for nurses in Havana, where experiments on yellow fever were being conducted. She nursed the victims of this disease through the spring of 1901. On June 4, 1901, she allowed herself to be bitten by a mosquito. She suffered a mild attack of yellow fever, recovered, and was bitten again on August 14. She had seriously doubted that the slight fever had given her immunity to the disease. The second attack proved fatal, and she died ten days later at the age of twenty-five.

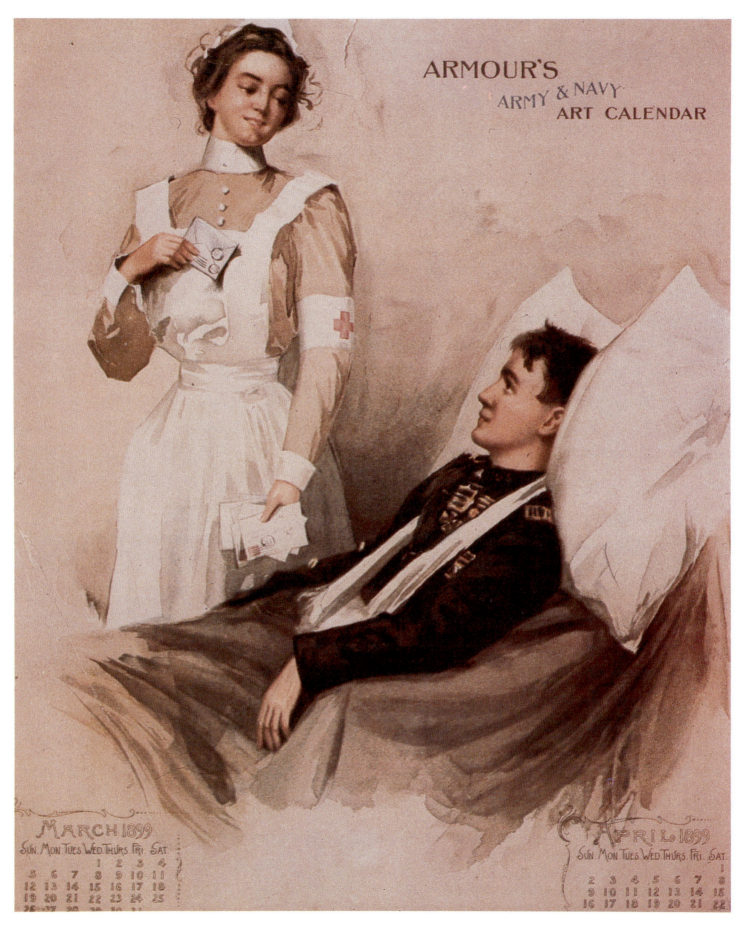

ARMOUR'S ARMY AND NAVY ART CALENDAR, *1899. Donahue Collection.*

Modern nursing movements followed the Spanish-American War, the first war in which graduate nurses served the armed forces.

Miss Maass was the only American and the only woman to die during the experiments. After her death the experiments were discontinued, and the disease was ultimately conquered. Miss Maass' body was sent to Fairmount Cemetery in Newark for burial with full military honors. In 1951 a commemorative stamp was issued in her honor by Cuba. In 1976 the United States issued a commemorative stamp in honor of her service to humanity. This was the first U.S. stamp to honor an individual nurse. In addition, a special medal commemorating the one-hundreth anniversary of Miss Maass' birth was struck by the Franklin Mint.

The war experience definitely proved the superiority of the trained nurse over the untrained volunteer and led to the initiation of a permanent nurse corps. Immediately following the war, both the Associated Alumnae, with the backing of influential citizens, and Dr. McGee proposed bills for the establishment of a nursing corps that would have the sanction and permanence of law. These bills were not passed. Finally in 1900, after a number of surgeons had spoken positively to the Congress about the work done by the nurses, the Army Reorganization Bill was presented. It provided a permanent Nurse Corps as part of the Medical Department of the Army; the corps would be composed of fully trained nurses (hospital school graduates) under an able director. An amendment stating that the superintendent of the Nurse Corps had to be a hospital school graduate was added before the bill was passed on February 2, 1901. The bill stated that the U.S. Army nurse's salary would be forty dollars per month for duty in the United States and fifty dollars per month for duty elsewhere. In 1918 the name was changed to the Army Nurse Corps (A.N.C.). Its motto has been "Where go the United States troops, there go the Army Nurses."

Since she was not a nurse, Dr. McGee was forced to resign when the Army Nurse Corps was established. She was succeeded by Dita H. Kinney, head nurse of the United States Army Hospital at Fort Bayard, New Mexico. The status of the Army nurse has shown slow but consistent improvement. Several events have assisted this process: Army nurses were accorded relative rank in 1920; they became eligible for retirement benefits in 1926; in 1947 Army nurses became part of the regular Army with full commission, pay, and other benefits as granted to male officers. A succession of leaders served in the position of superintendent, including Jane Delano, Isabel McIssac, and Dora Thompson, the first to have served in the military. In 1908 the U.S. Navy Nurse Corps was founded as an integral unit of the Navy.

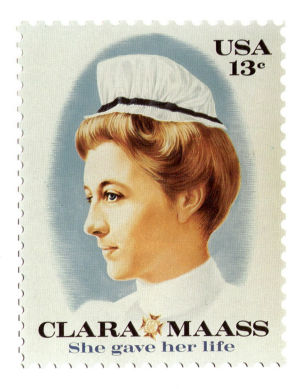

In 1976, the United States honored the first individual American nurse, Clara Maass, with a commemorative thirteen-cent stamp for her contribution to the nursing profession and humanity. The issuance marked the 100th anniversary of her birth. Courtesy of Howard B. Hurley.

■ EDUCATIONAL ADVANCEMENT FOR GRADUATE NURSES

By the end of the nineteenth century new educational opportunities became available for graduate nurses attending Teachers College, Columbia University. The Teachers College program was founded as a direct result of the efforts of the American Society of Superintendents of Training Schools for Nurses (renamed in 1912 the National League of Nursing Education and reorganized in 1952 under the present National League for Nursing). A special committee of the society, with Isabel Hampton Robb as its head, was created to investigate a

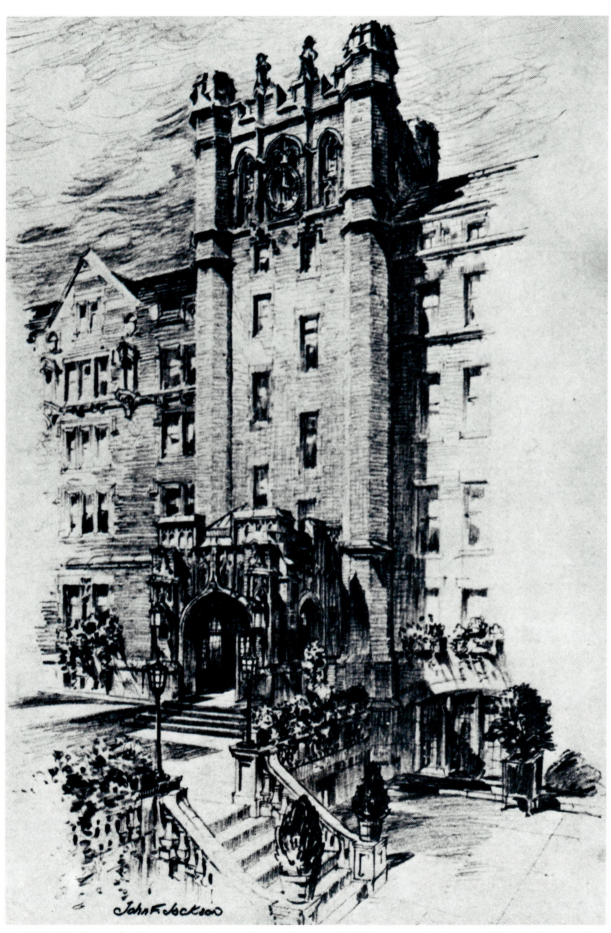

DODGE HALL. *From the Alumni Association Historic Statement, 1960. Special Collections, Milbank Memorial Library, Teachers College, Columbia University, New York.*

means to better prepare nurses for leadership in schools of nursing. According to one source, "It was useless to look to our own institutions for the solution of this problem, and the ordinary normal school or college was equally incapable of adjusting its facilities to our peculiar needs" (Stewart, 1909, p. 1). Teachers College, which had opened ten years earlier for the training of teachers, seemed the logical choice. The program was originally designed to prepare administrators of nursing service and nursing education. It was established as an eight-month course in hospital economics in 1899.

> The original course for nurses in hospital economics at Teachers College was at first rather heavily weighted with technical subjects in the household arts with some recognition of the sciences also present. Pedagogical subjects such as psychology and the philosophy of education were soon identified as valuable in the study of the problems of nursing education and were incorporated within the program. Additional lectures by leaders in the Society shared nursing experiences gained through accumulated years of practical service in hospitals and training-school work. In 1906, a new department of institutional administration was established in the college, the course in hospital economics becoming incorporated within its structure. From this time forward there was no longer any question as to the place of nursing in the general scheme of university education. The department continued to grow, broaden its educational program, emphasize the social and educational phases of the nurse's work, and include nursing specialties such as teaching and supervision, public health nursing, school nursing, and other related branches. Eventually, the name was changed to the Department of Nursing Education.
>
> *Donahue, 1981, pp. 41–42*

Mary Adelaide Nutting, former superintendent of nurses and principal of the Training School for Nurses at Johns Hopkins Hospital, came to Teachers College in 1907 and became the first nursing professor in the world. She was thus the first nurse to occupy a chair on a university faculty. Under her direction the department progressed and became a pioneer in education for nurses. The school became known as the "mother house" of collegiate education because it fostered the initial movements toward undergraduate and graduate degrees for nurses.

There is probably no ten-year span in nursing's history during which so many important events occurred or so many fateful decisions were made than in the period between 1890 and 1900. It was a time of unprecedented growth in American nursing, a period of emergence of several of our most important nursing leaders, an era of tremendous proliferation of schools of nursing, and the decade of the greatest organizational strides for the fledgling profession.

Teresa E. Christy

ADVANCING TOWARD NEW FRONTIERS

By the turn of the century, the trial period was over. The training school as well as the trained nurse were recognized and accepted by hospitals, medicine, and the general public. This revolution in nursing, combined with new developments in surgery and sanitary science, led to a tremendous expansion in hospitals. It was nursing that would ultimately make the application of these discoveries possible. Hospitals of all types sprang up, multiplied at an astonishing rate, and became independent entities because there was no regulating body of any type to set and enforce controls. It soon became apparent that a school of nursing was almost indispensable to the running of a hospital. Not only did nursing students improve the nursing service to patients, but also the cost of the improved service to the hospital was less. The students worked long hours and did hard physical labor in payment for the training they received. Most hospitals, therefore, set up their own schools or assumed control over schools that had been developed on an independent basis. The right of the hospital to set up a school was not questioned; nor was there any interference with the manner in which the school was run. In some instances hospitals had schools of nursing for the sole purpose of using the service contributed by students for the care of patients. The wide diversity among these schools and the exploitation of student nurses thus became important issues as the United States approached the twentieth century.

New frontiers beckoned to women and to nursing. Although still wanting to be useful, greater numbers of women also wished to be independent and free and find the means of demonstrating their intelligence and capabilities and proving their value as citizens. They wanted to have widening opportunities for respectable positions in the social order of the times. A number of individuals envisioned nursing as an area in which this could be accomplished. However, a change in the system of nursing education and practice was necessary to achieve this goal. Consequently, nursing leaders began to organize for the control of their own educational standards and for the improvement of nursing practice. They were beginning to see that their educational difficulties could not be solved by an isolated effort, that the united energies of all nurses and all schools would be needed in any serious attempt to attack the chaos that had been created in educational standards and ideals. According to Stewart (1943, p. 129), "nursing leaders banded together to support educational standards, to set up some legal controls to prevent the spread of poor schools, and to prevent unlimited expansion."

■ THE TURN OF THE CENTURY

The twentieth century has been referred to as "the century of social consciousness." The beginnings of social endeavors in the nineteenth century finally became reality with the development of a variety of social agencies. The states had begun to assume at least partial responsibility for the relief of the poor early in the nineteenth century. In 1863 Massachusetts, for example, had appointed a State Board of Charities that was charged with the care of the nonresident poor and with general supervision of state institutions. New York and Ohio created similar boards in 1867. By 1930 forty-one states had created boards for the supervision of relief. This movement for social reform brought about many changes that influenced health care and nursing.

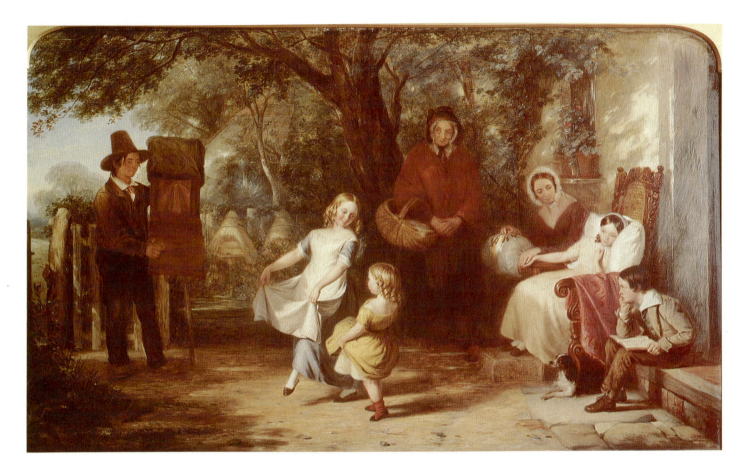

Thomas Webster, SICKNESS AND HEALTH, 1843. The Bridgeman Art Library Ltd./ Victoria and Albert Museum, London, England.

Attention began to be focused on specific dependents, such as the blind and the aged, but the provisions were totally inadequate for their maintenance. Child health received particular emphasis with the initiation of the first White House Conference on Child Welfare in 1910. Within two years the Children's Bureau was established (1912) by an act of Congress and placed within the Department of Labor. Its function was to investigate and report all matters that pertained to the welfare of children and child life among all classes of people. Studies of infant mortality, care available to mothers and infants in rural communities, and methods of instruction in hygiene were undertaken by this agency. Finally, federal aid for the reduction of infant mortality was suggested by Miss Julia Lathrop, chief of the Children's Bureau, in 1917. Her proposals were incorporated in the Sheppard-Towner Act of 1921, which authorized appropriations to provide grants-in-aid to states that would set up services for the welfare and hygiene of mothers and children.

Hundreds of nurses were employed to make home visits and supply health education and health screening of mothers and infants. These monies continued for seven years and stimulated the establishment of prenatal, infant, and preschool child health centers. Efforts were made to renew the Sheppard-Towner Act, but they were unsuccessful in the face of conservative forces. The continuation of this act was opposed by the American Medical Association:

> Resolved that the House of Delegates condemns as unsound
> in policy, wasteful and extravagant, unproductive of results and
> tending to promote communism, the federal subsidy system
> established by the Sheppard-Towner Maternity and Infancy Act
> and protests against a renewal of the system in any form.
>
> *American Medical Association, 1930*

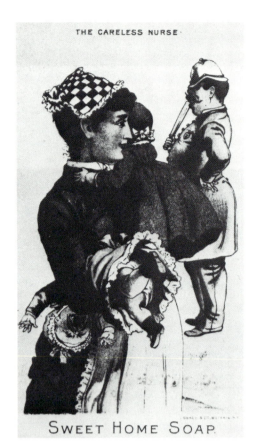

THE CARELESS NURSE.

SWEET HOME SOAP.

THE CARELESS NURSE. *The Bettmann Archive, New York.*

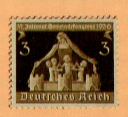

This 1936 postage stamp is one of a set of four issued by Germany in connection with the Sixth International Community Congress. It shows the nurse as symbol of community service. Courtesy of Howard B. Hurley.

Public health nurses, on the other hand, supported a renewal and watched with deep concern. When the federal aid ceased, the majority of the states continued to provide funds, although in decreased amounts.

The Settlement House Movement also became a popular cause. A "settlement house" frequently developed as a branch of the university, where intellectuals investigated the distressful conditions of the poor. The movement was started through the efforts of Arnold Toynbee, whose interest in the poor led him to establish university settlement projects. After his death, Oxford University students at Toynbee Hall (1875) in East London continued to study ways to alleviate community problems. Through their efforts the very poor had the opportunity to enrich their lives educationally, socially, and culturally. Every aspect of neighborhood and community welfare was met by social workers who lived among the people they served. The primary purpose of settlement work was to teach and assist wage earners to develop their potential in order to provide security and comfort for their families. Philanthropists who lived among the lower classes thus became their role models.

The first American settlement was developed on the Lower East Side of New York by Stanton Coit in 1886. Originally known as the "Neighborhood Guild," it was later called the "University Settlement." In 1889 Hull House was founded in Chicago by Jane Addams. This settlement came to be typical of ones that developed in other parts of America. The beginning of Hull House was a big old house that had been purchased by Jane Addams (1860–1935) and a friend, Ellen Gates. The doors were opened to the neighborhood, which was comprised of representatives of over thirty nationalities. Help of all types was offered for any situation. Miss Addams's neighbors clung to their customs, yet they wanted an education for their children and all the opportunities that America had to offer. Eventually, a day nursery, a kindergarten, and a library became essential components of Hull House. The community came to rely on Jane Addams, who also fought for suffrage and was the joint recipient of the 1931 Nobel Peace Prize (with Nicholas Murray Butler). By 1900 there were approximately 103 settlement houses in the United States.

Before the Civil War, another social agency was extended from England to America. The Young Men's Christian Association (YMCA) was established in London in 1844 and in the United States in 1851. Its initial function dealt with the spiritual, social, physical, and intellectual well-being of men, but it gradually expanded to include relief work, visiting of the sick, and employment assistance. The YMCA also provided specialized services in wartime. Several branches joined to form the United States Christian Commission to assist with the welfare of soldiers during the Civil War. Later, this commission cared for prisoners and provided recreation for soldiers in World War I. In World War II it cooperated with other agencies to form the United Service Organization (USO) for planned recreational programs for members of the armed forces. Corresponding with the development of the YMCA was a movement among women that resulted in the formation of the Young Women's Christian Association (YWCA).

The Salvation Army (1878), founded by William Booth (1829–1912), was originally organized as a mission for the poor in London. Booth and his associates eventually became known as the "Salvation Army," which was set up with a military structure from that time on.

340

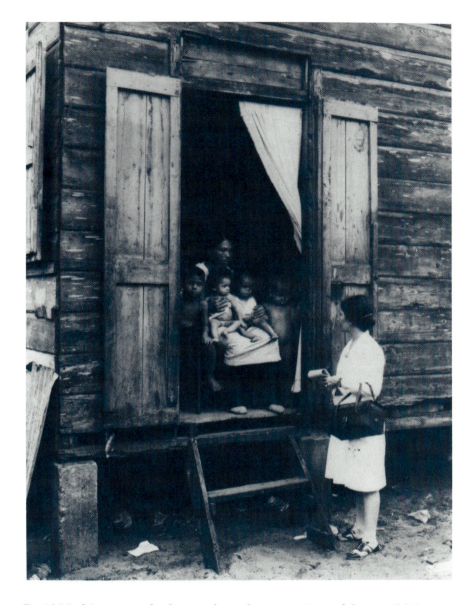

By 1893 this agency had spread to a large portion of the world. It, too, was interested in the physical and spiritual welfare of the individual. Christian living was practiced through the giving of food, clothing, and shelter to the poor. Those who were miserable could find a certain amount of protection through the organization.

Social services had no boundaries, and missionaries helped to establish hospitals, schools of nursing, and dispensaries wherever they were needed. Nurses helped with these reforms by traveling to lands wherever people were in need of care. The work of Sir Wilfred Grenfell (1865–1940) is just one example of the remarkable achievements. Sir Wilfred was an English medical missionary who went to Labrador in 1892 and built a chain of hospital centers. Physicians, nurses, and college students volunteered at this mission, which ultimately developed into a complete health service to cover both physical and spiritual needs.

Visiting Nursing

The apostolic deaconesses are considered to be the ancestors of the current visiting nurses. Early nursing orders, too, particularly the Sisters of Charity, visited the sick in their homes and became well

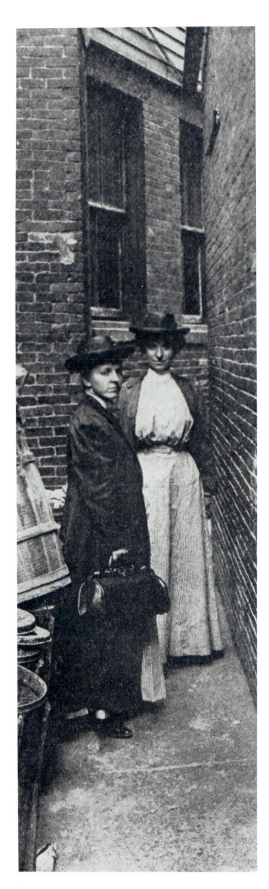

PHOTOGRAPH OF TWO VISITING NURSES
IN ALLEY WITH GARBAGE CANS, *January 1910.*
Mugar Memorial Library, Boston University,
Massachusetts. By permission from the
Visiting Nurse Association of Boston.

known for their efforts. During specific periods in history, home visits were the primary activity of nursing, until modern municipal hospitals were fully developed. The Protestant Sisters of Charity—organized by Elizabeth Fry—St. John's Home, the Order of St. Margaret, and other groups were initiated for this purpose. In addition, the deaconesses at Kaiserswerth received part of their nurses' training out in the community.

A formal structure for visiting nursing was established in Great Britain through the endeavors of William Rathbone, a wealthy citizen of Liverpool. His wife had died in 1859 after a long and painful illness during which she was cared for by a competent trained nurse. Mr. Rathbone pondered the fact that his wife, a woman who had everything that money could buy, had received relief from skilled nursing care. He concluded that the poor, whose illnesses were compounded by a lack of wealth and by inadequate surroundings, would be helped even more. Nurses, therefore, should be sent to the homes of the needy sick. Mr. Rathbone employed Mary Robinson, the nurse who had cared for his wife, for a trial period of three months to give nursing care and comfort to the poor of Liverpool. It is interesting to note that his plan was opposed on the basis of the unsanitary conditions often found in the homes of the poor. According to Rathbone, a contemporary physician made this statement:

> It is evident that the essential conditions of rational and successful sick nursing such as good air, light, warmth, bedding, good food, etc., are altogether wanting in the homes of the poor. Of what use are the gratuitous supply and regular giving of medicines, if every necessity is wanting for ordinary healthy living? It is not that the nurse shrinks from the privations and injurious influences existing in the cottages and hovels, but it is the impossibility of being useful under such circumstances that renders home nursing unattainable for the poor. One can comfort them in their cottages, and give them food and medicine, but to nurse and heal them there with any prospect of success cannot be done.
>
> *Rathbone, 1890, p. 7*

The general feeling was that if the poor were seriously ill, they should go to a hospital. However, Rathbone disagreed on the basis that many patients with serious illnesses were refused admission to general hospitals, that there would never be enough hospitals to take care of all serious illnesses among the poor, and that care given by the visiting nurse was less costly than that offered in the hospital. He soon hired additional nurses and began to train them at the school he founded at the Liverpool Royal Infirmary. His persistence resulted in the firm establishment of visiting nursing in Liverpool, which grew into a powerful organization. This experiment was soon followed by the emergence of other visiting nurses' societies.

Visiting nursing received a boost in 1887, when Queen Victoria celebrated her fifty-year jubilee. Of the 76,000 pounds raised by the women of England, the Queen donated 70,000 pounds to the cause of visiting nurses. This sum was augmented by other sources to establish the Queen Victoria Jubilee Institute for Nurses, which received its royal charter in 1889. Nurses in this organization were called the "Jubilee Institute Nurses," but they were also referred to as the "Queen's Nurses." Their example was followed by similar groups that developed throughout the Empire: the Victorian Order of Nurses

NURSES IN ACTION

*Wars of the
Twentieth Century*

It has often been said that nursing has made its greatest advances and notable achievements in connection with wars. In general, this statement is probably true, particularly when viewed from an historical perspective. One might wonder, however, why this has been the case, since injury and illness have always existed side by side with humanity. It seems that the truth of the statement lies in the fact that nations tend to recognize, respect, and value nurses when faced with the human tragedies of war. The unique circumstances of the war and the need for care of the wounded dramatically emphasize the value of nurses. Nurses are thus raised to a position of national stature.

Federal support of nursing and nursing education in the United States has been observed with each of the major wars, particularly World War II. This support has been demonstrated financially as well as through other means. In addition, the military has had a profound influence on nursing, the effects of which are still evident. Nursing, in turn, has affected the military. Its military members have shared a tradition of service; they have played an important role in the care of military personnel and their families both in times of peace and of war. Frequently they have assisted with the development of new techniques and innovations that have benefited medical and nursing

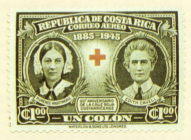

The Red Cross Society of Costa Rica was honored on its sixtieth anniversary in 1945 with a stamp portraying two of history's most famous nurses: Florence Nightingale, the angel of mercy, and Edith Cavell, the English nurse who was matron at Berkendael Medical Institute in Brussels. Cavell was arrested by German authorities in World War I for admittedly aiding Allied prisoners and assisting them to escape across the Dutch frontier. Despite efforts by the U.S. minister to Belgium to secure a reprieve, Edith Cavell was shot by the Germans on October 12, 1915, at the age of fifty. Courtesy of Howard B. Hurley.

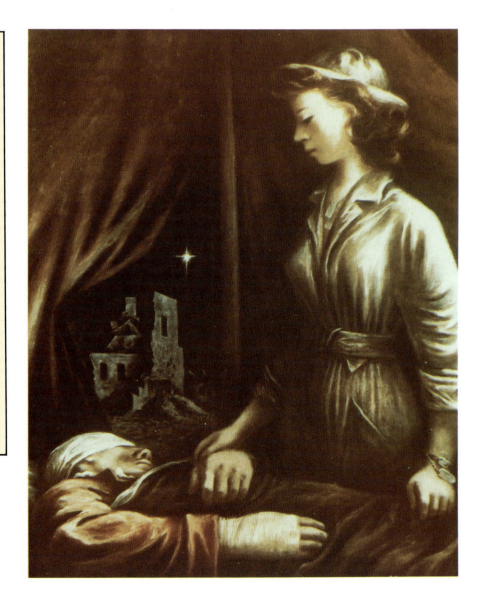

Fletcher Martin, G.I. ANGEL. *Defense Audiovisual Agency, Washington, D.C.*

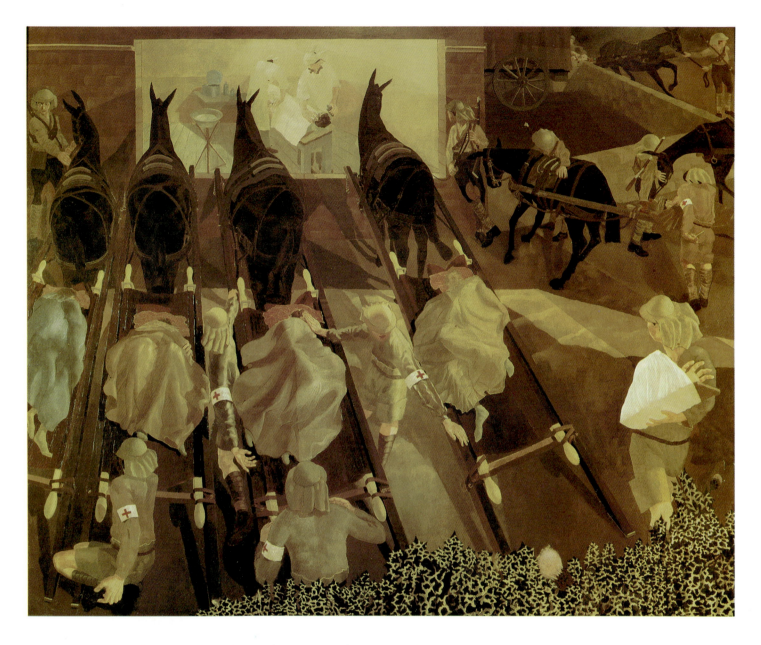

care for both soldiers and civilians. (For example, it was Air Force nurses who solved the problem of placement of food trays for litter patients.)

War brought a sharpened awareness of the nation's dependence on nurses and the urgent need to prepare them to meet the emergency. The speeding up of military and industrial defenses mandated adjustments in the number of nurses, in schools of nursing, and in nursing services. New programs were needed to expedite nursing preparedness, funds were needed for educational expansion, and intensified programs of publicity were necessary to increase the supply of applicants for nursing schools and to recruit nurses for military and other defense services. War placed heavy demands on nurses and nursing to meet the overall crises at home and abroad. Faced with an almost insurmountable task in time of war, nurses have always risen valiantly to the occasion. Particularly remarkable was the fact that in World War II a higher percentage of nurses volunteered for military service than did any other skilled or professional group, with the possible exception of physicians. Of 274,405 active graduate registered nurses, 75,000 applied for service (Editorial, *The Saturday*

Evening Post, 1945). This was one of the outstanding voluntary achievements of this war, and it spoke well for the "spirit of nursing." The fact that nurses *voluntarily* went overseas was acknowledged by hundreds of soldiers:

> To all Army nurses overseas: We men were not given the choice of working in the battlefield or the home front. We cannot take any credit for being here. We are here because we have to be. You are here because you felt you were needed. So, when an injured man opens his eyes to see one of you . . . concerned with his welfare, he can't but be overcome by the very thought that you are doing it because you want to . . . you endure whatever hardships you must to be where you can do us the most good. . . .

Quoted in Shields, editor, 1981, p. 27

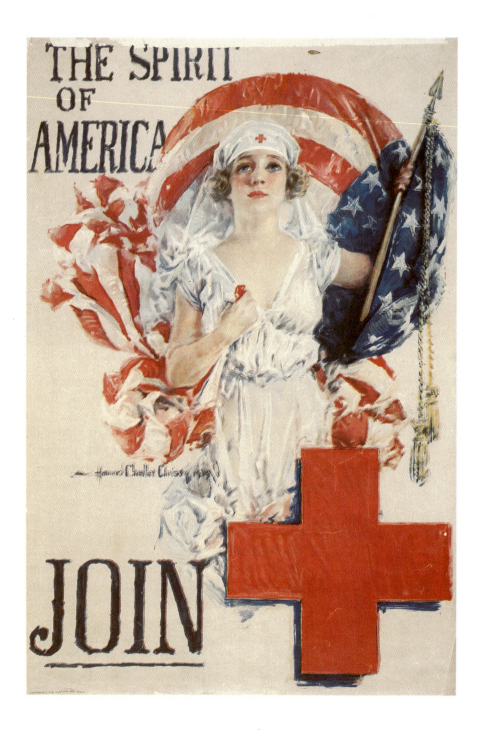

Howard Chandler Christy, THE SPIRIT OF AMERICA, *1919. Red Cross poster. Library of Congress, Washington, D.C.*

■ WORLD WAR I

A shot fired on June 28, 1914, in Sarajevo, in Serbia, killed the Archduke of Austria and his wife. This assassination was the precipitating factor of a series of events that ultimately forced the entrance of almost all of Europe and the world into a long and terrible war. One month later Austria declared war against Serbia, and a type of chain reaction followed: on August 1 Germany declared war on Russia and then on France; England declared war against Germany; declarations of war from nations all over the world were rapidly issued and continued through June 1918. In 1914 no one believed that the war would last longer than a few months; nor was anyone prepared for the cost in human lives or the vast expenditure in resources.

World War I created a large demand for nurses and taxed the medical and nursing resources of the entire world. The warring countries rapidly faced extreme shortages of physicians, nurses, medical supplies, and other resources necessary for adequate health care. At the outbreak of the war the American Red Cross sent units of physicians and nurses to assist in France, England, Germany, Austria, Serbia, and Russia. However, when America finally entered the war in April 1917, the American Red Cross Nursing Service became the reserve of the Army and the Navy. Under the able direction of Jane

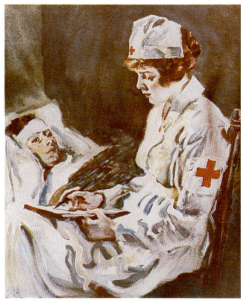

James Montgomery Flagg, ILLUSTRATION FOR THE AMERICAN RED CROSS, *World War I. Watercolor. Courtesy of Walter Reed.*

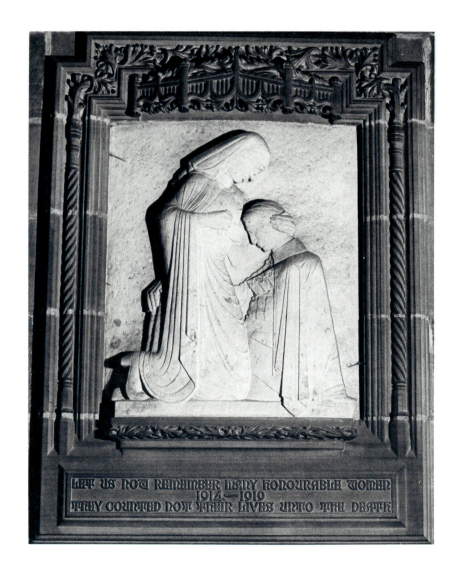

David Evans, LET US NOW REMEMBER MANY HONORABLE WOMEN. *Liverpool Cathedral, England.*

This memorial was dedicated to the nurses who died between 1914 and 1919 during World War I.

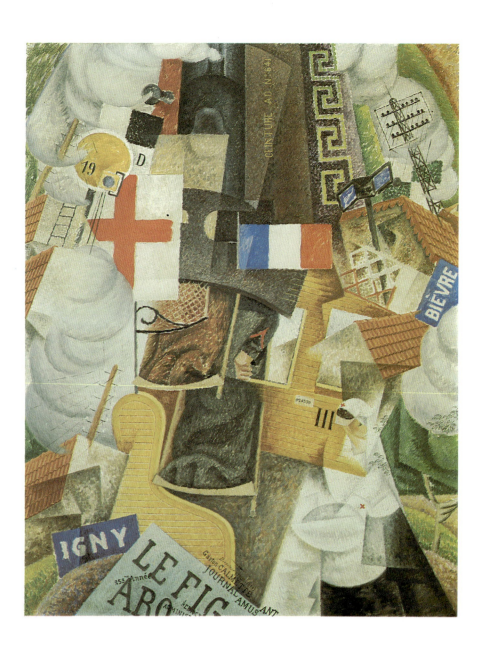

Gino Severini, TRAIN WITH WOUNDED SOLDIERS, *1914. Stedelijk Museum, Amsterdam, Netherlands. Copyright by A.D.A.G.P., Paris, 1985.*

Delano, it served as a procurement and recruitment agency and equipped nurses assigned to overseas duty. Through this agency, approximately 20,000 nurses were assigned to military service. Many of these Red Cross nurses remained in Europe and Asia after the war to assist with the relief programs of the stricken nations.

After a long struggle to maintain neutrality, the United States declared war on Germany on April 6, 1917, and many agencies were caught unprepared. Confusion and conflict arose, particularly in regard to the use of nurses' aides for service abroad. This issue was resolved by government authorities, who mandated that only trained nurses be sent to France with the Army (Stewart and Austin, 1963). As the war progressed, it became apparent that the supply of nurses was insufficient to meet both civilian and military needs. It was therefore strongly recommended by prominent medical, hospital, and lay spokesmen that the admission and graduation requirements of schools of nursing be drastically cut and that legal requirements be waived. To counteract these proposals and other problems that might ensue, M. Adelaide Nutting, Annie Goodrich, and Lillian Wald met on June 24, 1917, and formed the National Emergency Committee on

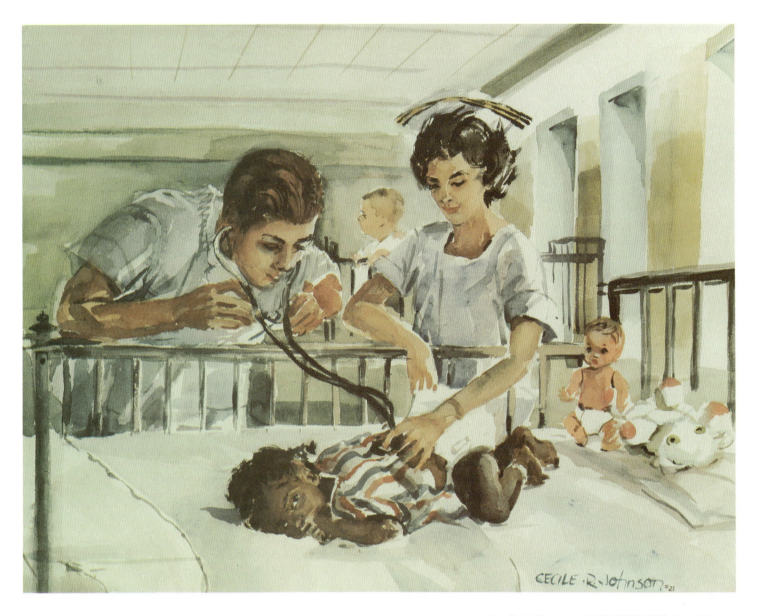

Cecile R. Johnson, PEDIATRIC UNIT AT A U.S. NAVAL HOSPITAL. *Defense Audiovisual Agency, Washington, D.C.*

Nursing. The stated purpose of this committee was to develop "the wisest methods of meeting the present problems connected with the care of the sick and injured in hospitals and homes; the educational problems of nursing; and the extraordinary emergencies as they arise" (U.S. Council of National Defense, 1917, pp. 1–5).

Vassar Training Camp

The National Emergency Committee on Nursing was eventually officially appointed by the federal government and became known as the Committee on Nursing of the General Medical Board of the Council of National Defense. A plan thus evolved for a three-month intensive theoretical training program for college graduates who wished to enter nursing schools. The original concept was proposed by Mrs. John Wood Blodgett, a trustee of Vassar, who partially financed the project. This program, known as the Vassar Training Camp of 1918, was soon under way at Vassar College under the chairmanship of Isabel M. Stewart. It was in actuality a preparatory course for college graduates seeking admission to schools of nursing. Over 400 college

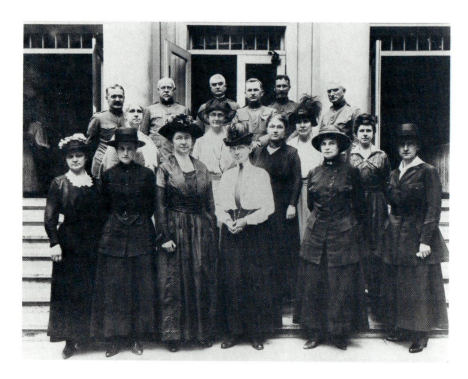

graduates participated in the program. At the completion of the intensive course, the college graduates entered some thirty-three affiliated schools of nursing for a period of two years and three months. The nursing schools had committed themselves to accepting a specified number of these students. Since the students wore the uniforms of the affiliated schools, they became known as "Vassar's Rainbow Division." Five other universities (Western Reserve University in Cleveland, University of Cincinnati, University of Iowa, University of Colorado, and University of California) offered similar programs. This cooperative effort between universities and schools of nursing provided a higher standard of teaching and the advantages of an institution of higher learning. The far-reaching contributions of the camp were reiterated by Katherine Densford Dreves, a member of this program who became an influential leader in nursing:

> First, the camp brought college recognition to nursing . . . the fact that prestigious Vassar College chose the camp for its major war effort helped (1) to bring nursing out of its hospital cloister into higher education and (2) to challenge colleges increasingly to accept responsibility for nurse preparation.
> Then, the camp helped immeasurably to interest college women in nursing. The camp brought into nursing the first very large group of well-educated, versatile women, almost half of whom went on to complete the entire nursing course. Also, the camp enlisted national recognition of nursing by the public and of the need for public and private support of nursing.
>
> *Dreves, 1975, p. 2002*

Army School of Nursing

In May 1918 the secretary of war authorized the establishment of the Army School of Nursing (also known as the Army Training School) at Walter Reed Hospital, Washington, D.C., with branches in other

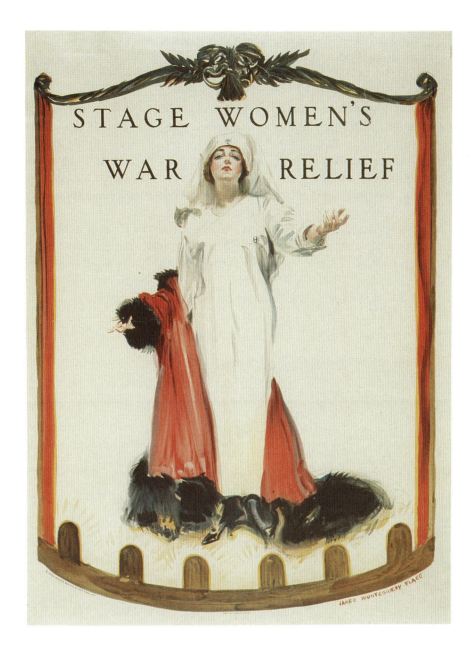

James Montgomery Flagg, STAGE WOMEN'S WAR RELIEF, *1918. Poster. Library of Congress, Washington, D.C.*

Nurses will always need to be organized and ready for service in times of disaster and national defense.

military hospitals across the country. The proponents of this school had presented the plan, prepared largely by the school's first dean, Annie W. Goodrich, before the twenty-fourth annual convention of the National League of Nursing Education (NLNE). Miss Goodrich had been appointed chief inspecting nurse of the Army hospitals at home and abroad and was charged with the evaluation of the quality of nursing services in military hospitals. Her unfavorable report was accompanied by the proposal for an Army School of Nursing. Viable arguments for the establishment of the school were presented:

> It would attract a high type of young women who would appreciate the opportunity to acquire a professional education while giving patriotic service; since the service of student nurses was an acceptable method of providing civilian hospitals with nursing service it could be assumed that such service could provide equally satisfactory care for military patients; because affiliations would be required for experience not available in military installations some civilian hospitals could anticipate sharing the

service of the Army school students; the graduates of the school, whether they remained in the ANC or not would constitute an important addition to the nursing resources of the nation.

Roberts, 1954, pp. 138–139

The convention voted its support, and a budget was approved in June 1918. The chief distinction of this school was that it was a separate educational unit with an independent federal fund budget that was specifically for educational purposes (Stewart, 1943). The course, based on the new *Standard Curriculum for Schools of Nursing,* covered three years and gave nine months' credit to college graduates. No tuition was required; board, lodging, laundry, and required textbooks were provided. Applications were received from thousands of enthusiastic women. The first graduating class (1921) numbered 500 students, probably the largest class of nurses ever graduated at one time. A total of 937 women completed the course before the school officially closed its doors in January 1933.

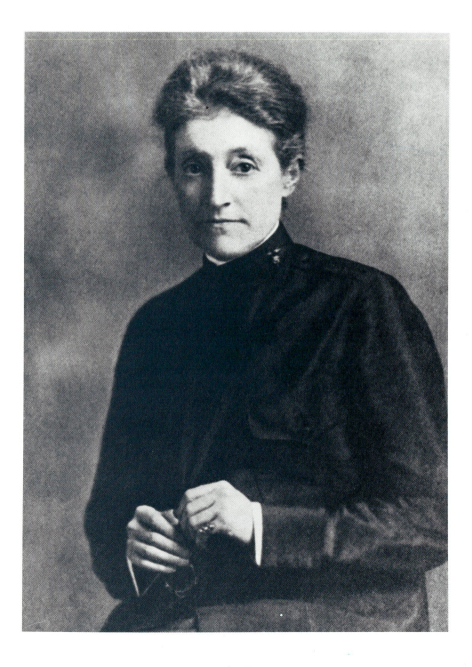

Portrait of ANNA W. GOODRICH, *Dean of the Army School of Nursing. National Library of Medicine, Bethesda, Maryland.*

402

Annie Warburton Goodrich (1866–1954) was the driving force behind many significant events in nursing. She was described as a crusader, statesman, dean of American nurses, most beloved of American nurses, and militant angel (Christy, 1970). Miss Goodrich was known nationally and internationally for her leadership ability, which facilitated the promotion of nursing toward a professional status. She received many honors and served as president of the ICN (1912–1915), the ANA (1916–1918), and the ACSN (1934–1936). A quote by Lillian Wald describes the strength of this almost legendary figure:

> Whether on platform or in committee or in conference, she inevitably suggests a torch, a spirit afire, and an apparently frail physique emphasizes this flaming attribute as the symbol of her genius. Though she seems to burn steadily she appears never to be consumed.
>
> *Quoted in Robinson, 1946, p. 349*

Annie Goodrich was designated as the third member of a group referred to as "the triumvirate" by Mary M. Roberts. M. Adelaide Nutting was the leader and occupied the tip of the pyramid; she was the educator who originated most ideas concerning developments in nursing schools; Lillian D. Wald, who occupied the second point in the triangle, was the practitioner and accepted founder of modern public health nursing; Annie W. Goodrich was the last of the trio, the skillful implementer who combined the ideas and desires of the other two (Christy, 1970). Miss Goodrich worked closely with Miss Wald while the latter was director of the Henry Street Settlement House in New York and simultaneously held the position of professor at Teachers College under Miss Nutting.

Miss Goodrich believed in collegiate nursing education and actively campaigned for that goal to be realized. Her positions as first dean of nursing at Yale University and at the Army School of Nursing epitomized this educational philosophy.

> It is desirable that nursing education should find its place in the university, which is another way of saying that it belongs where all educational expressions have been increasingly placed, and for the reason that universal knowledge is here assembled and distributed in accordance with the needs of the students as future builders of the community.
>
> *Goodrich, 1932, p. 173*

Her philosophy encompassed university preparation for not only teachers and administrators of nursing but also the practicing nurse. Throughout her lifetime Annie Goodrich fought the battle of educational standards for nursing along with other nursing leaders. Undoubtedly, her success at Yale University was the crowning achievement of her lifetime. Her dream of university preparation for *all* nurses, however, has still not been realized. In her eyes, therefore, nursing is not functioning to its fullest capacity: "Our place has been found in the institutions of the sick, but we shall never render our full service to the community until our place is also found in the University" (Proceedings of the Eighteenth Annual Convention of the American Society of Superintendents of Training Schools, 1912, p. 43).

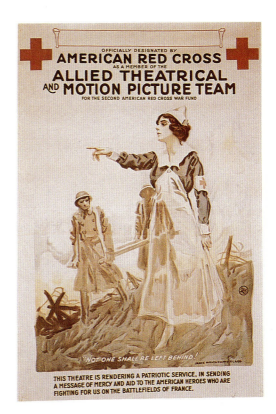

James Montgomery Flagg, NOT ONE SHALL BE LEFT BEHIND, *1918. Poster. Collection of the Library of Congress.*

Nurses, as well as other groups, answered the call for patriotic service during World War I.

Nursing at the Front

Conditions of warfare had changed a great deal since the time of the Spanish-American War. Military nursing needed to be revised and modernized to account for such things as submarine warfare, air attacks, shrapnel lacerations and wounds, poison gas, and trench warfare. The nurse's powers of observation and technical skills were challenged by shock, hemorrhage, communicable diseases, infected wounds, and the inhalation of poison gas. Hospitalization was the largest and most difficult of the problems associated with medical care in the American Expeditionary Forces. Great effort and the efficient use of resources were required to adequately care for the numbers of sick and wounded needing to be hospitalized.

A plan of organization for use during battles that lasted for days needed to be developed in order to care for the stream of sick and wounded. The American Army hospital service was divided into four stages. *Advanced dressing stations* (first aid stations) were located at the front lines in somewhat protected areas near the fighting lines. They were usually staffed by physicians and orderlies. Here emergencies were treated and the wounded were prepared for transport to the *field hospitals,* located a little farther back. (No women nurses served at the front in first aid stations and only occasionally did they serve in the field hospitals.) The wounded were then transported to *evacuation hospitals* (clearing stations) approximately ten miles back. Those wounded too seriously to travel farther remained here, where complete hospital services were available and care was given by nurses. Eventually all wounded were sent to *base hospitals,* usually by the trainload. These hospitals were located safely away from the front.

The peak strength of the Army and Navy Nurse Corps during World War I was nearly 23,000 (Chow, and others, 1978). Of the nurses who served, 260 died in the line of duty, some because of the

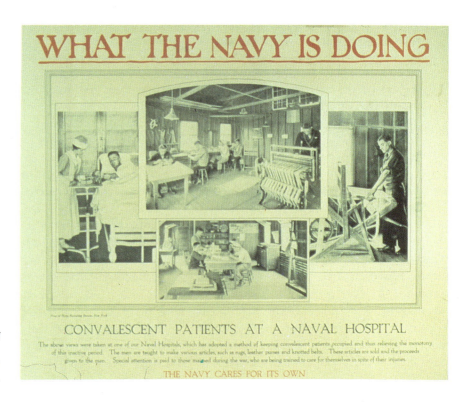

WHAT THE NAVY IS DOING, *c. 1919. Recruiting poster. National Archives and Records Service, Washington, D.C. This poster depicts a naval hospital for the care of war victims.*

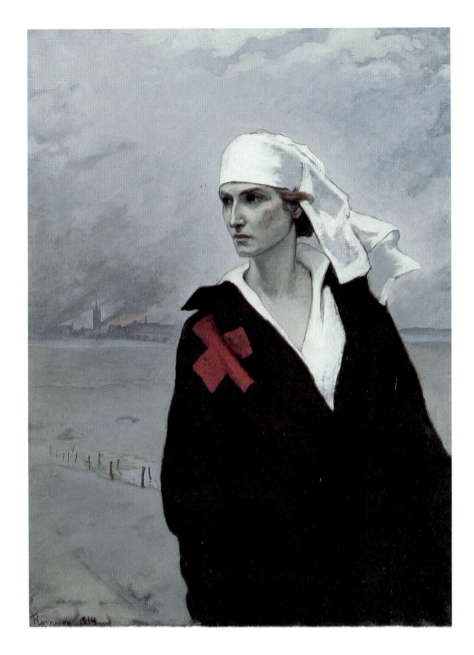

Romaine Brooks, LA FRANCE CROISÉE *(The Cross of France), 1914. Canvas, approx. 118.1 × 86.4 cm. National Museum of American Art, Smithsonian Institution, Washington, D.C., Gift of the Artist.*

influenza epidemic of 1918. None, however, died as a result of enemy action.

> The nurses who returned from their baptism of blood, after their familiarity with death, looked deeper into life. But all did not return. Nurses in war service died all over the country, in camps, on the way to camps, in hospital trains, base hospitals, and general hospitals. Several died in line-of-duty on foreign soil. The war-born pandemic of influenza took the lives of many nurses still in military service. A ship that reaches port with White Caps home from war is a thrilling sight, but always there are some who do not come back. In the first World War, many nurses were cited and decorated, but for others the last decoration was the wooden cross of the soldier for those who gave up their lives like soldiers.
>
> *Robinson, 1946, p. 327*

The Army was the largest single employer of nurses: 21,480 graduate nurses served in Army cantonments and hospitals; more

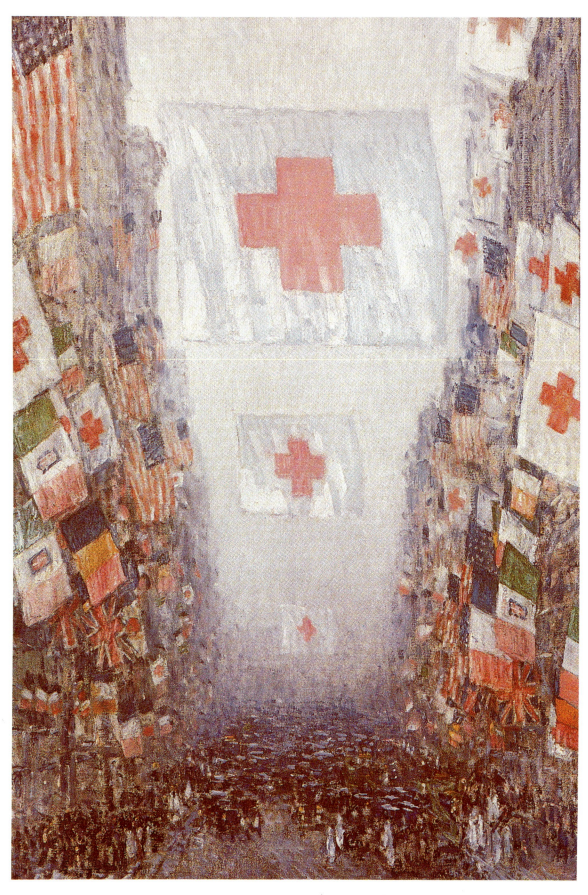

Childe Hassam, CELEBRATION DAY, *1918. Canvas, 90.2 × 59.7 cm. Christopher T. May, Trustee for Sterling, Meredith, and Laura May.*

In CELEBRATION DAY, *also known as* RED CROSS DAY, *the red and white banners of the Red Cross form a majestic processional as they recede up Fifth Avenue in New York City.*

than 10,000 served overseas (Vreeland, 1950). Awards presented to Army nurses included the Distinguished Service Cross (second only to the Medal of Honor, the highest combat decoration) to three nurses; the Distinguished Service Medal (highest noncombat decoration) to twenty-three; the French Croix de Guerre to twenty-eight nurses; the British Royal Red Cross to sixty-nine; and the British Military Medal to two nurses (Shields, editor, 1981). It was World War I that afforded the Navy Nurse Corps the first real opportunity to demonstrate the importance of its role. Navy nurses numbered 1224 in service in America and 327 who served abroad (Vreeland, 1950). The Navy Cross, the highest Navy decoration, was awarded to four Navy nurses during World War I, but an even greater honor was paid one of the four with the naming of a destroyer, the USS *Higbee* in January of 1945. This was the first time a fighting ship had been named after a woman in the service. That woman was Lenah S. Higbee, the second superintendent of the corps from 1911 to 1923. In accordance with the requirements of naval service, the Navy Nurse Corps was reduced after the war. By 1935, with the Government Economy Act, the number in the corps had dropped to 332.

American nurses on active duty faced not only the horrors and dangers of war but other types of conflicts and frustrations. These arose primarily because the nurses had no military rank. Army and Navy nurses had not been designated by Congress as either officers or enlisted men, although they had military status and were subject to military discipline. Consequently, the nurses could not assume the responsibilities for teaching and directing orderlies and corpsmen and for handling administrative problems as heads of wards and

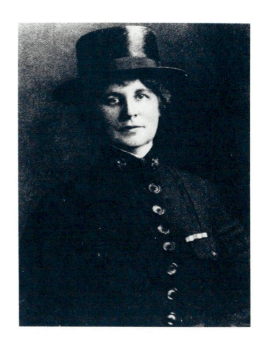

Portrait of MRS. L.H. SUTCLIFFE HIGBEE, *Second Superintendent of the Navy Nurses Corps, c. 1916. National Archives and Records Service, Washington, D.C.*

USS Higbee in Boston Harbor, May 1945. National Archives and Records Service, Washington, D.C.

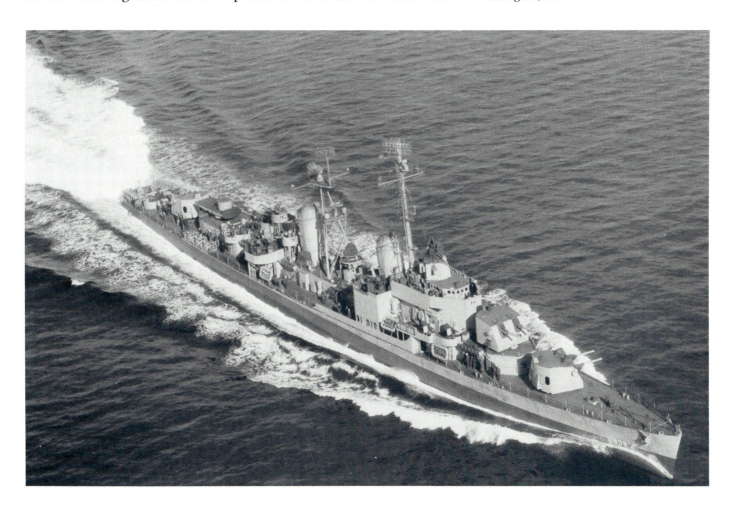

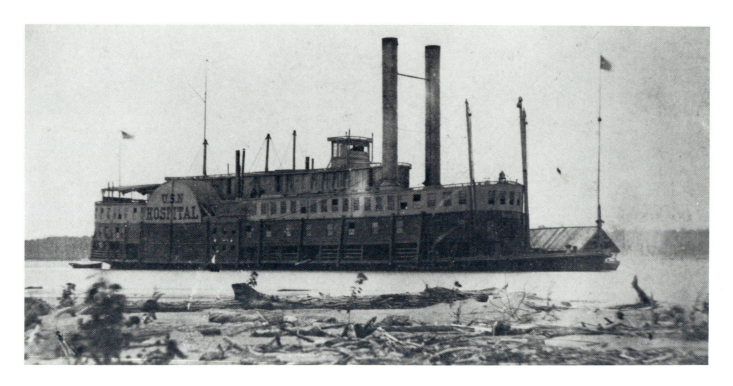

THE FIRST COMMISSIONED HOSPITAL SHIP, RED ROVER. *Naval Audiovisual Center, Washington, D.C.*

nursing services. Following the war, with the help of legal and other advisers and the support of the Votes for Women Amendment (passed 1920), nurses appealed to Congress. After a long, slow, and difficult battle, relative rank was granted to members of the Army Nurse Corps by amendment of the National Defense Act of June 4, 1920. At that time nurses were given officer status ranging from second lieutenant through major, but pay and allowances were not the same as for men. (In 1942 Navy nurses were accorded relative rank.) In 1944 nurses in both the Army and the Navy were given full military rank for the duration of World War II and six months longer. Finally, in 1947, full commissioned rank for nurses in the military services was permanently established. Florence A. Blanchfield became the first woman to be given the permanent commission of colonel in the regular Army. The Army-Navy Nurse Act of 1947 also provided for an Army Nurse Corps section in the Officers' Reserve Corps.

It is interesting to note that the first men were not commissioned as nurses until 1955—through the Bolton Amendment to the Army-Navy Nurse Act. Since that time, other legislative acts have improved the conditions of military nurses, including Public Law 90-130, which removed most promotional restrictions on the careers of nurse officers in the Army, Navy, and Air Force. Numerous rank and privilege "firsts" have occurred in military nursing and will continue at a steady pace.

The story of World War I cannot be left without at least mentioning one famous nurse heroine, Edith Cavell (1865–1915). She was an English nurse who founded a school of nursing in Brussels, Belgium, in 1909. Miss Cavell remained at the school when the war started and helped to organize an underground escape route for Allied soldiers. She also faithfully cared for sick Germans. Despite diplomatic efforts to obtain a reprieve for her, Edith Cavell was executed before a German firing squad on October 12, 1915. The charge was harboring British and French soldiers and assisting them with escape from Belgium. Miss Cavell did not deny the charges and faced her

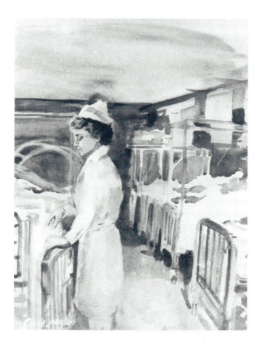

Cecile R. Johnson, NIGHT DUTY. *Defense Audiovisual Agency, Washington, D.C.*

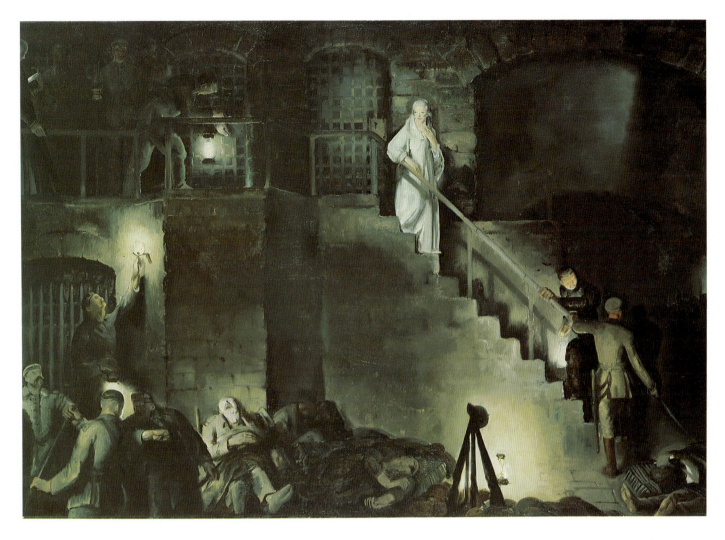

George W. Bellows, EDITH CAVELL DIRECTING THE ESCAPE OF SOLDIERS FROM PRISON CAMP, *1918. Canvas. Museum of Fine Arts, Springfield, Massachusetts, The James Philip Gray Collection.*

death with tremendous courage. It is reported that the following were her last words:

> I have no fear or shrinking; I have seen death so often that it is not strange or fearful to me. I thank God for this ten weeks' quiet before the end. Life has always been hurried and full of difficulty. This time of rest has been a great mercy. They have all been very kind to me here. But this I would say, standing as I do in view of God and eternity: I realize that patriotism is not enough. I must have no hatred or bitterness towards anyone.
>
> *Quoted in Judson, 1941, p. 281*

Edith Cavell, an English nurse, had organized the first school for nurses in Brussels, Belgium. There she cared for soldiers of all armies and directed the escape of Allied soldiers from prison camps during World War I. She was arrested by the Germans and executed on October 12, 1915.

■ WORLD WAR II

It took the second World War to bring the American nurse to her national stature. Serving in embattled lands whose names the public had never heard before, in hospital ships on all the seas, and in air ambulances evacuating the wounded by plane, the nurse came into her own as comforter and healer. Femininity in foxholes, with mud-caked khaki coveralls over pink panties, captured the imagination of the public and the fighting men of America.

Robinson, 1946, p. 358

The period between World War I and World War II was a time of great unrest because the defeated nations were dissatisfied with their lot. Depression on a worldwide scale led people to accept any type of leadership so long as it might restore them to prosperity. Bolshevism conquered Russia; Benito Mussolini and Fascism assumed control of Italy; Hitler and the National Socialist German Workers' Party (Nazis) steadily became more powerful in Germany; Spain underwent civil revolution; England and France were engaged in internal disagreements. It is no wonder that an era of dictatorship emerged and began to flourish in a number of nations. Major shifts in alignment also were observed as Italy and Japan, formerly in the Allied camp, joined with Germany in the so-called Axis, which opposed the United Nations.

The League of Nations had been established after World War I in an effort to preserve international peace. This organization was to act as a body of arbitration between nations. Members of the league would be committed to arbitration on all matters of dispute; hostilities would be postponed for three months after a decision was reached. The United States did not join this organization because of a traditional policy of remaining free from foreign entanglements. The league proved its value for a time but then began to weaken because it had no adequate means of enforcing its decisions.

During the late 1930s, as international relations slowly deteriorated, war broke out once again in Europe. From the time of the Treaty of Versailles, which had ended World War I, Germany had been denouncing the Polish Corridor. This strip of land had been awarded to the newly formed state of Poland, and the German city of Danzig had been placed under the League of Nations. In 1939 Hitler demanded that Danzig be returned to the Reich and that Germany be allowed to build a road across the Polish Corridor. A series of events occurred that terminated in the invasion of Poland by Germany without a formal declaration of war. Two days later Great Britain and France declared war on Germany. The United States had no desire to become involved in war. However, in 1940, anticipating the possibility that such a step might be unavoidable, it repealed the Neutrality Act of 1935. At this point America began to gear up for war. On December 7, 1941, the Japanese bombed Pearl Harbor, Hawaii, in a surprise air raid that ultimately changed the course of world events. On December 8, 1941, the United States declared war on Japan; two days later Germany and Italy retaliated and declared war against the United States. The world was immediately plunged into a terrifying conflict known as the "total war." Nursing and health services were once again radically affected as every man, woman, and child of belligerent countries became involved.

When war had been again threatening the country in 1940, Isabel Stewart wanted nursing to be prepared, to avoid mistakes and to profit from the achievements of World War I. That summer, according to Stella Goostray, she wrote to the president of the National League of Nursing Education and emphasized

the need of some official nursing committee or commission to think through the position that nursing should take with respect to national defense and the many adjustments that may be called for within the next few months.... I believe we should have such a commission or board that is representative of the nursing pro-

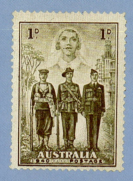

A set of four stamps, each in a different color, was issued by Australia in 1940 to commemorate her participation in World War II and particularly honoring her servicemen, represented by the sailor, soldier, and aviator. Her nurses have a prominent place of honor in this interesting design. Courtesy of Howard B. Hurley.

410

fession *as a whole* and that it should be at work *now*.... I do not want us to be stampeded into doing things we will be sorry for.

Goostray, 1954, p. 304

In July of 1940 the Nursing Council for National Defense was instituted at Miss Goostray's suggestion. The council included the six national nursing organizations (ANA, NLNE, NOPHN, ACSN, NACGN, AAIN), the federal nursing services, and representatives from such organizations as the American Hospital Association. Major Julia Stimson of the Army Nurse Corps was chairman of the council. With the declaration of war in 1942, the organization's name was changed to the National Nursing Council for War Service and Stella Goostray became its head. Plans were formulated to promote a national inventory of registered nurses, determine the role of nurses and nursing in the defense program, expand facilities of existing accredited schools of nursing, and supply supplementary nursing services to hospitals and public health agencies.

As more and more graduate nurses withdrew from civilian agencies to enlist in the Army and Navy Nurse Corps, the council tackled the problem of recruitment of students for schools of nursing. This work was assigned to the Committee on Education Policies and Resources. Isabel Stewart was appointed chairman of this committee, the first one constructed under the aegis of the council. The preliminary investigations of the committee indicated that financial aid to assist schools, to improve the preparation of faculty members, and to assist candidates who could not otherwise afford to enter nursing was a matter of primary importance.

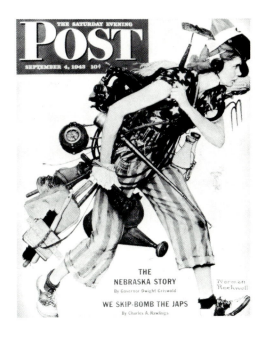

Norman Rockwell, "Rosie to the Rescue," cover of the SATURDAY EVENING POST, *September 4, 1943. Courtesy of Curtis Publishing Company, Indianapolis, Indiana.*

The United States Cadet Nurse Corps

Convinced of the possibility of getting a federal appropriation for nursing education for defense needs, Isabel Stewart began to pursue avenues through which such a goal might be achieved. Commissioner Studebaker of the United States Office of Education was sympathetic to the cause and invited her to Washington to prepare a plan for a request of funds. This she did with the assistance of nine other committee members. "The Proposal," as it came to be known, investigated the country's need for professional nursing services in both military and civilian situations, plans needed to meet that need, and the cost of such a program. It rapidly became apparent that nursing schools could not be expected to increase their enrollments, to increase instructional or housing facilities without financial assistance. The government needed to be persuaded that federal aid for nursing education was a legitimate and imperative defense measure. The committee soon made these findings:

> Uncle Sam was spending large sums in training his sons for national defense, but he had provided little or nothing for the preparation of his daughters who were to serve in the national forces. Apart from the experiment with the Army School of Nursing during the first World War, and the stipends to nurses given through the Social Security Act, practically no federal funds had

been appropriated for nursing education up to this time.... A plan was prepared and, after many vicissitudes, submitted in a lull to Congress. Finally, in June, 1941, with the assistance of friends of nursing education in Congress, a law was passed authorizing the expenditure of $1,200,000 for the current fiscal year to assist in the training of nurses for national defense. The administration of this fund was entrusted to the United States Public Health Service.

Stewart, 1943, p. 283

The first support for nursing education from federal funds specifically appropriated for that purpose thus occurred. The Appropriations Act for 1942 (effective July 1, 1941) was passed with inclusion of funds for nursing education through the efforts of Mrs. Frances Payne Bolton, a Congresswoman from Ohio and a friend of nursing. In July of 1942 this federal appropriation was increased to $3.5 million. This major feat resulted largely from the leadership of Miss Stewart, who served on the advisory committee for the initial proj-

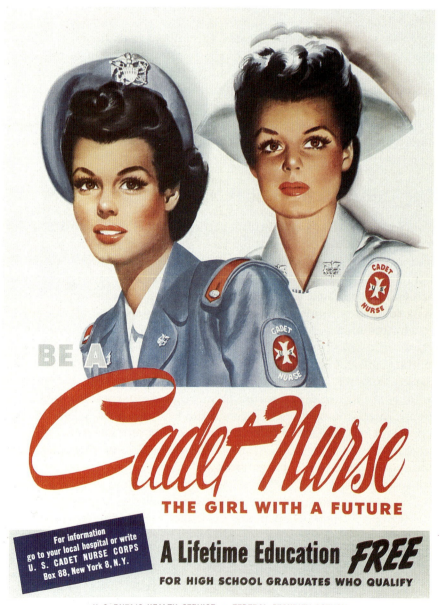

"CADET NURSE," THE GIRL WITH A FUTURE, 1944. *Poster. National Archives and Records Service, Washington, D.C.*

A recruitment poster emphasizing the wartime need and educational opportunities for those interested in nursing.

412

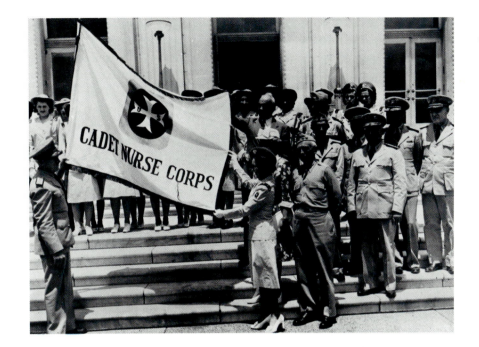

ect. The sum that was to be applied to "refresher," postgraduate, and basic programs was inadequate for existing needs, but it paved the way for future financial assistance to nursing schools.

Subsequently, a Nurse Training Act (Public Law No. 74, Seventy-Eighth Congress) was introduced into Congress in 1943 by Mrs. Frances Payne Bolton. A $60-million appropriation was voted at this time to cover the cost of an accelerated and expanded program of education for students entering approved schools of nursing, and later the amount was increased. The bill, commonly known as the Bolton Act, created the United States Cadet Nurse Corps. It provided for a thirty-month basic program, free tuition and fees, free uniforms, monthly stipends for students in approved basic schools of nursing, and grants for postgraduate work for graduate students.

The program of the Cadet Nurse Corps was administered by the United States Public Health Service, Division of Nursing Education, which was headed by Lucile Petry. (Miss Petry was appointed Assistant Surgeon General of the United States Public Health Service in 1949. She was the first woman to hold this position.) This program proved to be a major incentive for the improvement of standards in nursing education because schools had to meet requirements developed by the NLNE to obtain the federal monies. Nursing schools were also required to admit all qualified applicants, regardless of race or religion. An intensive publicity and recruiting campaign was launched. The desirability of a student reserve with benefits of an "attractive uniform," liberal scholarships, and subsistence grants was given wide press. Students who entered pledged themselves to serve where needed (military or civilian agencies) for the duration of the war and six months thereafter. The potential overcrowding of available space from the enormous influx of nursing students into this program was assisted by the passage of the Lanham Act (1941), which provided funds for dormitories, libraries, classrooms, and other physical facilities that were needed.

Quotas based on national nursing needs were established for the Cadet Nurse Corps: 125,000 for the first two years, with 65,000

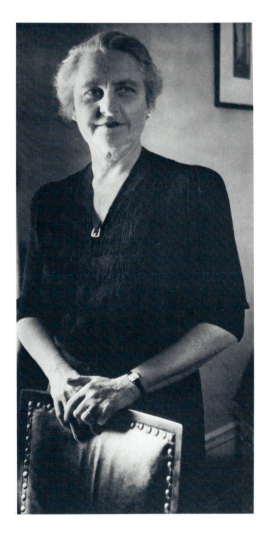

recruited during the first twelve months and 60,000 the following year. Both yearly quotas were exceeded, and the total number who joined the corps was 179,000. The program was a unique experiment that achieved remarkable success. In addition, from the start the National Nursing Council had ensured the removal of all barriers resulting from various forms of discrimination. Some important racial barriers were therefore removed. The way was paved for the acceptance of Black students into a greater number of nursing schools and for the enlistment of Black nurses into the Army and Navy. A committee of the council, the Coordinating Committee on Negro Nursing, was set up to assist with the recruitment of well-qualified Black students and the provision of better educational opportunities for these students. In 1944 the council also openly campaigned for racial equality in the military nursing services.

Nursing at the Front

The role of the nurse in war had been almost revolutionized since the time of Florence Nightingale in the Crimean War. By World War II, nurses constituted an integral part of the military structure. They were accustomed to organization, had a working knowledge of war that had been gained through personal experiences, and were prepared to meet the demands of modern warfare. By the end of this war, the romance between the nurse and the American G.I. would be real, built on mutual admiration and respect. The bravery of the nurses under the most rigorous and demanding situations was witnessed by many soldiers, who wrote of these experiences:

Franklin Boggs, NIGHT DUTY, *1945.*

Over 50,000 Army nurses served at the battlefront during World War II.

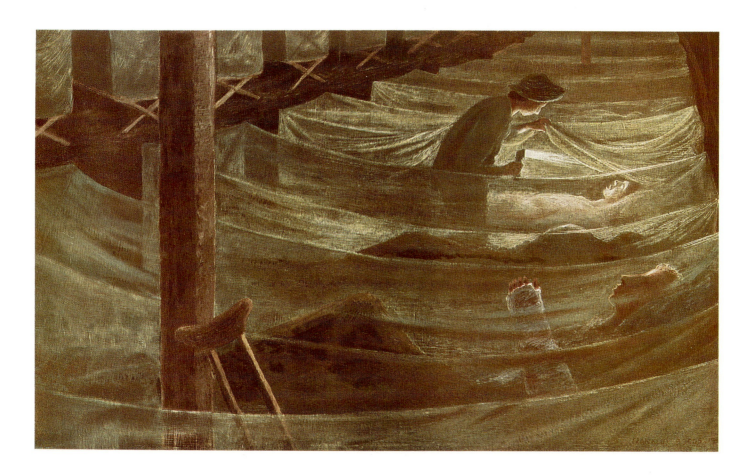

They were 24 hours with plenty of things dropping all around—planes being shot down. Let me tell you they quickly learned to dig fox holes. I have seen them digging them with a spoon—two things they soon learn to do—wear helmets and dig foxholes. . . . They were pretty hard put for food. They had no water except in their canteens when unloaded. [When I arrived with the equipment] . . . they welcomed the "old man" with food and equipment. They had no tents. Each nurse was given one blanket in half shelter tent, their "B" and "C" ration and a musette bag. They were wearing fatigues and steel helmets. They used the ground for their bed—but they were there ready to go and waiting for us. . . .

Quoted in Aynes, 1973, p. 245

The global scope of World War II presented a sharp challenge to military nurses. By the end of the war, nurses had been stationed on the soil of approximately fifty nations scattered over the face of the globe. They worked and lived in the installations of the Army and the Navy, in hotels and other adapted structures, in cantonment barracks, in tent hospitals, and in Quonset and other prefabricated huts. Speed in rendering care was probably the biggest factor that kept the death rate below that of World War I.

The sulfonamides, the advent of penicillin, DDT, new developments in antimalarial therapy, and the ready availability of blood and blood derivatives, plus the heroism and ingenuity of the medical corpsmen, were among the factors which contributed to that favorable result.

Roberts, 1954, p. 344

Nursing care also contributed to the statistics and made a great difference in the recovery of sick and wounded soldiers.

The peak strength of the Army and Navy Nurse Corps was nearly 69,000 during World War II. These nurses gave care in front-line situations, field hospitals, evacuation hospitals, base hospitals,

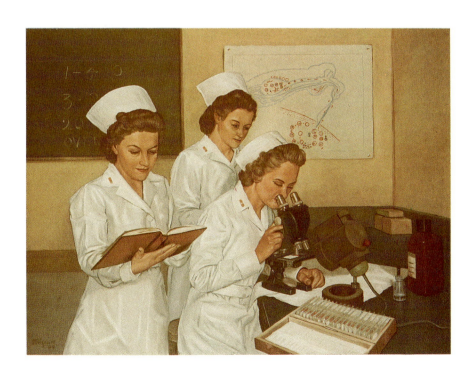

Manuel Tolegian, LABORATORY WARFARE, *1945.*

415

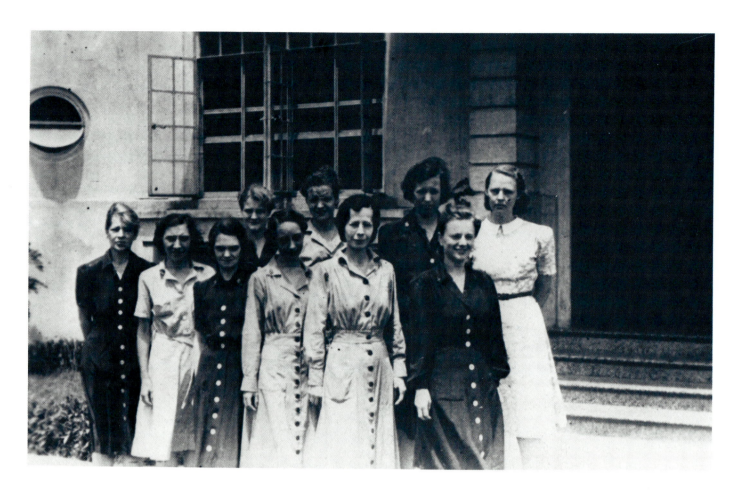

NAVAL NURSES AT SANTO TOMAS INTERNMENT CAMP, *September 1942. Dorothy Terrill Collection, Baton Rouge, Louisiana.*

hospital ships, trains, and in the air. Army nurses served at nine stations and fifty-two areas. Navy nurses served on a dozen hospital ships and in over 300 naval stations. Both served wherever the American soldier could be found. More than 1600 nurses were decorated for meritorious service and bravery under fire. They received honors that included the Distinguished Service Medal, Silver Star, Distinguished Flying Cross, Soldier's Medal, Bronze Star Medal, Air Medal, Legion of Merit, Army Commendation Medal, Purple Heart, and Gold Star. A total of 201 nurses died; 16 of these deaths were the result of enemy action. Throughout the war, nurses in both the Army and the Navy were held as prisoners by the Japanese in the Philippines at Santo Tomas civilian prison camp near Manila. They continued to give nursing care under terrific hardships until their release in 1945. Eleven Navy nurses were interned for a period of thirty-seven months.

A new field of military nursing opened up in World War II— flight nursing. Both the Army and the Navy instituted flight nurse programs for assistance with the extended use of air transport for the evacuation of wounded soldiers. Nurses were specially trained to give nursing care to the wounded on stretchers piled three tiers deep on either side of a cargo plane that had been converted into a rough ambulance. They were also taught to perform duties related to ground medical installations. Admittance to the program began with application for commission in the Army Nurse Corps; this was followed by a minimum of six months in the Army Air Force unit hospital. Application could then be made for admittance to the flight nursing school. After completion of these requirements, an automatic designation of "flight nurse" was still not granted. The nurse needed

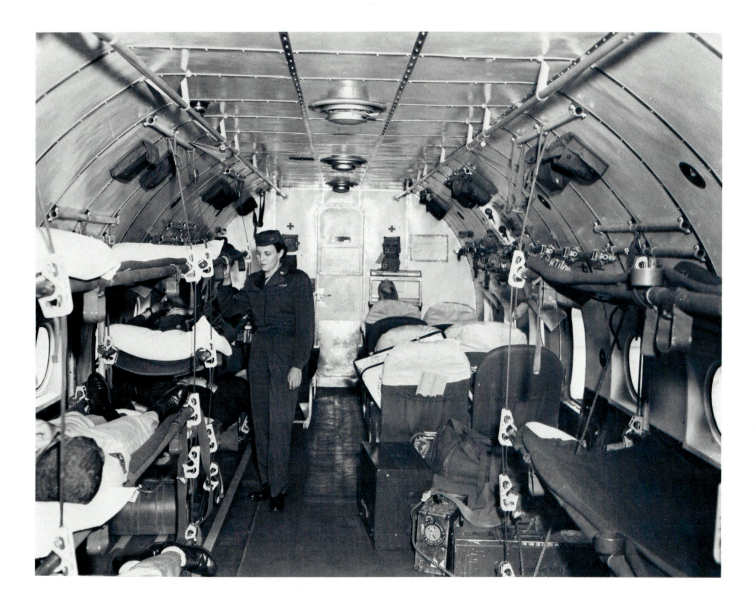

Flight nurse talking with patients aboard a C-54 air evacuation plane prior to takeoff from Andrews Air Force Base. U.S. Air Force Photo.

to submit a request to the commanding general of the Army Air Forces for the designation. The first class of Army Nurse Corps flight nurses was graduated from the School of Air Evacuation at Bowman Field, Kentucky, on February 18, 1943. Many nurses desired entrance to the program because flight nurses represented the elite of the corps.

Music had frequently been used in the military to relieve tension and boost morale. The "Song of the Army Nurse Corps" was officially adopted by January 1944. "The marching music was composed by Lou Singer and the lyrics written by Hy Zaret, a professional doing his bit as a private in the Special Services in New York. . . . Army bands at home and overseas played it . . ." (Aynes, 1973, p. 243):

> We march along with faith undaunted beside our gallant fighting men;
> Whenever they are sick or wounded, we nurse them back to health again;
> As long as healing hands are wanted, You'll find the nurses of the Corps,
> On ship, or plane, on transport train, at home or on a far off shore;
> With loyal heart we do our part, for the Army and the Army Nurse Corps.

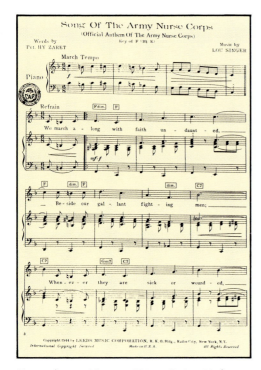

THE SONG OF THE ARMY NURSE CORPS, *by*
Hy Zaret and Lou Singer. Mugar Memorial
Library, Boston University, Massachusetts.
Copyright 1944 by MCA Music, A Division of
MCA Inc., New York. All Rights Reserved.

This achievement occurred through the effort of Edith A. Aynes and was supported by Colonel Blanchfield, who wrote the foreword:

> There is no burden so heavy, no night so long that it cannot be eased by music. The members of the Army Nurse Corps should be encouraged to sing, for in song there is a contentment that means happier times, good fellowship, better care for their patients and a more optimistic outlook for the entire Corps.
>
> *Aynes, 1973, p. 243*

A final newcomer in the federal nursing services was the Air Force Nurse Corps, established within the Air Force Medical Service in July 1949. An Army–Air Force Regulation was published on June 8, 1949, that provided for the separation of certain Air Force activities that were formerly the responsibility of the Army Medical Department (Vreeland, 1950). The purpose of this enforcement was twofold: the complete separation of Army and Air Force medical activities and the establishment of the Air Force Nurse Corps. Procedures were developed whereby nurses in the Army who were on duty with the Air Force and nurses who were stationed at Army in-

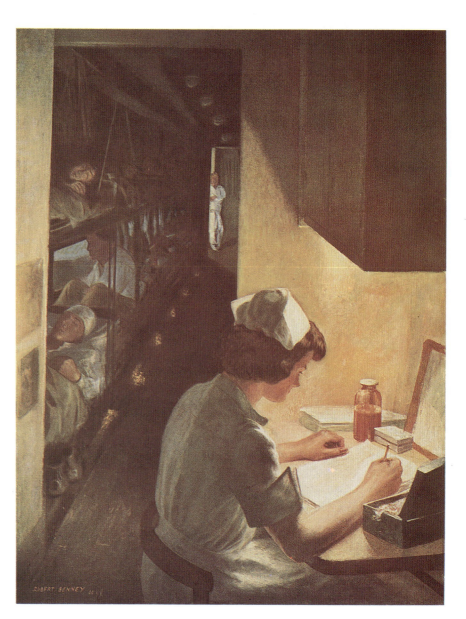

Robert Benney, NIGHT VIGIL, *1945.*

The Army nurse checks the patients' charts while aboard a hospital train in World War II.

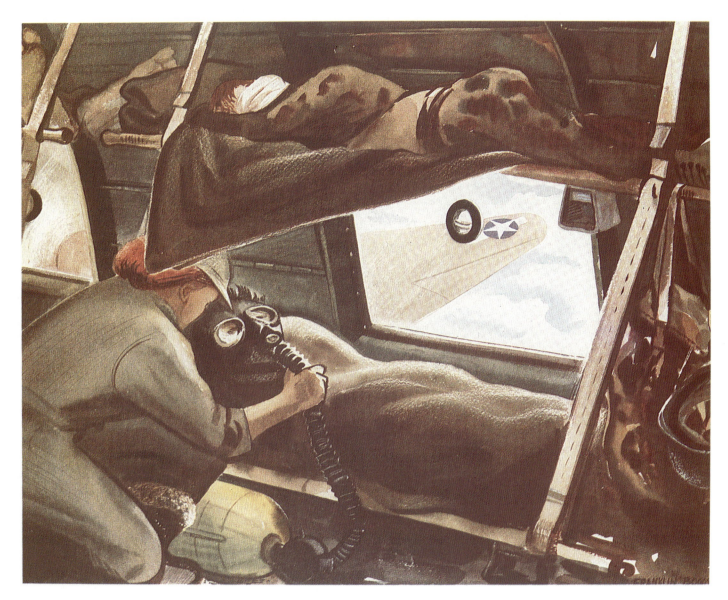

Franklin Boggs, AIR EVACUATION, *1945.*

stallations could request to be transferred to the Air Force Nurse Corps. A total of 1199 Army nurses on active duty transferred from the Army to the Air Force, becoming the nucleus for the Air Force Nurse Corps. One year later the corps prepared to assist with the air evacuation of battle casualties from the Korean area. This was to become a vital key to the survival of the soldier wounded in the Korean War.

The Nurse Draft Bill

The large number of graduate nurses engaged in military service was still not enough; voluntary enlistments were not meeting anticipated needs. During what was to become the closing months of the war, steps began to be taken to draft nurses into military service. An article by the well-known columnist Walter Lippmann, which appeared on December 19, 1944, included a charge of gross neglect against the Army. Lippmann contended that the Army had not provided adequate numbers of nurses to care for wounded soldiers:

> The last thing our people will put up with is that sick and wounded American soldiers should suffer because the Army cannot find enough women to nurse them. Yet, I am reporting

419

only the stark truth, which is well known to the Army and to the leaders of the medical profession, when I say that in military hospitals at home and abroad our men are not receiving the nursing care they must have, and that with casualties increasing in number and in seriousness, this will mean for many of the men brought in from the battlefields that their recovery is delayed, and even jeopardized.

Lippmann, 1944

It was not long before President Roosevelt, in his State of the Union message on January 6, 1945, came forth with an unprecedented request for a draft of women nurses. The ANA went on record as approving such a move provided that the Selective Service legislation include *all women.* The Nurse Draft Bill quickly passed the House of

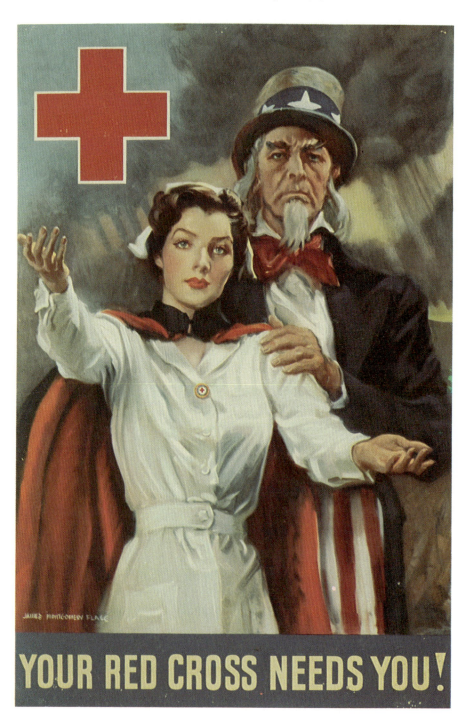

James Montgomery Flagg, YOUR RED CROSS NEEDS YOU, *1942. Poster. Library of Congress, Washington, D.C.*

The Red Cross Nursing Service was planned on a large scale by the voluntary affiliation of the American Nurses' Association with the Red Cross officials.

YOUR RED CROSS NEEDS YOU!

420

Representatives but became bogged down in the Senate. The threat of the draft initiated an overwhelming mass of applications from nurses for war service, and the result was an excess of nurses in the military. The conclusion of the war on the European front made the draft bill virtually unnecessary, and it was quietly withdrawn in May 1945.

■ THE KOREAN WAR

The Korean War broke out on June 25, 1950, and thrust nurses once again into service in combat areas. The nurses of the armed forces—Army, Navy, and Air Corps—were called upon as a result of the invasion of South Korea. Although this action was not officially designated as a "war," the realities of casualties were nonetheless harsh. The United States was essentially forced to play a role in a situation created by the conflicting ideologies of the freedom-loving Western world and Communism. Fears of an acute nursing shortage prompted the Joint Committee on Nursing in National Security, along with representatives of the six national nursing organizations, to recommend the following:

> That all possible means be developed for recruiting more students for schools of nursing.
>
> That as many practical nurses be trained and employed to help professional nurses as hospitals and other community agencies could utilize to good advantage.
>
> That nurses be withdrawn systematically from the civilian services for military duty according to a plan that ensured their employment at the highest level of skill for which they were prepared.
>
> That state and local advisory boards of nurses be organized and be given the authority by the government to review assignment of nurses to the armed forces and to civilian agencies.
>
> That, if there was total mobilization, nurses be redistributed within the fields of nursing and within community agencies so that the most essential civilian needs would be taken care of first.
>
> That major effort be directed to improving sound basic nursing education and to increase enrollment in schools of nursing that offered effective programs.
>
> That selected nurses be encouraged to prepare for responsibilities as teachers, supervisors, and administrators, as well as for the special fields, in order to safeguard essential nursing service.
>
> That administration of nursing services be improved so that nursing skills would be used to the best advantage and their full value would reach more people.
>
> That nursing service be stabilized as much as possible and turnover of staff held to a minimum through the adoption and application of sound personnel policies for nurses and allied workers.
>
> *Joint Committee on Nursing in National Security, 1951, pp. 78–79*

During World War II the Army had experimented with and demonstrated the need for a new type of hospital that would be located as close to the front as was relatively safe, about eight to twenty

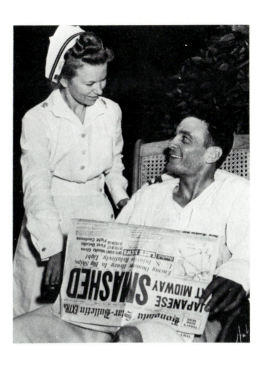

BATTLE OF MIDWAY, *June 1942. National Archives and Records Service, Washington, D.C.*

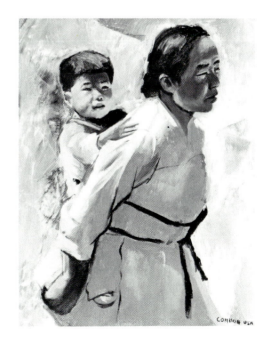

Russell Connor, KOREAN MOTHER AND CHILD. *Defense Audiovisual Agency, Washington, D.C.*

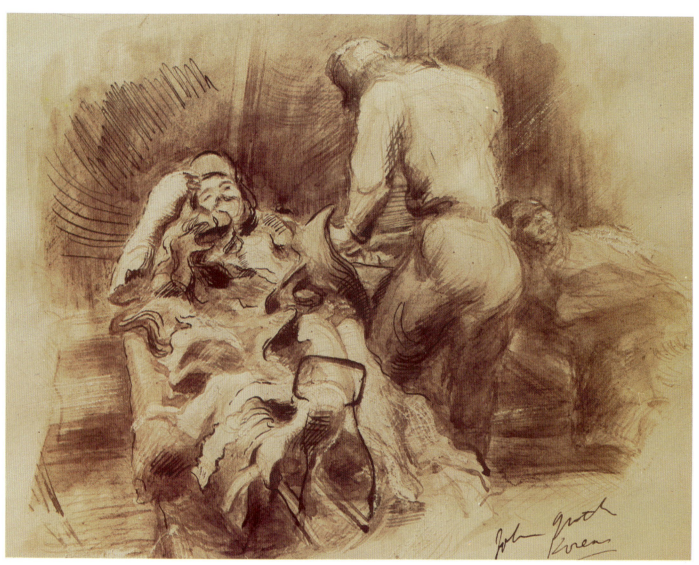

John Groth, A NURSE AT WORK, *Korean War. Watercolor. Defense Audiovisual Agency, Washington, D.C.*

miles. This new unit first appeared in late November 1942 and was tried out under actual combat conditions in Korea. The Mobile Army Surgical Hospital (MASH) could be moved at a moment's notice. It was basically a sixty-bed unit with the flexibility to expand five or six times beyond its standard bed capacity. Within a few hours several hundred patients could be admitted and treated. The hospital was usually staffed by ten physicians, twelve nurses (two were anesthetists), and ninety corpsmen. It could be set up in any type of location that was available—a barn, church, schoolhouse, or in the tents that were carried with it (*American Journal of Nursing,* 1951, p. 387). An Army helicopter detachment was attached to each MASH unit to provide for immediate evacuation for the critically ill.

The MASH unit became the first hospital to which the wounded were sent and was a great factor in maintaining morale.

The proximity of the unit to the front, its trained personnel, its adequate supply of whole blood, and its rapid helicopter and ambulance evacuation services all contributed greatly to the reduction of mortality rates in Korea as compared with those during World War II: the mortality rate among wounded soldiers who reached hospitals in Korea was half the corresponding rate during World War II.

Kalisch and Kalisch, 1978, p. 543

422

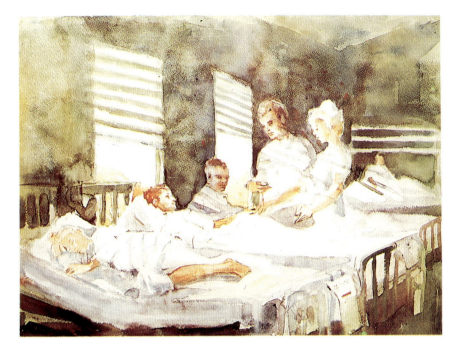

Cecile R. Johnson, EVENING ROUNDS. *Defense Audiovisual Agency, Washington, D.C.*

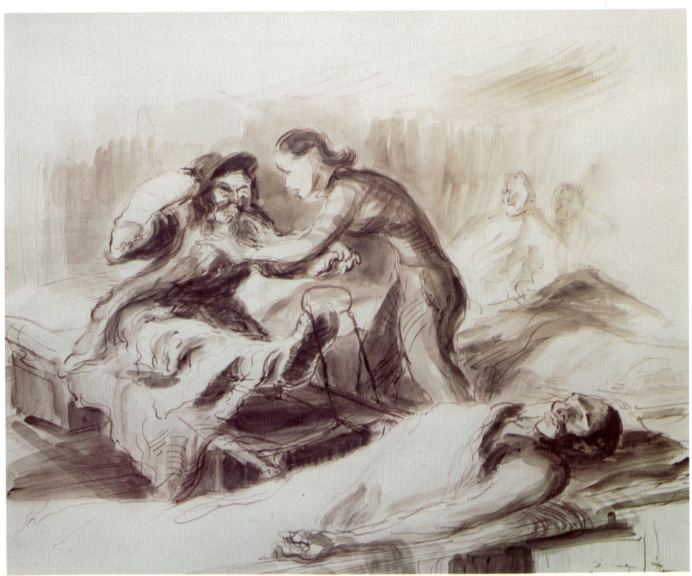

John Groth, RECEIVING TENT, *Korean War. Watercolor. Defense Audiovisual Agency, Washington, D.C.*

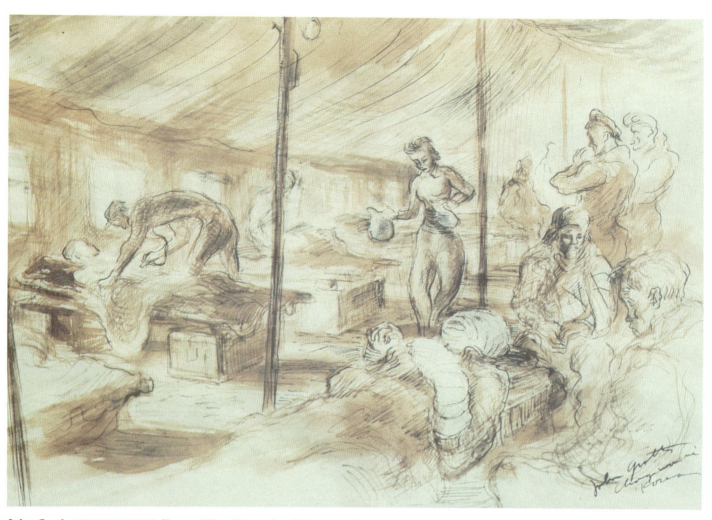

John Groth, RECOVERY TENT, *Korean War. Watercolor. Defense Audiovisual Agency, Washington, D.C.*

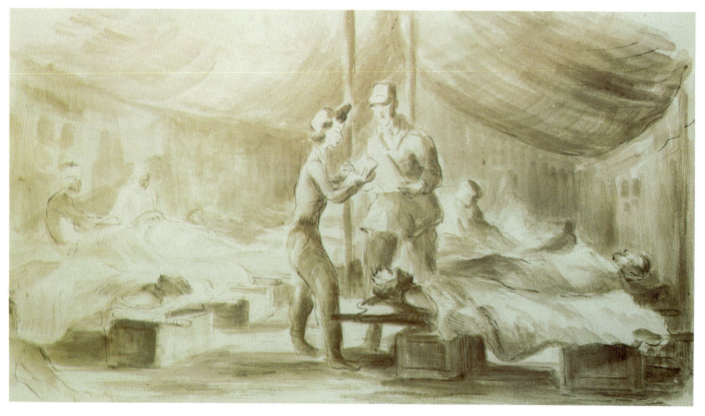

John Groth, FIELD HOSPITAL WARD, *Korean War. Watercolor. Defense Audiovisual Agency, Washington, D.C.*

424

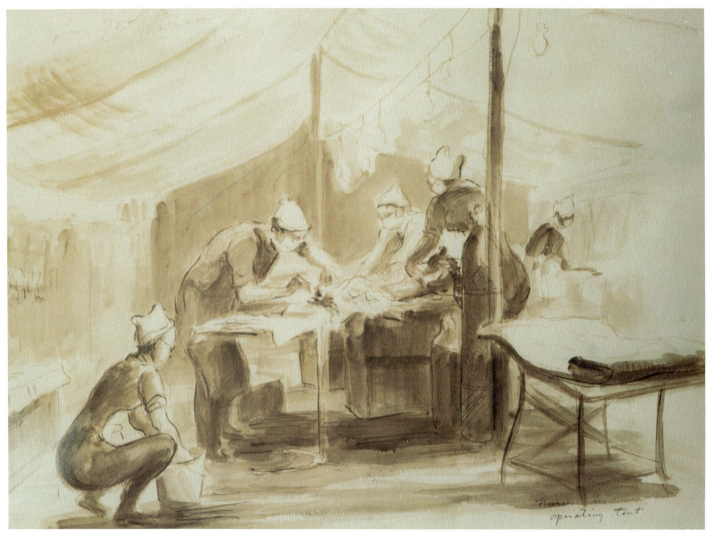

John Groth, NURSES IN THE OPERATING TENT, *Korean War. Watercolor. Defense Audiovisual Agency, Washington, D.C.*

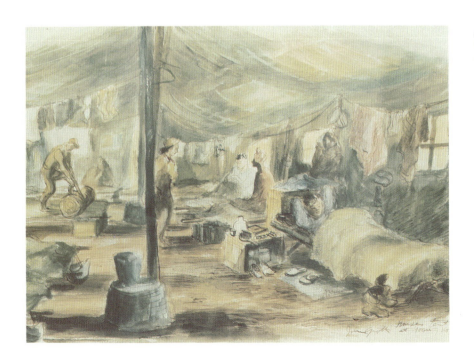

John Groth, NURSES' TENT, *Korean War. Watercolor. Defense Audiovisual Agency, Washington, D.C.*

A pattern of action was followed as patients were admitted: pulses and blood pressures were taken and recorded on tags attached to each litter; whole blood was started; penicillin was given to everyone with an open wound; clothing was cut away and wounds exposed; critical cases were identified; and patients were sorted on the basis of treatment. Chest, abdominal, or extremity injuries comprised the majority of cases.

The fledging Air Force Nurse Corps faced its first major test during this war. The members' primary responsibility was the care of patients airlifted during the Korean conflict. The volume of patients was staggering. As many as 3925 patients were aeromedically evacuated on one day, December 5, 1950 (Chow and others, 1978). The corps had mobilized its resources and accelerated training programs. By the end of the war, over 350,000 patients had been evacuated by propeller-driven cargo aircraft.

Throughout the ground fighting and during the prolonged peace negotiations that lasted for two years, until July 27, 1953, nurses served throughout the Korean peninsula. Nurses had once again made a tremendous contribution to advances in the delivery of care to the wounded.

■ THE VIETNAM WAR

The Vietnam War became the longest conflict in which American troops were committed in the history of the United States. It was a war like no other that evoked conflict and controversy initially at home. It was an extremely unpopular war, and thousands of people marched in protest and hundreds were arrested trying to storm the Pentagon. Student unrest erupted on campuses across the country as the war dragged on and American casualties escalated. The futility of American intervention was felt, and this resulted in problems never before experienced by veterans of other wars. "There was widespread resistance to fighting, extensive drug usage, and racial conflict among American troops. Profound guilt, feelings of stasis, impotence, psychic numbness, and a deeply embedded antiestablishment anger were common" (Kalisch and Kalisch, 1978, pp. 634–635). Deep and lasting wounds occurred that were not always caused by enemy action. An appropriate name for this conflict could well be the "forgotten war" because there is a silence, and at times a mystique, that pervades discussions of this war. This is consistent with published accounts in the nursing literature, which are fewer in number than those of either World War I or World War II.

America's interest in Southeast Asia began in 1950. At that time President Truman sent a thirty-five-man military advisory team to assist the French with their fight against the North Vietnamese. In 1954 the French garrison at Dien Bien Phu fell to communist forces; this was followed by a subsequent agreement between France and North Vietnam to partition Vietnam. The agreement was, however, contingent on free reunification elections. South Vietnam believed that free elections were impossible in North Vietnam and refused to prepare for them. Other events occurred, including President Eisenhower's offer of economic aid and training for the South Vietnamese army. By 1960 North Vietnam had formed the National Liberation Front (Viet

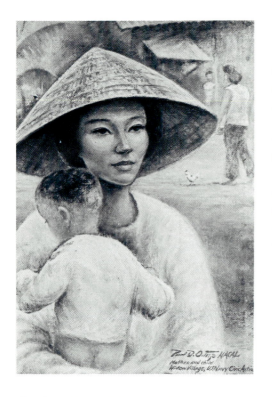

Paul Ortlip, MOTHER AND CHILD—WIDOW VILLAGE, VIETNAM, *1967. Defense Audiovisual Agency, Washington, D.C.*

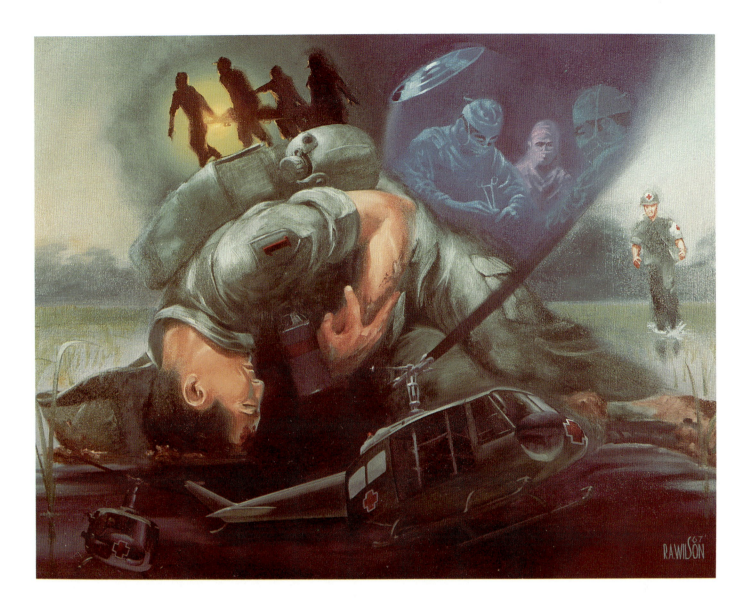

Sgt. Ronald A. Wilson, ANATOMY OF A DUSTOFF, *Vietnam, 1967.* Defense Audio-visual Agency, Washington, D.C.

The term "dustoff" was derived from the speed of landing, unloading the wounded, and the quick takeoff causing lots of dust. A medical corpsman accompanied the patients.

Cong) of South Vietnam. The number of American "military advisers" steadily grew in proportion to increased terrorism in South Vietnam. The involvement of American military nurses did not begin until March 1962.

The first contingent to arrive in the Republic of Vietnam were ten Army nurses assigned to the 8th Field Hospital, Nha Trang. By February of 1966, 300 military nurses of the Army, Navy, and Air Force were serving. More than 200 were members of the Army, 37 (not including flight nurses assigned aboard medical air evacuation aircraft) were Air Force, and 39 were Navy, including the 29 serving aboard the hospital ship *Repose.* This ship was later joined by the *Sanctuary.* Both were equipped to give optimal medical and nursing care to the wounded. Between March 1962 and March 1973 more than 5000 nurses served in Vietnam (Shields, 1981).

Nurse casualties also occurred in Vietnam. The only nurse and only woman, however, to die as a result of hostile fire was First Lieutenant Sharon A. Lane of Canton, Ohio. Lieutenant Lane died from shrapnel wounds during an enemy rocket attack on June 8, 1969, while on duty at the 312th Evacuation Hospital, Chu Lai. Her memory and spirit will live along with that of the thousands of men killed in action in Vietnam and elsewhere. The essence of her being is

427

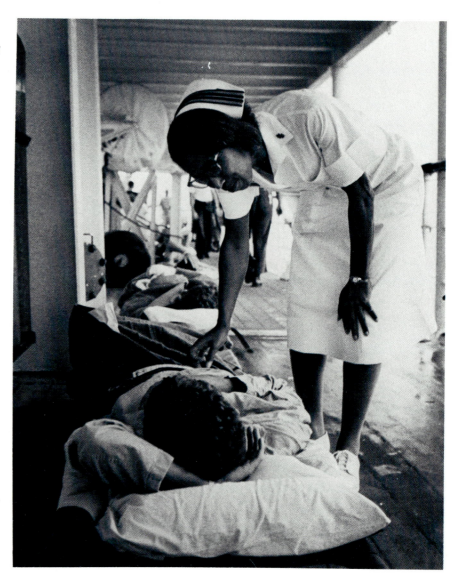

poignantly described by Colonel Maude M. Smith, ANC (ret.), in an imaginary monologue:

Message from Sharon

A Reading

I am Lieutenant Lane. Do you remember me?
I was taken from your midst beyond the China Sea
Yes! I am Sharon Lane and I am here with them
The very many thousand valiant young men
Yes! I am with them now where it's evermore serene
Indeed! I am treated regally—as if I were a queen
We were sad to leave you though little was our choice
But lasting peace is ours now we say with one voice
We rest in summer meadows that are always green
The beauty that surrounds us is bright fresh and clean
Friendly birds sing songs amid heavenly flowers
And time is not measured in mere moments or in hours
Butterflies flit gently over clover that is sweet
And joy and love abound on the paths where we all meet
We do not dwell in sorrow on the days missed of our youth
In the cause of freedom—in man's epic search for truth
We only plead that you will think it carefully through
Before another brutal war claims other young folk too

428

I was caring for a soldier
Leaning over his bed
A bit of shrapnel pierced my neck
In seconds I was dead
I didn't even have a chance
To breathe a quick good-bye
To gesture — to scream
Or to say a prayer or cry
It happened very suddenly
A long time ago
And I am not regretful
I do want you to know

That all of us up here have received the answers now
To our souls' burning questions that suffice somehow
Enjoy earth's awesome wonder the while that you are there
But accept in your hearts that here too it is fair
The ones who are so dear to you abiding here with me
We know you're only human and can't see as we now see
We have learned these lessons well so early in life's game
That death is not the end of thought and all men are the same
We are part of a unity in which mortal beings share
A mystical oneness of which we're quite aware
We also know our sacrifice shall not have been in vain
If it has meant that nevermore shall war destroy again
Please keep the sacred trust of peace that we all place in you
The sort of trust you put in us—the faith that we kept too
Yes! I am Sharon Lane. Love binds me to you yet
As it does the gallant men. Lest you forget!

Smith, 1984, p. 3

The appointment of male nurses to the regular forces of the Army, Navy, and Air Force Nurse Corps was made possible by a Congressional bill in 1966. Mrs. Francis P. Bolton, Representative from Ohio, had initially introduced the bill in 1961 and resubmitted it in 1963. She again introduced legislation in January 1965, which was followed by an identical bill by Samuel S. Stratton, Representative from New York, in May 1965. As a result, the number of male nurses in the services steadily rose. At one point all-male nursing units were

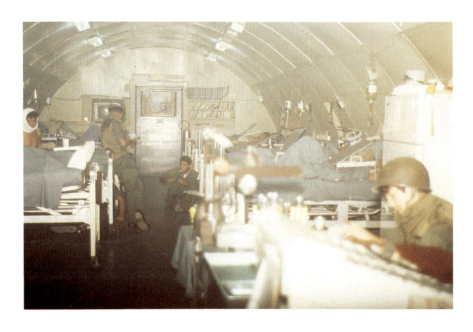

WARD B-8 DURING TET OFFENSIVE, *CuChi, Republic of Vietnam, 1967. Courtesy of Lt. Col. (Ret.) Sarah A. Balkema.*

An Air Force nurse checks the identification of an injured man during the Strike Command exercise, Goldfire I, designed to test newly developed Air Force tactical support techniques against current conventional Army–Air Force techniques in 1964. U.S. Air Force Photo.

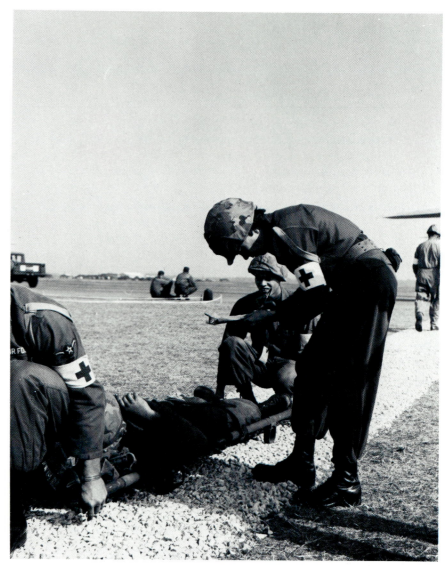

ARRIVAL OF PATIENT EVACUATED BY AMBULANCE, *CuChi, Republic of Vietnam, 1967. Courtesy of Lt. Col. (Ret.) Sarah A. Balkema, U.S. Army.*

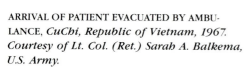

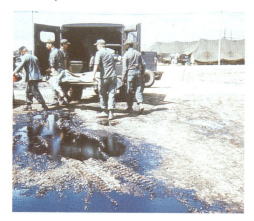

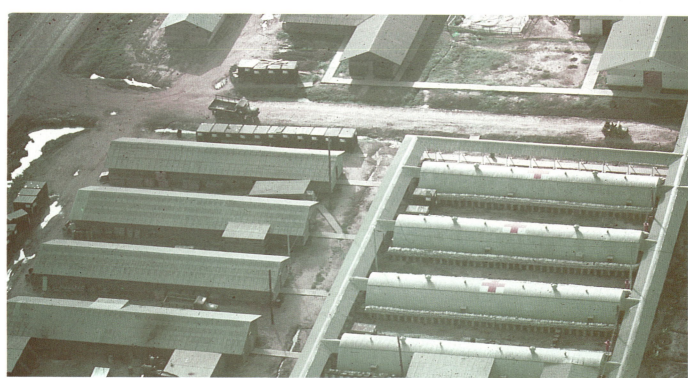

12TH EVACUATION HOSPITAL OF THE U.S. ARMY, *CuChi, Republic of Vietnam, 1967. Courtesy of Lt. Col. (Ret.) Sarah A. Balkema.*

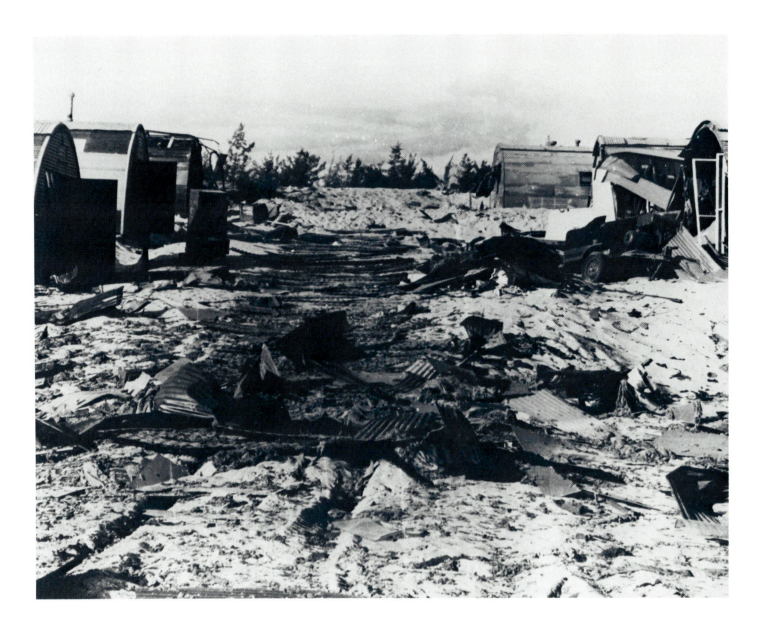

NAVAL HOSPITAL, *Da Nang, Vietnam, 1965.*
Naval Audiovisual Center, Washington, D.C.

View of the main street of the hospital
compound after the 1965 attack by the Viet
Cong. Surgery was once performed on the
left, and the labs were originally located
on the right.

established. These were dissolved as the presence of the female nurse was again recognized as an important morale booster.

No front lines in the traditional sense existed in Vietnam; nor were there secure road networks in combat areas. The hospitals, therefore, could not follow and support tactical operations, and ground evacuation was next to impossible. All hospitals became fixed installations, and helicopters became the primary means of evacuation. Inflatable rubber shelters known as MUST (Medical Unit, Self-contained, Transportable) hospitals became operational in Vietnam. They, too, were fixed but could have been moved under proper conditions. These semipermanent structures were equipped with integral electrical power, air conditioning, heating, hot and cold water, and waste disposal. Sophisticated medical equipment and facilities combined with quality nursing resulted in the best care ever available to those in combat.

A massive exodus of Vietnamese refugees took place at the end of the Vietnam War in April 1975. Military nurses worked diligently to provide nursing care to these homeless people in refugee camps and during air evacuation to the United States. They also contributed to the teaching of Vietnamese nurses and physicians while aiding in the health care of Vietnamese villagers.

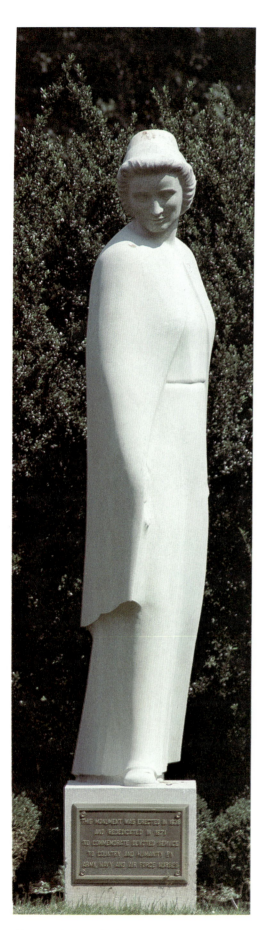

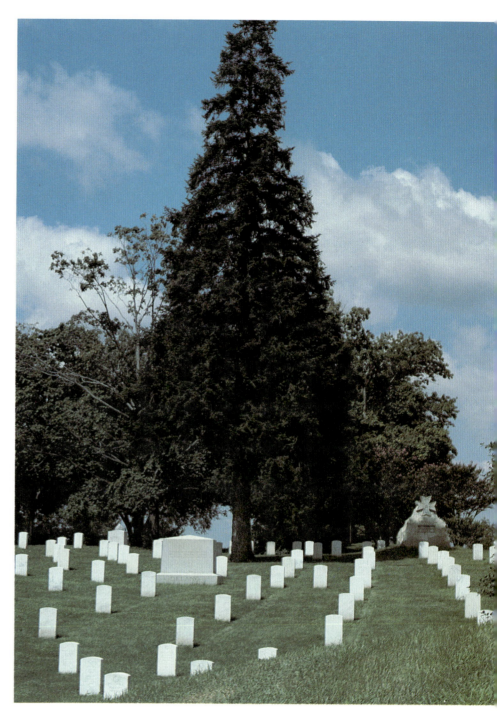

Frances Luther Rich, SPIRIT OF NURSING, *1938. Tennessee marble. Arlington National Cemetery, Arlington, Virginia. Courtesy of Morton Broffman.*

■ IN HONOR OF . . .

A considerable number of memorials have been dedicated to nurses and nursing. The majority can be categorized as ecclesiastical, military, or educational. Those related to military nursing bear testimony to the strong relationship between war and nursing. They represent a variety of methods for bestowing honor, such as through statues, cornerstones, scholarships and loan funds, buildings, chapels, hospital ships, and stained glass windows. One of the most impressive is the Nurses' Monument in Arlington National Cemetery. This monument, which symbolizes the "Spirit of Nursing," was dedicated to Army and Navy nurses. Carved by Frances Luther Rich, the daughter of actress Irene Rich, the monument is made of Tennessee marble. At the unveiling ceremonies on November 8, 1938, Julia C. Stimson,

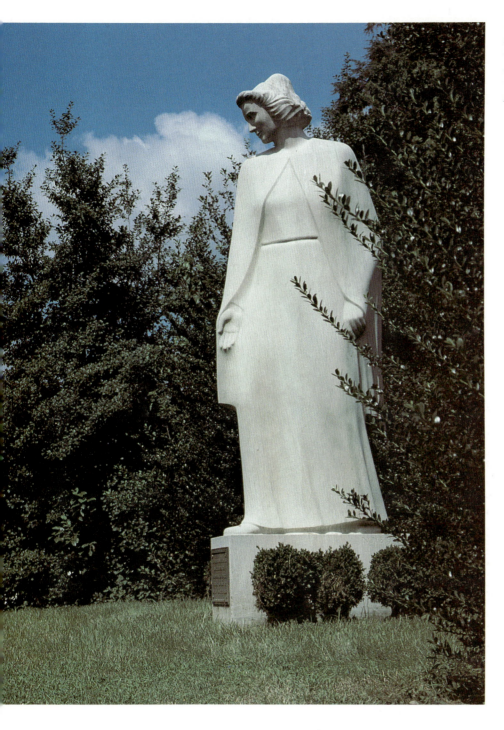

The SPIRIT OF NURSING *monument, which looks over the graves at Arlington National Cemetery, stands as a constant reminder of the compassion and bravery of the nation's military nurses. Courtesy of Morton Broffman.*

superintendent of the Army Nurse Corps (ret.) and current president of the ANA, made the dedication: "Their tenderness and compassion, their competence, courage and human qualities . . . the spirit of nursing of the past, of today, and of the years to come" (*American Journal of Nursing,* 1939, p. 90). The Nurses' Monument, which overlooks the graves from the top of a "hilly slope," was rededicated on March 11, 1971, by the chiefs of the Army, Navy, and Air Force.

A *Biblical Fable on Our Origins*

In the beginning, God created nursing.
He (or She) said, I will take a solid, simple,
significant system of **education** *and an adequate,*
applicable base of clinical **research,** *and*
On these rocks, will I build My greatest gift
to Mankind—nursing practice.
On the seventh day, He—threw up His hands.

And has left it up to us.

Margretta M. Styles

NURSING

The State of the Art

As the end of the twentieth century is approaching, nursing stands poised between the past and the future. The question of what lies ahead is open to speculation as the state of nursing's art is ever changing and responsive to societal needs. The twentieth century has been marked by many changes in the healing arts, some of which are in striking contrast to earlier epochs in history. Yet many of the extraordinary innovations that have occurred are continuations of contributions from the past. These changes have resulted from an interplay of numerous factors that have arisen in an increasingly technological age.

There is little doubt that nursing practice has been forced to make severe accommodations within this larger societal context as knowledge has continued to increase and attitudes and values have shifted. Nursing practice has expanded and extended in both horizontal and vertical directions. Some believe that this expansion has been too great and that professional growth comes by limiting functions rather than by extending them; they believe that the focus of concentration should be on the functions that are of a professional nature and integral to nursing. They argue that nursing has gone too

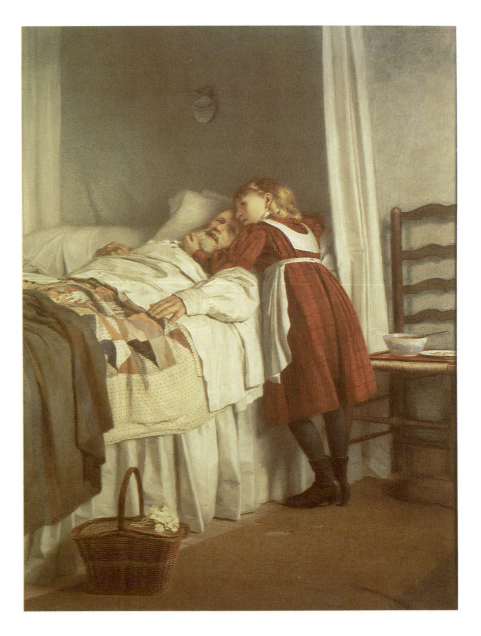

James Hayllar, GRANDFATHER'S LITTLE NURSE. *The Bridgeman Art Library Ltd./Galerie George, London, England.*

436

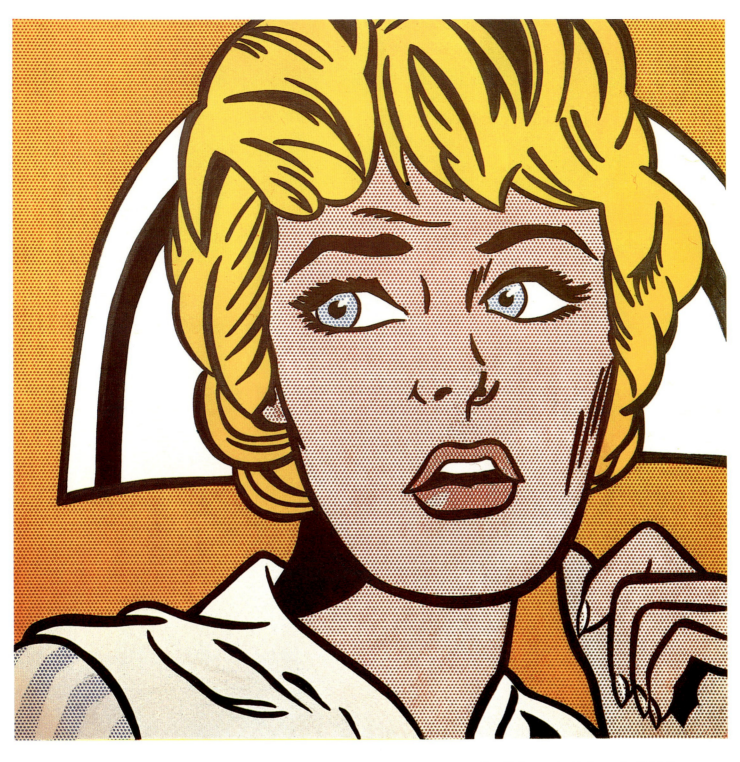

far and that it has begun to encroach on the medical domain. Others believe that the expanded roles in nursing fulfill a vital need and provide health care services where either none exist or are limited. In addition, the assumption of additional functions by nurses is viewed as necessary in order that the best possible care be rendered. Whatever the case, the changing environment has called for an education to keep pace with the modern world. Yet the struggle for the inclusion of educational programs for nursing in institutions of higher learning still continues at a time when education is needed more than ever to develop individuals who can deal with the problems of adjustment in modern life. Alfred North Whitehead, a scien-

Roy Lichtenstein, THE NURSE, *1964. Canvas. Hessisches Landesmuseum Darmstadt, Federal Republic of Germany, Collection of Karl Ströher.*

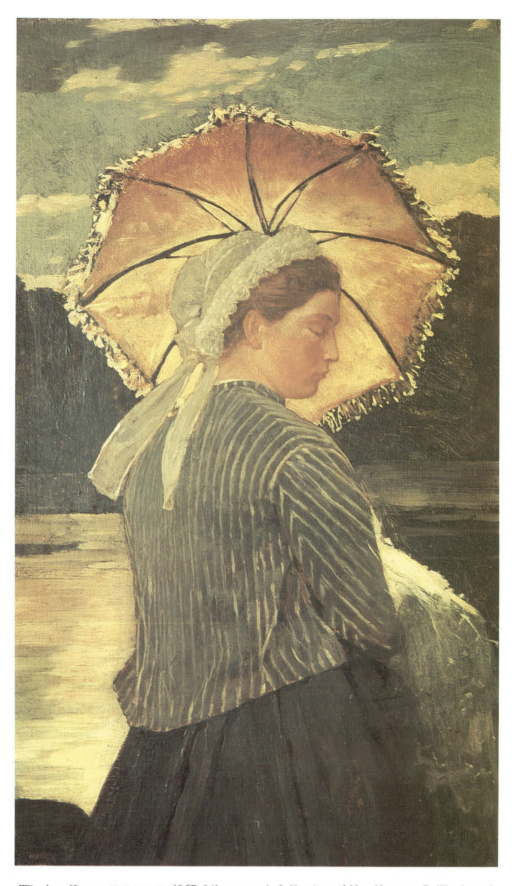

Winslow Homer, THE NURSE, *1867. Oil on wood. Collection of Mrs. Norman B. Woolworth, New York.*

The connotations of the word "nurse" have changed throughout history. A woman who cares for and tends young children became synonymous with a nurse. Homer's painting originally included a baby looking over the woman's shoulder.

tist and philosopher, issued a warning in 1929 that is relevant to nursing's educational situation of today:

In the conditions of modern life, the rule is absolute, the race which does not value trained intelligence is doomed. Not all your heroism, not all your social charm, not all your wit, not all your victories on land or at sea can move back the finger of fate. Today we maintain ourselves. Tomorrow science will have moved forward yet one more step, and there will be no appeal from the judgment which will then be pronounced on the uneducated.

Whitehead, 1929, p. 22

The education of nurses for the future must provide for the society of the future. At the same time the full potentialities of individual nurses and nursing at large must not be sacrificed.

The scientific, technological, and societal movements of the twentieth century have had a significant effect on the development of health care and on the direction of nursing services. A wide spectrum of change has occurred and catapulted society from the horse-and-buggy era to the space age. Diseases such as smallpox, diphtheria, and cholera, which virtually devastated populations in the past, are now rare or nonexistent. Scientific advances have made it possible for man to prolong life: sophisticated diagnostic methods permit visualization

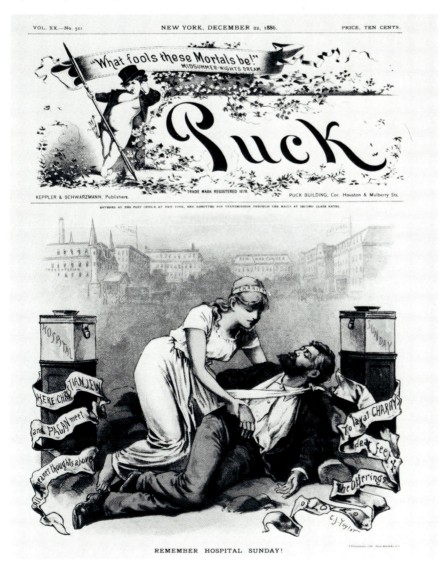

REMEMBER HOSPITAL SUNDAY!

C.J. Taylor, REMEMBER HOSPITAL SUNDAY. *Cover from* PUCK, *December 22, 1886. Library of Congress, Washington, D.C.*

This cover appeared as a plea for public support of volunteer hospitals. The woman helping the injured man is wearing a hair band with the word "charity" written across it.

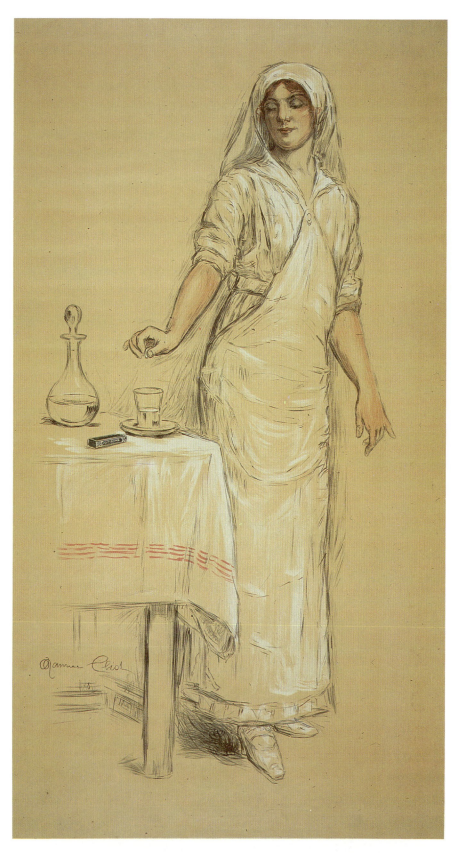

of the most minute internal structures of the human body; anesthetic agents and improved asepsis enhance surgical practice; grafts and transplants of healthy structures or even mechanical devices are used to replace diseased organs; miracle drugs wipe out formerly hopeless infections and bacterial diseases; the inner workings of the cell are open to scrutiny through physical and chemical means; and the hospital has moved from pesthouse to comprehensive health center.

Other current events and social issues were also influencing, either directly or indirectly, the health care delivery system and the roles and functions of its providers. During the first fifty years of the twentieth century many factors gave impetus to the progress of nursing: two world wars, self-organization of nurses, government and nursing legislation, problems of social welfare, support of health fields by national foundations, and the complexities of medicine. In the latter part of the century other social movements profoundly influenced health care and nursing; these included the rise of consumerism (the increased awareness and expectations of the patient for quality in health care delivery), changes in work-leisure patterns, the fight for civil rights, progress in public health, the development of voluntary and governmental health organizations, and the struggle for equal rights for women. All these factors—combined with the internal forces in nursing of consciousness raising, role innovation, and the drive for professionalization—shaped the role of the nurse and nursing (Reeder, 1978).

As the twentieth century witnessed improvements in the general standard of living, significant progress in transportation, communications, and other areas, and the lengthening of the life span, industrialization transformed rural America into an urban society. The social scene was marked by increasing change and complexity in nearly every field of endeavor. Urban centers rapidly became overcrowded because of an unprecedented population expansion and the unrestricted immigration of millions of poor Europeans. Health problems were aggravated, and problems in the provision of adequate

Artist's depiction of the complex of The University of Iowa Hospitals and Clinics. Courtesy of The University of Iowa Hospitals and Clinics, Department of Nursing, Iowa City, Iowa.

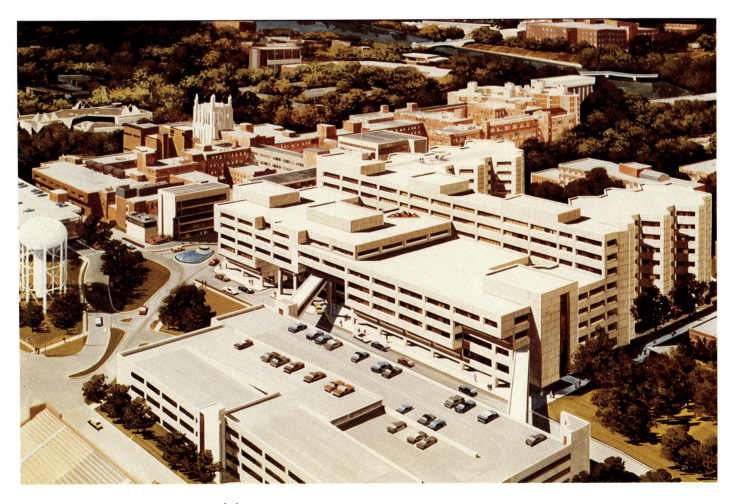

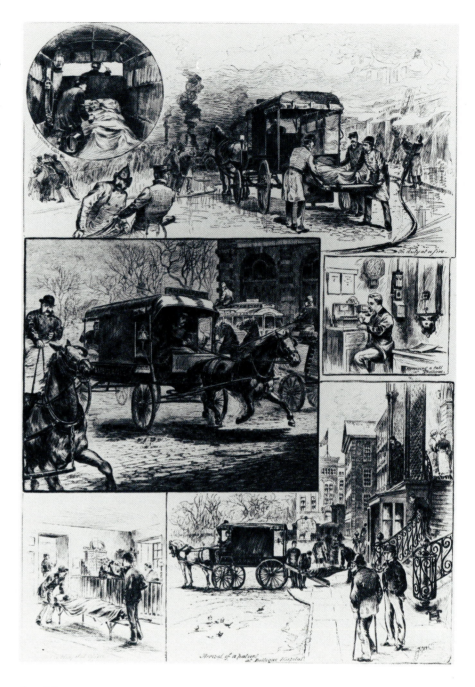

health care were intensified. Hospital services were broadened to provide for middle class patients as well as the indigent and homeless. Consequently, the whole concept of nursing had to be reevaluated and changed to fit the needs of this age of reform.

■ THE CHANGING SCENE IN NURSING

Numerous changes have occurred in nursing throughout the course of the twentieth century. The advent of new drugs, new techniques, and new technologies has placed new responsibilities on nurses and has mandated radical changes in nursing care. The patient care of today is of necessity different from that given at the time of Florence Nightingale, since nurses are expected to perform many tasks formerly done by physicians. Before the 1930s few graduate nurses

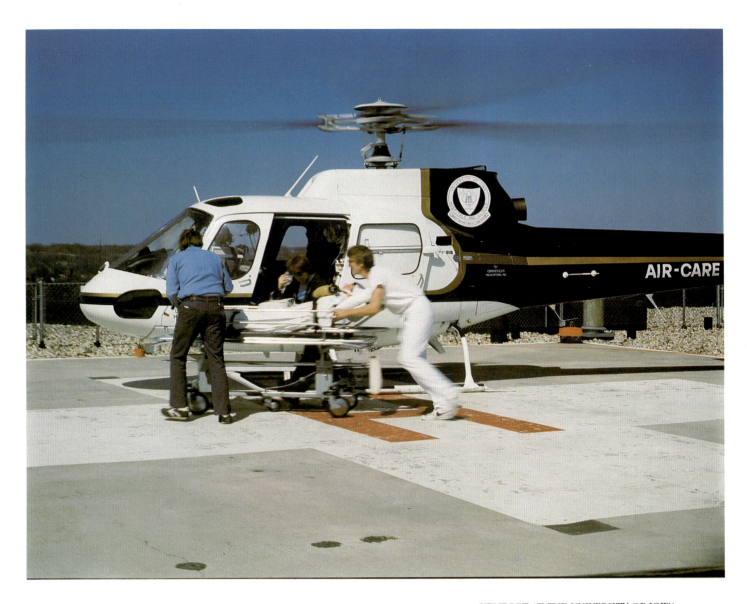

HELIPORT AT THE UNIVERSITY OF IOWA HOSPITAL. *Courtesy of The University of Iowa Hospitals and Clinics, Department of Nursing, Iowa City, Iowa.*

were employed by hospitals because most nursing care was done by nursing students. At that time "nursing" included a variety of non-nursing tasks, such as scrubbing floors, carrying trays, and cleaning equipment, in addition to the so-called routine care of patients. The students were left with relatively little time to give adequate nursing care—let alone incorporate an holistic approach to that care.

By the 1940s many more tasks and procedures were being done by nurses as a result of the introduction of new innovations in health care. Nurses' functions then included blood pressure measurement, suctioning in a variety of conditions, transfusion assistance, oxygen administration, medication injection, and other more sophisticated techniques. Nurses were also assisting in operating rooms, delivery rooms, and outpatient facilities. More and more individuals were being admitted to hospitals to have greater numbers of procedures performed as these institutions became safer and more efficient. This phenomenon was significantly enhanced by the advent of hospitalization insurance and prepayment plans for hospital care. In *Nursing for the Future* Esther Lucile Brown reported that in one large teaching hospital over 100 procedures (exclusive of operating, obstetrical,

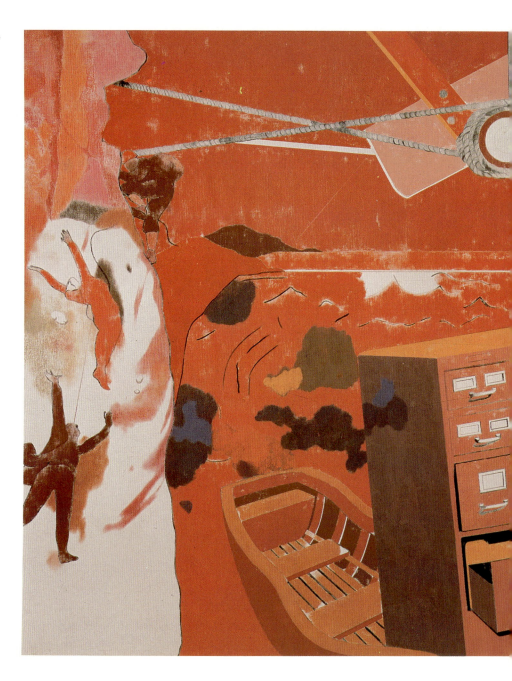

R.B. Kitaj, ERIE SHORE, *1966. Nationalgalerie, Berlin, Federal Republic of Germany.*

and outpatient services) were being done. This finding is substantiated by Dennison:

> [Nurses] managed the apparatus for Wangensteen suction, tidal irrigation, and bladder decompression. They irrigated eyes, cecostomies, colostomies, and draining wounds. They did artificial respiration, applied sterile compresses, and painted lesions. . . . They did catheterizations, sitz baths, and turpentine stupes. They gave insulin and taught the patient or his relatives to give the drug and examine urine. They administered approximately 1500 medications daily, by mouth or hypodermic. They assisted with lumbar punctures, thoracenteses . . . and phlebotomies.
>
> *Dennison, 1942, p. 777*

Nursing shortages occurred periodically throughout the twentieth century. Even the belief that there would be an oversupply of nurses for civilian work after World War II was dashed. Many nurses stopped practicing to devote time to their family responsibilities.

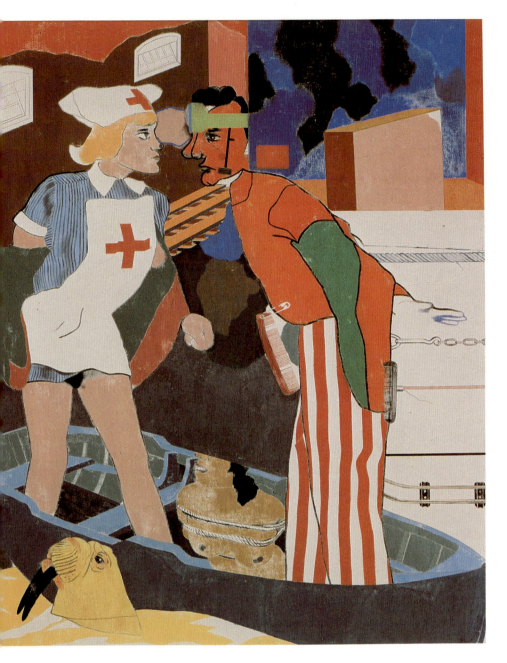

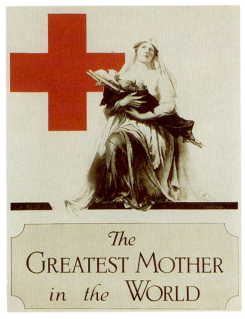

A.E. Foringer, THE GREATEST MOTHER IN THE WORLD, *World War I poster. Lithograph. Defense Audiovisual Agency, Washington, D.C.*

Many nurses did not return to practice, their answer to an authoritarian and paternalistic system in which they had no participation in planning or decision making. Many refused to be involved in a work structure that offered few rewards, long hours, hard physical labor, and very low salaries.

Compounding this situation were other significant events that led to the gradual development of a new organizational pattern for hospital care. The demonstrated success of resuscitation stations on the front lines in World War II led to the emergence of special units for patient care. Postanesthesia and recovery rooms were established to prevent postoperative complications. Eventually this was to transfer to a broader concept, the intensive care unit, after the use of MASH units in the Korean conflict. Progression from the intensive care unit to the intermediate, self-care, long-term care, and home care units was thus possible. This concept of "progressive patient care" was set into motion and in operation by the middle 1950s (Haldeman and

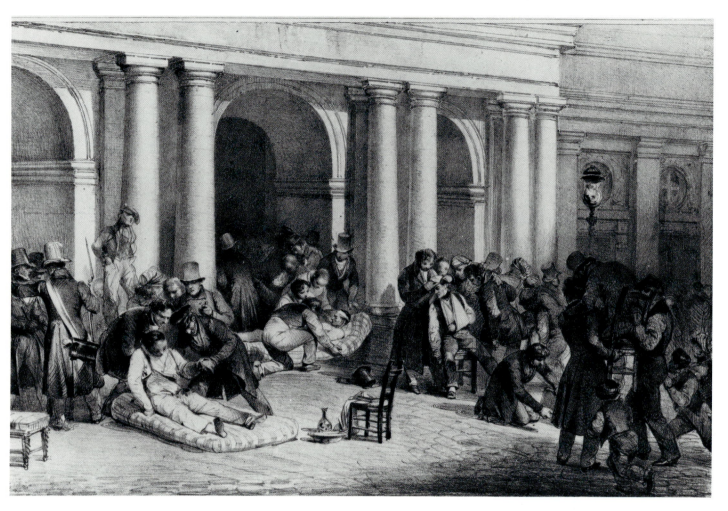

EMERGENCY TREATMENT IN THE COURT OF THE PALAIS ROYAL. *National Library of Medicine, Bethesda, Maryland. During the Revolution in July 1830, the court of the Palais Royal was used to treat the casualties of the revolt.*

Abdellah, 1959). This development of specific types of units, although advantageous in many respects, created the need for specialized nursing skills and varying nurse-patient ratios in some areas, which contributed further to the nursing shortage.

As the ranks of nurses continued to diminish and new nursing demands increased, "team nursing" was introduced. This new and different method of assignment used fewer well-prepared personnel. It was designed to fit particular assignments to the background and expertise of the provider of service. Philosophically, team nursing was a system whereby different types of hospital nursing personnel could be placed into teams to provide quality nursing care for groups of patients. The professional nurse would directly supervise all patients and team members. In addition, team conferences would be held for planning and evaluation, nursing care plans would ensure continuity of care, and in-service education and on-the-job training would be provided as necessary (Lambertsen, 1953). Unfortunately, the quality of nursing care and patient satisfaction diminished as fewer registered professional nurses were giving direct care to patients. The work was indeed coordinated, but the nursing care was fragmented. This was particularly disastrous as major advances in diagnostic and treatment procedures and the development of sophisticated technology continued. The 1950s and 1960s were a revolutionary time for health care:

> A sampling of major advances during the two decades includes the development of the heart-lung machine, open heart surgery, cardiac catheterization, renal dialysis, laser surgery, high-

446

frequency implements for blood coagulation, and new vaccines, pharmaceuticals, and monitoring devices. The expanding field of medical science had made nursing care increasingly more complex and had made demands of increasing gravity on nurses as well. To effectively give care, nurses needed to be able to identify very subtle changes in patients' status, learn new sophisticated treatment techniques, increase their ability to interpret laboratory data, recognize delicate physiological interrelationships, and closely monitor the efficacy of potent and sometimes experimental forms of drug therapy.

Fitzpatrick, 1983, pp. 34–35

It became clear that a different approach to nursing care was needed, one that would provide both quality and an holistic framework. A movement was begun in the 1960s to close the gap between the professional nurse and the patient. It was initiated as an important innovation in 1963 through the efforts of Lydia Hall, who was the inspiration behind the philosophy and work of the Loeb Center for Nursing and Rehabilitation at Montefiore Hospital in New York. The overall purpose of this center is to provide continuous quality nursing care that emphasizes the facilitation of healing, prevention of complications, promotion of health, and prevention of recurrences and new illnesses. Nursing care is given solely by professional nurses in a setting that enhances the movement of the patient from the general hospital to home. The nurse is the *primary factor* in patient care and coordinates the combined efforts of the patient, the family, and the nurse in the solving of problems that might hinder ultimate recovery. Medicine and allied fields are viewed as ancillary treatment. In this structure the assumption is made that less medical care is needed; more professional nursing care and teaching are needed (Hall, 1963). Slowly, other such attempts were made by acute care hospitals under the guise of "comprehensive" or "total" nursing care. However, nurses were frustrated in their efforts by inadequate staffing, emphasis on efficiency, and lack of regard for patient orientation.

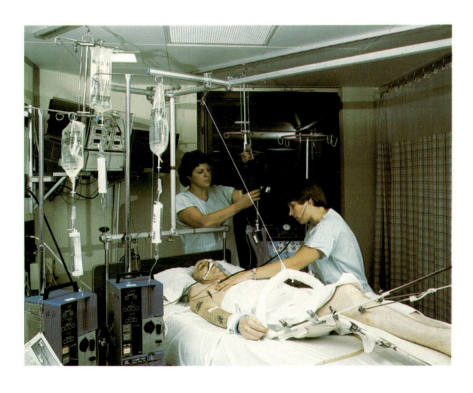

INTENSIVE CARE UNIT. *Courtesy of The University of Iowa Hospitals and Clinics, Department of Nursing, Iowa City, Iowa.*

447

It was not until the 1970s, however, that the combined goal of nursing care by professional nurses and total patient care (holistic approach) began to be realized with the advent of *primary nursing*. The primary nurse is responsible for the patient's total care for the entire hospitalization period, twenty-four hours a day, seven days a week. High-quality nursing care is promoted through this modality because the primary nurse assumes responsibility for the entire spectrum of functions, including teaching, consultation, comprehensive care with continuity, planning and evaluation of care, documentation of progress, discharge planning, and referrals to ancillary services or agencies (Marram, Barrett, and Bevis, 1979). When the primary nurse is not physically present, an associate nurse follows the plan of care. In this system nurses truly can be patients' advocates, they can be accountable for their own practice, and they can make decisions based on available data.

Although primary nursing has been growing in popularity since its inception, its success depends on adequate staffing, administrative support, and technically and educationally prepared nurses. It has been received favorably by patients, and it is hoped that it will gain total recognition and acceptance by health care delivery systems. The best argument for the implementation of primary nursing is that it has the greatest potential for placing the patient in an environment conducive to the attainment of wellness.

Some primary nurses now engage in private practice or share a private practice with a physician. One such "independent practitioner," M. Lucille Kinlein, hung out her shingle in May 1971. Others engage in various alternative methods of care. For example, Dr. Delores Krieger, a professor of nursing at New York University, has repopularized the theory of therapeutic touch. She has achieved national recognition for her expertise in this area and has taught many nurses and other individuals to use this therapy.

Although great strides have been made in nursing, problems continue. Working conditions and environments are still sources of conflict. Nurses are now voicing their concerns regarding inadequate staffing, low wages, long hours, unsafe practices, nurses' inability to use their own knowledge, judgment, and decision-making abilities, and other circumstances that prohibit the rendering of high-quality nursing care. In those situations where all attempts at communication have failed, nurses have turned to organization through local units of the state professional organization or other types of bargaining units.

The nurses of today are expected to be many things to many people and to function in a variety of settings. They are to be excellent caregivers, adequate researchers, seekers of knowledge, and thinkers grounded in scientific and logical thought. Nurses are involved with scientific and technical advances and with all types of new roles that have broadened their opportunities but increased their scope of responsibilities. They are slowly but steadily moving toward a goal of holistic treatment for *all* individuals in a sructure that is not always supportive. Nurses will continue to meet the challenges of the future identified by Florence Nightingale:

> No system can endure that does not march. Are we walking
> to the future or to the past? Are we progressing or are we
> stereotyping? We remember that we have scarcely crossed the

threshold of uncivilized civilization in nursing; there is still so much to do. Don't let us stereotype mediocrity. We are still on the threshold of nursing.

In the future, which I shall not see, for I am old, may a better way be opened! May the methods by which every infant, every human being will have the best chance of health, the methods by which every sick person will have the best chance of recovery, be learned and practiced! Hospitals are only an intermediate state of civilization never intended, at all events, to take in the whole sick population.

Nightingale, 1860

Nursing Research and Theory

Nursing research is new, yet old. Florence Nightingale is generally regarded as the first "nurse researcher," since her nursing reforms were based on careful investigation. In recognition of her great contribution to the field of social statistics, she was made a fellow in the Royal Statistical Society in 1858 and was granted an honorary membership in the American Statistical Society in 1874. Sir Francis Galton acknowledged her preeminence in statistics. Queen Victoria deplored the fact that she could not have Miss Nightingale in the War Office. One author's comments illustrate her deep commitment to this field of endeavor:

Miss Nightingale's attitude towards the application of statistics in the field of social dynamics was very similar to that of Thomas Buckle; they both deplored the fact that a wealth of data was available, but unapplied. Her typically practical philosophy demanded that if statistics were to be useful, they must be used. They must aid in the establishment of preventive measures. . . .

Florence Nightingale was determined to make statistics an active reality which would influence the general welfare as well as the health of man. . . .

Newton, 1949, p. 33

Although the Nightingale tradition of education was transmitted to America, the approach to and use of research was not. In addition, the "training schools" in America were not conducive to the development of critical thinking or problem solving. Inquiring minds were not fostered through the prevailing atmosphere of rigid discipline and unquestioning obedience. These elements, which were strong influences within nursing schools, reduced individualism, creativity, critical thinking, and assertiveness. They served to place students and graduate nurses in a subservient role, a position where they have remained for many years.

The environment in which nursing operated was not conducive to nursing research; nor were nurses prepared with the skills to pursue it. However, the need for nursing research was recognized by the early leaders, who were committed to the scientific method of collecting and interpreting data to generate new knowledge for the improvement of nursing care. Probably the earliest research report, done by M. Adelaide Nutting, was *The Educational Status of Nursing* (1912). A comprehensive analysis of nursing during this period, it revealed the appalling practices and conditions under which student

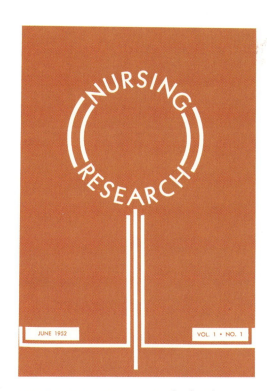

NURSING RESEARCH, *cover to the first issue, 1952. By permission from the American Journal of Nursing Company, New York.*

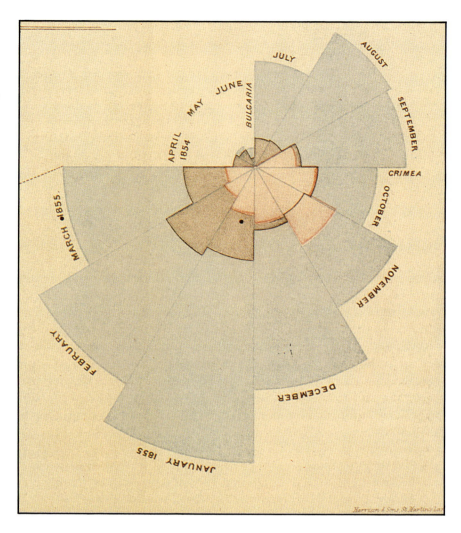

Florence Nightingale's "coxcomb" diagram for April 1854 to March 1855 showing the extent of needless deaths in British military hospitals during the Crimean War. Each colored wedge is proportional to the number of casualties being represented. From her book NOTES OF MATTERS AFFECTING THE HEALTH, EFFICIENCY AND HOSPITAL ADMINISTRATION OF THE BRITISH ARMY, *1858. By permission of the Houghton Library, Harvard University, Cambridge, Massachusetts.*

nurses functioned. Other reports followed during the first half of the twentieth century, as did studies of nursing practice, nursing services, nursing education, nursing service administration, and virtually every field related to nursing. The majority of these were done by individuals who were not nurses.

Leadership ability in the area of nursing research was demonstrated early by Isabel M. Stewart. Although her activities and interests in this area were not widely known, they were nonetheless significant. Intrigued by the time and motion studies for improvement of efficiency in industry and home economics, Miss Stewart began to investigate the potential of this technique for nursing. She visited Dr. and Mrs. Frank Gilbreth, who set up beds in the living room of their home in Providence, Rhode Island, for use as a laboratory. This was the beginning of Isabel Stewart's attempt at an activity analysis of nursing to differentiate between nursing and non-nursing functions. This minimal study still provides standards of nursing care useful in current nursing practice. From this meagre beginning, Miss Stewart continued her pursuits and conducted research in nursing and nursing education. She studied philosophical, educational, and historical research methods and incorporated these into her books and other writings. Eventually she published the Teachers College *Nursing Education Bulletin,* possibly the first research journal in nursing. This was done in the face of opposition from other nurses, whose concept of research was limited to test-tube methods. In an editorial in 1929 Isabel Stewart explained her position:

450

If nursing is ever to justify its name as an applied science, if it is ever to free itself from these old superficial, haphazard methods, some way must be found to submit all our practices as rapidly as possible to the most searching tests which modern science can devise. Not only bacteriological and physiological and chemical tests are needed, but economic and psychological and sociological measurements also, if they are appropriate and workable. There is not much use waiting for someone outside our own body to recognize our critical situation and to offer to do the work for us. Some help may be secured from physicians and from experts in other fields, but most of the experimentation that is done will have to be carried on in all probability by our own members. Nurses may not be prepared to make the more difficult studies at once, but if a few will prepare themselves to start in a small way and to show what can be done, others will undoubtedly become interested, and in time, resources will be found, if the results warrant them.

Stewart, 1929, p. 3

Miss Stewart firmly believed that students should receive a research orientation, and she involved them in studies and projects that needed or were under investigation. Thus she incorporated research training into the program of graduate study in nursing education. She recognized, however, that not all individuals were "fitted" for investigation, and so she proposed that a few minds could take a lead in such activities. With that goal in mind, Miss Stewart consistently urged that graduate students have more advanced preparation in research. Student reaction was positive, as described by Dr. McManus:

Inspired, prodded and encouraged by Miss Stewart, an increasing number of students did undertake doctoral study. Without her interest, support, and patient understanding, I know I could and would not have persevered toward that goal; I am sure this is true of many others of her students. . . .
  Miss Stewart laid the firm foundation for nursing research and research preparation in the Division of Nursing Education at Teachers College.

McManus, 1962, p. 6

As a lasting tribute to her impact on nursing research, Teachers College in 1961 opened a fund with a goal of $400,000 to establish the Isabel Maitland Stewart Research Professorship in Nursing and Nursing Education.

A series of events eventually transpired that led to a decided commitment to the incorporation of nursing research in the overall structure of nursing. Sigma Theta Tau initiated a research fund in the 1930s to develop an awareness of the need for research. The Association of Collegiate Schools of Nursing (ACSN) sponsored a special forum on nursing research in 1941. The ANA House of Delegates approved a research program in 1950. This program was designed as a long-term research project to study (1) nursing functions in a variety of settings and geographical locations and (2) nurses' relationships with their co-workers and associates. Teachers College established the Institute of Research and Service in Nursing Education during the early 1950s to provide a full-time mechanism for studying and developing nursing education through research. Launching of the journal

Nursing Research in 1952 was evidence of nursing's promotion and communication of research and scholarly productivity. In 1955 the American Nurses' Foundation was organized as a membership corporation of the ANA. The purpose of this foundation was to provide research grants to graduate nurses for scientific and educational projects; conduct studies, surveys, and research; provide grants to public and private nonprofit educational institutions; and publish scientific, educational, and literary work. This was followed by the establishment of a Commission on Nursing Research (1970) and a Council of Nurse Researchers (1972) in the ANA.

Governmental funds for nursing research began to be allocated at the end of World War II. Between 1940 and 1956, small grants were awarded to numerous individuals and institutions for various research projects through the Department of Health, Education and Welfare. An extramural grant program in nursing research was originated in the United States Public Health Service's Division of Nursing Resources in fiscal year 1956. Monies were awarded to qualified researchers for projects in nursing. This was the first time grants from federal sources were made available for nursing research. Federal support of research training for nurses was also provided in a twofold approach: through special predoctoral fellowships established by the Division of Nursing Resources and through nurse-scientist graduate training grants to both assist institutions with development of nursing research competence and provide stipends for graduate nursing students preparing for research. Finally, the integration of research in nursing into all nursing collegiate educational programs was accomplished in the 1970s.

The value of nursing research which has already been demonstrated, will become even more important as nursing continues its march toward professional status and excellence in performance. Research has proven to be a mechanism of generating new knowledge for nursing that will ultimately ensure quality of nursing care. A growing acceptance of nursing research has occurred as this area has become recognized as an effective method for cost containment. The most efficient and most effective modes of nursing can be identified through nursing research.

Nursing is one of several "semi-professions" involved in an extensive campaign to achieve full professional status. One characteristic associated with established professions is the acquisition of a unique body of scientific knowledge through vigorous training. Discussions regarding the development of nursing theories to assist with this generation of knowledge and to assist with the definition and identification of the unique role and functions of nursing have taken place since the middle 1960s and early 1970s. The origins of nursing theories, however, go back much farther. Some individuals in nursing identify Florence Nightingale as the first nursing theorist. She, indeed, followed principles related to cleanliness, fresh air, good food, rest, sleep, and exercise. She was the first individual to define and describe nursing in her *Notes on Nursing.* She did have significant thoughts, ideas, and principles, though at times they were disjointed. Yet one must systematically analyze these according to defined criteria to establish whether they constituted a theory.

The struggle to clearly identify a unique knowledge base for nursing (nursing science) has been continuous, particularly in relation to defining and describing the functions of nursing. Definitions of these functions were published by the ANA in 1932, 1937, and 1955. However, they lacked specificity and prompted individual nurses to write their own. Two of the pioneers in this area were Virginia Henderson and Hildegard Peplau. Miss Henderson's definition of nursing was first published in 1955, and it was revised in 1966.

> The unique function of the nurse is to assist the individual (sick or well), in the performance of those activities contributing to health or its recovery (or to peaceful death) that he would perform unaided if he had the necessary strength, will, or knowledge. And to do this in such a way as to help him gain independence as rapidly as possible.
>
> *Henderson, 1966, p. 15*

In 1952 Dr. Peplau published *Interpersonal Relations in Nursing,* which described four phases of the nurse-client relationship and led to numerous studies in the communication area. She brought interpersonal theories from psychiatry into nursing as a basis for the analysis of these interactions in terms of therapeutic quality. It is pos-

Theodore Gericault, AFTER DEATH, *1818. Canvas, approx. 45.7 × 55.9 cm. The Art Institute of Chicago, Illinois, A.A. Munger Collection.*

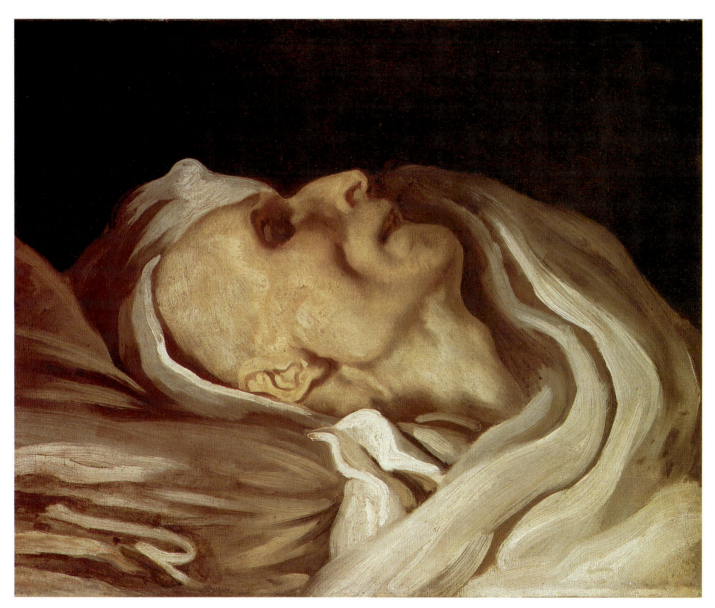

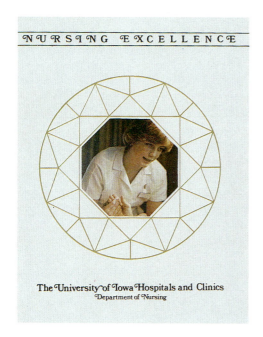

sible that this work was one of the first proposed theoretical frameworks for nursing. Ida J. Orlando (1961) offered communications theory for the description of what she labeled "a deliberate nursing approach." Imogene M. King (1971) later began to explain the intricate transactional process between nurse and patient.

A significant catalyst in the movement for the development of nursing theory was Dr. Martha E. Rogers, whose work was a vivid testimony for nursing to be recognized as a science:

> The science of nursing is an emergent—a new product. The inevitability of its development is written in nursing's long commitment to human health and welfare. With today's rapid and unprecedented changes, new urgency has been added to the critical need for a body of scientific knowledge specific to nursing. Only as the science of nursing takes on form and substance can the art of nursing achieve new dimensions of artistry.
>
> The science of nursing aims to provide a body of abstract knowledge growing out of scientific research and logical analysis and capable of being translated into nursing practice.
>
> *Rogers, 1970, pp. 83, 86*

The need for and development of nursing theories were prominent issues in the 1970s. Several theories and conceptual frameworks emerged through the diligence of such individuals as Sister Callista Roy, Martha E. Rogers, Imogene M. King, Dorothea Orem, and Margaret A. Newman.

Nursing is beginning to be recognized as a legitimate science, but a continuing momentum is necessary to achieve this goal. The united efforts of nurse scholars and practitioners of nursing are needed to assist with the identification of a knowledge base for nursing and to formulate a theory or theories to validate professional practice.

Educational Advancement

The history of master's education in nursing is rather vague because information about these programs was not available until the mid-century. What is known about the earlier programs is that they differed in organization and structure, varied in requirements, admitted students at differing times throughout the year, and used a variety of labels. Even more significant is the fact that initially all the post-diploma programs were considered to be "postgraduate education" and were identified as such. It was therefore difficult to differentiate between some baccalaureate and master's level programs.

The growth of university nurse educational programs sparked graduate study in nursing. The lack of prepared nurses for teaching and administrative positions was apparent, and the need to rectify this weakness was pressing. Master's degree programs were thus initiated and soon became viewed as the level for specialization for teaching and administration. Dr. M. Louise Fitzpatrick (1983) describes the following four phases in this development that incorporate primary influences and changes.

Origins: 1939–1952. This phase relates to the difficulty in tracing the development of nurse education programs. However, several important events were occurring. Baccalaureate programs of

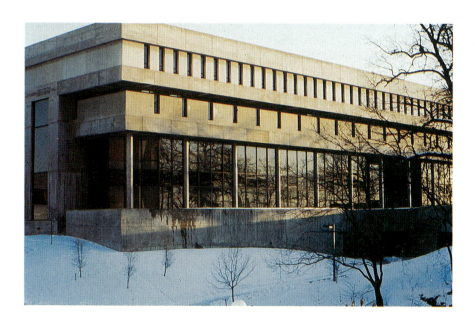

varying types were increasing in number. *Nursing for the Future* (1948) was published, and an accreditation system was established in 1949—both of which promoted the elucidation of the nature of collegiate education. An informal group of representatives from five area New York schools was convened by Dr. R. Louise McManus. This group proposed baccalaureate education as a beginning level and the master's as the specialized degree.

Transitional Stage: 1953–1964.

It was during these eleven years that master's education was recognized as the advanced level of nursing education. A conference on graduate education was sponsored by the NLN in 1954 and 1955. Guidelines were formulated for organization, administration, curriculum, and testing, and a Subcommittee on Graduate Education in Nursing (of the NLN) was created. The emphasis in master's content vacillated and moved from both clinical and functional role preparation in all programs for teachers, administrators, and clinical specialists to the elimination of double preparation in the late 1960s as clinical specialization became extremely popular. A shift is once again occurring in the 1980s, as the position in favor of double preparation is gaining momentum.

Regionalization.

Regional planning in graduate education was begun in the 1950s with the development of two organizations: the Southern Regional Educational Board (SREB) and the Western Interstate Commission on Higher Education (WICHE). Both were committed to better nursing through strong master's programs to prepare faculty. The Western Interstate Commission for Higher Education in Nursing (WICHEN) was begun in the Western area of the country in 1955 to promote graduate and professional education in the health fields. These programs contributed greatly to graduate education that was research based.

Maturing of Master's Education: 1964–1975.

Master's education in nursing matured and became an important credential for nurses in leadership positions during these years. Increased interest in research and an expanding number of graduate programs in clinical specialties occurred. The Nurse Training Act of 1964 (Title

VIII of the Public Health Service Act) provided a comprehensive financial package for construction, faculty development, student grants, and loans. Between 1964 and 1971, over $334 million was appropriated by Congress for nursing education.

Master's graduate study has become firmly entrenched in the structure of nursing education. There are continuing discussions regarding both the purpose and the product of such an education. Consequently, the emphasis in content periodically shifts in relation to prevailing philosophies, nursing care needs, and social forces. However, educational upgrading is apparent, since the number of nurses attaining master's degrees is rapidly increasing.

Social forces that have affected the development of nursing have also influenced the development of doctoral education in nursing. Although the first graduate courses and graduate programs of study originated in 1899 at Teachers College, many years passed before a bona fide doctoral program came into being. The first doctoral program in nursing was initiated at Teachers College, Columbia University, about 1920 and led to an Ed.D. in nursing education. The evolution of additional programs was a slow process directly related to nursing's continuing struggle for respect, credibility, recognition, and power. One author has summarized the difficulty of this growth in the following way:

> The evolution of the nursing profession has occurred within a political context that has placed many constraints upon the developmental process. Conflicts within administrative hierarchy, the effects of sexism, and circumscribed roles for women are but a few of the constraints. In this context, doctoral education *for* nurses and *in* nursing is but another step in the overall struggle for independence and recognition of worth.
>
> *Grace, 1978, p. 114*

Other factors inhibited a rapid growth in doctoral preparation for nurses: nursing was perceived solely as a practice discipline; there was a fear that nurses might become too knowledgeable and pose a threat to the medical hierarchy; a retarded growth in master's programs resulted in an inadequate pool of doctoral candidates until the 1960s; the nature, orientation, and direction of the nursing doctorate was not clearly defined; and a body of scientific knowledge was lacking.

In 1934 New York University followed Teachers College with a Ph.D. and an Ed.D. in nursing. In 1954 the University of Pittsburgh established a Ph.D. in nursing. The first D.N.S. (doctorate in nursing science) in psychiatric nursing was initiated at Boston University in 1960. Since there were so few doctoral programs in nursing before 1960, the majority of nurses who sought doctoral preparation were forced to pursue degrees in other fields. Education was the most popular field; the natural, behavioral, and biologic sciences were the other chosen areas of study.

According to Styles (1977), the history of doctoral education divided itself into two logical components: the early years, which were dominated by doctoral education *for* nurses, and the current years, with their emphasis on doctoral education *in* nursing. This is consistent with Grace's discussion (1978) of the evolution of specific forms of doctoral programs in nursing. The first form was that of the functional specialty, with an emphasis on the methodologies and knowledge base necessary for teaching and administration. The second form involved preparation in basic scientific disciplines upon which the science and art of nursing rest. This movement was greatly enhanced by the nurse-scientist program of the federal government in which grants were awarded to finance the education of nurses in closely related disciplines. The intent was for these graduates to return to faculty positions and provide input into basic science and research content in nursing. The third and current form is doctoral programs *in* nursing.

Two doctoral degree programs *in* nursing are now offered: the Ph.D., or academic doctorate with emphasis on nursing research, and the D.N.S., or professional doctorate with emphasis on nursing practice. There is disagreement as to which type will best prepare a nurse to assume power and position and to exert influence in the health care system. Which will better prepare the nurse for the generation and application of new knowledge? Which will better enable the nurse to conduct and use nursing research? "Inasmuch as the problem also has plagued every other scholarly discipline and profession, the question of which is the appropriate doctoral degree for a nurse has never found and continues to find little consensus" (Metarazzo and Abdellah, 1971, p. 404).

The Age of Specialization

The concept of nursing specialties was literally unheard of before the influence of Florence Nightingale and the advent of modern nursing. Each nurse was expected to provide for patients no matter what illness caused the need for nursing care. In hospitals patients were not segregated according to diseases until the early decades of the twentieth century. This change may have been the initiating factor in the movement toward specialization, since patients were placed in specific areas according to medical diagnoses. Yet until World War II the majority of nurses worked as general staff nurses in hospitals, as pub-

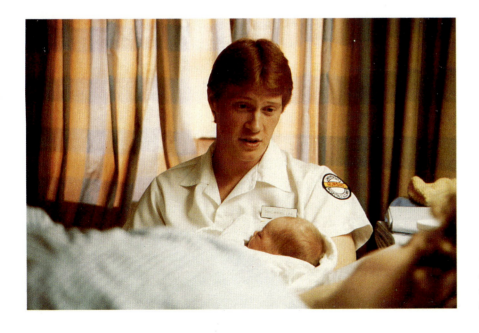

NURSE WITH A NEWBORN BABY. *Courtesy of The University of Iowa Hospitals and Clinics, Department of Nursing, Iowa City, Iowa.*

lic health nurses, and as private duty nurses. The scientific and medical advances made during and after this war resulted in a vast body of knowledge that gave impetus to medical specialties. These were deemed necessary so that expansion and utilization of the knowledge could occur.

Eventually the trend toward specialized care units gained momentum and various nursing roles evolved. These roles became known as *expanded* roles and *extended* roles. Although the terms are frequently used interchangeably, there is a difference between the two. The extended role refers to a physician extender with a cure orientation; the physician retains authority and decision-making power. The expanded role is an expansion or broadening of care-oriented nursing in which the nurse collaborates with the physician when indicated.

The first nursing specialists have existed since the late nine-

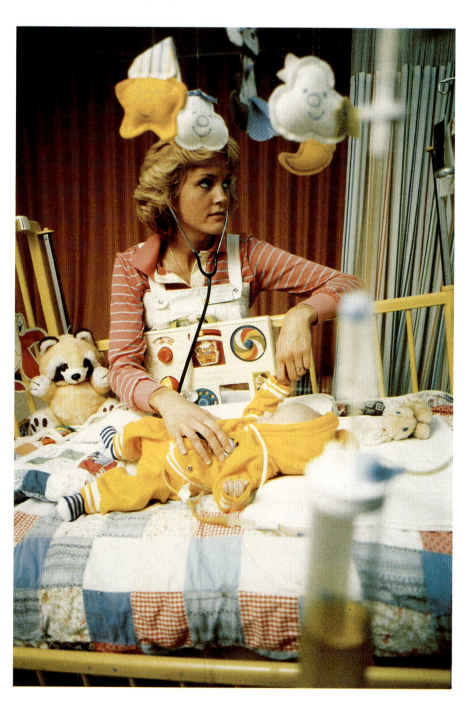

NURSE CHECKING THE HEARTBEAT OF A YOUNG CHILD ON A COLORFUL PATCHWORK BLANKET. *Courtesy of The University of Iowa Hospitals and Clinics, Department of Nursing, Iowa City, Iowa.*

teenth and early twentieth centuries: the nurse midwife and the nurse anesthetist. The training of nurse-midwives was a direct response to the need for improvement in maternal child care, the unregulated practice of untrained midwives, and the unavailability of obstetricians in poor rural areas. The role of nurse anesthetist developed as part of the increasing sophistication in surgery in the early 1900s, when it was recognized that trained assistants were needed to administer anesthetics. No longer was it safe or satisfactory to have untrained medical students or attendants administering anesthesia. These early specialists were recruited from the available pool of trained nurses to meet very specific societal demands and needs. Opposition from particular specialty groups in medicine and legal barriers to practice were among their greatest struggles. Unfortunately, the same struggles are occurring with current nursing specialization.

> Although nurse anesthetists and nurse midwives were initially trained and supervised by physicians, the development of autonomous clinical specialization in nursing has not been well received by medical groups. Opposition to the training and clinical practice of nurse midwives and nurse anesthetists continues to be an issue. . . . the nurse midwifery and nurse anesthetist conflicts have resulted in underutilization and inappropriate use of these highly skilled nurse specialists. Debate and ambivalence regarding their role continues to confuse the American public. The resolution of territorial disputes between nursing and medicine is long overdue. However, it can be anticipated that debate and conflict will continue as long as highly skilled nurse specialists are perceived as a "threat to the other groups' social and/or financial status or its power or base of control."
>
> *Krampitz, 1981, p. 62*

The need for legal restrictions on nursing practice or the placement of nursing practice under the direct supervision of medicine are concerns heard consistently in discussions of specialization in nursing. This is not surprising, since it has been documented historically that physicians have often tried to keep nursing under restraint. Now as before do nurses need to define and control their nursing practice and heed the words of Lavinia Dock:

> Nothing, I think dear Editor, is more trying to one's toleration than to see men—most of whom never did and never can comprehend what a woman's work really is, what its details are, or how it ought to be done—undertaking to instruct and train women in something so unquestionably her own special field as nursing. I do not limit this statement to men only, but will say that physicians, be they men or women, cannot teach nursing, any more than nurses can teach medicine. Medicine and nursing are not the same; and how-ever much we may learn from the physician about disease and its treatment, the whole field of nursing—as nursing is realized by the *patient* (the centre of the question)—is unknown to him. I agree that he can criticise nursing intelligently, but he cannot show how it ought to be done or do it himself, except in rare instances.
> We need, then, to recognize those qualities and characteristics in our work which are superior to what men can teach us, and to hold firmly to them, refusing to give them up, and most unremittingly should we resist all attempts to take our right

459

of teaching our own work out of our hands, putting nurses out of their true relation to their own calling, and bringing up a set of imperfect imitators of pseudoscientific men, mere satellites of the medical profession, who will be neither doctor nor nurse.

Dock, editorial, 1901

One other early nurse specialist bears mentioning—the industrial nurse. This specialty arose in response to the hazards and abnormal health conditions in shops, factories, and other fields of industrial labor. Initially, little concern was given to the care of injuries. In its early stages industrial nursing was a home visiting service; patient referrals were initiated by physicians. Ada Mayo Stewart was the first nurse in this specialty. She was hired by Fletcher D. Proctor in 1895 to act as a visiting nurse for the families of the employees of his Vermont Marble Company. The growth of industrial nursing was a slow one until the massive boom in the defense industry during World War II. Nurses were then rapidly employed in all types of manufacturing plants, a practice that in most instances was continued even after the war.

The 1960s witnessed another distinct growth period of specialization in nursing that has continued to the current time. All types of specialty areas—coronary care units, surgical intensive care units, medical intensive care units, burn units, dialysis units, oncology units—were developed in hospitals and necessitated the changing of nursing roles. In addition, gaps identified in the health care system of America in this era led nursing to experiment with the role of "clini-

MOBILE CRITICAL CARE UNIT. *Courtesy of The University of Iowa Hospitals and Clinics, Department of Nursing, Iowa City, Iowa.*

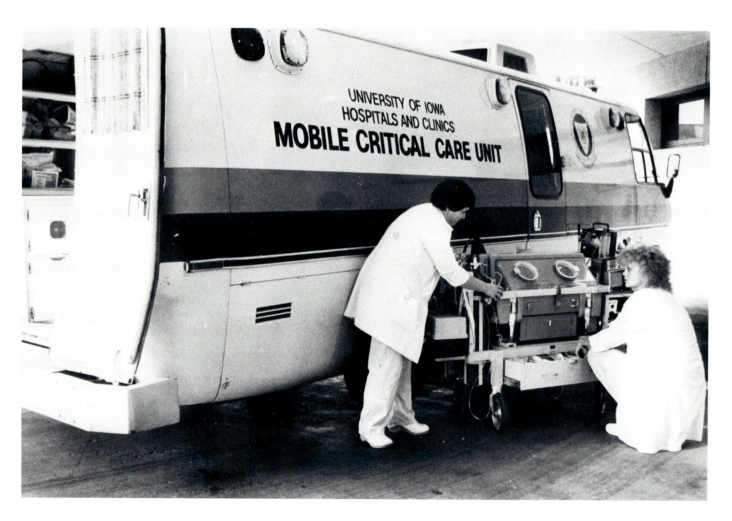

cal specialist" or "nurse clinician." This new concept allowed nurses to use their expertise, based on in-depth knowledge, for advanced nursing practice. Once again, nursing efforts were partially thwarted as hospital administrations frequently would not pay for such services and would assign responsibilities to the specialist head nurse or staff nurse. The specialist was thus prohibited or prevented from functioning in the clinician role. All obstacles to this role have not yet been overcome, but clinical specialists currently function in a variety of settings, including hospitals, outpatient facilities, in conjunction with individual or groups of physicians, and in private or joint practice with other nurse specialists and/or physicians. In 1954 the first *graduate* level program to prepare clinical specialists was developed by Hildegard E. Peplau at Rutgers University; the specialty area of the program was psychiatric nursing.

The "nurse practitioner" was also introduced in this period as the result of a specific demonstration funded by the Commonwealth Foundation at the University of Colorado in 1965. Dr. Henry Silver, a pediatrician, and Dr. Loretta Ford, a public health nurse of the University of Colorado, collaborated in this venture. This demonstration project resulted in the establishment of the pediatric nurse practitioner program, which was designed to prepare nurses to give comprehensive well-child care in ambulatory settings. The nurses were further taught to make judgments about acute or chronic conditions in children and to perform as primary practitioners in childhood emergencies. One effect of these innovations was the development of numerous new titles in nursing, such as *nurse clinician, clinical nurse specialist,* and *nurse practitioner.* All of these differed in meaning, requirements for preparation, and expected performance. It is clear that standard titles are lacking, as demonstrated by a list of over eighty different titles for nurse practitioners generated by Grippando (1977, p. 253). In addition, about twenty-seven organizations now represent various types of specialized nursing practice, and the list continues to grow. The American Nurses' Association, however, defined its position on the issue through a social policy statement:

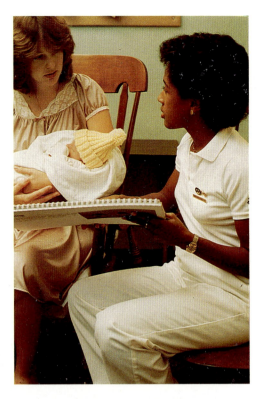

NURSE TALKING WITH A PATIENT. *Courtesy of The University of Iowa Hospitals and Clinics, Department of Nursing, Iowa City, Iowa.*

> The specialist in nursing practice is a nurse who, through study and supervised practice at the graduate level (master's or doctorate), has become expert in a defined area of knowledge and practice in a selected clinical area of nursing. Specialists in nursing practice are also generalists, in that they hold a baccalaureate in nursing, and therefore are able to provide the full range of nursing care. In addition, upon completion of a graduate degree in a university graduate program with an emphasis on clinical specialization, the specialist in nursing practice should meet the criteria for specialty certification through nursing's professional society.
>
> *American Nurses' Association, 1980*

The role of the nurse is constantly changing, and nursing practice is becoming more sophisticated. New theories, techniques, skills, and tools are being used in practice to meet the current needs of a society that is highly technological, complex, and dynamic. Specialization has led to the development of revised or new curricula in basic educational programs and the establishment of new programs in graduate education to prepare nurses to acquire the knowledge, skills, and responsibilities consistent with this role.

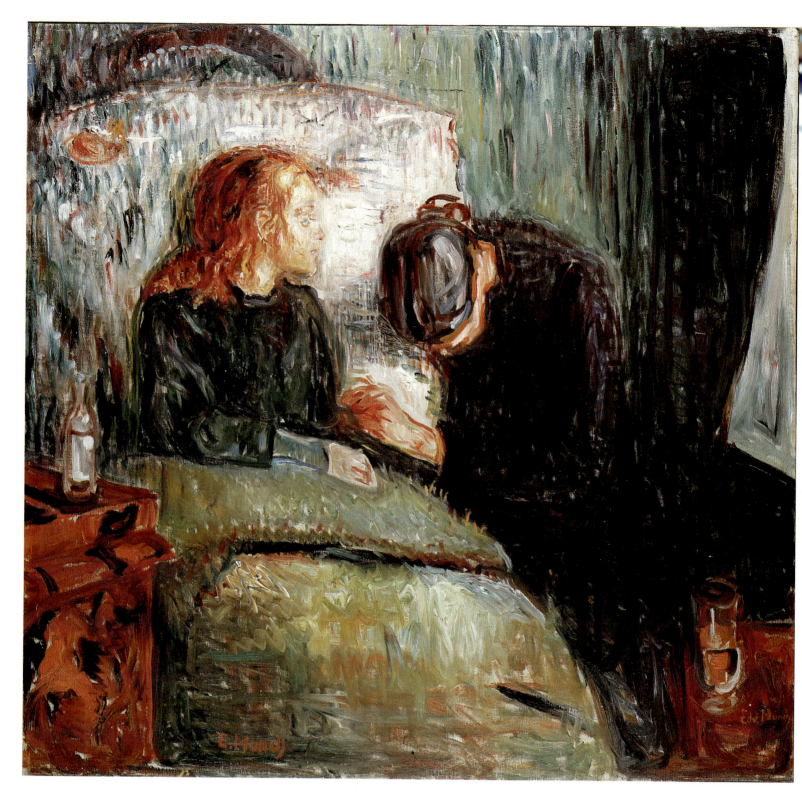

Edvard Munch, THE SICK CHILD, *1906–07.*
The Tate Gallery, London, England.

■ CONTINUED GROWTH OF ORGANIZATIONS

The American Nurses' Association and the National League for Nursing have continued to represent the interests of nursing since the restructuring process in 1952. Their combined achievements and contributions are many. Each has served to promote and improve conditions in nursing service, practice, education, research, and a

462

number of other related areas. Each has undergone some reorganization in programs in an attempt to keep pace with societal changes and demands. This period of change has resulted in advantages and disadvantages for both organizations.

The NLN adopted a new structure in 1967 to provide greater flexibility so that the national board of directors and the constituent leagues could enjoy a closer working relationship. The membership continued to include individuals and agencies in addition to the Assembly of Constituent Leagues for Nursing with six regional assemblies for planning, coordination, and implementation of programs — the councils of Associate Degree Programs, Baccalaureate and Higher Degree Programs, Diploma Programs, Practical Nursing Programs, Hospital and Related Institutional Nursing Services, Home Health Agencies and Community Health Services. Other changes occurred, including the hiring of a commercial firm to develop a new licensing examination for professional nurses (the State Board Test Pool of the NLN was relieved of this activity). Various issues that arose were dealt with in the most feasible manner possible. One action that evoked a tremendous response from agency members was an historic statement entitled "Nursing Roles — Scope and Preparation," issued by the NLN in February 1982. Through this statement the importance of a baccalaureate degree was recognized and accepted as an important credential for professional nursing.

The ANA has continued its efforts on behalf of individual nurses through its programs on economic and general welfare, its certification of practitioners, the development of standards for practice, and other significant activities in the service, practice, education, and research areas. Although the organization's classic "position paper" issued in 1965 did much toward the advancement of nursing, it also intensified controversy over the future direction of the hospital diploma program. This paper, prepared by the ANA Committee on Education, was adopted as a proposal for study by the ANA House of Delegates in 1964. It was released in 1965, proposed and approved by the ANA membership in 1966, and reaffirmed in 1978 when the ANA passed the Entry into Practice Resolution at the national convention. The statement and resolution, predicated on the need for improved nursing practice, concluded that:

> The education for all of those who are licensed to practice
> nursing should take place in institutions of higher education;
> minimum preparation for beginning professional nursing practice
> should be a baccalaureate degree; minimum preparation for
> beginning technical nursing practice should be an associate
> degree in nursing; education for assistants in the health service
> occupations should be short, intensive preservice programs in
> vocational education rather than on-the-job training.
>
> *American Nurses' Association, 1965*

At the 1982 ANA convention the House of Delegates voted for a major bylaw change that mandated the restructuring of the ANA commencing in 1984. The essence of this change was that state nurses' associations would be the units of membership in the ANA; the individual member would belong to ANA through state membership. Two objectives were to be achieved through this "federation model": the strengthening of ANA while allowing for flexibility and the granting of autonomy of state nurses' associations.

All nursing organizations have served to effect some aspect of change and provide the necessary communication for collective action. Consolidation of the organizations was achieved in 1952 to increase efficacy and efficiency and to ensure collaboration. Since that time, additional associations have arisen, usually in response to a major issue facing either a group or the entire profession. The current proliferation of nursing organizations may serve to dilute the profession and create disunity. Therefore caution must be exercised and measures taken to prevent this from occurring. The newer organizations are added testimony of the complexities and technologies that are being experienced within the society.

National Black Nurses' Association

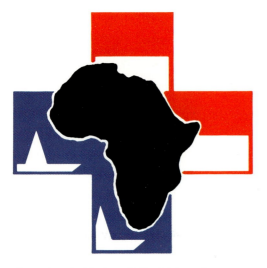

Logo for the National Black Nurses' Association. Courtesy of the National Black Nurses' Association, Boston, Massachusetts.

The National Association of Colored Graduate Nurses existed for almost four decades, until the ANA House of Delegates in 1948 voted to rapidly remove all barriers that prevented full participation of racial minority nurses in the association. To bypass some state associations, the ANA offered individual membership to Black nurses, and in 1949 approximately 634 Black nurses belonged to the organization. A special committee was also set up to explore comparable functions of the NACGN and the ANA.

> Encouraged by the developments on the national level, the black nurses voted in 1949 to dissolve NACGN, and formal dissolution occurred on January 31, 1951. The struggle for professional parity, they thought, was over. The dream of recognition and equality was finally to be realized.
>
> *Smith, 1975, p. 225*

The intent of Black nurses was to become a part of the mainstream of organized nursing and of the ANA. This was apparently not the total answer for Blacks and other minorities. "In many sections of the country, nurses are organizing in ethnically identifiable associations, because they have not felt they were integrated into the professional association" (Shaw, 1975, p. 8). Thus the emergence of the National Black Nurses' Association, Inc., in 1971, a structure that would not duplicate the functions of the ANA but would complement them so as to meet the special needs of Black nurses. This organization was begun through the efforts of Dr. Lauranne Sams, as the vehicle to assist with voiced concerns of Black nurses. Some of these concerns were the absence of Black nurses in positions of leadership; limited opportunities for Black nurses to share in shaping ANA policies and priorities; loss of identity of Black nurses; and limited recognition of their contribution to nursing. Membership was open to all licensed nurses (R.N. and L.P.N.) and nursing students. "Its future is uncertain, as would seem to be true of other emergent nursing organizations organized around race, sex, specialization, and division of labor" (Smith, 1975, p. 226).

American Association of Colleges of Nursing

Developments among the professional nursing associations included the establishment of the American Association of Colleges of Nursing (AACN) in 1969. This organization, which is a national association of nursing deans from colleges and universities, was created to provide administrators of baccalaureate and graduate degree nursing programs with an outlet for review of developments in the health field. Its numerous activities are executed to improve the practice of professional nursing by elevating the quality of degree programs. Schools of nursing are represented by their respective deans, who discuss common concerns. Through a concerted effort, the AACN has continually influenced public policy related to nursing and nursing education.

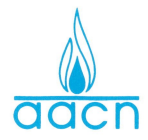

Logo for the American Association of Colleges of Nursing. Courtesy of the American Association of Colleges of Nursing, Washington, D.C.

National Federation for Specialty Nursing Organizations and the ANA

As nursing specialty organizations increased in the early 1970s, the numerous groups expressed the desire for unity and communication. They were dissatisfied with the ANA and believed that it was not concerned with the needs of the specialty groups. The American Association of Critical-Care Nurses called for a meeting in January 1972 to provide a forum to communicate and seek mechanisms for support and cooperation. The First National Congress in Nursing, as the meeting was called, was held at the Western White House in San Clemente, California.

At about the same time, in April 1972, the ANA board of directors decided to call a similar meeting "to explore how the organizations can work toward more coordination on areas of mutual interest" (National Federation for Specialty Nursing Organizations, 1984, p. 3). They invited the presidents and staff of nursing organizations, and mutual concerns were identified.

The First National Congress in Nursing was an historic event in which support and cooperation between specialty groups and the ANA were sought. It was decided that the group convened by the ANA and the National Nurses' Congress would merge. A third meeting was held in Denver in June of 1972. The title of the organization was determined to be The Federation of Specialty Nursing Organizations, and the ANA and twelve specialty groups became charter members. This organization has more than doubled its charter membership since its inception in 1973. It currently represents over 360,000 nurses throughout the United States who have differing clinical backgrounds. The name of the organization was changed to the National Federation for Specialty Nursing Organizations (NFSNO) in 1981.

American Academy of Nursing

The American Academy of Nursing was established in 1973 under the auspices of the American Nurses' Association. Membership in this academy is limited to those graduate nurses who are members of the ANA. A nurse who becomes a Fellow in the American Academy of Nursing (F.A.A.N.) has provided documentation of outstanding contributions to nursing. Potential members are nominated and voted upon by current members. Election to this group is considered an honor because members represent a selected group of leaders in the profession.

Nurses' Coalition for Action in Politics

Nurses for Political Action was started in 1972 as the first national organization of nurses to enter the political arena. It soon became affiliated with the ANA and has been regarded as its legislative and political action arm (Kalisch and Kalisch, 1978). The name was eventually changed to Nurses' Coalition for Action in Politics (N-CAP). N-CAP was organized as a nonpartisan and nonprofit association. Its expressed goal is the attainment of substantial political influence on national policy related to health care delivery. This group encourages and assists nurses to become social and political activists. It continues to strive for support for nursing from legislators and government officials.

American Association for the History of Nursing

Early American nursing leaders supported and promoted the study of nursing history and advocated its incorporation into curricula of schools of nursing. In particular, M. Adelaide Nutting, Lavinia L. Dock, and Isabel M. Stewart even became known as authorities on nursing history through the publication of their classic works on the subject. Dedicated to fostering greater understanding of and respect for nursing's past, they were committed to the belief that to understand and deal with problems and trends in nursing education and nursing practice nurses needed to be familiar with their history. These leaders believed that no one can get a true picture of present-day situations without finding out how the issues developed and what their underlying causes were. This general philosophy was expressed by Stewart:

> History can often help individuals to deal more effectively with persistent issues and conflicts by throwing light on their origins, and by indicating long-term trends that show the general direction in which things are moving. Educators who know something of the historical foundations of a system of education are also in a better position to evaluate the materials that have gone into it, to capitalize its assets and to eliminate what is no longer useful.
>
> *Stewart, 1943, p. viii*

Unfortunately, there has been no consistent support for historical inquiry. In fact, emphasis on the historical foundations of nursing decreased over time to the point that few nursing history courses are currently available in schools of nursing. Nor are there sufficient nursing faculty available who are prepared to teach them. In an effort to revive an interest in nursing history, a small number of interested nurses and historians began meeting as an historical methodology interest group in 1978 as part of a federally funded project for the development of nursing research in the Midwest. Originally called the International History of Nursing Society, the name of the group was changed in 1980 to the American Association for the History of

466

Nursing. The membership is comprised of individuals, nurses and non-nurses, who are interested in achieving the purpose of the association—to educate the public about the history and heritage of the nursing profession by:

a. Stimulating interest and national/international collaboration in promoting the history of nursing.
b. Encouraging research in the history of nursing.
c. Promoting the development of centers for preservation and use of materials of historical importance to nursing.
d. Serving as a resource for information related to nursing history.
e. Producing and distributing to members of the public educational materials regarding the history and heritage of the nursing profession.

AAHN, Bylaws, May 1983

The movement, although slow, has begun to return nursing history to the curricula of schools of nursing, to foster historical research and to collect, restore, and preserve historical materials relevant to nursing's rich heritage.

■ . . . IN CONCLUSION

Early and contemporary leaders in nursing consistently refer to nursing as an art as well as a science. Art in this context, however, is more than a static and linear concept. It involves a type of perception that is active, dynamic, and developing. An emotional quality guides the transformation of the material in art, but the role of intelligence or thinking is stressed. Art is thus a form of qualitative inquiry that draws its substance from the esthetic insight. Isabel M. Stewart frequently wrote about nursing as an art. She stressed that the nurse as a "true artist" was essential to the progression of nursing into something other than a highly skilled trade. Miss Stewart realized that numerous individuals thought of art and technique as a single entity, but she emphasized that a piece of work could be technically perfect and yet fall short of being a work of art. Technique, soul, mind, and imagination were all essential in the formation of a true artist.

> The real essence of nursing, as of any fine art, lies not in the mechanical details of execution, nor yet in the dexterity of the performer, but in the creative imagination, the sensitive spirit, and the intelligent understanding lying back of these techniques and skills. Without these, nursing may become a highly skilled trade, but it cannot be a profession or a fine art. All the rituals and ceremonials which our modern worship of efficiency may devise, and all our elaborate scientific equipment will not save us if the intellectual and spiritual elements in our art are subordinated to the mechanical, and if the means come to be regarded as more important than ends.
>
> *Stewart, 1929, p. 1*

The heritage of nursing is a rich one. Its history is a record of pioneering that reflects new advancements with each generation. Al-

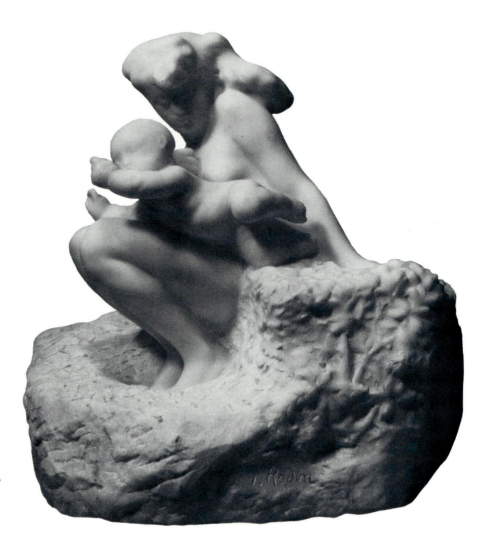

Auguste Rodin, WOMAN AND CHILD. *Marble, 43.2 × 44.5 × 33 cm. National Gallery of Art, Washington, D.C., Gift of Mrs. John W. Simpson 1942.*

though the entire story of the development of nursing has not been told in these pages, it is hoped that the reader will be able to envision the beauty and essence of its art as captured by some of the greatest masters in the world. This wide range of artwork adds significantly to an understanding of nursing itself because the history of nursing portrayed through art demonstrates the most valuable aspect of nursing: care and caring. Caring is the essence of nursing—caring for, caring with, and caring about. The pages of this book, through discussion and artwork, reflect the history of that caring as it has varied according to societal events and needs throughout the ages. No one, however, through pen or canvas, will ever be able to entirely capture the true art and the caring spirit of nursing. Both defy expression!

Nursing is an art; and if it is to be made an art,
it requires as exclusive a devotion, as hard
  a preparation, as any painter's or sculptor's
  work;
for what is the having to do with dead
  canvas or cold marble,
compared with having to do with the living
  body—the temple of God's spirit?
It is one of the Fine Arts;
I had almost said,
  the finest of the Fine Arts.

Florence Nightingale

LIST OF PLATES

472

473

475

REFERENCES

Unit 1

Alexander, W.: The history of women from earliest antiquity to the present time, London, 1782, C. Dilly.

Berdoe, E.: The origin and growth of the healing art, London, 1893, Swan, Sonnenschein & Co.

Catlin, G.: North American Indians, vol. 1, Edinburgh, John Grant, 1926.

Davison, W.C.: Nursing as the foundation of medicine, North Carolina Medical Journal, April 1943, p. 141.

Dock, L.L., and Stewart, I.M.: A short history of nursing, ed. 2, New York, 1925, G.P. Putnam's Sons.

Dolan, J.A., Fitzpatrick, M.L., and Hermann, E.K.: Nursing in society: a historical perspective, ed. 15, Philadelphia, 1983, W.B. Saunders Co.

Jamieson, E.M., and Sewall, M.F.: Trends in nursing history, Philadelphia, 1950, W.B. Saunders Co.

Mason, O.T.: Woman's share in primitive culture, New York, 1894, D. Appleton & Co.

Nutting, M.A., and Dock, L.L.: A history of nursing, vol. 1, New York, 1937, G.P. Putnam's Sons.

Robinson, V.: White caps: the story of nursing, Philadelphia, 1946, J.B. Lippincott Co.

Shryock, R.H.: The history of nursing: an interpretation of the social and medical factors involved, Philadelphia, 1959, W.B. Saunders Co.

Stewart, I.M.: How can we help to improve our teaching in nursing schools? Canadian Nurse 22:1593, 1918.

Stewart, I.M.: Popular fallacies about nursing education, The Modern Hospital 18:1, November 1921.

Stewart, I.M., and Austin, A.L.: A history of nursing, ed. 5, New York, 1962, G.P. Putnam's Sons.

Unit 2

Berdoe, E.: The origin and growth of the healing art, London, 1893, Swan, Sonnenschein & Co.

Bhishagratna, K.K.L., trans.: The sushruta samhita, Calcutta, 1907, J.N. Bose.

Castiglioni, A.: A history of medicine, ed. 2, trans. E.B. Krumbhaar, New York, 1947, Alfred A. Knopf.

Dolan, J.A., Fitzpatrick, M.L., and Hermann, E.K.: Nursing in society: a historical perspective, ed. 15, Philadelphia, 1983, W.B. Saunders Co.

Edwards, A.B.: Pharaohs, fellahs, and explorers, New York, 1892, Harper & Brothers.

Frank, C.M., Sr.: The historical development of nursing, Philadelphia, 1953, W.B. Saunders Co.

Goodnow, M.: Nursing history, Philadelphia, 1942, W.B. Saunders Co.

Hermann, P.: Conquest by man, New York, 1954, Harper & Brothers.

Jamieson, E.M., and Sewall, M.F.: Trends in nursing history, Philadelphia, 1950, W.B. Saunders Co.

Jones, W.H.S.: Malaria and Greek history, Manchester, 1909, Manchester University Press.

Kaviratna, A.C., trans.: Charaka-Samhita, Calcutta, n.d.

Lewis, F.: Quantum mechanics of politics—and life, Des Moines Sunday Register, November 13, 1983, p. 1C.

Lyons, A.S.: Ancient China. In Lyons, A.S., and Petrucelli, R.J.: Medicine: an illustrated history, New York, 1978, Harry N. Abrams, Inc.

Lyons, A.S.: Ancient Hebrew medicine. In Lyons, A.S., and Petrucelli, R.J.: Medicine: an illustrated history, New York, 1978, Harry N. Abrams, Inc.

Lyons, A.S.: Hippocrates. In Lyons, A.S., and Petrucelli, R.J.: Medicine: an illustrated history, New York, 1978, Harry N. Abrams, Inc.

Lyons, A.S.: Medicine in Roman times. In Lyons, A.S., and Petrucelli, R.J.: Medicine: an illustrated history, New York, 1978, Harry N. Abrams, Inc.

Nutting, M.A., and Dock, L.L.: A history of nursing, vol. 1, New York, 1937, G.P. Putnam's Sons.

Reinach, S.: Orpheus: a history of religions, New York, 1930, Liveright, Inc.

Rosen, G.: A history of public health, New York, 1958, M.D. Publications, Inc.

Sellew, G., and Nuesse, C.J.: A history of nursing, St. Louis, 1946, The C.V. Mosby Co.

Seymer, L.R.: A general history of nursing, London, 1932, Faber & Faber Ltd.

Shryock, R.H.: The history of nursing: an interpretation of the social and medical factors involved, Philadelphia, 1959, W.B. Saunders Co.

Stewart, I.M., and Austin, A.L.: A history of nursing, ed. 5, New York, 1962, G.P. Putnam's Sons.

Taylor, H.O.: Greek biology and medicine, Boston, 1922, Marshall Jones Co.

Unit 3

Christy, T.E.: Historical perspectives on accountability. In Williamson, J.A., editor: Current perspectives in nursing education, St. Louis, 1976, The C.V. Mosby Co.

Dock, L.L., and Stewart, I.M.: A short history of nursing, ed. 2, New York, 1925, G.P. Putnam's Sons.

Dolan, J.A., Fitzpatrick, M.L., and Hermann, E.K.: Nursing in society: a historical perspective, ed. 15, Philadelphia, 1983, W.B. Saunders Co.

Frank, Sister C.M.: The historical development of nursing, Philadelphia, 1953, W.B. Saunders Co.

Garrison, F.H.: An introduction to the history of medicine, Philadelphia, 1913, W.B. Saunders Co.

Goodnow, M.: Nursing history, Philadelphia, 1942, W.B. Saunders Co.

Haeser, H.: Geschichte Christlicher Krankenpflege und Pflegerschaften, Berlin, 1857, Anmerkungen.

Jamieson, E.M., and Sewall, M.F.: Trends in nursing history, Philadelphia, 1950, W.B. Saunders Co.

Kingsley, C.: Hypatia, New York, n.d., Lovell, Coryell & Co.

Lord, J.: Beacon lights of history, vol. 5, Great women, New York, 1885, Fords, Howard, & Hulbert.

Lyons, A.S.: Medicine under Islam (Arabic medicine). In Lyons, A.S., and Petrucelli, R.J.: Medicine: an illustrated history, New York, 1978, Harry N. Abrams, Inc.

Nutting, M.A., and Dock, L.L.: A history of nursing, vol. 1, New York, 1937, G.P. Putnam's Sons.

Petrucelli, R.J.: The dark ages. In Lyons, A.S., and Petrucelli, R.J.: Medicine: an illustrated history, New York, 1978, Harry N. Abrams, Inc.

Putnam, E.J.: The lady, New York, 1921, G.P. Putnam's Sons.

Robinson, V.: White caps: the story of nursing, Philadelphia, 1946, J.B. Lippincott Co.

Saint Jerome: Letters. In Nicene and post-Nicene fathers of the Christian church, vol. 6, New York, 1893, The Christian Literature Co.

Sellew, G., and Nuesse, C.J.: A history of nursing, St. Louis, 1946, The C.V. Mosby Co.

Seymer, L.R.: A general history of nursing, London, 1932, Faber & Faber Ltd.

Shryock, R.H.: The history of nursing: an interpretation of the social and medical factors involved, Philadelphia, 1959, W.B. Saunders Co.

Stewart, I.M.: The education of nurses, New York, 1943, The Macmillan Co.

Stewart, I.M., and Austin, A.L.: A history of nursing, ed. 5, New York, 1962, G.P. Putnam's Sons.

Tuker, M.A.R., and Malleson, H.: Handbook to Christian and ecclesiastical Rome, New York, 1900, The Macmillan Co.

Walsh, J.J.: The history of nursing, New York, 1929, P.J. Kenedy & Sons.

Unit 4

Austin, A.L.: History of nursing source book, New York, 1957, G.P. Putnam's Sons.

Butler, A.: The lives of the saints, 12 vols, ed. and rev. by Thurston and Attwater, London, 1934, Burns, Oates & Wasbourne, Ltd.

Chesterton, G.K.: St. Francis of Assisi, New York, 1924, George H. Doran Co.

Eckenstein, L.: Women under monasticism, Cambridge, 1896, Cambridge University Press.

Frank, Sister C.M.: The historical development of nursing, Philadelphia, 1953, W.B. Saunders Co.

Fuller, J.: The days of St. Anthony's fire, New York, 1968, Macmillan Publishing Co., Inc.

Garrison, F.H.: An introduction to the history of medicine, Philadelphia, 1913, W.B. Saunders Co.

Griffin, G.J., and Griffin, H.J.: History and trends of professional nursing, St. Louis, 1973, The C.V. Mosby Co.

Haggard, H.W.: Devils, drugs, and doctors, New York, 1929, Harper & Brothers.

Jamieson, E.M., and Sewall, M.F.: Trends in nursing history, Philadelphia, 1950, W.B. Saunders Co.

Lamb, H.: The crusades: iron men and saints, New York, 1930, Doubleday, Doran & Co.

Nutting, M.A., and Dock, L.L.: A history of nursing, vol. 1, New York, 1937, G.P. Putnam's Sons.

Robinson, V.: White caps: the story of nursing, Philadelphia, 1946, J.B. Lippincott Co.

Sellew, G., and Nuesse, C.J.: A history of nursing, St. Louis, 1946, The C.V. Mosby Co.

Seymer, L.R.: A general history of nursing, London, 1932, Faber & Faber Ltd.

Shryock, R.H.: The history of nursing: an interpretation of the social and medical factors involved, Philadelphia, 1959, W.B. Saunders Co.

Zinsser, H.: Rats, lice and history, New York, 1934, Blue Ribbon Books, Inc.

Unit 5

Cohen, I.B.: Florence Nightingale, Scientific American **250**:128, March 1984.

Cook, Sir Edward: The life of Florence Nightingale, vols. 1 and 2, London, 1914, The Macmillan Co.

Devane, R.S.: The failure of individualism, Dublin, 1948, Browne & Nolan, Ltd.

Dickens, C.: Martin Chuzzlewit, New York, 1910, The Macmillan Co.

Dolan, J.A., Fitzpatrick, M.L., and Hermann, E.K.: Nursing in society: a historical perspective, ed. 15, Philadelphia, 1983, W.B. Saunders Co.

Evans, A.D., and Howard, L.G.R.: The romance of the British voluntary hospital movement, 1930.

Frank, Sister C.M.: The historical development of nursing, Philadelphia, 1953, W.B. Saunders Co.

Goldsmith, M.: Florence Nightingale: the woman and the legend, London, 1937, Hodder & Stoughton.

Haggard, H.W.: Mystery, magic and medicine, New York, 1933, Doubleday, Doran & Co., Inc.

Howard, J.: An account of the principal lazarettos in Europe, London, 1791, Johnson, Dilly & Cadel.

Hunt, L.: Essays—the monthly nurse, London, 1889, Fredericke Warne & Co.

Jamieson, E.M., and Sewall, M.F.: Trends in nursing history, Philadelphia, 1950, W.B. Saunders Co.

Nightingale, F.: Notes on nursing, New York, 1860, D. Appleton & Co.

Nutting, M.A., and Dock, L.L.: A history of nursing, vol. 1, New York, 1937, G.P. Putnam's Sons.

Nutting, M.A., and Dock, L.L.: A history of nursing, vol. 1, New York, 1937, G.P. Putnam's Sons.

Petrucelli, R.J.: Art and science. In Lyons, A.S., and Petrucelli, R.J.: Medicine: an illustrated history, New York, 1978, Harry N. Abrams, Inc.

Robinson, V.: White caps: the story of nursing, Philadelphia, 1946, J.B. Lippincott Co.

Sellew, G., and Nuesse, C.J.: A history of nursing, St. Louis, 1946, The C.V. Mosby Co.

Seymer, L.R.: A general history of nursing, London, 1932, Faber & Faber Ltd.

Shryock, R.H.: The history of nursing: an interpretation of the social and medical factors involved, Philadelphia, 1959, W.B. Saunders Co.

Smith, F.B.: Florence Nightingale: reputation and power, London, 1982, Croom Helm.

Stewart, I.M.: Florence Nightingale—educator, Teachers College Record **41**:208, December 1939.

Strachey, G.L.: Florence Nightingale. In Eminent victorians, London, 1918, G.P. Putnam's Sons.

Whitney, J.: Elizabeth Fry, Boston, 1936, Brown & Co.

Woodham-Smith, C.: Florence Nightingale, New York, 1951, McGraw-Hill Book Co.

Works of Charles Lamb: On the genius and character of Hogarth, vol. 1, 1818.

Unit 6

Andrews, C.M.: The fathers of New England, vol. 6, The chronicles of America, New Haven, Conn., Yale University Press.

Ashley, J.: Hospitals, paternalism, and the role of the nurse, New York, 1976, Teachers College Press.

Austin, A.L.: History of nursing source book, New York, 1957, G.P. Putnam's Sons.

Baker, N.B.: Cyclone in calico: the story of Mary Ann Bickerdyke, Boston, 1952, Little, Brown & Co.

Boardman, M.T.: Under the Red Cross flag at home and abroad, Philadelphia, 1915, J.B. Lippincott Co.

Bradford, S.: Harriet Tubman: the Moses of her people, New York, 1961, Corinth Books.

Carlisle, R.: An account of Bellevue Hospital, New York, 1893, Society of Alumni of Bellevue Hospital.

Cheney, E.D., editor: Louisa May Alcott: her life, letters, and journals, Boston, 1889, Little, Brown & Co.

Dock, L.L.: History of the reform in nursing in Bellevue Hospital, American Journal of Nursing 2:90, 1901.

Donahue, M.P.: Isabel Maitland Stewart's philosophy of education, doctoral dissertation, 1981, The University of Iowa.

Frank, Sister C.M.: The historical development of nursing, Philadelphia, 1953, W.B. Saunders Co.

Gibbon, J.M., and Mathewson, M.S.: Three centuries of Canadian nursing, Toronto, 1947, The Macmillan Co. of Canada Ltd.

Goodnow, M.: Nursing history, Philadelphia, 1942, W.B. Saunders Co.

Grippando, G.M.: Nursing perspectives and issues, Albany, N.Y., 1983, Delmar Publishers, Inc. Reproduced by permission.

Hahn, R.E.: A history of nursing scrapbook, American Journal of Nursing 27:279, 1927.

Hale, S.: Lady nurses, Godey's Lady's Book and Magazine 82:188, 1871.

Henrietta, Sister: A famous New Orleans hospital, American Journal of Nursing 39:249, March 1939.

Jamieson, E.M., and Sewall, M.F.: Trends in nursing history, Philadelphia, 1950, W.B. Saunders Co.

Kane, J.N.: Famous first facts, New York, 1934, The H.W. Wilson Co.

Kenton, E., editor: The Jesuit relations and allied documents (1610–1791), New York, 1925, A. & C. Boni.

Lyons, A.S.: The nineteenth century (The beginnings of modern medicine). In Lyons, A.S., and Petrucelli, R.J.: Medicine: an illustrated history, New York, 1978, Harry N. Abrams, Inc.

Miller, H.S.: The history of Chi Eta Phi Sorority, Inc., 1932–1967, Washington, D.C., 1968, Negro Life and History, Inc.

Munson, H.W.: Linda Richards, American Journal of Nursing 48:552, 1948.

Nutting, M.A., and Dock, L.L.: A history of nursing, vol. 2, New York, 1907, G.P. Putnam's Sons.

Preston, A.: Nursing the sick and the training of nurses, Philadelphia, 1863, King & Baird.

Proceedings of the American Medical Association, New Orleans, May 1869. Reprinted in Medical News 20:339, 351, 1869.

Robinson, V.: White caps: the story of nursing, Philadelphia, 1946, J.B. Lippincott Co.

Roddis, L.H.: The U.S. Hospital Ship *Red Rover* (1862–1865), Military Surgeon 77:92, August 1935.

Selections from Leaves of Grass by Walt Whitman, New York, 1961, Avenel Books (Crown Publishers, Inc.).

Shryock, R.H.: The history of nursing: an interpretation of the social and medical factors involved, Philadelphia, 1959, W.B. Saunders Co.

Sigerist, H.E.: American medicine, New York, 1934, W.W. Norton & Co., Inc.

Stewart, I.M.: The hospital economics course from the students' standpoint, Paper presented before the Maryland Nurses' Association, 1909.

Stimson, J.C.: Earliest known connection of nurses with Army hospitals in the United States, American Journal of Nursing 25:18, 1925.

Walsh, J.J.: The history of nursing, New York, 1929, J.P. Kenedy & Sons.

Unit 7

American Nurses' Association: Proceedings of convention, 1950.

American Nurses' Association: The A.N.A. and you, New York, 1941, The Association.

Ashley, J.: Nursing and early feminism, American Journal of Nursing 75:1465, September 1975.

Association of Collegiate Schools of Nursing: Proceedings of the tenth annual meeting, 1943.

Brown, E.L.: Nursing for the future, New York, 1948, Russell Sage Foundation.

Christy, T.E.: Cornerstone for nursing education, New York, 1969a, Teachers College Press.

Christy, T.E.: Portrait of a leader: M. Adelaide Nutting, Nursing Outlook 17:20, January 1969b.

Christy, T.E.: Portrait of a leader: Isabel Maitland Stewart, Nursing Outlook 17:44, October 1969c. Copyright 1969, American Journal of Nursing Company. Reprinted with permission.

Christy, T.E.: The fateful decade, 1890–1900, American Journal of Nursing 75:1163, July 1975. Copyright 1975, American Journal of Nursing Company. Reprinted with permission.

Committee for the Study of Nursing Education: Nursing and nursing education in the United States, New York, 1923, The Committee.

Committee on the Grading of Nursing Schools: Nurses, patients, and pocketbooks, New York, 1928, The Committee.

Dock, L.L., and Stewart, I.M.: A short history of nursing, ed. 4, New York, 1938, G.P. Putnam's Sons.

Dolan, J.A., Fitzpatrick, M.L., and Hermann, E.K.: Nursing in society: a historical perspective, ed. 15, Philadelphia, 1983, W.B. Saunders Co.

Fitzpatrick, M.L.: Prologue to professionalism, Bowie, Md., 1983, Robert J. Brady Co.

Gibbon, J.M., and Mathewson, M.S.: Three centuries of Canadian nursing, Toronto, 1947, The Macmillan Co. of Canada Ltd.

Kansas State Nurses' Association: Lamps on the prairie: a history of nursing in Kansas, Kansas, 1942, Emporia Gazette Press.

Mollett, W.: On the necessity of legal registration for nurses, London, Nursing Record, June 28, 1888.

Nutting, M.A.: American Journal of Nursing 5:654, 1905.

Nutting, M.A.: Greetings. In Souvenir programme of the annual convention of the New York State Nurses' Association, the New York State League for Nursing, the New York Organization for Public Health Nursing, Albany, N.Y., October 27–29, 1925.

Nutting, M.A.: A sound economic basis for schools of nursing, New York, 1926, G.P. Putnam's Sons.

Nutting, M.A., and Dock, L.L.: A history of nursing, vol. 3, New York, 1912, G.P. Putnam's Sons.

Rathbone, W.: History and progress of district nursing, New York, 1890, The Macmillan Co.

Roberts, M.M.: American nursing: history and interpretation, New York, 1954, The Macmillan Co.

Roberts, M.M.: Lavinia Lloyd Dock—nurse, feminist, internationalist, American Journal of Nursing 56:176, February 1976.

Robinson, V.: White caps: the story of nursing, Philadelphia, 1946, J.B. Lippincott Co.

Seymer, L.R.: A general history of nursing, London, 1932, Faber & Faber Ltd.

Stewart, I.M.: Popular fallacies about nursing education, The Modern Hospital 18:1, November 1921.

Stewart, I.M.: The education of nurses, New York, 1943, The Macmillan Co.

Stewart, I.M.: Reminiscences of Isabel M. Stewart, New York, 1961, Oral History Research Office, Columbia University.

Stewart, I.M., and Austin, A.L.: A history of nursing, ed. 5, New York, 1962, G.P. Putnam's Sons.

Wald, L.D.: The house on Henry Street, New York, 1915, Henry Holt & Co.

Woolf, S.J.: Miss Wald at 70 sees her dreams realized, New York Times Magazine, March 7, 1937.

Unit 8

Aynes, E.A.: **From Nightingale to eagle**, Englewood Cliffs, N.J., 1973, Prentice-Hall, Inc.

Bureau of Medicine and Surgery: Navy Nurse Corps observes forty-fifth anniversary (release), Military Surgeon 113:45, July 1953.

Chow, R.K., and others: Historical perspectives of the U.S. Air Force, Army, Navy, Public Health Service, and Veterans Administration Nursing Services, Military Medicine 143:457, July 1978.

Christy, T.E.: Portrait of a leader: Annie Warburton Goodrich, Nursing Outlook 18:46, 1970.

Dreves, K.D.: Nurses in American history: Vassar Training Camp for nurses, American Journal of Nursing 75:2000, November 1975.

Flikke, J.O.: Nurses in action: the story of the Army Nurse Corps, Philadelphia, 1943, J.B. Lippincott Co.

Goodrich, A.W.: The school of nursing and the future, Proceedings of the thirty-eighth annual convention of the National League of Nursing Education, New York, 1932, National Headquarters.

Goostray, S.: Isabel Maitland Stewart, American Journal of Nursing 54:302, March 1954.

Joint Committee on Nursing in National Security: Mobilization of nurses for national security, American Journal of Nursing 51:78, February 1951. Copyright 1951, American Journal of Nursing Company. Reprinted with permission.

Judson, H.: Edith Cavell, New York, 1941, The Macmillan Co.

Kalisch, P.A., and Kalisch, B.J.: The advance of American nursing, Boston, 1978, Little, Brown & Co.

Lippmann, W.: American women and our wounded men, Washington Post, December 19, 1944. Reprinted in the Congressional Record as an extension of the remarks of Hon. Edith Nourse Rogers, December 19, 1944.

The nurses have not lagged behind, editorial, The Saturday Evening Post, April 28, 1945.

Nurses monument unveiled in Arlington, American Journal of Nursing 39:90, 1939.

Proceedings of the eighteenth annual convention of the American Society of Superintendents of Training Schools for Nursing, New York, 1912, The Society.

Roberts, M.M.: American nursing: history and interpretation, New York, 1954, The Macmillan Co.

Robinson, V.: White caps: the story of nursing, Philadelphia, 1946, J.B. Lippincott Co.

Shields, E.A., editor: Highlights in the history of the Army Nurse Corps, Washington, D.C., 1981, U.S. Army Center of Military History.

Smith, M.M.: Message from Sharon—a reading, The Connection 8:3, June 1984.

Song of the Army Nurse Corps. Music by Lou Singer. Words by Hy Zaret. Copyright 1944 by MCA Music, a division of MCA Inc., 445 Park Avenue, New York, New York 10022.

Stewart, I.M.: The education of nurses, New York, 1943, The Macmillan Co.

Stewart, I.M., and Austin, A.L.: A history of nursing, ed. 5, New York, 1962, G.P. Putnam's Sons.

U.S. Council of National Defense: First annual report of the Council of National Defense, fiscal year, 1917, Washington, D.C., 1917, U.S. Government Printing Office.

Vreeland, E.M.: Fifty years of nursing in the federal government nursing services, American Journal of Nursing 50:626, October 1950.

With the Army Nurse Corps in Korea, American Journal of Nursing 51:387, June 1951.

Unit 9

American Nurses' Association: First position paper on education for nurses, American Journal of Nursing 65:106, 1965.

American Nurses' Association: Nursing: a social policy statement, Kansas City, Mo., 1980, The Association.

Dennison, C.: Nursing service in the emergency room, American Journal of Nursing 42:777, July 1942.

Dock, L.L.: Editorial, American Journal of Nursing, vol. 2, December 1901.

Fitzpatrick, M.L.: Prologue to professionalism, Bowie, Md., 1983, Robert J. Brady Co.

Grace, H.K.: The development of doctoral education in nursing: a historical perspective. In Chaska, N.L., editor: The nursing professional—views through the mist, New York, 1978, McGraw-Hill Book Co.

Grippando, G.M.: Nursing perspectives and issues, Albany, N.Y., 1977, Delmar Publishers, Inc.

Haldeman, J.C., and Abdellah, F.G.: Concepts of progressive patient care, Hospitals 33:38, 1959.

Hall, L.: A center for nursing, Nursing Outlook 11:805, 1963.

Henderson, V.: The nature of nursing, New York, 1966, Macmillan Publishing Co., Inc.

Kalisch, P.A., and Kalisch, B.J.: The advance of American nursing, Boston, 1978, Little, Brown & Co.

King, I.M.: Toward a theory of nursing, New York, 1971, John Wiley & Sons, Inc.

Krampitz, S.D.: Clinical specialization: historical antecedents of today's issues. In McCloskey, J.C., and Grace, H.K.: Current issues in nursing, Boston, 1981, Blackwell Scientific Publications, Inc.

Lambertson, E.C.: Nursing team organization and functioning, New York, 1953, Teachers College, Columbia University.

Marram, G., Barrett, M., and Bevis, E.: Primary nursing: a model for individualized care, ed. 2, St. Louis, 1979, The C.V. Mosby Co.

McManus, R.L.: Isabel M. Stewart—foremost researcher, Nursing Research **2**:6, Winter 1962.

Metarazzo, J.D., and Abdellah, F.H.: Doctoral education for nurses in the United States, Nursing Research **20**:404, 1971.

National Federation for Specialty Nursing Organizations Public Relations Committee: NFSNO: the first ten years, Washington, D.C., 1984, The Federation.

Newton, M.E.: Florence Nightingale's philosophy of life and education, unpublished dissertation, 1949, Leland Stanford Junior University.

Nightingale, F.: Notes on nursing, New York, 1860, D. Appleton & Co.

Reeder, S.J.: The social context of nursing. In Chaska, N.L., editor: The nursing profession: views through the mist, New York, 1978, McGraw-Hill Book Co.

Rogers, M.E.: An introduction to the theoretical basis of nursing, Philadelphia, 1970, F.A. Davis Co.

Shaw, E.: The black nurse—then, now, and ? Paper presented for continuing education, Nashville, Tenn., 1973, Meharry Medical College.

Smith, G.R.: From invisibility to blackness: the story of the National Black Nurses' Association, Nursing Outlook **23**:225, April 1975.

Stewart, I.M.: The science and art of nursing, editorial, Nursing Education Bulletin **2**:1, Winter 1929.

Styles, M.M.: Doctoral education in nursing: the current situation in historical perspective. In National Conference on Doctoral Education in Nursing, Philadelphia, 1977, University of Pennsylvania.

Styles, M.M.: On nursing: toward a new endowment, St. Louis, 1982, The C.V. Mosby Co.

Whitehead, A.N.: The aims of education and other essays, New York, 1929, The Macmillan Co.

SELECTED BIBLIOGRAPHY

Abdellah, F.G., and Levine, E.: Better patient care through nursing research, New York, 1979, Macmillan Publishing Co., Inc.

Abdellah, F.G., and others: Patient centered approaches to nursing, New York, 1960, Macmillan Publishing Co., Inc.

Adams, F.: The genuine words of Hippocrates, Baltimore, 1939, Williams & Wilkins Co.

Addams, J.: Forty years at Hull House, New York, 1935, The Macmillan Co.

Albert, J.: Air evacuation from Korea—a typical flight, Military Surgeon 112:256, 1953.

Alcott, L.M.: Hospital sketches, Boston, 1885, Roberts Brothers.

Alcott, L.M.: Hospital sketches, camp and fireside stories, Boston, 1963, James Redpath.

Alexander, W.: The history of women from earliest antiquity to the present time, London, 1782, C. Dilly.

Alger, R.A.: The Spanish-American War, New York, 1901, Harper & Brothers.

American Foundation for Mental Hygiene: The mental hygiene movement: origin, objects and work of the National Committee and of the American Foundation for Mental Hygiene, New York, 1938, The Foundation.

American Journal of Nursing: The story of the journal, New York, 1950, The Journal.

American Nurses' Association: The A.N.A. and you, New York, 1941, The Association.

American Nurses' Association: Proceedings of convention, 1950.

American Nurses' Association: First position paper on education for nurses, American Journal of Nursing 65:106, 1965.

American Nurses' Association: Nursing: a social policy statement, Kansas City, Mo., 1980, The Association.

Andrews, C.M.: The fathers of New England, vol. 6, The chronicles of America, New Haven, Conn., Yale University Press.

Armstrong, G.: The summer of pestilence: a history of yellow fever, Philadelphia, 1856, J.B. Lippincott & Co.

Ashley, J.: Nursing and early feminism, American Journal of Nursing 75:1465, September 1975.

Ashley, J.: Hospitals, paternalism, and the role of the nurse, New York, 1976, Teachers College Press.

Association of Collegiate Schools of Nursing: Proceedings of the tenth annual meeting, 1943.

Auel, J.M.: The clan of the cave bear, New York, 1980, Bantam Books, Inc.

Austin, A.L.: History of nursing source book, New York, 1957, G.P. Putnam's Sons.

Austin, A.L.: The Woolsey sisters of New York: 1860–1900, Philadelphia, 1971, American Philosophical Society.

Aynes, E.A.: From Nightingale to eagle, Englewood Cliffs, N.J., 1973, Prentice-Hall, Inc.

Bache, D.: The place of the female nurse in the Army, Journal of the Military Service Institution 25:307, 1899.

Bacon, F.: Founding of the Connecticut training school for nurses, Trained Nurse 15:187, 1895.

Baker, N.B.: Cyclone in calico: the story of Mary Ann Bickerdyke, Boston, 1952, Little, Brown & Co.

Baker, R.: The first woman doctor: the story of Elizabeth Blackwell, M.D., New York, 1944, Julian Messner.

Baker, R.: America's first trained nurse, Linda Richards, New York, 1959, Julian Messner.

Barrus, C.: Nursing the insane, New York, 1908, The Macmillan Co.

Barton, G.: Angels of the battlefield: an history of the labors of the Catholic sisterhoods in the late Civil War, Philadelphia, 1897, Catholic Publishing Co.

Barton, W.E.: Life of Clara Barton, Boston, 1922, Houghton-Mifflin Co.

Bedford, W.K.R., and Holbeche, R.: The order of the Hospital of St. John of Jerusalem, London, 1902, F.E. Robinson & Co.

Berdoe, E.: The origin and growth of the healing art, London, 1893, Swan, Sonnenschein & Co.

Bessey, M.: Magic and the supernatural, London, 1966, Spring Books.

Bhishagratna, K.K.L., trans.: The sushruta samhita, Calcutta, 1907, J.N. Bose.

Billings, J.S., and Hurd, H.M., editors: Hospitals, dispensaries, and nursing, International Congress of Charities, Correction and Philanthropy, sec. 3, Baltimore, 1894, Johns Hopkins Press.

Blackwell, E.: Pioneer work in opening the medical profession to women: autobiographical sketches, New York, 1895, Longmans, Green & Co.

Boardman, M.T.: Under the Red Cross flag at home and abroad, Philadelphia, 1915, J.B. Lippincott Co.

Boyd, L.C.: State registration for nurses, ed. 2, Philadelphia, 1915, W.B. Saunders Co.

Bradford, S.: Harriet Tubman: the Moses of her people, New York, 1961, Corinth Books.

Brainard, A.M.: The evolution of public health nursing, Philadelphia, 1922, W.B. Saunders Co.

Breasted, J.H.: The conquest of civilization, New York, 1938, Harper & Brothers.

Breay, M., and Fenwick, E.G.: The history of the International Council of Nurses, 1899–1925, Geneva, 1931, The International Council of Nurses.

Breckinridge, M.: Wide neighborhood, New York, 1952, Harper & Brothers.

Bridges, D.C.: A history of the International Council of Nurses, 1899–1964, Philadelphia, 1967, J.B. Lippincott Co.

Bridgman, M.: Collegiate education for nursing, New York, 1953, Russell Sage Foundation.

Brown, A.F.: Research in nursing, Philadelphia, 1958, W.B. Saunders Co.

Brown, E.L.: Nursing as a profession, New York, 1936, Russell Sage Foundation.

Brown, E.L.: Nursing for the future, New York, 1948, Russell Sage Foundation.

Brown, E.L.: Nursing reconsidered: a study of change. I. The professional role in institutional nursing, Philadelphia, 1970, J.B. Lippincott Co.

Brown, E.L.: Nursing reconsidered: a study of change. II. The professional role in community nursing, Philadelphia, 1971, J.B. Lippincott Co.

Bulwer-Lytton, E.: The last days of Pompeii, New York, 1834, Dodd, Mead, & Co.

Bureau of Medicine and Surgery: Navy Nurse Corps observes forty-fifth anniversary (release), Military Surgeon 113:45, July 1953.

Burgess, M.A.: Nurses, patients and pocketbooks, New York, 1928, National League of Nursing Education.

Burgess, M.A.: Nursing schools today and tomorrow, New York, 1934, National League of Nursing Education.

Butler, A.: The lives of the saints, 12 vols., ed. and rev. by Thurston and Attwater, London, 1934, Burns, Oates & Wasbourne, Ltd.

Caldwell, T.: Dear and glorious physician, New York, 1959, Doubleday & Co.

Carlisle, R.: An account of Bellevue Hospital, New York, 1893, Society of Alumni of Bellevue Hospital.

Carnegie, M.E.: Historical perspectives of nursing research, Boston, 1976, Nursing Archive of Boston University.

Castiglioni, A.: A history of medicine, ed. 2, trans. E.B. Krumbhaar, 1947, Alfred A. Knopf.

Catlin, G.: North American Indians, vol. 1, Edinburgh, John Grant, 1926.

Caulfield, E.: The infant welfare movement in the eighteenth century, New York, 1931, Paul B. Hoeber.

Cheney, E.D., editor: Louisa May Alcott: her life, letters, and journals, Boston, 1889, Little, Brown & Co.

Chesterton, G.K.: St. Francis of Assisi, New York, 1924, George H. Doran Co.

Chow, R.K., and others: Historical perspectives of the U.S. Air Force, Army, Navy, Public Health Service, and Veterans Administration Nursing Services, Military Medicine 143:457, July 1978.

Christy, T.E.: Cornerstone for nursing education: a history of division of nursing education of Teachers College, Columbia University, 1899–1947, New York, 1969, Teachers College Press.

Christy, T.E.: Portrait of a leader: Isabel Hampton Robb, Nursing Outlook 17:26, 1969.

Christy, T.E.: Portrait of a leader: Isabel Maitland Stewart, Nursing Outlook 17:44, 1969.

Christy, T.E.: Portrait of a leader: Lavinia Lloyd Dock, Nursing Outlook 17:72, 1969.

Christy, T.E.: Portrait of a leader: M. Adelaide Nutting, Nursing Outlook 17:20, 1969.

Christy, T.E.: Portrait of a leader: Annie Warburton Goodrich, Nursing Outlook 18:46, 1970.

Christy, T.E.: Portrait of a leader: Lillian D. Wald, Nursing Outlook 18:50, 1970.

Christy, T.E.: Equal rights for women: voices from the past, American Journal of Nursing 71:288, 1971.

Christy, T.E.: The fateful decade, 1890–1900, American Journal of Nursing 75:1163, July 1975.

Christy, T.E.: Historical perspectives on accountability. In Williamson, J.A., editor: Current perspectives in nursing education, St. Louis, 1976, The C.V. Mosby Co.

Christy, T.E.: Clinical practice as a function of nursing education: a historical analysis, Nursing Outlook 28:493, 1980.

Churchill, F.: On the theory and practice of midwifery, Philadelphia, 1851, Blanchard & Lea.

Clay, R.M.: Medieval hospitals of England, London, 1909, Methuen & Co.

Cohen, I.B.: Florence Nightingale, Scientific American 250:128, March 1984.

Commission on Nursing Research, American Nurses' Association:

Priorities for research in nursing, Kansas City, Mo., 1976, The Association.

Committee on Nursing and Nursing Education in the United States: Nursing and nursing education in the United States, New York, 1928, The Macmillan Co.

Committee on the Structure of National Nursing Organizations: New horizons in nursing, New York, 1950, The Macmillan Co.

Cook, Sir Edward: The life of Florence Nightingale, vols. 1 and 2, London, 1914, The Macmillan Co.

Cooper, P.: Navy nurse, New York, 1946, McGraw-Hill Book Co.

Cope, Z.: Florence Nightingale and the doctors, Philadelphia, 1958, J.B. Lippincott Co.

Crawford, R.: The plague and pestilence in literature and art, New York, 1914, Oxford University Press.

Cunningham, J.T.: Clara Maass—a nurse—a hospital—a spirit, New Jersey, 1976, Rae Publishing Co.

Curtayne, A.: St. Catherine of Siena, New York, 1935, Sheed & Ward.

Curtis and Denny: Early history of the Boston Training School, American Journal of Nursing 2:331, 1902.

Damel-Rops, H.: Monsieur Vincent, New York, 1961, Hawthorn Books.

Davison, W.C.: Nursing as the foundation of medicine, North Carolina Medical Journal, April 1943, p. 141.

Defoe, D.: A journal of the plague year (1721), New York, 1966, Penguin Books.

Delano, J.A.: Nursing as it relates to the war, American Journal of Nursing 18:1064, 1918.

Delano, J.A.: How American nurses helped win the war, Modern Hospital 12:7, 1919.

Dennison, C.: Nursing service in the emergency room, American Journal of Nursing 42:777, July 1942.

Deutsch, A.: Mentally ill in America: a history of their care and treatment from colonial times, New York, 1937, Doubleday.

Deutsch, A.: The mentally ill in America, ed. 2, New York, 1946, Columbia University Press.

Devane, R.S.: The failure of individualism, Dublin, 1948, Browne & Nolan, Ltd.

Dickens, C.: A tale of two cities, New York, 1859, E.P. Dutton & Co.

Dickens, C.: Martin Chuzzlewit, New York, 1910, The Macmillan Co.

Dock, L.L.: Textbook of materia medica for nurses, New York, 1890, G.P. Putnam's Sons.

Dock, L.L.: Editorial, American Journal of Nursing, vol. 2, December 1901.

Dock, L.L.: History of the reform in nursing in Bellevue Hospital, American Journal of Nursing 2:90, 1901.

Dock, L.L.: Hygiene and morality, New York, 1912, G.P. Putnam's Sons.

Dock, L.L., and others: History of American Red Cross nursing, New York, 1922, The Macmillan Co.

Dock, L.L., and Stewart, I.M.: A short history of nursing, ed. 2, New York, 1925, G.P. Putnam's Sons.

Dock, L.L., and Stewart, I.M.: A short history of nursing, ed. 4, New York, 1938, G.P. Putnam's Sons.

Dolan, J.A., Fitzpatrick, M.L., and Hermann, E.K.: Nursing in society: a historical perspective, ed. 15, Philadelphia, 1983, W.B. Saunders Co.

Donahue, M.P.: Isabel Maitland Stewart's philosophy of education, doctoral dissertation, 1981, The University of Iowa.

Douglas, M., editor: Witchcraft: confessions and accusations, London, 1970, Tavistock Publications.

Dreves, K.D.: Nurses in American history: Vassar Training Camp for nurses, American Journal of Nursing **75**:2000, November 1975.

Duffus, R.L.: Lillian Wald, neighbor and crusader, New York, 1938, The Macmillan Co.

Eckenstein, L.: Women under monasticism, Cambridge, 1896, Cambridge University Press.

Edwards, A.B.: Pharaohs, fellahs, and explorers, New York, 1892, Harper & Brothers.

Ehrenreich, B., and English, D.: Witches, midwives, and nurses: a history of women healers, New York, 1973, The Feminist Press.

Elgood, C.: A medical history of Persia, London, 1951, Cambridge University Press.

Elmore, J.A.: Black nurses: their service and their struggle, American Journal of Nursing **76**:435, 1976.

Evans, A.D., and Howard, L.G.R.: The romance of the British voluntary hospital movement, 1930.

Faddis, M.O.: A school of nursing comes of age, Cleveland, 1973, The Alumni Association of The Frances Payne Bolton School of Nursing.

Faulkner, H.V.: The quest for social justice, 1899–1914, New York, 1931, The Macmillan Co.

Faxon, N.W.: The hospital in contemporary life, Cambridge, Mass., 1949, Harvard University Press.

Fiske, A.: Structure and functions of the body: a handbook of anatomy and physiology for nurses and others desiring a practical knowledge of the subject, Philadelphia, 1911, W.B. Saunders Co.

Fitzpatrick, M.L.: The National Organization for Public Health Nursing, 1912–1952: development of a practice field, New York, 1975, National League for Nursing.

Fitzpatrick, M.L.: Prologue to professionalism, Bowie, Md., 1983, Robert J. Brady Co.

Flanagan, L.C.: One strong voice: the story of the American Nurses' Association, Kansas City, Mo., 1976, The Association.

Flikke, J.O.: Nurses in action: the story of the Army Nurse Corps, Philadelphia, 1943, J.B. Lippincott Co.

Foran, J.K., and Morrissey, S.H.: Jeanne Mance; or, the angel of the colony, Montreal, 1931, Sisters of the Hotel Dieu.

Frank, Sister C.M.: The historical development of nursing, Philadelphia, 1953, W.B. Saunders Co.

Fuller, J.: The days of St. Anthony's fire, New York, 1968, Macmillan Publishing Co., Inc.

Garrison, F.H.: An introduction to the history of medicine, Philadelphia, 1913, W.B. Saunders Co.

Gelinas, A.: Nursing and nursing education, New York, 1946, The Commonwealth Fund.

Gibbon, E.: The decline and fall of the Roman Empire, New York, Viking Press.

Gibbon, J.M., and Mathewson, M.S.: Three centuries of Canadian nursing, Toronto, 1947, The Macmillan Co. of Canada Ltd.

Ginzberg, E.: A pattern of hospital care, New York, 1949, Columbia University Press.

Giordani, I.: Catherine of Siena, Milwaukee, 1959, Bruce Publishing Co.

Goldsmith, M.: Florence Nightingale: the woman and the legend, London, 1937, Hodder & Stoughton.

Goodnow, M.: Nursing history, Philadelphia, 1942, W.B. Saunders Co.

Goodrich, A.W.: The school of nursing and the future, Proceedings of the thirty-eighth annual convention of the National League of Nursing Education, New York, 1932, National Headquarters.

Goodrich, A.W.: The social and ethical significance of nursing, New York, 1932, The Macmillan Co.

Goostray, S.: Isabel Maitland Stewart, American Journal of Nursing **54**:302, March 1954.

Grace, H.K.: The development of doctoral education in nursing: a historical perspective. In Chaska, N.L., editor: The nursing professional—views through the mist, New York, 1978, McGraw-Hill Book Co.

Grattan, J.H.G., and Singer, C.: Anglo-Saxon magic and medicine, New York, 1952, Oxford University Press.

Griffin, G.J., and Griffin, H.J.: History and trends of professional nursing, St. Louis, 1973, The C.V. Mosby Co.

Grippando, G.M.: Nursing perspectives and issues, Albany, N.Y., 1977, Delmar Publishers, Inc.

Grosvenor, G., and others: Everyday life in ancient times, Washington, D.C., National Geographic Society.

Haeser, H.: Geschichte Christlicher Krankenpflege und Pflegerschaften, Berlin, 1857, Anmerkungen.

Haggard, H.W.: Devils, drugs, and doctors, New York, 1929, Harper & Brothers.

Haggard, H.W.: Mystery, magic and medicine, New York, 1933, Doubleday, Doran & Co., Inc.

Hahn, R.E.: A history of nursing scrapbook, American Journal of Nursing **27**:279, 1927.

Haldeman, J.C., and Abdellah, F.G.: Concepts of progressive patient care, Hospitals **33**:38, 1959.

Hale, S.: Lady nurses, Godey's Lady's Book and Magazine **82**:188, 1871.

Hall, L.: A center for nursing, Nursing Outlook **11**:805, 1963.

Hampton, I.A.: Nursing: its principles and practice for hospital and private use, Philadelphia, 1893, W.B. Saunders Co.

Hampton, I.A., and others: Nursing of the sick—1893, New York, 1949, McGraw-Hill Book Co.

Hanaford, P.: Daughters of America, or women of the century, Augusta, Me., 1882, True & Co.

Harnack, A.: Luke, the physician, New York, 1909, G.P. Putnam's Sons.

Henderson, V.: The nature of nursing, New York, 1966, Macmillan Publishing Co., Inc.

Henrietta, Sister: A famous New Orleans hospital, American Journal of Nursing **39**:249, March 1939.

Hermann, P.: Conquest by man, New York, 1954, Harper & Brothers.

Hill, D.: Magic and superstition, London, 1968, Hamlyn Publishing Group.

Hobson, W.: World health and history, Bristol, 1963, John Wright & Sons.

Holland, M.A.: Our Army nurses, Boston, 1895, B. Wilkins & Co.

Howard, J.: An account of the principal lazarettos in Europe, London, 1791, Johnson, Dilly & Cadel.

Hughes, E.C., Hughes, H.M., and Deutscher, I.: Twenty thousand nurses tell their story, Philadelphia, 1958, J.B. Lippincott Co.

Hunt, L.: Essays—the monthly nurse, London, 1889, Frederick Warne & Co.

Jacobs, J.B.: Elizabeth Fry, Pastor Fliedner and Florence Nightingale, Annals of Medical History **3**:17, 1921.

Jamieson, E.M., and Sewall, M.F.: Trends in nursing history, Philadelphia, 1950, W.B. Saunders Co.

Johns, E., and Pfefferkorn, B.: An activity analysis of nursing, 1934, New York Committee on the Grading of Nursing Schools.

Johns, E., and Pfefferkorn, B.: The Johns Hopkins Hospital School of Nursing, 1889–1949, Baltimore, 1954, Johns Hopkins University Press.

Joint Committee on Nursing in National Security: Mobilization of nurses for national security, American Journal of Nursing **51**:78, February 1951.

Jolly, E.R.: Nuns of the battlefield, Providence, R.I., 1927, Providence Visitor Press.

Jones, W.H.S.: Malaria and Greek history, Manchester, 1909, Manchester University Press.

Judson, H.: Edith Cavell, New York, 1941, The Macmillan Co.

Kalisch, P.A., and Kalisch, B.J.: The advance of American nursing, Boston, 1978, Little, Brown & Co.

Kane, J.N.: Famous first facts, New York, 1934, The H.W. Wilson Co.

Kansas State Nurses' Association: Lamps on the prairie: a history of nursing in Kansas, Kansas, 1942, Emporia Gazette Press.

Kavanagh, J.: Women of Christianity, New York, 1852, D. Appleton Co.

Kaviratna, A.C., trans.: Charaka-Samhita, Calcutta, n.d.

Kellogg, F.S.: Mother Bickerdyke as I knew her, Chicago, 1907, Unity Publishing.

Kelly, H.A.: Walter Reed and yellow fever, New York, 1923, G.P. Putnam's Sons.

Kenton, E., editor: The Jesuit relations and allied documents (1610–1791), New York, 1925, A. & C. Boni.

Kernodle, P.B.: Red Cross nurse in action: 1882–1948, New York, 1949, Harper & Brothers.

Kimber, D.C., and Gray, C.E.: Anatomy and physiology for nurses, New York, 1893, The Macmillan Co.

King, I.M.: Toward a theory of nursing, New York, 1971, John Wiley & Sons, Inc.

King, L.S.: The medical world of the eighteenth century, Chicago, 1958, University of Chicago Press.

Kingsley, C.: Hypatia, New York, n.d., Lovell, Coryell & Co.

Kramer, M.: Reality shock: why nurses leave nursing, St. Louis, 1974, The C.V. Mosby Co.

Krampitz, S.D.: Clinical specialization: historical antecedents of today's issues. In McCloskey, J.C., and Grace, H.K.: Current issues in nursing, Boston, 1981, Blackwell Scientific Publications, Inc.

Lamb, H.: The crusades: iron men and saints, New York, 1930, Doubleday, Doran & Co.

Lambertsen, E.C.: Nursing team organization and functioning, New York, 1953, Teachers College, Columbia University.

Lambertsen, E.C.: Education for nursing leadership, Philadelphia, 1958, J.B. Lippincott Co.

Lazaro, A.R.: The role of the flight nurse in air evacuation, Military Surgeon **105**:60, 1949.

Leake, C.D.: The old Egyptian medical papyri, Lawrence, 1952, University of Kansas Press.

Lee, E.: History of the School of Nursing of the Presbyterian Hospital, 1892–1942, New York, 1942, G.P. Putnam's Sons.

Lesnik, M.J., and Anderson, B.L.: Legal aspects of nursing, Philadelphia, 1947, J.B. Lippincott Co.

Lewis, E.P.: A collection of editorials from Nursing Outlook 1971–1980, American Journal of Nursing Company, 1980.

Lewis, F.: Quantum mechanics of politics—and life, Des Moines Sunday Register, p. 1C, November 13, 1983.

Lin, Y.: The wisdom of China and India, New York, 1942, Random House.

Link, E.P.: Elizabeth Blackwell, citizen and humanitarian, Woman Physician **26**:451, 1971.

Lippmann, W.: American women and our wounded men, Washington Post, December 19, 1944. Reprinted in the Congressional Record as an extension of the remarks of Hon. Edith Nourse Rogers, December 19, 1944.

Longmore, T.: The sanitary contrasts of the British and French armies during the Crimean War, London, 1883, C. Griffin & Co.

Lord, J.: Beacon lights of history, vol. 5, Great women, New York, 1885, Fords, Howard, & Hulbert.

Lowenfels, W.: Walt Whitman's Civil War, New York, 1961, Alfred A. Knopf, Inc.

Lyons, A.S.: Ancient China. In Lyons, A.S., and Petrucelli, R.J.: Medicine: an illustrated history, New York, 1978, Harry N. Abrams, Inc.

Lyons, A.S.: Ancient Hebrew medicine. In Lyons, A.S., and Petrucelli, R.J.: Medicine: an illustrated history, New York, 1978, Harry N. Abrams, Inc.

Lyons, A.S.: Hippocrates. In Lyons, A.S., and Petrucelli, R.J.: Medicine: an illustrated history, New York, 1978, Harry N. Abrams, Inc.

Lyons, A.S.: Medicine in Roman times. In Lyons, A.S., and Petrucelli, R.J.: Medicine: an illustrated history, New York, 1978, Harry N. Abrams, Inc.

Lyons, A.S.: Medicine under Islam (Arabic medicine). In Lyons, A.S., and Petrucelli, R.J.: Medicine: an illustrated history, New York, 1978, Harry N. Abrams, Inc.

Lyons, A.S.: The nineteenth century (The beginnings of modern medicine). In Lyons, A.S., and Petrucelli, R.J.: Medicine: an illustrated history, New York, 1978, Harry N. Abrams, Inc.

Lyons, A.S., and Petrucelli, R.J.: Medicine: an illustrated history, New York, 1978, Harry N. Abrams, Inc.

Mannino, A.J.: Men in nursing, American Journal of Nursing **51:**198, 1951.

Marram, G., Barrett, M., and Bevis, E.: Primary nursing: a model for individualized care, ed. 2, St. Louis, 1979, The C.V. Mosby Co.

Marshall, H.E.: Dorothea Dix, forgotten Samaritan, Chapel Hill, 1937, University of North Carolina Press.

Marshall, H.E.: Mary Adelaide Nutting, Baltimore, 1972, Johns Hopkins University Press.

Mason, O.T.: Woman's share in primitive culture, New York, 1894, D. Appleton & Co.

Maynard, T.: Apostle of charity: the life of St. Vincent de Paul, New York, 1939, Dial Press.

Maynard, T.: St. Benedict and his monks, London, 1956, Staples Press.

McIsaac, I.: Bacteriology for nurses, New York, 1909, The Macmillan Co.

McKenzie, J.L., and Chrisman, N.L.: Healing herbs, gods and magic, Nursing Outlook **25**:326–329, 1977.

McMahon, N.: The story of the Hospitallers of St. John of God, Westminster, Md., 1959, Newman Press.

McManus, R.L.: Isabel M. Stewart—foremost researcher, Nursing Research **2**:6, Winter 1962.

Mead, K.C.: History of women in medicine, New York, 1938, Haddam Press.

Merejkowski, D.: The romance of Leonardo da Vinci, New York, 1902, Random House.

Merton, R.K.: Issues on the growth of a profession, New York, 1958, American Nurses' Association.

Metarazzo, J.D., and Abdellah, F.H.: Doctoral education for nurses in the United States, Nursing Research **20**:404, 1971.

Middleton, J., editor: Magic, witchcraft and curing, New York, 1967, The Natural History Press.

Miller, H.S.: The history of Chi Eta Phi Sorority, Inc., 1932–1967, Washington, D.C., 1968, Negro Life and History, Inc.

Mollett, W.: On the necessity of legal registration for nurses, London, Nursing Record, June 28, 1888.

Montag, M.L.: The education of nursing technicians, New York, 1951, G.P. Putnam's Sons.

Montag, M.L.: Community college education for nursing: an experiment in technical education for nursing, New York, 1959, McGraw-Hill Book Co.

Morison, S.E.: The Oxford history of the American people, New York, 1965, Oxford University Press.

Morison, S.E., and Commager, H.S.: The growth of the American republic, vols. 1 and 2, New York, 1942, Oxford University Press.

Morten, H.: Nurse's dictionary of medical terms and nursing treatment, Philadelphia, 1894, W.B. Saunders Co.

Morton, T.G.: The history of the Pennsylvania Hospital, 1751–1895, Philadelphia, 1897, Times Printing House.

Mumey, H.: Hygiene for nurses, St. Louis, 1918, The C.V. Mosby Co.

Munson, H.W.: Linda Richards, American Journal of Nursing 48: 552, 1948.

Munson, H.W., and Stevens, K.: Story of the National League of Nursing Education, Philadelphia, 1934, W.B. Saunders Co.

NACGN—four decades of service, New York, 1945, The National Association of Colored Graduate Nurses.

National Commission for the Study of Nursing and Nursing Education: an abstract for action, New York, 1970, McGraw-Hill Book Co.

National Federation for Specialty Nursing Organizations Public Relations Committee: NFSNO: the first ten years, Washington, D.C., 1984, The Federation.

National League of Nursing Education: Standard curriculum for schools of nursing, New York, 1917, The League.

National League of Nursing Education: Curriculum for schools of nursing, New York, 1927, The League.

National League of Nursing Education: A curriculum guide for schools of nursing, New York, 1937, The League.

Newcomb, C.: St. John of God, New York, 1958, Dodd, Mead & Co.

Newman, M.A.: Theory development in nursing, Philadelphia, 1979, F.A. Davis Co.

Newton, M.E.: Florence Nightingale's philosophy of life and education, unpublished dissertation, 1949, Leland Stanford Junior University.

Nightingale, F.: Notes on nursing, New York, 1860, D. Appleton & Co.

Nightingale, F.: Notes on hospitals, ed. 3, London, 1867, Longmans.

The nurses have not lagged behind, editorial, The Saturday Evening Post, April 28, 1945.

Nurses monument unveiled in Arlington, American Journal of Nursing 39:90, 1939.

Nutting, M.A.: American Journal of Nursing 5:654, 1905.

Nutting, M.A.: Educational status of nursing, U.S. Bureau of Education Bulletin 7:1, 1912.

Nutting, M.A.: Greetings. In Souvenir programme of the annual convention of the New York State Nurses' Association, the New York State League for Nursing, the New York Organization for Public Health Nursing, Albany, N.Y., October 27–29, 1925.

Nutting, M.A.: A sound economic basis for schools of nursing, New York, 1926, G.P. Putnam's Sons.

Nutting, M.A., and Dock, L.L.: A history of nursing: the evolution of nursing systems from earliest times to the foundations of the first English and American training schools for nurses, 4 vols., New York, 1907 and 1912, G.P. Putnam's Sons.

Ogden, Brother Daniel: Of valiant men: a chronicle of the congregation of Alexian Brothers, Wisconsin, 1957, The Novitiate Press.

O'Malley, I.B.: Florence Nightingale, 1820–1856, London, 1931, Thornton Butterworth.

On the genius and character of Hogarth. In The works of Charles Lamb, 1818.

Orlando, I.J.: The dynamic nurse-patient relationship: function, process, and principles, New York, 1961, G.P. Putnam's Sons.

Orum, D.: Nursing: Concepts of practice, New York, 1971, McGraw-Hill Book Co.

Osler, Sir William: Aequanimitas, Philadelphia, 1932, Blakiston Co.

Oursler, F.: The greatest book ever written, New York, 1951, Doubleday & Co., Inc.

Oursler, F.: The greatest story ever told, New York, 1949, Doubleday & Co., Inc.

Pachter, H.: Paracelsus: magic into science, New York, 1961, Collier Books.

Paget, S.: Ambrose Paré and his times, New York, 1897, G.P. Putnam's Sons.

Parker, W.W.: Woman's place in the Christian world: superior morally, inferior mentally to man: not qualified for medicine or law; the contrariety and harmony of the sexes, Transactions of the Medical Society of Virginia 23:86, 1892.

Parton, J., and others: Eminent women of the age, Hartford, Conn., 1868, S.M. Betts Co.

Payne, G.H.: The child in human progress, New York, 1916, G.P. Putnam's Sons.

Pennock, M., editor: Makers of nursing history, New York, 1940, Lakeside Publishing Co.

Peplau, H.: Interpersonal relations in nursing, New York, 1952, G.P. Putnam's Sons.

Petrucelli, R.J.: Art and science. In Lyons, A.S., and Petrucelli, R.J.: Medicine: an illustrated history, New York, 1978, Harry N. Abrams, Inc.

Petrucelli, R.J.: The dark ages. In Lyons, A.S., and Petrucelli, R.J.: Medicine: an illustrated history, New York, 1978, Harry N. Abrams, Inc.

Poole, E.: Nurses on horseback, New York, 1935, The Macmillan Co.

Power, E.: Medieval people, New York, 1924, Barnes & Noble.

Powers, E.J.: Hospital pencilings, Boston, 1866, Edward L. Mitchell.

Preston, A.: Nursing the sick and the training of nurses, Philadelphia, 1863, King & Baird.

Proceedings of the American Medical Association, New Orleans, May 1869. Reprinted in Medical News 20:339, 351, 1869.

Proceedings of the eighteenth annual convention of the American Society of Superintendents of Training Schools for Nursing, New York, 1912, The Society.

Pugh, G.F., and Fisher, A.J.B.: Ethics and health in late Victorian society, London, 1970, Arundel.

Putnam, E.J.: The lady, New York, 1921, G.P. Putnam's Sons.

Quinn, N.K., and Somers, A.R.: The patient's bill of rights: a significant aspect of the consumer revolution, Nursing Outlook 22:240, 1974.

Rathbone, W.: History and progress of district nursing, New York, 1890, The Macmillan Co.

Rathbone, W.: Sketch of the history and progress of district nursing from its commencement in the year 1859 to the present date, New York, 1890, The Macmillan Co.

Ravenel, M.R., editor: Half century of public health, New York, 1921, American Public Health Association.

Rayfield, S.: A study of Negro public health nursing, Public Health Nursing 22:525, 1930.

Reeder, S.J.: The social context of nursing. In Chaska, N.L., editor:

The nursing profession: views through the mist, New York, 1978, McGraw-Hill Book Co.

Reinach, S.: Orpheus: a history of religions, New York, 1930, Liveright, Inc.

Riesman, D.: The story of medicine in the Middle Ages, New York, 1936, Harper & Brothers.

Robb, I.H.: Some of the lessons of the late war and their bearing upon trained nursing, Cleveland Medical Gazette **14**:463, 1898–1899.

Robb, I.H.: Nursing ethics: for hospital and private use, Cleveland, 1900, Koeckert.

Robb, I.H.: Nursing as a profession, Albany Medical Annals **21**:491, 1900.

Robb, I.H.: The affiliation of training schools for nurses for educational purposes, American Journal of Nursing **5**:670, 1905.

Robb, I.H.: Educational standards for nurses, with other addresses on nursing subjects, Cleveland, 1907, Koeckert.

deRobeck, N.: Saint Elizabeth of Hungary, Milwaukee, 1953, Bruce Publishing Co.

Roberts, M.M.: American nursing: history and interpretation, New York, 1954, The Macmillan Co.

Roberts, M.M.: Lavinia Lloyd Dock—nurse, feminist, internationalist, American Journal of Nursing **56**:176, February 1976.

Robinson, V.: White caps: the story of nursing, Philadelphia, 1946, J.B. Lippincott Co.

Rockefeller Foundation and nursing education, American Journal of Nursing **20**:525, 1920.

Rockefeller Foundation, Division of Medical Education: Nursing education and schools of nursing, New York, 1932, The Foundation.

Rodabaugh, J.H., and Rodabaugh, M.J.: Nursing in Ohio: a history, Columbus, 1951, The Ohio State Nurses Association.

Roddis, L.H.: The U.S. Hospital Ship *Red Rover* (1862–1865), Military Surgeon **77**:92, August 1935.

Rogers, M.E.: An introduction to the theoretical basis of nursing, Philadelphia, 1970, F.A. Davis Co.

Rosen, G.: A history of public health, New York, 1958, M.D. Publications, Inc.

Rosenberg, C.: The cholera years, Chicago, 1962, The University of Chicago Press.

Roy, Sister Callista: Introduction to nursing: an adaptation model, Englewood Cliffs, N.J., 1967, Prentice-Hall, Inc.

Saint Jerome: Letters. In Nicene and post-Nicene fathers of the Christian church, vol. 6, New York, 1893, The Christian Literature Co.

Saint Thomas Aquinas: Basic writings, New York, Random House.

Sandwith, F.M.: The nursing and care of the sick prior to 1850, Hospitals **56**:273, 1914–1915.

Schermerhorn, E.: On the trial of the eight pointed cross: a study of the heritage of the Knights Hospitallers in feudal Europe, New York, 1940, G.P. Putnam's Sons.

Scovil, E.R.: In the sickroom: the art of nursing, New York, 1888, Montgomery.

Seaman, V.: The midwives monitor, and mothers mirror, being three concluding lectures of a course of instruction on midwifery; containing directions for pregnant women; rules for the management of natural births, and for early discovering when the aid of a physician is necessary; and cautions for nurses, respecting both the mother and child. To which is prefixed, a syllabus of lectures on that subject, New York, 1800, I. Collins.

Seelye, Rev. L.C.: The need of a collegiate education for women, North Adams, Mass., 1874, American Institute of Instruction.

Selections from Leaves of Grass by Walt Whitman, New York, 1961, Crown Publishers.

Sellew, G., and Nuesse, C.J.: The history of nursing, St. Louis, 1946, The C.V. Mosby Co.

Seymer, L.R.: A general history of nursing, London, 1932, Faber & Faber Ltd.

Seymer, L.R.: Florence Nightingale, London, 1940, Faber & Faber Ltd.

Shaw, E.: The black nurse—then, now, and ? Paper presented for continuing education, Nashville, Tenn., 1973, Meharry Medical College.

Shields, E.A., editor: Highlights in the history of the Army Nurse Corps, Washington, D.C., 1981, U.S. Army Center of Military History.

Shryock, R.H.: The history of nursing: an interpretation of the social and medical factors involved, Philadelphia, 1959, W.B. Saunders Co.

Sigerist, H.E.: American medicine, New York, 1934, W.W. Norton & Co., Inc.

Simmons, L.W.: The role of the aged in the primitive society, New Haven, Conn., 1945, Yale University Press.

Smith, F.B.: Florence Nightingale: reputation and power, London, 1982, Croom Helm.

Smith, G.R.: From invisibility to blackness: the story of the National Black Nurses' Association, Nursing Outlook **23**:225, April 1975.

Smith, M.M.: Message from Sharon—a reading, The Connection **8**:3, June 1984.

Smith-Rosenberg, C., and Rosenberg, C.: The female animal: medical and biological views of woman and her role in nineteenth century America, Journal of American History **60**:332, 1973.

Song of the Army Nurse Corps. Music by Lou Singer. Words by Hy Zaret. Copyright 1944 by MCA Music, a division of MCA Inc., 445 Park Avenue, New York, New York 10022.

Spalding, H.S.: Talks to nurses: the ethics of nursing, New York, 1920, Benziger.

Staupers, M.K.: No time for prejudice, New York, 1961, Macmillan Publishing Co., Inc.

Steuer, R.O., and Saunders, J.B. de C.M.: Ancient Egyptian and Cnidian medicine, Berkeley, 1959, University of California Press.

Stevens, E.F.: American hospital of the twentieth century: a treatise on the development of medical institutions, both in Europe and in America, since the beginning of the present century, ed. 2, New York, 1928, Architectural Record Co.

Stevens, R.: American medicine and the public interest, New Haven, Conn., 1971, Yale University Press.

Stewart, H.R.: The value of the public health nurse to the community, Modern Medicine **1**:429, 1919.

Stewart, I.M.: The hospital economics course from the students' standpoint, Paper presented before the Maryland Nurses' Association, 1909.

Stewart, I.M.: How can we help to improve our teaching in nursing schools? Canadian Nurse **22**:1593, 1918.

Stewart, I.M.: Popular fallacies about nursing education, The Modern Hospital **18**:1, November 1921.

Stewart, I.M.: The science and art of nursing, editorial, Nursing Education Bulletin **2**:1, Winter 1929.

Stewart, I.M.: Florence Nightingale—educator, Teachers College Record **41**:208, December 1939.

Stewart, I.M.: The education of nurses, New York, 1943, The Macmillan Co.

Stewart, I.M.: Reminiscences of Isabel M. Stewart, New York, 1961, Oral History Research Office, Columbia University.

Stewart, I.M., and Austin, A.L.: A history of nursing, ed. 5, New York, 1962, G.P. Putnam's Sons.

Stimson, J.C.: Earliest known connection of nurses with Army hospitals in the United States, American Journal of Nursing **25**:18, 1925.

Stimson, J.C.: History and manual of the Army Nurse Corps, Carlisle, Pa., 1937, Army Medical School.

Stirling, M., and others: Indians of the Americas, Washington, D.C., 1955, National Geographic Society.

Stobart, J.C.: The glory that was Greece, rev. ed., Boston, 1934, Beacon Press.

Storer, H.: Nurses and nursing, Boston, 1868, Lee & Shepard.

Strachey, G.L.: Florence Nightingale. In Eminent victorians, London, 1918, G.P. Putnam's Sons.

Strachey, R.: The cause, a short history of the women's movement in Great Britain, London, 1928, G. Bell & Sons.

Struthers, L.R.: The school nurse, New York, 1917, G.P. Putnam's Sons.

Styles, M.M.: Doctoral education in nursing: the current situation in historical perspective. In National Conference on Doctoral Education in Nursing, Philadelphia, 1977, University of Pennsylvania.

Styles, M.M.: On nursing: toward a new endowment, St. Louis, 1982, The C.V. Mosby Co.

Talley, C.: Ethics: a textbook for nurses, New York, 1925, G.P. Putnam's Sons.

Taylor, E.J.: The school of nursing at the Yale University, American Journal of Nursing **25**:9, 1925.

Taylor, H.O.: Greek biology and medicine, Boston, 1922, Marshall Jones Co.

Thatcher, V.S.: History of anesthesia with emphasis on the nurse specialist, Philadelphia, 1953, J.B. Lippincott Co.

Thibodeau, J.A.: Nursing models: analysis and evaluation, Belmont, Calif., 1983, Wadsworth Health Sciences.

Thompson, J.: The ANA in Washington, Kansas City, Mo., 1972, American Nurses' Association.

Thompson, M.: The cry and the covenant, New York, 1954, Doubleday & Co.

Thoms, A.B.: Pathfinders: a history of the progress of colored graduate nurses, New York, 1929, Kay Printing House.

Thoms, A.B., and Bullock, C.E.: Developing of facilities for colored nurse education, Trained Nurse and Hospital Review **80**:722, 1928.

Thorwald, J.: Science and secrets of early medicine, New York, 1963, Harcourt, Brace, & World, Inc.

Tiffany, F.: Life of Dorothea Lynde Dix, Boston, 1937, Houghton.

Tinkham, C., and Voorhees, E.: Community health nursing—evolution and process, New York, 1972, Appleton-Century-Crofts.

Tuker, M.A.R., and Malleson, H.: Handbook to Christian and ecclesiastical Rome, New York, 1900, The Macmillan Co.

Tuttle, G.T.: The male nurse, American Journal of Insanity **63**:192, 1906.

Uhlhorn, G.: Christian charity in the ancient church, New York, 1883, Charles Scribner.

U.S. Council of National Defense: First annual report of the Council of National Defense, fiscal year 1917, Washington, D.C., 1917, U.S. Government Printing Office.

Vallery-Radot, D.: Life of Pasteur, Garden City, N.Y., 1923, Doubleday.

Van Doren, M.: Walt Whitman, New York, 1945, Viking Press.

Van Loon, H.W.: R.V.R.: the life and times of Rembrandt, New York, 1931, Liveright Publishing Co.

Vreeland, E.M.: Fifty years of nursing in the federal government nursing services, American Journal of Nursing **50**:626, October 1950.

Wakeford, C.: The wounded soldiers' friends: the story of Florence Nightingale, Clara Barton, and others, London, 1917, Headley-Brothers.

Wald, L.D.: The house on Henry Street, New York, 1915, Henry Holt & Co.

Wald, L.: Windows on Henry Street, Boston, 1934, Little, Brown & Co.

Walsh, J.J.: The history of nursing, New York, 1929, P.J. Kenedy & Sons.

Waltari, M.: The Egyptian, New York, 1949, G.P. Putnam's Sons.

Waters, Y.: Visiting nursing in the United States, New York, 1909, Charities Publication Committee.

Weeks-Shaw, C.S.: A textbook of nursing of the use of training schools, families, and private students, New York, 1885, Appleton.

Weinreb, N.: The Babylonians, New York, 1953, Doubleday & Co.

Wells, C.: Bones, bodies, and disease, New York, 1964, Frederick A. Praeger.

West, M., and Hawkins, C.: Nursing schools at the mid-century, New York, 1950, National Committee for the Improvement of Nursing Services.

Wheeler, H.: Deaconesses, ancient and modern, New York, 1889, Hunt & Eaton.

Whitehead, A.N.: The aims of education and other essays, New York, 1929, The Macmillan Co.

Whitman, W.: The works of Walt Whitman, New York, 1968, Funk & Wagnall's, Inc.

Whitman, W.: The wound-dresser, a series of letters written from the hospitals in Washington during the war of the rebellion, Boston, 1898, Small, Maynard.

Whitney, J.: Elizabeth Fry, Boston, 1936, Brown & Co.

Wilson, F.: Crusader in crinoline: the life of Harriet Beecher Stowe, Philadelphia, 1941, J.B. Lippincott Co.

With the Army Nurse Corps in Korea, American Journal of Nursing **51**:387, June 1951.

Woelful, N.: Molders of the American mind, New York, 1933, Columbia University Press.

Wong, K.C., and Wu, Lieu-Teh: History of Chinese medicine, Shanghai, 1936, National Quarantine Service.

Woodham-Smith, C.: Florence Nightingale, New York, 1951, McGraw-Hill Book Co.

Woody, T.: A history of women's education in the United States, 2 vols., New York, 1929, The Science Press.

Woolf, S.J.: Miss Wald at 70 sees her dreams realized, New York Times Magazine, March 7, 1937.

Woolley, L.: History unearthed, London, 1963, Ernest Benn Ltd.

Woolsey, J.S.: Hospital days, New York, 1868, Van Nostrand.

Wylie, W.G.: Hospitals: their history, organization and construction, New York, 1877, Appleton.

Zielger, P.: The black death, New York, 1969, John Day Co.

Zimmermann, A.: ANA: its record on social issues, American Journal of Nursing **76**:588, 1976.

Zinsser, H.: Rats, lice and history, New York, 1934, Blue Ribbon Books, Inc.

INDEX

Numbers in italics refer to illustrations.

494

499

501

504

This book was typeset in eleven point ITC Garamond Book by Village Typographers, Inc., Waterloo, Illinois. Color separations and film preparation were provided by Colorific Litho, Inc., St. Louis, Missouri. The book was printed and bound in St. Louis and Jefferson City, Missouri, by Von Hoffmann Press, Inc., on Stirling Offset Enamel. The cover material is Centennial Buckram, supplied by Joanna Western Mills. The design is by The Quarasan Group, Inc., Northfield, Illinois.

in Canada; the King Edward VII Order in South Africa; the Bush Nursing Association in South Africa; and the Plunket Nurses in New Zealand.

Although organized attempts at the development of visiting nursing occurred quite early in the history of the United States, the momentum needed for its progression was slow in coming. The earliest visiting nurse services were connected with denominational groups participating in religious and charitable works. Nondenominational societies were established in 1877 in New York (the Women's Branch of the New York City Mission), in 1886 in Boston and Philadelphia, and in 1889 in Chicago. These visiting nurse associations (V.N.A.), which employed trained nurses chiefly for the care of the sick in their homes, were often called "Instructive District Nursing Associations." Teaching, as the name indicates, was also a vital function of the home care of the sick; principles of hygiene and sanitation were taught in addition to specific aspects of health and illness. Isabel Hampton commented on the association name in an address to the International Congress of Nurses in 1893:

> In District Nursing we are confronted with conditions which require the highest order of work, but the actual nursing of the patient is the least part of what her work and influence should be among the class which the nurse will meet with. To this branch of nursing no more appropriate name can be given than "Instructive Nursing," for educational in the best sense of the word it should be.

The Henry Street Settlement

The "nursing settlement" was one of the factors that assisted with the expansion of the scope of visiting nursing into the larger field of public health nursing. However, it approached social problems from the point of view of nursing. The work environment, low wages, the neighborhood environment, the cultures and customs of the people, and other variables were examined and evaluated for their particular influence on health. The first of these was the world-famous Henry Street Settlement, which was opened as a cooperative and partially self-supporting neighborhood service in 1893. Its history is vividly described in two books authored by Lillian Wald. *The House on Henry Street* (1915) and *Windows on Henry Street* (1934).

Lillian D. Wald (1867–1940), a wealthy young woman of high ideals, became interested in the need for nursing and social services among the poor soon after she graduated from the New York Hospital School of Nursing in 1891. Born in Cincinnati, Ohio, and raised in Rochester, New York, she was of Polish-German-Jewish stock. Lillian Wald was educated at Miss Crittenden's English and French Boarding and Day School for Young Ladies and Little Girls. Influenced by her physician relatives, however, she left to become a nurse. After her graduation she spent a year nursing at the New York Juvenile Asylum, but then she entered Woman's Medical College in New York. During her medical school days Miss Wald was asked to go to New York's Lower East Side to instruct immigrant mothers on the care of the sick. She was profoundly shocked by what she found there.

At the turn of the century the Lower East Side of New York was a wilderness of overcrowded tenements where the sick lay unattended. Groups of immigrants of different nationalities filtered into

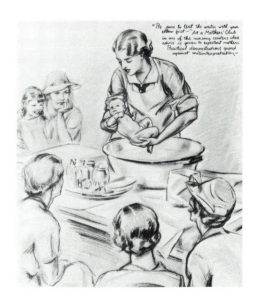

Cyrus Leroy Baldridge, BE SURE TO TEST THE WATER WITH YOUR ELBOW FIRST. *Drawing from the 1938 pamphlet the* HENRY STREET VISITING NURSE SERVICE. *Mugar Memorial Library, Boston University, Massachusetts. By permission from the Henry Street Settlement Urban Life Center.*

343

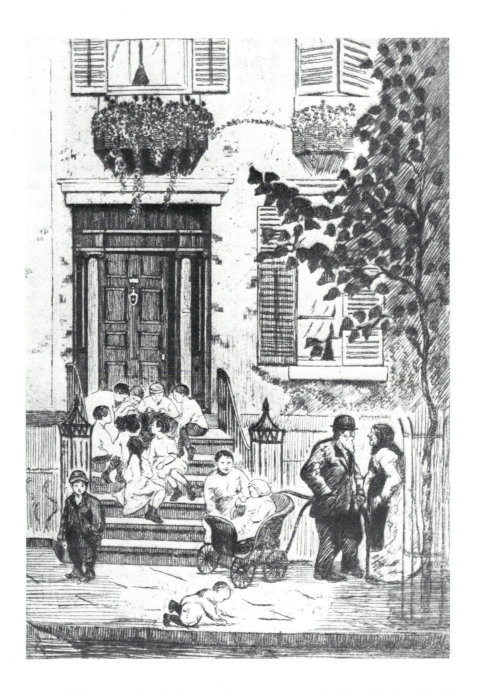

the neighborhood and lived under great physical hardships. Death and morbidity rates were extremely high, and those who were fortunate moved to better neighborhoods before they succumbed to the health hazards of the slum. Lillian Wald soon personally experienced these dreadful conditions when a child approached her for help as she was teaching a group of mothers. She described this turning point in her life in the following way:

> From the schoolroom where I had been giving a lesson in bed-making, a little girl led me one drizzling March morning. She had told me of her sick mother, and gathering from her incoherent account that a child had been born, I caught up the paraphernalia of the bed-making lesson and carried it with me.
> The child led me over broken roadways ... between tall, reeking houses ... past odorous fish-stands for the streets were a market-place, unregulated, unsupervised, unclean, past evil-smelling, uncovered garbage cans, and perhaps worst of all, where so many little children played. ...

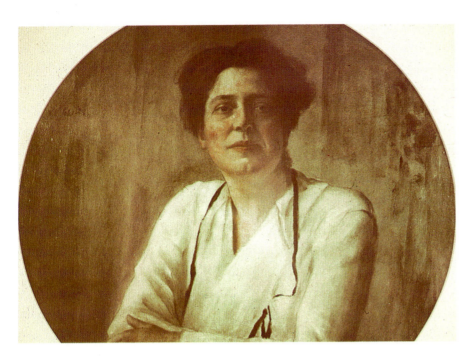

The child led me on through a tenement hallway, across a court where open and unscreened closets were promiscuously used by men and women, up into a rear tenement, by slimy steps whose accumulated dirt was augmented that day by the mud of the streets, and finally into the sickroom.

All the maladjustments of our social and economic relations seemed epitomized in this brief journey and what was found at the end of it. The family to which the child led me was neither criminal nor vicious . . . and although the sick woman lay on a wretched, unclean bed, soiled with a hemorrhage two days old, they were not degraded human beings. . . .

It would have been some solace if by any conviction of the moral unworthiness of the family I could have defended myself as a part of society which permitted such conditions to exist . . . miserable as their state was, they were not without ideals for the family life, and for society, of which they were so unloved and unlovely a part.

That morning's experience was a baptism of fire. Deserted were the laboratory and the academic work of the college. I never returned to them. . . . To my inexperience it seemed certain that conditions such as these were allowed because people did not *know,* and for me there was a challenge to know and tell. When early morning found me still awake, my naive conviction remained that, if people knew things,—and "things" meant everything implied in the condition of this family,—such horrors would cease to exist, and I rejoiced that I had a training in the care of the sick that in itself would give me an organic relationship to the neighborhood in which this awakening had come.

Wald, 1915, pp. 4–8

In 1893 Miss Wald persuaded a classmate, Miss Mary Brewster, to go into the tenement district with her to live and work. The two nurses rented the top floor of a tenement house on Jefferson Street and began to carry on whatever nursing and social work fell their way. As their workload increased, the house at 265 Henry Street was

Cyrus Leroy Baldridge, PUBLIC HEALTH NURSES FROM FOREIGN COUNTRIES. *Drawing from the 1938 pamphlet, the* HENRY STREET VISITING NURSE SERVICE. *Mugar Memorial Library, Boston University, Massachusetts. By permission from the Henry Street Settlement Urban Life Center.*

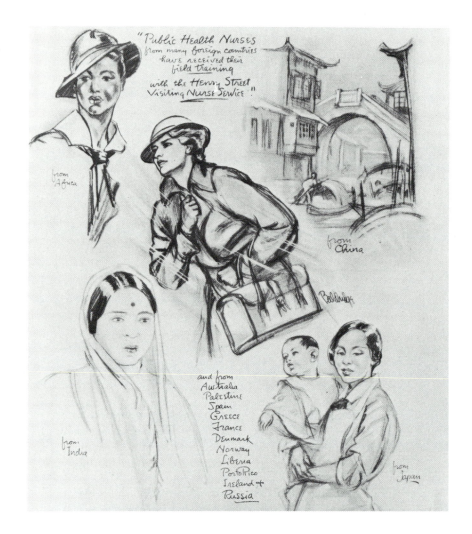

acquired with the help of Jacob H. Schiff, a banker and philanthropist, and others. This "House on Henry Street" became the Henry Street Visiting Nurse Service and eventually encompassed nursing service, social work, and an organized program of social, cultural, and educational activities. The scope of the settlement went far beyond the care of the sick and the prevention of disease. It aimed at rectifying those causes that were responsible for the poverty and misery itself. In keeping with this aim, Lillian Wald battled for legislative reforms that would ensure some measure of justice for the "unfortunates." Her initiative and skill in securing support for new ideas and new plans made her one of the most influential health workers of her day (Stewart and Austin, 1962).

Lillian Wald is regarded as the founder of what is now called public health or community nursing. She coined the phrase "public health nursing" and transformed the stereotyped visiting nursing of her time into the community movements that ultimately widened the horizons of modern nursing (Robinson, 1946). She created a system whereby patients had direct access to nurses and nurses had direct access to patients. Miss Wald insisted that the nurses should be at the call of people who needed them, without the intervention of a medical man (Woolf, 1937). When warranted, however, a patient would be referred to a physician at one of the free dispensaries. No distinction was made between those who could pay and those who could not; services were available to all who sought them.

346

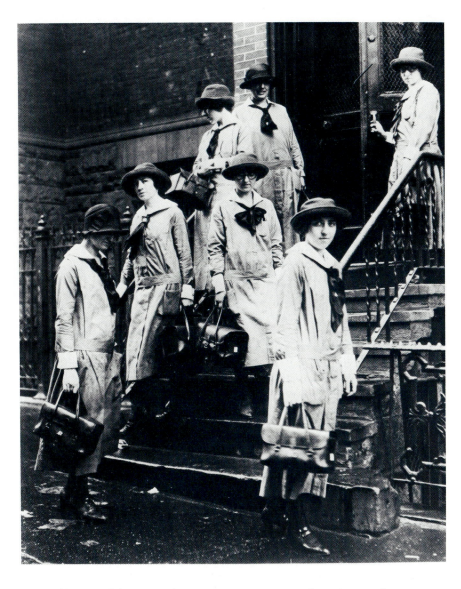

Lillian Wald's contributions to nursing and society at large were numerous and included the following:

1893 Supplied sputum cups and disinfectants to pioneer tuberculosis nurses.

1895 Made adjoining backyards into a neighborhood playground (Bunker Hill of Playgrounds).

1897–1909 Investigated unemployment, cases of dispossessed tenants, New York midwives, children out of school because of physical defects, working fourteen-year-old children, labor and construction camps in New York, working conditions of girls in department stores, factories, and canneries.

1899 Assisted with the development of lectures on public health nursing at Teachers' College, Columbia University. By 1913 she and Mary Adelaide Nutting had established an educational program in public health nursing in which nurses would receive theoretical coursework at Teachers' College and practical experience at the Henry Street Settlement.

1902 Initiated public school nursing in America.

1905 Served on the mayor's Pushcart Commission.

1908 Served on the State Immigration Commission.

1909 Initiated nursing service for industrial policyholders of the Metropolitan Life Insurance Company.

1912 The United States Children's Bureau was created by act of Congress as part of the Department of Commerce and Labor. Miss Wald is credited with the idea for this federal bureau.

1912 Established the Rural Nursing Service of the American Red Cross. (The name was changed in the following year to the Town and Country Nursing Service.)

1912 Became the first president of the National Organization for Public Health Nursing.

With the death of Lillian D. Wald, the nation had truly lost a unique citizen. Throughout her lifetime she had opposed political and social corruption and supported those measures that would improve the health, welfare, and happiness of humanity.

> She had stirred the melting-pot on her adopted block, and it became a community undertaking. In the amalgamation of the multitudes that came to these shores, in the eternal warfare against prejudice, she was a steadfast guide. Amid the darkness of ignorance and poverty, she pointed the path to the light. An American who devoted her life to those of foreign birth, this descendant of immigrants walked the ways of democracy. Her work was an international rainbow of friendship across humanity's sky. . . . Presidents, governors, senators, have paid her appropriate tribute. The credo of the Visiting Nurse Service of the Henry Street Settlement is Lillian D. Wald's finest epitaph: Response to every call for help, without regard to race or creed or color.
>
> *Robinson, 1946, p. 296*

The Henry Street Settlement paved the way for the foundation of nursing settlements in other American cities. The earliest among these were in Richmond, Virginia (1900), San Francisco, California (1900), and Orange, New Jersey (1903).

The Frontier Nursing Service

There is a striking contrast between the development of midwifery in Europe and in the United States. Midwifery was always considered an important specialty in Europe, with a two-year course usually required. Nearly all state-registered nurses in England were at one time registered midwives who had six months or more of specialized training. Yet in the United States the training of nurses in the area of midwifery had been prevented primarily by the attitudes of physicians. The physicians held the view that every woman should be assisted in delivery by a physician, an attitude that continued to be prominent into the 1930s. This opposition was related to the belief that nurse-midwifery represented an intrusion on the field of medical practice. It ignored the fact that the maternal death rate was high; a large number of untrained, ignorant midwives were practicing; and thousands of women employed incompetent midwives.

The use of midwives was customary among the foreign born in the cities and among Blacks, particularly those in the rural regions of

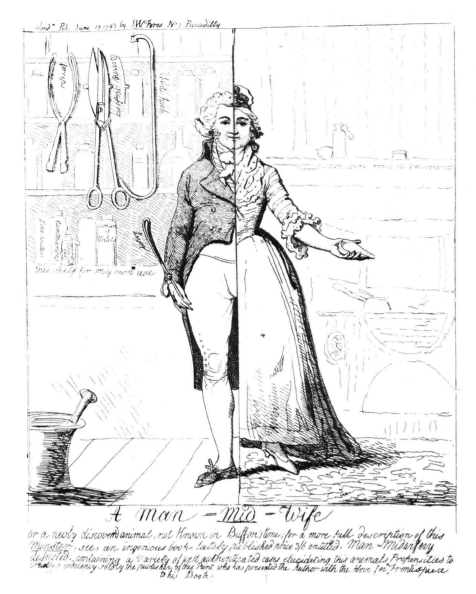

Within the image, handwritten label text:
Lond.º Pub. June 15 1793 by S W Fores N.º 3 Piccadilly

A Man = Mid = Wife

or a newly discovered animal, not known in Buffon's time; for a more full description of this Monster; see, an ingenious book lately published price 3/6 entitled, Man = Midwifery dissected, containing a Variety of well authenticated cases elucidating this animals Propensities to cruelty & indecency solely the publisher, by this Prent who has presented the Author with the Above for Frontispiece to his Book.

Cartoon of A MAN-MID-WIFE OR A NEWLY DISCOVERED ANIMAL, *depicting a midwife bisected into male and female halves. From S.W. Fores,* MAN-MIDWIFERY DISSECTED, *London, 1793. Wellcome Institute for the History of Medicine, London, England.*

the South. In many instances medical care for these women was non-existent. Although many of the midwives had practical experience that was an asset in normal deliveries, injury or death to the mother or child (or both) often occurred with abnormal or difficult deliveries. Early in the 1900s studies were undertaken that began the long march to reform in the care of mothers and babies. In addition, some nurses began to advocate the training and use of nurse-midwives in America, particularly in those areas where medical care was lacking. However, this movement lacked support from physicians, nurses, and the general public and therefore did not have a strong impact.

A few schools for nurse-midwives were finally developed. In 1911 Bellevue Hospital established a school of midwifery that continued until 1935. This school was specifically designed to aid the 40,000 New York women who were being assisted in delivery by untrained women. It was discontinued when the majority of women entered hospitals for delivery. The founding of centers that offered courses and granted certificates in nurse-midwifery followed. Such institutions included the Maternity Center Association (which opened the first school for nurse-midwives in the United States) in connection with the Lobenstine Clinic in New York; the Tuskegee Institute in Alabama (a short-lived school for Black nurse-midwives assisted by

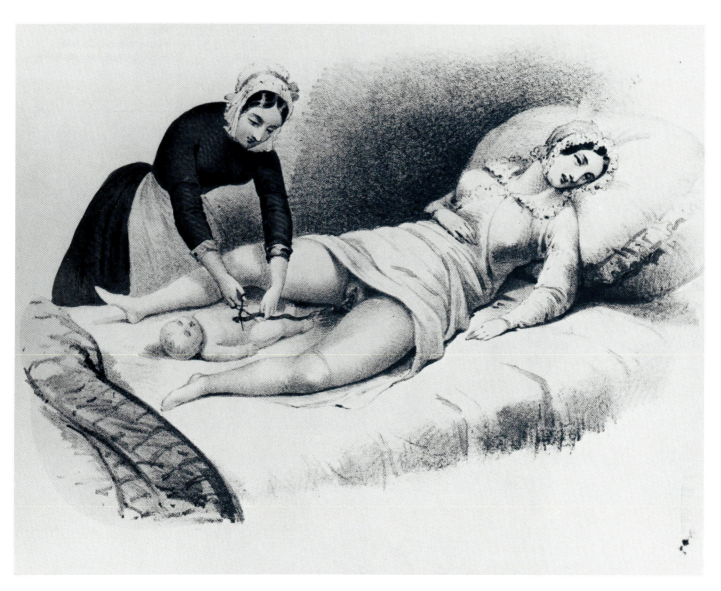

A NURSE-MIDWIFE CUTS THE CORD OF A
NEWBORN INFANT LYING BETWEEN THE LEGS
OF THE MOTHER ON THE BED, *c. 1850. Col-
ored lithograph. From Beach's* IMPROVED
SYSTEM OF MIDWIFERY. *National Library of
Medicine, Bethesda, Maryland.*

federal funds during the war); the Frontier Nursing Service in Kentucky; and the Catholic Maternity Institute in New Mexico. Finally,
certificates in nurse-midwifery were offered in conjunction with a
master's degree at Yale University, Johns Hopkins University, New
York Medical College, Catholic University, Columbia University, and
the University of Utah (Dolan, Fitzpatrick, and Hermann, 1983).

The Frontier Nursing Service provided the first organized midwifery service in this country. It was founded in 1925 by Mary Breckinridge, the daughter of a family distinguished in American history.
Although married twice, she retained her maiden name. Her only
children, Breckie and Polly, died in infancy, and this was thought to
be the catalyst for her interest and involvement in midwifery. Mary
Breckinridge graduated from St. Luke's Hospital Training School in
New York (1910) and later from the British Hospital for Mothers and
Babies, Woolwich, London (1925), where she received her certificate
in midwifery. For several years (1919–1923), she became occupied
with public health activities in devastated France and actually organized public health nursing there.

Mary Breckinridge recognized the need for a rural midwifery
service in the Appalachian Mountains of Kentucky, where for centuries both nursing and midwifery had been practiced under almost
medieval conditions by the "granny women." These "midwives"

were generally illiterate, had no formal training in midwifery, knew little about prenatal or postnatal care, and were often superstitious. They rarely called a physician, even when faced with serious complications. Their practices ranged from the use of soot as a medication to the placing of an axe, blade side up, under the bed as a preventive measure.

The people who settled in these hills became isolated from the rest of the country because of their location. They maintained the old customs of early marriage and large families. The Appalachian area was part of the "cradle of the nation" and had one of the highest birth rates in the United States.

Mary Breckinridge, who had witnessed midwifery services first-hand in England, New Zealand, and Australia, was determined to initiate a similar plan for the care of mothers, babies, and children in these foothills. To accomplish her goal she was forced to use English-trained midwives for many years, since there were so few trained midwives in America.

The members of the Frontier Nursing Service worked in Leslie County, Kentucky, where the lack of highways necessitated travel by horse or mule. The area was divided into eight districts of approximately seventy-eight square miles each. Two nurses lived in the middle of each district and were responsible for the health of all those

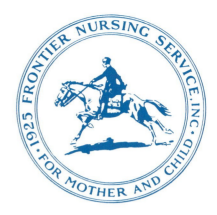

Logo for the Frontier Nursing Service, a demonstration in family centered primary health care since 1925. Frontier Nursing Service, Hyden, Kentucky.

MARY BRECKINRIDGE ON HORSEBACK, c. 1938. Founder of the Frontier Nursing Service, Hyden, Kentucky.

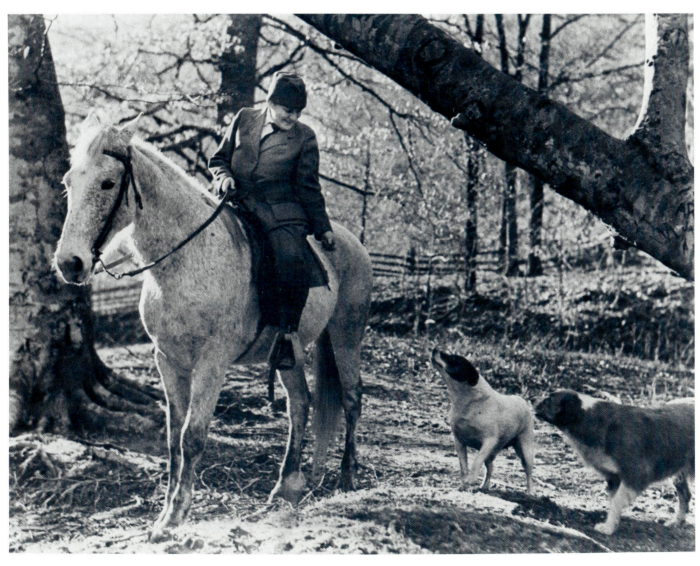

who lived there. A primary form of health care was provided in which a family-centered approach was emphasized. Each of the "nurses on horseback" had certification as a nurse-midwife, and they gave antepartal, intrapartal, and postpartal care to the women in their districts. They performed normal deliveries but called a physician in the event of a complicated case. A study of the first 1000 cases showed that the proportion of complications during pregnancy and delivery was lower among patients cared for by the service than among the general population. Mary Breckinridge and her staff had demonstrated the usefulness of such a service in areas where physicians were not readily accessible.

By 1935 a small twelve-bed general hospital, the Hyden Hospital and Health Center, was founded and functional. The medical director not only was responsible for the hospitalized patients but also responded to the nurses in the several districts. The advent of World War II prompted the establishment of a Graduate School of Midwivery, since the British nurses wished to return home to care for their own people. This school was founded by the Frontier Nursing Service in 1939 at Hyden, Kentucky.

In recent years a growing number of nurses have begun to specialize in the practice of nurse-midwifery. It involves a definite return to or reintroduction of past techniques. For example, the practices of home delivery and natural childbirth, the use of the sit-

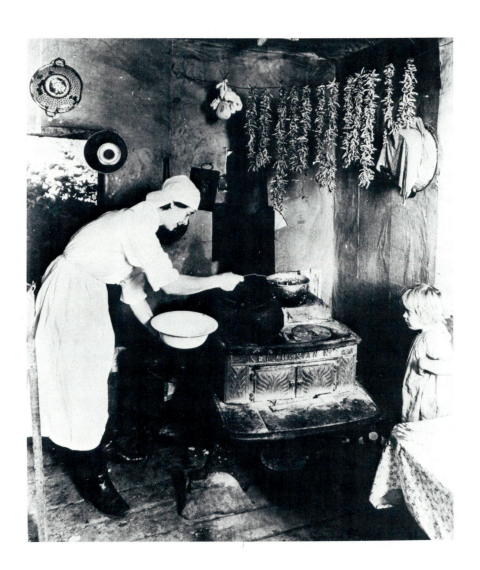

A member of the Frontier Nursing Service is preparing to attend a childbirth as a youngster watches. The Bettmann Archive, New York.

ting position on "obstetrical chairs" or "birthing chairs," and the employment of nurse-midwives are on the rise. In some respects this has been fostered by third-party insurance reimbursement for midwifery services and the development of birthing centers in hospitals and free-standing maternity centers.

The Status of Women

The history of nursing is essentially the story of women. From primitive times nursing has been inextricably bound to the female of the species; and even today the majority of nurses are still women. Robinson vividly depicts the origin of the mother-nurse in a rather simplistic summary. Yet the description serves to emphasize the close bond that occurred between the two roles:

> Biology made the female the nurse of the species. The first mother who leaned over the first cradle of leaves in the primitive forest was the first nurse—and back of this fat-hipped woman with the hanging breasts, the projecting face, and the heavy eyebrow ridges, stretched countless ages of her prehuman ancestry. In the purposeful efforts of animals to aid their young and injured are found the rudiments of medicine and nursing. The utter helplessness of the human infant, even after he has mastered the difficult art of holding his overgrown head erect, developed a prolonged connection between mother and child. Before the dawn of agriculture, the male stepped out of his cave or rock-shelter, club in hand, the hunter of all living things; the female remained behind, the nurse of the young and the sick.
>
> *Robinson, 1946, p. 360*

The development of nursing, therefore, parallels and reflects the women's movement. For a long period in history, the position of women in society left much to be desired. The role of women remained passive, although statements about the equality of women with men were heard periodically. Throughout the centuries women were generally regarded as the property of men and had no legal rights or power. (Rare exceptions can be cited, such as the position of the Roman matron at the start of the Christian era.) For example, the Code of Hammurabi stated that women were the exclusive property of men. Ancient norms regarding women were enforced, particularly during the time of the Reformation. Yet some glimmers of potential for change began to surface as early as the beginning of the seventeenth century. A group of courageous and persistent women emerged to champion the cause of their sex and earn the title of "feminists." These women advocated equal rights for women that would include legal and academic privileges, marriage reform that would allow for preference rather than arrangement, and the right to vote, own property, and hold office. Although they met vehement opposition to their cause, they continued their struggle toward the emancipation of women. Through their efforts the position of women slowly began to improve.

Books, essays, and articles that dealt with women's rights began to appear. Works written by the early feminists included "The Excellencies of Women and the Errors of Men" by Lucretia Marinelli of Italy; *The Learned Maid,* a book by Anna von Schurman of Holland;

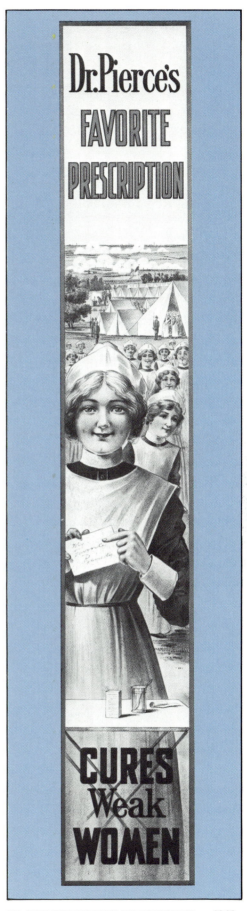

DR. PIERCE'S FAVORITE PRESCRIPTION, *c. 1918. Poster. Philadelphia Museum of Art, Pennsylvania, Gift of William H. Helfand.*

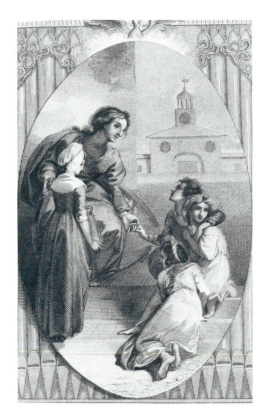

Designed by Thomas Stothard, R.A., ASYLUM FOR FEMALE ORPHANS, *c. 1785. Engraving. British Museum, London, England.*

"A Serious Proposal to the Ladies" by the English feminist, Mary Astell; two volumes on *The Strictures on Female Education* by another Englishwoman, Hannah More. This movement owed much to Mary Wollstonecraft's epic book, *A Vindication of the Rights of Women,* written in 1792. The "rights" that were discussed in this work were simply human rights that should have been impartially applied to women. This author argued against the existing double standard of morality that was prevalent in the society. Mary Wollstonecraft was indeed a fitting example of her beliefs. She had acquired an education and entered the business world as a translator for a publisher in London. Supporters of her ideas turned them into action.

Successful and powerful novels also began to be published by women. Among these were *Evelina* by Fanny Burney; *Pride and Prejudice* by Jane Austen; *Jane Eyre* and *Wuthering Heights* by Charlotte Brontë; *The Mill on the Floss* by George Eliot; and *Uncle Tom's Cabin* by Harriet Beecher Stowe.

Women became reformers, educators, and developers—making their voices heard in any way possible. They rallied to advance their right of suffrage when they discovered that social reforms could be achieved through the power of the vote. Prominent in the American women's movement was Susan B. Anthony (1820–1906). English women later began suffrage efforts and met with comparable resistance. Even Queen Victoria voiced her protest:

> this mad, wicked folly of Woman's Rights, with all its attendant horrors. Lady —— ought to get a *good whipping*. It is a subject which makes the Queen so furious she cannot contain herself.

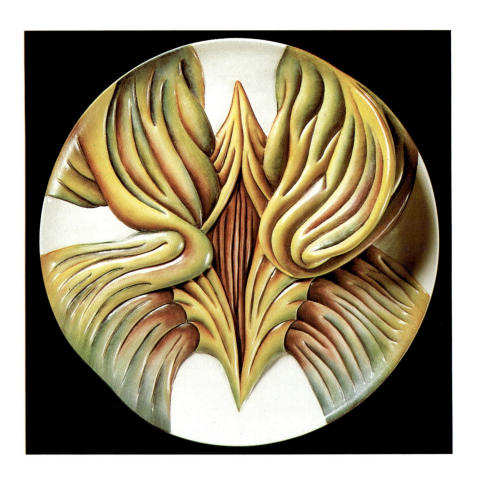

Judy Chicago, "Mary Wollstonecraft," plate from THE DINNER PARTY, *1979. China-painted porcelain, 35.6 cm diameter. Through the Flower, Benicia, California.*

354

Tennyson has some beautiful lines on the difference of men and women in *The Princess*. Woman would become the most hateful, heartless, and disgusting of human beings were she allowed to unsex herself; and where would be the protection which man was intended to give the weaker sex?

Quoted in Robinson, 1946, p. 365

After nearly seventy-five years of frustration and struggle, the United States Constitution was amended in 1920 to allow women to vote.

Nursing leaders were involved in women's rights as well as in human rights. Nurses were found among the marchers in the pilgrimages of the suffragettes. The most colorful and zealous suffragist was Lavinia Lloyd Dock (1858–1956), one of nursing's greatest leaders and a radical feminist. She was actively engaged in social protest, picketing and parading for women's rights, and protesting against war, which were not regarded as "nurselike" or "ladylike" activities. She also voiced her opinions and concerns about social issues whenever an opportunity arose. At one point "Little Dockie" was to speak about the history of nursing in Europe to a group of nursing students at Teachers College. Miss Nutting was away and the incident was described by Isabel Stewart:

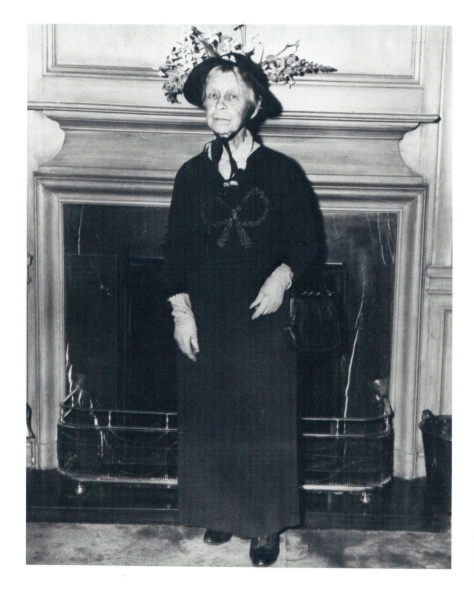

Portrait of LAVINIA L. DOCK. *Special Collections, Milbank Memorial Library, Teachers College, Columbia University, New York.*

355

> I was quite young and I'd never seen Miss Dock. . . . I was sure
> I'd know her when I met her, because she'd be tall and angular
> and intellectual looking. Who should turn up at the door but this
> small, short sort of roly-poly little person with curly hair. She'd
> just been at a suffrage meeting, and had "Votes for Women"
> across her hat and "Votes for Women" across her chest. She said,
> "Now what am I going to talk about?" I said . . . "you were to talk
> about nursing on the Continent." "Oh," she said, "very bad. It'll
> not be any better till they get the suffrage. I'll talk about
> suffrage."
>
> *Stewart, 1961, pp. 139–140*

Miss Stewart continued:

> This suffrage thing—it was the whole thing for her; she wanted
> not only to work for it but really to suffer for it. She went over
> to Britain to work with Mrs. Pankhurst, and she wanted above all
> things to go to jail. Oh, she got there all right . . . that was during
> the war, at the beginning of the First World War. She was a
> member of the advanced wing of the Suffrage Party, and they
> were having a meeting in Washington at the time that Wilson
> was beginning to think of the possibility of war. They discussed
> it, and a friend of mine who was there at the time tells me that
> Lavinia got up and seized the flag which was there and said,
> "Youth to the Colors!" and on she marched, out of the door, and
> they followed her, and she went right to the White House, and
> they picketed the White House!
>
> She is about this high, you know. . . . Anyway, they all went
> into the cooler for the night. I think it just pleased her no end.
>
> *Stewart, 1961, p. 275*

Lavinia L. Dock, one of six children in a cultured and affluent family, was born in Harrisburg, Pennsylvania. Both of her parents were well educated and insisted upon equal education for both their sons and daughters. Lavinia was an accomplished organist and pianist, but she decided to enter Bellevue Hospital Training School for Nurses, from which she graduated in 1886. She became a night supervisor at Bellevue Hospital, where she wrote one of the first textbooks for nurses, *Materia Medica for Nurses.* She was aware of the problems the students encountered in learning about drugs and solutions and wrote this book to aid them in the mastery of this content. Since the publisher was unwilling to make the original investment, Lavinia's father advanced the necessary amount. According to Roberts (1956), this investment paid off handsomely; over 100,000 copies of several editions were sold.

During her lifetime Miss Dock held various positions in nursing. She became an assistant to Isabel Hampton Robb at Johns Hopkins Hospital for a time. After leaving Johns Hopkins, she was appointed superintendent of nurses at the Illinois Training School in Chicago. She regarded this brief venture as a failure and left there wondering how they had put up with her. She then joined the Henry Street Settlement to work with Lillian Wald. Miss Dock considered the work at the settlement suited to her and she was happiest there.

Lavinia Dock was concerned with the many problems that were plaguing nursing. She questioned the serious and long-term effects of women's subjugation to men. She believed that male dominance in the health field was the major problem confronting the nursing profession. In 1903 Miss Dock spoke of those developments that would almost ensure male dominance and, in turn, have a major impact on the development of nursing. Her pleas for caution went unheeded, and nurses became accomplices to their own subordination.

> Nursing leaders ignored all her warnings and in the second decade of the century actually became nonvoting members of the American Hospital Association. They worked with physicians and administrators on joint committees, expecting their oppressors to help them solve nursing problems. They sought approval from men, not liberation. As a result, from the first decade of the century onward, physicians and hospital administrators have remained in positions of dominance and control over nursing and health care.
>
> *Ashley, 1975, p. 1466*

Finally, the oppression of nurses was built into the law and the educational system through the legalization of paternalism and the institutionalization of apprenticeship. The threats became a reality as male domination progressed to a state of completion. A powerful combination of male domination and sexual discrimination surfaced and prevented the recognition of nurses as professional equals of physicians with the right to practice independently. Unfortunately, even at present, inequality in the health care field continues to be a serious impediment to the development of the highest potential of nursing.

Lavinia Dock served nursing in numerous elected capacities. Her keen and versatile mind was respected by her colleagues at home and abroad, who looked to her for guidance. She conducted a study of professional organization bylaws and was instrumental in the establishment of the American Society of Superintendents of Training Schools for Nurses. Miss Dock became this organization's first secretary as well as the first secretary of the International Council of Nurses (1899). She is regarded as the chief American influence in the organization of the nurses of the world. Lavinia Dock was active in the movement to effect passage of legislation for the control of nursing practice.

Outspoken on the then-taboo subject of venereal disease, Miss Dock published a book in 1910, *Hygiene and Morality,* which shocked some people. The world of nursing profited by her numerous articles that appeared in the early issues of the *American Journal of Nursing.* The four-volume *History of Nursing* (vols. 1 and 2, 1907; vols. 3 and 4, 1912), written in collaboration with M. Adelaide Nutting became *the* classic text on nursing history. The condensed version, *A Short History of Nursing,* was coauthored with Isabel M. Stewart. Finally, the *History of American Red Cross Nursing* was a massive and comprehensive work. These studies made Miss Dock one of the foremost of nursing historians—

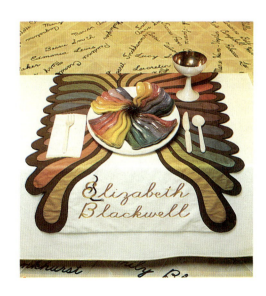

Judy Chicago, "Elizabeth Blackwell," plate from THE DINNER PARTY, 1979. China-painted porcelain, 35.6 cm diameter. Through the Flower, Benicia, California.

> a result achieved by the vitality of her style, knowledge of languages, command of facts, international outlook, an intelligence that would not compromise with stupidity, and a character that scorned to appease evil howsoever intrenched.
>
> *Robinson, 1946, p. 301*

At the turn of the century, some strides had indeed been made toward the achievement of equality and freedom for women. A particular milestone occurred with the readmission of women into the medical field. Elizabeth Blackwell (1821–1910) was the pioneer who was admitted to Geneva Medical College in Geneva, New York, in 1847. Unable to obtain a hospital staff appointment after graduation, she established the New York Infirmary for Women and Children. She also was responsible for the founding of the Women's Medical College of that institution.

However, the women's movement continues even today, and it experiences periodic defeats as well as intermittent successes. The ideal embodied in the efforts of these early nursing leaders has yet to be achieved. The nursing movement mirrors this journey.

■ THE RISE OF ORGANIZED NURSING

Modern nursing was still very young when a few farsighted leaders spurred the movement toward organizational developments. These leaders realized that a group was stronger than an individual, that an organization could accomplish things an individual could not, and that from unity came strength. They believed nursing's real power and potential could be realized through the united efforts of individual members striving to promote its interests. Their commitment to organized nursing was fostered by serious conditions that jeopardized both the recipients and the providers of nursing care. The primary concern of these leaders was, therefore, twofold: protection of the public from poorly trained nurses and the lack of standardization in nurse training.

Lack of endowments had placed the training schools under the control of medicine and hospital administration. The schools provided cheap service to the hospital and thus became profitable enterprises for the institutions. The education of the students was incidental; the students' chief responsibility was to provide care for the hospital, to provide service. The exploitation of nurses occurred as hospitals relied on the inexpensive student labor force to staff the units. With no standards or controls, training schools proliferated at an alarming rate. Consequently, inferior schools also developed and no standards of practice existed to protect the public from unsafe care. The biggest problems facing nursing at the beginning of the twentieth century were those dealing with the setting of standards. These conditions were depicted graphically in a history of nursing in Kansas:

> Lacking a model, the majority of the hospital founders conceived of the trained hospital nurse as a substitute for the competent mother or neighbor who cares for the sick in the home. Primarily she should be a "good housekeeper" of the neighborly type. Since the average housewife of Kansas was still scrubbing her own floors and doing the family washing, it was assumed that these and similar chores were part of the work of a nurse. Even after it became apparent that there was much waste in using educated women for such labors, hospitals continued to spend every available cent to add to their number of student nurses... the students, promised an education, would work for little or for nothing except room and board.... Humanitarians, quite as much as the physicians who founded hospitals as money-making

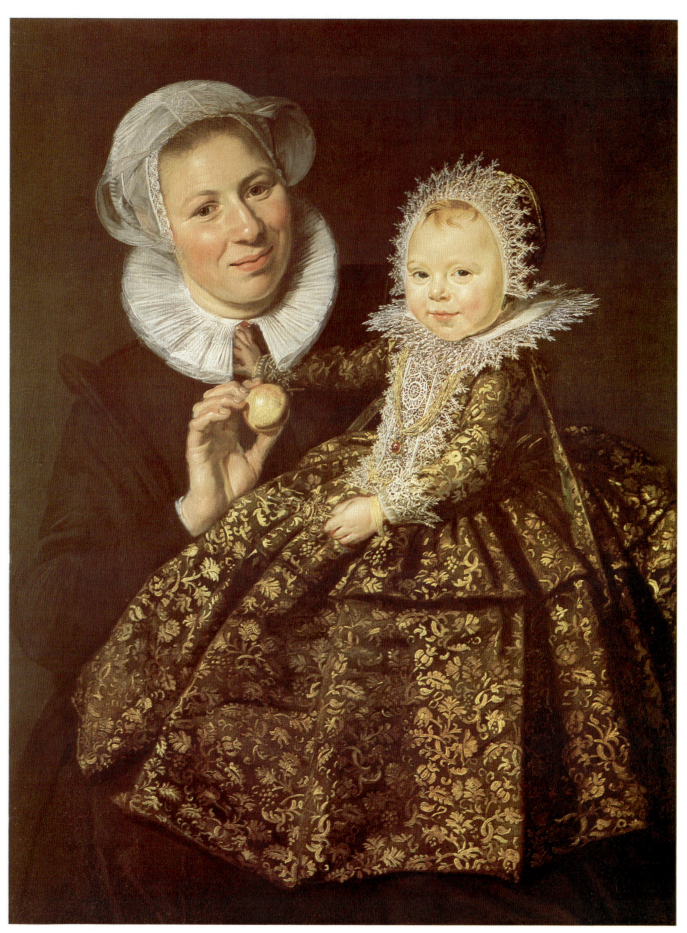

Frans Hals, NURSE AND CHILD, *c. 1620. Berlin-Dahlem, Staatliche Museen Preussischer Kulturbesitz, Berlin, Federal Republic of Germany.*

ventures, shared in the exploitation. . . . It simply did not occur to them that they were perpetuating one wrong in correcting another.

Kansas State Nurses' Association, 1942, p. 93

Organizations for Nurses

Conditions had reached a critical point by the end of the nineteenth century, and an organizational structure was viewed as the one mechanism whereby changes could be attained in nursing education and nursing practice. The first attempt to establish an organization of nurses took place in England. Mrs. Bedford Fenwick, an internationally prominent leader from London, began a campaign in 1887 for nurse registration. This idea was not well accepted, even though the quality of nursing care was inconsistent and frequently inferior in Britain. Mrs. Fenwick was, however, convinced that standards were necessary to improve nursing, and she founded the British Nurses' Association in 1888 to achieve legal sanction. This association was the first of its type anywhere in the world. It grew rapidly and its members numbered 1000 by the end of one year. Membership was not limited to graduate nurses but included some physicians (a few were honorary officers!). Although there was opposition to this organization, eventually it obtained a royal charter in 1892 under the title of The Royal British Nurses' Association. Similar societies developed in other countries as the advantages from such a united endeavor were demonstrated. The overall aim of each of the organizations was similar—to improve the education and status of nurses and to secure for them state recognition (Seymer, 1932).

The earliest nurses' association in America, of which there is scant information, was the Philomena Society. It was started in New York in 1886 but lasted only one year. As nursing schools developed, however, alumnae associations were formed to foster fellowship and mutual support and to provide economic assistance when necessary. These groups became convenient units for amalgamation, which later proved to be beneficial when the national organization emerged. The first alumnae associations were formed at Bellevue Hospital in New York (1889), Illinois Training School of Cook County Hospital in Chicago (1891), Johns Hopkins Hospital in Baltimore (1892), Massachusetts General Hospital in Boston (1895), and Boston City Hospital (1896).

American Society of Superintendents of Training Schools for Nurses. The year 1893 marks the "debut" of American nursing and the beginning of a new era in nursing education. At the World's Fair in Chicago in that year, the International Congress of Charities, Corrections and Philanthropy was held. A part of this congress was devoted to hospitals and dispensaries. Through the encouragement of Mrs. Bedford Fenwick, Dr. John S. Billings, chairman of the congress, agreed that nursing should occupy a place on the program. The subsection on nursing was chaired by Isabel Adams Hampton, superintendent of nurses at Johns Hopkins Hospital. The meeting was attended by both American and Canadian nurses, and papers were read that reflected and frankly presented the major nursing issues and concerns. In addition, the need for a national union was urged. The papers were eventually compiled in a publication, *Nursing of the Sick, 1893,* and were viewed as an historical record of the progress made and the problems encountered in the two decades following the opening of the first training school.

The day after the nursing program had taken place, Miss Hampton arranged for a meeting with a small group to discuss the possibilities for a nursing organization. This meeting was attended by directors of nursing schools and resulted in the formation of the American Society of Superintendents of Training Schools for Nurses as a binational organization. Membership was restricted to those nurses associated with nurse training; thus, in effect, it became an accrediting agency for schools of nursing in the United States and Canada (Stewart and Austin, 1962). The aim of the society was to develop high educational standards for schools of nursing through the establishment of universal requirements for admission, a sound program of theory and practice, and improved working conditions. A curriculum committee was promptly appointed, and a report was published two years later. In 1907 Canadian members formed their own independent organization, the Canadian Society of Superintendents of Training Schools, with Mary Agnes Snively as its first president. In 1912 the American society became known by a new name, the National League of Nursing Education, and still later as the National League for Nursing.

The society was occupied for the first two years with the development of a national association of graduate nurses in order that the practice of all types of nursing might be represented. This effort was led by Isabel Hampton Robb, M. Adelaide Nutting, and Lavinia L. Dock, all of whom were at Johns Hopkins. Miss Dock carefully studied the laws under which professional organizations could operate and how they could be formulated. Her report to the society at the 1896 convention proposed that alumnae associations be the mode of entrance to the new organization; the development of local and state units would follow. A committee was appointed to prepare a constitution and bylaws for a national nurses' organization; it was instructed to meet with a number of delegates from the oldest alumnae associations.

Nurses' Associated Alumnae of the United States and Canada. The committee of the society and the delegates of the alumnae associations met in New York in September 1896. The following year the constitution and bylaws that had been prepared by this group were accepted and a national nurses' association was established. This second organization, created for the rank and file in nursing, was called the Nurses' Associated Alumnae of the United States and Canada. The original purposes of this association in 1897 were: "(1) To establish and maintain a code of ethics; (2) to elevate the standards of nursing education; (3) to promote the usefulness and honor, the financial and other interests of the nursing profession" (American Nurses' Association, 1941, p. 2). A primary objective was to secure legislation to differentiate between the trained and the untrained nurse, since the title of "trained nurse" had come to mean all grades of training and all grades of women.

When the association sought to incorporate, it was found that New York law prohibited foreign membership. It was therefore necessary to eliminate the words "and Canada," which prohibited fur-

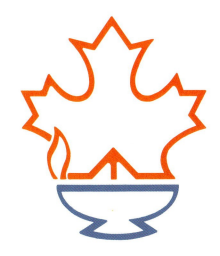

Logo for the Canadian Nurses Association. Courtesy Canadian Nurses Association, Ottawa, Ontario.

ther Canadian participation. Canadian nurses withdrew from the organization as early as 1900. In 1908 the Provisional Organization of the Canadian National Association of Trained Nurses was formed. The name was changed to the Canadian Nurses Association at the 1924 convention. In the early years of this association, "the recurring problems under discussion were education of student nurses, improvement of nursing care of patients, amelioration of conditions for nurses, and the need for state registration of nurses as a safeguard to the public" (Gibbon and Mathewson, 1947, p. 348). By the time the association was renamed the American Nurses' Association in 1911 and chartered by the state of New York, Canadian membership had been discontinued.

The first president of the Nurses' Associated Alumnae was Isabel Adams Hampton Robb (1859–1910). One author described her as "the radiant center of the magnetic force which brought the two national organizations into existence before 1900" (Roberts, 1954, p. 26). Another has called her the "architect of American nursing organizations" (Fitzpatrick, 1983). Whatever titles are used to describe her, Mrs. Robb was undoubtedly one of the greatest early leaders in American nursing and perhaps the best loved. She was a forceful and farsighted individual, yet she demonstrated a gentle force that was considered a main characteristic of her leadership:

> With great practical ability in details, Miss Hampton had a power of seeing the future which was like that of a sibyl. She had visions of nursing growth, organization, and activities, which came first as hazy, indefinite pictures, gradually taking form until all was clear and vivid, filling her with joy and enthusiasm, eager interest, and untiring energy . . . filled with the highest belief in the mission of women as the superior moral force, and in the possibility of universal happiness. . . .
>
> *Nutting and Dock, vol. 3, 1912, pp. 123–124*

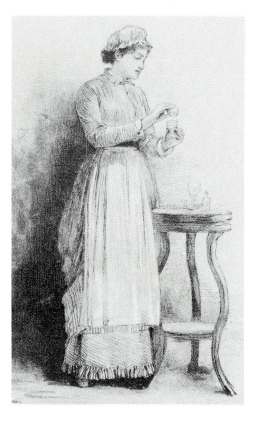

THE NURSE, *Isabel A. Hampton, Bellevue Hospital, 1882. Sketched from life for* CENTURY MAGAZINE, *November 1882, in "A New Profession for Women." The Bettmann Archive, New York.*

Isabel Adams Hampton was born in Canada (Welland, Ontario). She attended the Collegiate Institute of St. Catharine's, Ontario, after which she taught at the Merriton School for approximately three years. In 1881 she was admitted to the Bellevue Hospital Training School for Nurses and graduated in 1883. For a brief period Miss Hampton served as a relief supervisor at Women's Hospital in New York, followed by two years as a staff nurse at St. Paul's Hospice in Rome, Italy. Upon her return to the United States, she became superintendent of nurses at Illinois Training School in Chicago, where she introduced several innovations of educational import. Miss Hampton implemented a graded system of theory and practice, terminated the practice of students doing private duty as part of their education (she believed this practice to be an exploitation of the students, since the hospital received the fees), and originated the concept of affiliation, whereby students could gain necessary experiences not available in their home institutions. These innovations were undoubtedly influenced by her experience as a teacher and by her grounding in educational theory.

Miss Hampton was not yet thirty when she was chosen to organize the school of nursing of Johns Hopkins Hospital. It is said that she created quite a sensation upon her arrival because of her serenity and beauty. William Osler, a fellow Canadian, supposedly stated that

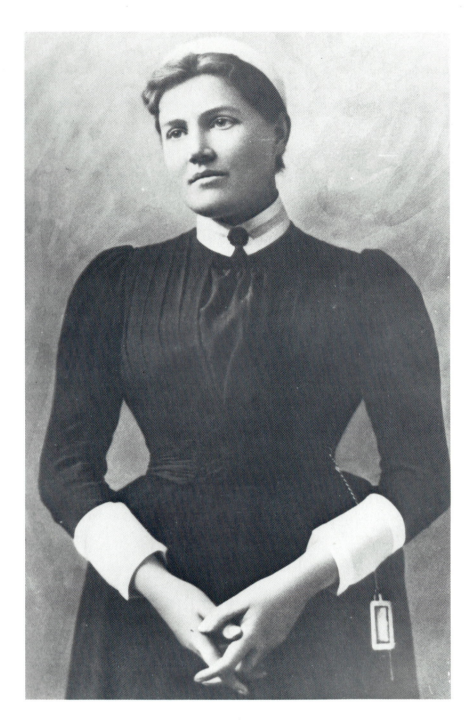

Sergeant Kendall, ISABEL A. HAMPTON, *first Superintendent of Nurses of the Johns Hopkins Hospital Training School for Nurses, c. 1890. The Alan Mason Chesney Medical Archives, Johns Hopkins Medical Institutions, Baltimore, Maryland.*

she entered Hopkins like "an animated Greek statue." She was likened to Venus by both men and women. Lavinia Dock expressed the overall sentiment:

> I thought I had never seen a more beautiful or majestic figure except on the pedestal of some classic sculpture. Miss Hampton's color was rich and fresh, her eyes the clearest blue, unusually large and beautifully set and opened; her voice was one of her greatest charms, being very sweet and quiet, yet with a certain thrill in it when she was in earnest. Her hands were also extremely beautiful, displaying her character and power of organization. They were perfect enough to have been modeled.
>
> *Quoted in Robinson, 1946, p. 173*

More innovations were attempted. Miss Hampton became a "principal" rather than a "superintendent," and policies for a twelve-hour day were established that included time for meals, recreation, rest and study periods. She also recognized the need for nursing publications and authored three influential books: *Nursing: Its Principles and Practice for Hospital and Private Use* (1894), *Nursing Ethics* (1900), and *Educational Standards for Nurses* (1907). It was at Johns Hopkins that Miss Hampton met Dr. Hunter Robb, who had been a resident in gynecology. They were married at St. Margaret's, Westminster, London, on July 12, 1894, with the bride carrying flowers sent by Florence Nightingale. Dr. Robb was not well liked by Isabel's colleagues because they believed that he was not an equal match for her in either intellectual ability or physical appearance. The Robbs settled in Cleveland, Ohio, where they eventually had two sons.

Mrs. Robb continued her activities in nursing and made her greatest contributions after her marriage. She helped found the two national nursing organizations, shouldered the burden for the launching of the program for graduate nurses at Teachers College, was one of the original members of a committee to found the *American Journal of Nursing,* and was essentially the central force in the early development of professional nursing in the United States. One wonders how much more she would have accomplished had she not died prematurely in a traffic accident on April 15, 1910.

Mary Adelaide Nutting (1858–1948) was a nursing leader who was greatly influenced by Isabel Hampton Robb and, in fact, became her successor at Johns Hopkins. Miss Nutting, too, was born in Canada (Quebec), and she received special instruction in music and art in private schools in Montreal, Boston, and Ottawa. An alumna of the first graduating class of Johns Hopkins, Miss Nutting translated Miss Hampton's dreams of a three-year course and an eight-hour day into reality. However, Adelaide Nutting was an innovator in her own right. According to Christy (1969b), she was second only to Florence Nightingale in overall contributions to nursing. "Her influence as an educational experimenter and a creative thinker went far beyond the two institutions in which her main work was done, the second being Teachers College, Columbia University" (Stewart, 1943, p. 143).

During her tenure in Baltimore, Miss Nutting initiated and developed the preliminary course, tuition fees, and scholarships at Johns Hopkins. She helped with the organization of the Maryland State Nurses Association, served as its first president, and facilitated the efforts of the nurses in their quest for state registration. She also began collecting materials and books for an historical collection for the nursing school. These later became the basis for the first two volumes of the four-volume *A History of Nursing* written with Lavinia Dock. Miss Nutting wrote many articles, some of which were published as a collection in *A Sound Economic Basis for Schools of Nursing.* She prepared two influential reports on nursing education that were issued through the United States Bureau of Education. Her letters, speeches, and published works demonstrated her belief in a broad education for nurses that would prepare them for great responsibilities in all life situations. Her lifelong dream was to see basic education for nurses firmly established in institutions of higher learning—in universities.

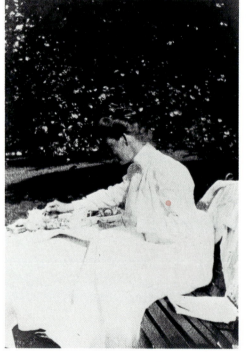

M. ADELAIDE NUTTING, *1905. The Alan Mason Chesney Medical Archives, Johns Hopkins Medical Institutions, Baltimore, Maryland.*

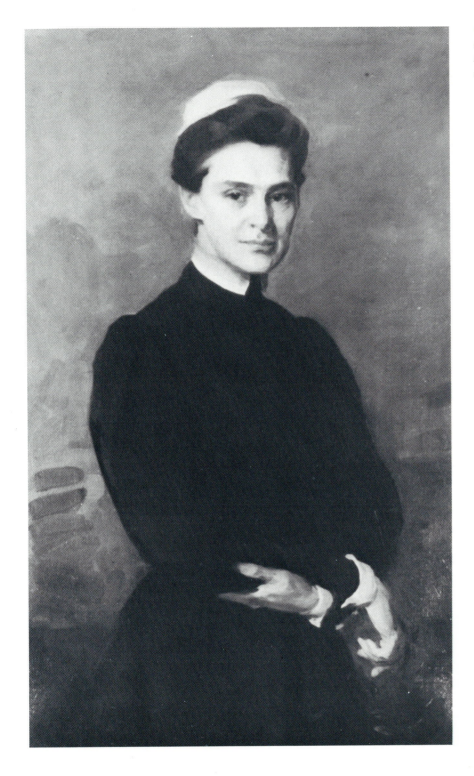

Cecilia Beaux, M. ADELAIDE NUTTING, *1906.*
Special Collections, Milbank Memorial
Library, Teachers College, Columbia Univer-
sity, New York.

In 1907 M. Adelaide Nutting took charge of the hospital economics course at Teachers College and became the first professor of
nursing in the world. Her original title was Professor of Domestic
Administration, but it was changed to Professor of Nurses Education
in 1910. She remained at Teachers College until her retirement in
1925. In addition to her administrative and educational responsibilities at this institution, Miss Nutting participated in many nursing activities, including organizational work, committee work, government
projects, the war effort, publications, and international endeavors.
She was the prime instigator in the establishment of the Vassar

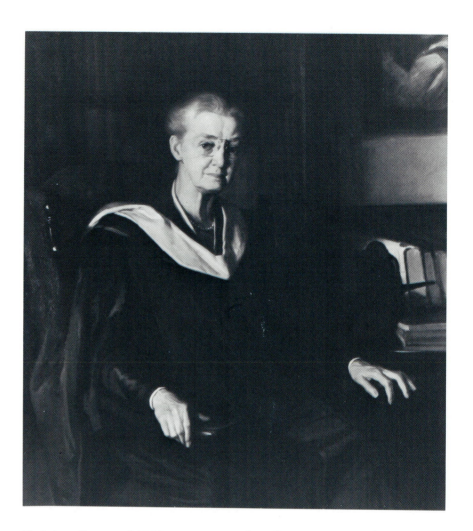

Stanislav Rembski, M. ADELAIDE NUTTING IN ACADEMIC ROBES, *c. 1932. Special Collections, Milbank Memorial Library, Teachers College, Columbia University, New York.*

Training Camp of 1918, a program that drew women who were college graduates into nursing.

Miss Nutting received many awards in recognition of her deep and lasting commitment and service to nursing. She was granted an honorary master of arts degree from Yale in 1921, the Liberty Service Medal for humanitarian and patriotic services, and the Adelaide Nutting Medal for Leadership in Nursing Education in 1944. This medal was designed by the National League of Nursing Education. The Adelaide Nutting Historical Nursing Collection at Teachers College was dedicated to her memory and outstanding leadership. Miss Nutting died on October 3, 1948, after a long illness. She was a visionary whose words will long be remembered as being forever relevant:

> We need to realize and to affirm anew that nursing is one of the most difficult of arts. Compassion may provide the motive, but knowledge is our only working power. Perhaps, too, we need to remember that growth in our work must be preceded by ideas, and that any conditions which suppress thought, must retard growth. Surely we will not be satisfied in perpetuating methods and traditions. Surely we shall wish to be more and more occupied with creating them.
>
> *Nutting, 1925*

American Nurses' Association. The American Nurses' Association became the successor to the Nurses' Associated Alumnae of the United States in 1911. The original federation of alumnae asso-

366

ciations proved less workable as nurses became more mobile and began to move from state to state. A national organization with participation through state associations or through individual membership seemed more feasible, particularly because by 1912 thirty-nine state nurses' associations had been organized. The original body remained a federation of alumnae associations until the convention of 1916, when it was decided to establish membership through the state associations. State associations would eventually provide the means for achieving legal regulation. Unity of nurses within specific states, therefore, was essential to the passage of any licensing laws.

The ANA is *the* professional organization for registered nurses in the United States, and as such it holds membership in the International Council of Nurses. In the early years of the organization, state registration was a major concern. The purposes of the ANA have always been to foster high standards of nursing practice, to promote the welfare of nurses, and to improve the general working conditions of nurses.

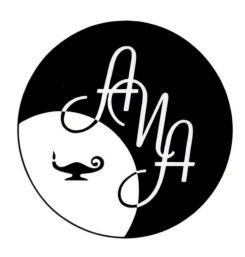

Logo for the American Nurses' Association. Courtesy of the American Nurses' Association, Inc., Kansas City, Missouri.

International Council of Nurses.

The International Council of Nurses, established in 1899, is the oldest of all international organizations for professional workers. It was founded by Mrs. Bedford Fenwick in cooperation with nursing leaders from many countries. In 1900 the council's constitution was adopted, and the first meeting was held at the World Exposition in Buffalo, New York, in 1901. Membership was open to self-governing national nurses' associations rather than to individuals (as such, it is an association of associations). Its established purposes were to provide a means of communication between the nurses of all nations and to offer opportunities for nurses from all parts of the world to meet and confer on questions relating to patient welfare and the nursing profession. The International Council of Nurses stands for the full development of the human being and citizen in every nurse and ever higher standards of education, professional ethics, public usefulness, and civic spirit.

National Association of Colored Graduate Nurses.

Although the nursing organizations never expressed any racial prejudice, Black nurses realized they had problems of their own that would be best served by a separate organization. They needed to break down discriminatory practices that occurred because of the hue of their skin and with no consideration for their nursing proficiency. Black nurses were also denied membership in some state and local nursing organizations.

The National Association of Colored Graduate Nurses (NACGN) was established in 1908. Its founding was the direct result of the vision, wisdom, and initiative of Martha Franklin, a graduate of the school of the Woman's Hospital of Philadelphia. Miss Franklin had conducted a study of the status of Black nurses before sending out letters to explore interest in the formation of a national organization. A meeting was held in August 1908 in New York under the sponsorship of the alumnae of Lincoln School for Nurses and its president, Adah Thomas. By the end of this meeting the association had been formed and its objectives determined: to achieve higher professional standards; to break down discriminatory practices facing Negro nurses in schools, in jobs, and in organizational activities; to develop Negro nurse leadership. Miss Franklin was named the first president of this association.

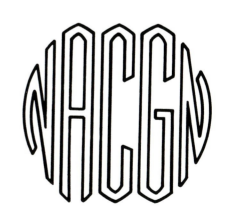

Logo for the National Association of Colored Graduate Nurses. Courtesy of Schomburg Center for Research in Black Culture, The New York Public Library, New York.

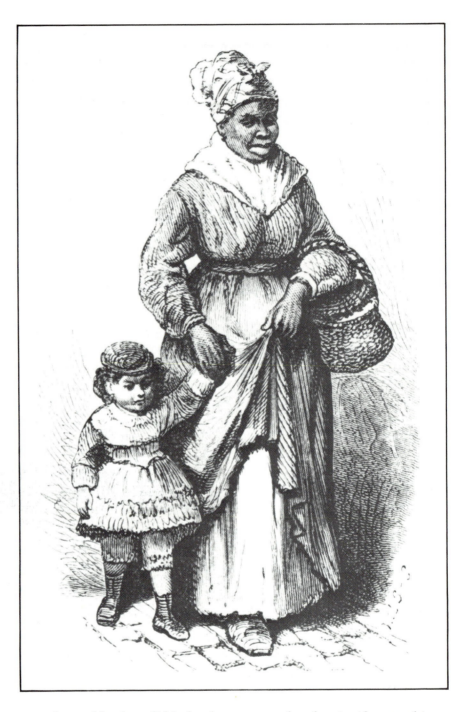

"The Negro Nurses Stroll on the Sidewalks, Chattering in Quaint French to the Little Children," New Orleans, 1873. Schomburg Center for Research in Black Culture, The New York Public Library, New York.

Several leaders did indeed emerge and make significant achievements. Adah Thomas led the campaign for the acceptance of Black nurses in the Red Cross. These nurses served with the Army Nurse Corps in World War I. Miss Thomas also founded a registry for Black nurses in New York (1918) and authored the first book on Black nursing history. Estelle Massey (Osborne) was the first Black nurse to serve on the ANA board of directors, was awarded the NACGN scholarship for advanced study, and was the first Black nurse to earn a master's degree with a major in nursing from Teachers College. Mabel K. Staupers served as executive officer of the NACGN from 1934 to 1949, was elected the last president of the association, and chronicled the history of the organization in *No Time for Prejudice* (1961).

The NACGN continued to make valuable contributions to nursing. It brought the concerns of Blacks in America to the attention of

368

both nurses and the general public. In 1949 the organization believed it had accomplished its purpose and voted for dissolution. The program was phased out gradually over the next two years. In 1950 the ANA committed itself to assume responsibility for the functions of the NACGN by virtue of a platform adopted by the ANA house of delegates. The platform supported "full participation of minority groups in association activities . . . and the elimination of discrimination in job opportunities, salaries, and other working conditions" (American Nurses' Association, 1950).

National League of Nursing Education.

With the change of membership and scope of functions, the American Society of Superintendents of Training Schools was renamed the National League of Nursing Education (NLNE) in 1912. The membership was expanded to include those individuals whose greatest interest and training was in the field of nursing education, directors of public health nursing, members of state boards of nurse examiners, and those directly concerned with teaching and supervising in nursing schools. The goal of uniform standards now was seen to be impractical, since minimum requirements for state registration varied from state to state. The league decided to assist schools of nursing to achieve professional status comparable with that of similar professional groups. Therefore special attention was given to increased financial support for nursing schools, sounder educational programs, and closer associations with institutions of higher learning. In 1932 the league became the Department of Education of the ANA, as voted upon by both organizations. It was therefore necessary to hold membership in the ANA in order to be a member of the NLNE. The National League of Nursing Education was the organization most active in shaping educational thinking and practice in nursing for many years; its annual reports became a major asset to nursing.

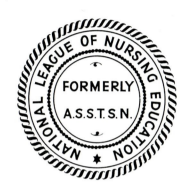

Seal for the National League of Nursing Education. Donahue Collection. By permission of the National League for Nursing, New York.

The National Organization for Public Health Nursing.

The third national nursing association, the National Organization for Public Health Nursing (NOPHN), was established in 1912. By this time, district and visiting nursing had expanded rapidly to keep pace with the growth of new social services. National standards were urgently needed for one of the most promising movements of modern society. In addition, the care given by the nurse in the community differed from that given by the nurse in the hospital. A joint committee of the two national organizations, with Lillian D. Wald as chair and Mary S. Gardner as secretary, was appointed. The committee arranged for representatives of agencies employing visiting nurses to attend a meeting to be held in conjunction with the ANA and NLNE convention in Chicago in 1912. As a result, this organization came into being, but it was different in the makeup of its membership:

> The name was selected with the utmost care to emphasize the fact that the new organization was not composed solely of nurses and that it would be concerned with the development of *nursing*. Three classes of membership were agreed upon: corporate (agency), individual (active public health nurses), and associate. The associate members would be non-public health nurses and lay persons, privileged to participate in discussions

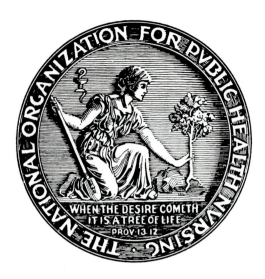

Seal for The National Organization for Public Health Nursing. Donahue Collection. Courtesy of the National League for Nursing, New York.

The seal symbolically represents the public health nurse, who plants the tree of life with the hope for better health in the community. "When the desire cometh it is a Tree of Life."

but with no voting power. That restriction was removed at an early date when fear of lay domination or interference with strictly professional matters had been found to be quite groundless.

Roberts, 1954, p. 88

Lillian D. Wald was destined to become the first president of the new organization. Her social vision, excellent facility in public relations, and extraordinary gift for friendship were definite assets in the overall public health movement. Miss Wald led the members in the enormous task of establishing standards for public health nurses, arranging courses to prepare them for their work, increasing the numbers of public health nurses, and building up organized voluntary and official agencies for home and community visiting nurse services. Two other officers were equally prominent: Mary S. Gardner, a pioneer in visiting nursing and author of a book on public health nursing, and Ella Phillips Crandall, director of the first public health nursing program at Teachers College. *Public Health Nursing* was the official journal of the organization. Although the three major organizations had somewhat different functions, they also had common purposes and interests and worked closely together.

Sigma Theta Tau. Sigma Theta Tau was founded in 1922 at Indiana University. As the national honor society of nursing, this organization promotes nursing research and leadership. Its members, who are selected on the basis of scholarly achievement and professional leadership, include baccalaureate degree students, graduate students in nursing programs, and community nursing leaders.

The Association of Collegiate Schools of Nursing. The Association of Collegiate Schools of Nursing (ACSN) was organized in 1933 to represent schools or departments of nursing associated with universities. In 1932 a decision had been made by representatives of more than twenty schools in San Antonio to proceed with such an organization. The following January a conference was held at Teachers College, and it was decided to form the association. The standards or purposes adopted in 1935 were:

1. To develop nursing education on a professional and collegiate level.
2. To promote and strengthen relationships between schools of nursing and institutions of higher learning.
3. To promote study and experimentation in nursing service and nursing education.

ACSN, 1943, p. 30

Membership standards were established, and membership was extended to schools that met specific criteria. The association did not originally consider itself an accrediting agency, but it visited and evaluated schools that applied for membership and thus was regarded by many as an accrediting body.

The ACSN was engaged in many activities related to higher education during its existence. It constantly emphasized the need for research in nursing and the preparation of nurse researchers. Both would be mandatory if nursing was ever to qualify on an equal basis

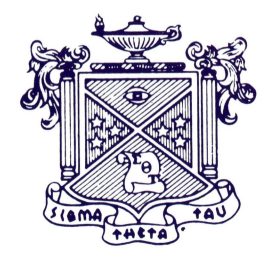

Shield for the nursing honor society, Sigma Theta Tau, established in 1922 at the University of Indiana in Indianapolis.

with other departments in colleges and universities. In 1950 the association's Committee on Research recommended that the American Journal of Nursing Company be asked to publish a periodical that would focus on research in nursing. This was the beginning step toward the publication of *Nursing Research.*

When changes in organized nursing ultimately occurred, the decision was made that the responsibilities of the ACSN would be assumed by the Department of Baccalaureate and Higher Degrees of the new NLN. The association had indeed proven its value to nursing and nursing education in a very short time span.

■ A NEW LOOK FOR ORGANIZED NURSING

The numerous changes that had been occurring in nursing service and education mandated changes for organized nursing. The particular challenges of the Depression and World War I had forced some modification of their structure and activities. Increased numbers of nurses were needed to meet the World War II effort, and yet no one nursing association could speak or act for nursing as a whole. A commission representing all nursing interests was thus established to facilitate the efforts of both nursing and the national defense. Originally called the Nursing Council on National Defense, it was reorganized in late 1940 and renamed the National Nursing Council for War Service. The initial voting members of the council included the ANA, NLNE, NOPHN, ACSN, NACGN, and the Red Cross Nursing Service. As soon as the American Association of Industrial Nurses (AAIN) organized in 1942, it gained membership. In addition, representatives of the Army and Navy Nurse Corps, United States Public Health Service (USPHS), Veterans Administration, Children's Bureau, Office of Indian Affairs, American Hospital Association, and the Canadian Nurses Association were ex officio members.

The representatives of these prestigious agencies were able to secure access to important sources of advice and information that greatly assisted the program. The council's preliminary work was financed by nursing. Later, beginning in 1942, the W.K. Kellogg Foundation became the council's principal source of income and contributed over $300,000. (Allocations for special projects were received from other foundations and private sources.) For the duration of the war, state nurses' associations carried most of the local expenses of council-sponsored projects. The council was responsible for developing nursing programs to meet wartime needs:

1. It reviewed wartime projects in relation to the functions of the member agencies and recommended new projects to appropriate agencies.
2. It administered projects which did not fall within the scope of any one member agency.
3. Under the changing conditions of war, it outlined projects which seemed to be beyond the scope of any voluntary agency and referred them to the Government's Subcommittee.

Roberts, 1954, p. 358

371

When the war finally ended, the council decided to continue functioning until such time as another body replaced it or another method was recommended for continued coordination among the nursing associations. Esther Lucile Brown was engaged "to direct a study of the organization, administration, and support of professional and practical nursing as a basis for influencing the quality of nursing for the public" (Fitzpatrick, 1983, p. 169). The council also appointed a committee to plan for an accrediting agency for nursing education, and the National Nursing Accrediting Service was established in 1948. The council dissolved in that same year.

The accomplishments of the council during the war and several years after it proved that unified planning could be done by nursing, that cooperative efforts could and did improve the efficiency of organized nursing. The leaders of the associations were convinced that a permanent measure was necessary to ensure continued collaboration. A special committee, the Promoting Committee for the Structure of National Professional Nursing Organizations, began its study under Amelia Grant in 1945. This resulted in a "Report on the Structure of Organized Nursing," which was delivered at the biennial convention of 1946. It was determined that the six organizations in the study—the ANA, NLNE, NACGN, NOPHN, ACSN, and AAIN—were divided on three main points: non-nurse membership, special interests, and program emphasis. Considering the import of these issues, two alternative plans for organized nursing were proposed. The first

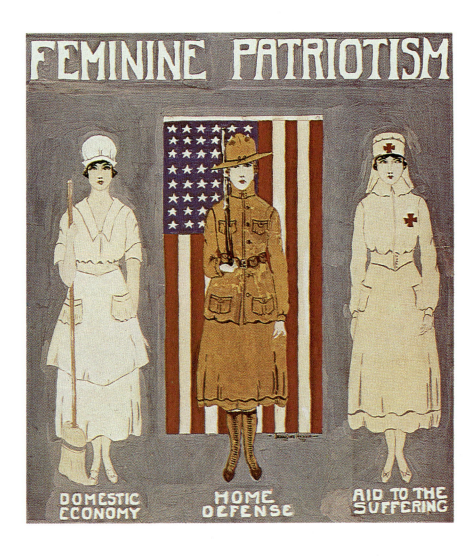

FEMININE PATRIOTISM, *American poster.*
National Archives and Records Service,
Washington, D.C.

suggested a single organization, the ANA, composed of five types of membership—professional nurses, public members, allied professionals, nursing schools and service agencies, and non-nursing organizations. The second plan was a two-organization system. One organization, the ANA, would accept only nurses. The other would be a national organization for nursing service composed of nurses, lay persons, allied professionals, and agency members. Cooperation would evolve through a joint commission for common concerns and a national nursing center with representatives from both organizations on its board.

After long months of deliberation by all concerned associations and individuals, more committee work, and the development of other plans, the ANA House of Delegates cast a majority vote for a two-organization plan at the 1950 Biennial Convention. The structure called for two distinct organizations: first, a somewhat reorganized American Nurses' Association (ANA), comprised entirely of nurses and able to speak for the profession, and second, the National League for Nursing (NLN), comprised of nurses and non-nurses, individual and corporate members and representing those responsible for sound development and support of nursing services and nursing schools. Between 1950 and 1952, staffing and bylaws were developed. The new structure was adopted at the Biennial Convention in Atlantic City, June 15 to 20, 1952. That historic meeting was attended by over 9000 individuals. The two associations, under the direction of their newly elected presidents, Elizabeth K. Porter (ANA) and Ruth Sleeper (NLN), immediately initiated steps for the reorganization of state associations and the establishment of headquarters in New York. Several organizations were absorbed by the National League for Nursing: National League of Nursing Education, National Organization for Public Health Nursing, Association of Collegiate Schools of Nursing, Joint Committee on Practical Nurses and Auxiliary Workers in Nursing Services, Joint Committee on Careers in Nursing, National Committee for the Improvement of Nursing Services, and National Nursing Accrediting Service.

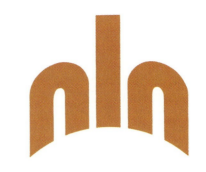

Logo for the National League for Nursing. Courtesy of the National League for Nursing, New York.

■ THE CAMPAIGN FOR LEGISLATION AND REGISTRATION

The first published words regarding licensure for nurses came from a physician, Sir Henry W. Acland, in 1860. A regius professor of medicine at Oxford University, he wrote that nurses should be centrally registered, should follow a recognized curriculum of study, and should be able to meet a minimum standard of proficiency (Mollett, 1888). British nurses, however, did not begin to organize for state regulation of nursing practice until 1887. The first registration or licensing law for nurses was actually passed in Cape Colony, South Africa, in 1891. Although it was not a distinct nursing law, but one incorporated as part of a medical and pharmacy act, it nonetheless gave hope to the British nurses who were having a difficult campaign. It was not until 1919, after a struggle commonly referred to as the "Thirty Years' War," that these nurses were able to succeed in their efforts. In 1901 New Zealand passed a Nurses' Registration Act, which was the first true nursing act. Similar laws were adopted in five other countries, including Canadian provinces, by 1914. Meanwhile American nurses had begun a campaign of their own for a proposed program of legislation. They believed that the protection of the public and the welfare of the individual nurse were primary issues of concern.

The need for professional controls that would protect nursing standards was made evident by the proliferation of schools of nursing. The maintenance of these standards, however, was not purely a nursing problem, since the public safety and welfare were involved. The continued development of poorly qualified schools jeopardized the public by the perpetuation of "unqualified" or "improperly trained" nurses. The newly formed nursing associations thus focused attention on acquiring a mechanism that would secure legal recognition for graduate nurses. Legislation that would distinguish between graduate and nongraduate personnel was desired. Control of education and professional practice in America came under the states, not under the federal government. State organizations were, therefore, being formed to carry on what proved to be a long and bitter fight for nurse registration. Active campaigns were launched and appeals for action were made by state nurses' associations to state legislatures. The force of opposition came from outside groups who were financially interested in preventing nurses from achieving state recognition.

In 1898 a public statement on nurse licensure was made by Sophia Palmer before the New York State Federation of Women's Clubs. The idea was endorsed by the federation in the form of a resolution, and the campaign for legislation and registration was actively begun. This work was carried on for many years by the associations and the leaders in nursing. Finally, in a span of less than two months, the states of North Carolina, New Jersey, New York, and Virginia achieved licensure laws in 1903. An *American Journal of Nursing* editorial of November 1903, presumably written by Sophia Palmer, clearly and succinctly defined the issue:

IMPROVING THE IMAGE OF NURSING, *reproduced in the* AMERICAN JOURNAL OF NURSING, *January 1983. Courtesy of the artist Kristine Boyd.*

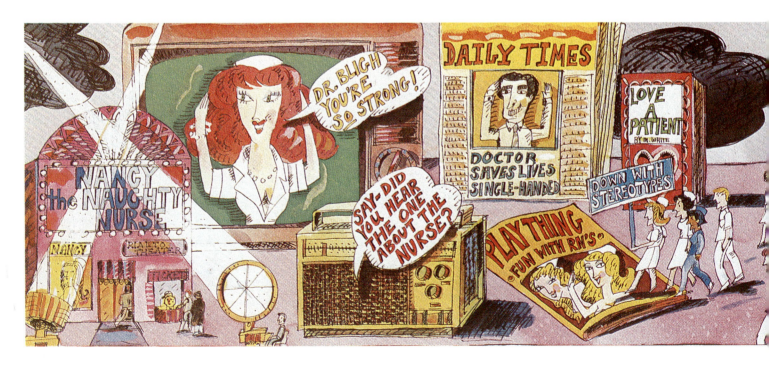

The A,B,C of State Registration

It would seem as if every nurse in the land must, after all that has been said and written, understand the reasons for State registration, and comprehend something of how such registration will affect the nurse already in practice, but we frequently hear from or talk with nurses who we realize have failed to grasp . . . the reasons for this great movement. . . .

This movement . . . is a purely educational one; it is the first great concerted effort of nurses for the advancement, elevation, and protection of the nurses of the future. . . .

Nurses cannot realize even with all the advance that has been made . . . the trained nurse of today has no legal standing. . . . She does not belong to a profession, she is not classed even with the graduates of a technical school, and the woman who has taken up nursing without any training, or who has been discharged from a training school for serious cause, has the same right to call herself a trained nurse before the law as she who has given three years of hard work and hard study.

How long will nurses permit such conditions to exist when only a strong, concerted action is needed to improve the educational standard, to protect the public and nurses themselves against imposters, and to give trained nursing a place among the honorable professions!

Twenty years later, legislation regulating nurses' training was implemented in forty-eight states, Hawaii, and the District of Columbia. This provided for the licensing of nurses after examination and for nurse representation on examining boards. Boards of nurse examiners of the respective states were authorized by law to judge the competency of nurses applying for registration and licensing. Although the state laws were similar, they varied in their requirements and the power behind them. They were permissive, not mandatory; denied the untrained the use of the RN title; specified a time period when qualified trained nurses were eligible for registration without examination. The conditions of the early nurse licensure laws, the

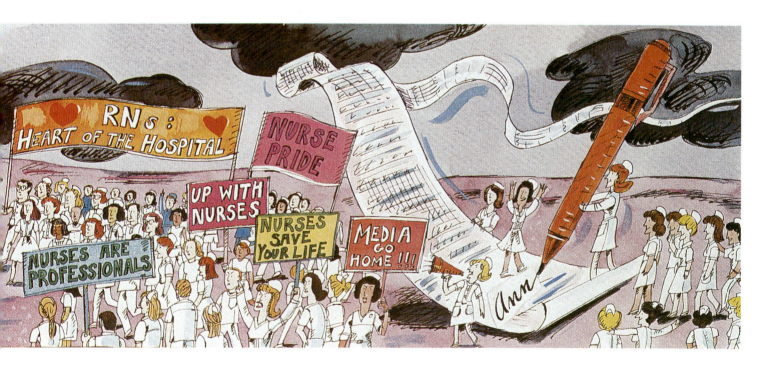

first nurse practice acts, were very weak and left much to be desired. Yet registration had positive results, such as accreditation and a movement toward uniformity in nursing schools. In addition, the campaign and struggle for state laws did much to strengthen and unite the whole of nursing.

■ EDUCATIONAL TRENDS AND DEVELOPMENTS

Following 1900, the increasing complexity of nursing services exerted continual pressure for the improvement of nursing schools. Most schools continued under hospital control; most operated on a subprofessional level. Nursing organizations, nurses, foundations, committees, agencies, and hospital groups began to conduct surveys and studies of nurses and nursing. Consequently, recommendations began to be made relevant to educational standards and practices. The influence of newer educational viewpoints surfaced in experiments and innovations. Continued support for upgrading nursing education was being demonstrated. In *A Sound Economic Basis for Schools of Nursing,* M. Adelaide Nutting emphasized the subordination of the educational program:

> Heavy demands of the wards made it impossible for all students to attend their weekly lecture and it was always arranged that some students would choose to take very full notes and read them later to the assembled group of less fortunate. Lectures came under the category of privileges like "hours off duty" to be granted "hospital duties permitting."
>
> *Nutting, 1926, pp. 339–340*

What must be remembered is that the progressive development in educational reforms in schools of nursing was intertwined with aspects of life in the United States at the turn of the century.

> With the frontier gone, the continent subdued, and the nation now proud of its designation as a world power, a new era of mature consolidation was at hand. The democratic political foundations upon which the nation had been established remained intact, indeed were broadened by the termination of Negro slavery. Tens of millions of Europeans of many races and peoples had been absorbed without any serious social consequences and population had increased from five to seventy-six million. The national wealth in the last half of the nineteenth century had increased from seven to eighty-eight million dollars, and the standard of living for the common man was better than almost anywhere in the world. Great strides had been made in agriculture and industry, through the utilization of limited government assistance, cheap labor, plentiful natural resources, and "clever Yankee inventions." These factors made possible the rise . . . and the upgrading of the nursing profession which accompanied it in the new era now opening.
>
> The objectives of Americans were not merely utilitarian. Free public education and freedom of religion were deeply cherished and influential ideals. In literature, the arts, and the sciences,

there was tremendous enthusiasm, growing pride, and substantial achievement, and traditional reformism, aimed at removing or reducing the ills of society, remained strong and vigorous. In place of slavery and illiteracy, industrial monopoly, farm tenancy, unequal rights for women, and epidemic disease became the new targets for change.

Christy, 1969a, pp. 3–4

Some improvements were being made, particularly in the better schools of nursing. An early preparatory course was started in Scotland at the Glasgow Infirmary in 1893. Mrs. Rebecca Strong, then superintendent, with the assistance of Dr. McEwen, who was one of Lister's students, succeeded in having nursing students enter St. Mungo's College for a short course of theoretical instruction followed by practical training in the hospital. This was the first connection of any kind that nursing students had with an institution of higher learning. The inception of preparatory or preliminary courses made these programs more like those of educational institutions rather than a strict apprenticeship system. The first such course in America was developed in 1901 through the efforts of Miss Nutting at Johns Hopkins. This preparatory course was six months long and offered basic sciences as well as nursing principles and practice, the latter experience being on the hospital wards. The primary difference in this instance was that the clinical experience was for the purpose of education, not service.

A number of schools adopted this plan, but many of them found it difficult to supply the theoretical and practical courses required. A few developed preparatory courses in affiliation with technical schools such as Drexel Institute, Pratt, and Simmons College.

Dock and Stewart, 1938, p. 178

Within ten years, approximately eighty-six schools had preparatory courses that averaged three to four months in length.

Other improvements and changes were also occurring. Terminology used to describe the individual in a nursing program was

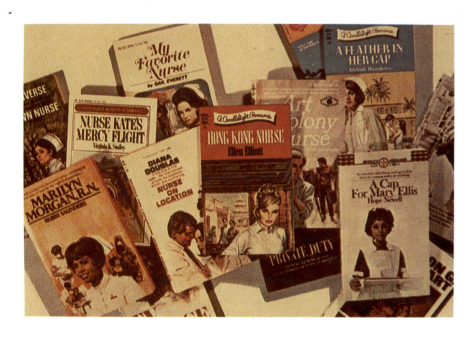

A collage of books illustrating the typical image of the nurse in romantic fiction. Donahue Collection.

altered from "pupil nurse" to "student nurse." This change was significant because "pupil" implies intellectual immaturity and guardianship, whereas "student" describes a more mature, independent, self-directed learner. The title of "Principal of the School of Nursing" was being adopted to portray the nursing program as educational. Teachers and lecturers were being referred to as "nursing school faculty." A greater interest in pedagogical methods was observed. Efforts were also being made to introduce student government as a way to tone down the militaristic discipline, to treat students as adults. Other educational experiments begun at Johns Hopkins and later adopted in other schools were payment of tuition fees by pupils, payment of lecturers from university staffs, the three-year course, full-time instructors, separate nursing school announcements outlining a fully organized course of study, high school graduation as a requirement for admission, use of scholarships, and the eight-hour day (adopted by Johns Hopkins in 1895). It is clear that nurses were beginning to broaden their concept of the meaning and responsibility of the title "profession," as pointed out by Miss Nutting in 1905:

> We claim, and I think justly, the status of a profession; we have schools and teachers, tuition fees and scholarships, systems of instruction from preparatory to postgraduate; we are allied with technical schools on one hand and here and there a university on the other; we have libraries, a literature, and fast-growing numbers of periodicals owned, edited, and published by nurses; we have societies and laws. If therefore we claim to receive the appurtenances, privileges, and standing of a profession, we must recognize professional responsibilities and obligations which we are in honor bound to respect and uphold.
>
> *Nutting, 1905, pp. 654–655*

Nursing literature was expanding in several ways. A great increase in text and reference books had occurred as well as other types of nursing literature. Nurses themselves had begun to produce a large portion of this material, either individually or through their organizations. When the schools of nursing were established, textbooks were urgently needed. Clara Weeks Shaw wrote the first American nursing text in 1885, *A Textbook of Nursing for the Use of Training Schools, Families and Private Students.* She was joined by other reputable authors, including Isabel Hampton, author of *Nursing: Its Principles and Practice for Hospital and Private Use,* Diana Kimber, who wrote *Anatomy and Physiology,* and Lavinia Dock, author of *Textbook on Materia Medica for Nurses.* By 1930 there were approximately 700 textbooks for nurses. Most of them had been written by nurses and published in the United States.

Journals also became necessary for establishing a means of communication between nurses in various locations. *The Trained Nurse and Hospital Review* (renamed *The Nursing World*), established in 1888, was the first national nursing and hospital journal. It was eventually combined with the *Journal of Practical Nursing, The Nightingale, The Nurse, The Nursing World,* and *The Nursing Record.* One of the first activities of the Associated Alumnae was to consider and investigate the possibility of establishing a professional journal that would be its official magazine.

On October 1, 1900, the first issue of the *American Journal of*

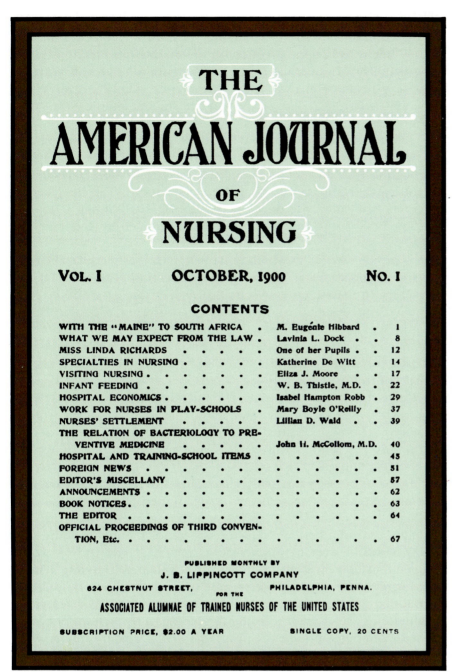

THE AMERICAN JOURNAL OF NURSING

VOL. I | OCTOBER, 1900 | NO. I

CONTENTS

WITH THE "MAINE" TO SOUTH AFRICA	M. Eugénie Hibbard	1
WHAT WE MAY EXPECT FROM THE LAW	Lavinia L. Dock	8
MISS LINDA RICHARDS	One of her Pupils	12
SPECIALTIES IN NURSING	Katherine De Witt	14
VISITING NURSING	Eliza J. Moore	17
INFANT FEEDING	W. B. Thistle, M.D.	22
HOSPITAL ECONOMICS	Isabel Hampton Robb	29
WORK FOR NURSES IN PLAY-SCHOOLS	Mary Boyle O'Reilly	37
NURSES' SETTLEMENT	Lillian D. Wald	39
THE RELATION OF BACTERIOLOGY TO PREVENTIVE MEDICINE	John H. McCollom, M.D.	40
HOSPITAL AND TRAINING-SCHOOL ITEMS		45
FOREIGN NEWS		51
EDITOR'S MISCELLANY		57
ANNOUNCEMENTS		62
BOOK NOTICES		63
THE EDITOR		64
OFFICIAL PROCEEDINGS OF THIRD CONVENTION, Etc.		67

PUBLISHED MONTHLY BY
J. B. LIPPINCOTT COMPANY
624 CHESTNUT STREET, PHILADELPHIA, PENNA.
FOR THE
ASSOCIATED ALUMNAE OF TRAINED NURSES OF THE UNITED STATES

SUBSCRIPTION PRICE, $2.00 A YEAR — SINGLE COPY, 20 CENTS

THE AMERICAN JOURNAL OF NURSING, *cover to the first issue, October 1900. Mugar Memorial Library, Boston University, Massachusetts. By permission from the American Journal of Nursing Company, New York.*

Nursing appeared through the particular efforts of Miss Mary E.P. Davis and Miss Sophia F. Palmer. Individual nurses and alumnae associations had bought shares of stock to finance the original enterprise. By 1912 the ANA became the sole owner of *Journal* stock; some of it had been donated, but the majority of it had been purchased. Miss Palmer served as editor until her death in 1920, when she was succeeded by Mary M. Roberts. The first "office" of the *American Journal of Nursing* was a trunk kept in the home of Miss Palmer where manuscripts and other materials related to the magazine were stored. This publication became the official organ of the ANA and one of the leading professional journals in the country.

Mary Roberts was also committed to this journal's success, and she secured special preparation in journalism. Under her leadership the American Journal of Nursing Company was formed and slowly moved toward expansion in publications. Miss Roberts, an historian in her own right (*American Nursing: History and Interpretation,* 1954), fostered the "story of nursing" in the pages of the *Journal.* Nell V. Beeby was appointed editor upon the retirement of Miss Roberts in 1949. Under Miss Beeby's administration two new journals went into production: *Nursing Outlook,* the official organ of the NLN, and *Nursing Research,* the vehicle for communication of all types of studies relating to nursing.

Affiliations between hospitals for the purpose of rounding out the students' clinical experience were also begun. These were often extended in time and set as a condition for registration, particularly for the smaller and more specialized institutions. The first formal program of affiliation was developed at the Illinois Training School in Chicago; Bellevue in New York was also a recognized leader in this regard.

A trend emerged in which university hospitals were established in various geographical locations in connection with medical departments. In a sense nursing schools thus became a part of the general university system. In most instances, however, the educational program was not classified as a university program, nor were the student nurses considered students of the university. An attempt was made to accomplish this in 1897, when the University of Texas assumed control over the John Sealy Hospital of Galveston and established it as a university hospital. The nursing school was recognized as a regular school of the medical department, and the superintendent of nurses occupied a place on the university committee of instruction. The school, however, was not required to meet the standards of the university.

In 1909, through the influence of Dr. Richard Olding Beard, the School of Nursing of the University of Minnesota became the first nursing school organized as an integral part of a university. Nursing students were admitted and registered as regular students of the university with all university requirements and privileges. "It was not an independent unit, however, since both hospital and nursing school functioned under the college of medicine and surgery. Nor did it offer at that time a college degree" (Stewart, 1943, p. 175). Ten years of pioneering effort went into the upgrading of the school before it offered a degree-granting basic program (1919). Similar schools were established in the Universities of Indiana and Cincinnati and later in several other colleges and universities.

In 1916, two five-year bachelor's degree programs were established at Teachers College, New York, in cooperation with Presbyterian Hospital and the University of Cincinnati's School of Nursing and Health. Within seven years similar programs were instituted in thirteen universities and three colleges (Committee for the Study of Nursing Education, 1923). A combined academic and professional course of five, or sometimes four, years led to both a college degree and the nursing diploma. In general, an attempt was made to mix occupational preparation with a liberal arts education.

Another significant innovation in nursing education occurred with the development of associate degree programs in community colleges. These schools exhibited a phenomenal growth, but their nursing programs evoked a great deal of controversy. It was felt that this community college connection equated nursing education with vocational training at a time when a professional status was being sought for nursing. This model of education was developed by Dr.

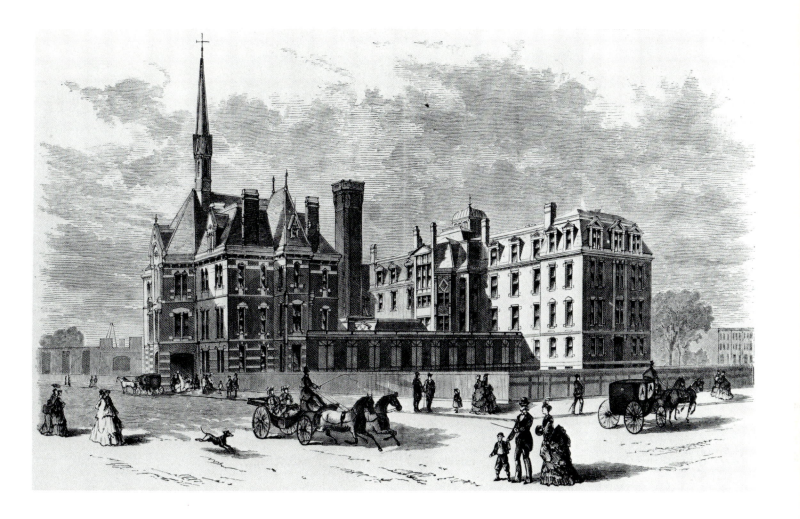

Presbyterian Hospital, New York City. From HARPER'S WEEKLY, *November 16, 1872. Courtesy of the New-York Historical Society, New York.*

Mildred Montag of Teachers College in 1949 as a result of planned research and eventual controlled experimentation. The original pilot project began in 1952 with seven junior and community colleges and one hospital from each of six regions of the United States. The program was administered by Teachers College, and Dr. Montag directed it. The product of this new type of program was to be the *nurse technician,* who operated somewhat below the professional nurse but above the practical nurse. The project concluded in 1957 and was followed by the rapid proliferation of community college nursing programs.

The first steps in the evolution of schools of nursing from hospitals to universities had occurred. As time went on, the superior educational opportunities afforded by a university or a college became abundantly clear. As an integral part of the university—with its liberal education, physical facilities, resources, and level of instruction—a school of nursing would be primarily an educational undertaking.

> Hardly less valuable is the effect of the university atmosphere
> and surroundings on the student "morale." Ambition reacts to
> the atmosphere of intellectual competition; the student nurse is
> stimulated to do her best and take her place with credit among
> her fellow students of the various schools. She feels, too, a new
> sense of dignity and of the importance of her work through her
> recognition as a member of an educational institution.
>
> *Committee for the Study of Nursing Education,*
> *1923, p. 483*

■ STUDIES OF NURSING AND NURSING EDUCATION

The first comprehensive and critical survey of schools of nursing in the United States was *The Educational Status of Nursing* (1912). It was sponsored by the Federal Bureau of Education and directed by M. Adelaide Nutting, who developed the questionnaire and interpreted the data. The majority of the 1100 schools that responded were classified as mediocre educationally and utilitarian in purpose. It was noted in the report that the "exceptional" schools had an adequate supply of applicants; the "poor" schools complained of a continual shortage of applicants. Several recommendations were offered: that standards in nursing schools be raised; that schools of nursing secure financial independence; that the schools become educational institutions in fact, not just in name. This study set a precedent for future investigations that soon followed.

The need for alterations in nursing and nursing education became apparent as the nation absorbed changes in its social, political, and economic structures. Rapid developments in medical science, technological advances in hospitals, and increased demands for health care highlighted this need. It was World War I, however, that particularly dramatized the indispensable role played by nursing and the need for more and better prepared nurses. A pamphlet by Isabel M. Stewart, *Developments in Nursing Education Since 1918* (1921), summed up the impact of the war years on the nursing profession:

> Many of the old barriers of precedent and tradition were broken down, and there was a greater willingness to try new methods and to combine forces with others to conserve limited strength and other resources. Some of these war experiments . . . have been incorporated in our present system and promise to be of permanent value.
>
> Probably the greatest contribution of the war experience to nursing lies in the fact that the whole system of nursing education was shaken for a little while out of its well-worn ruts and brought out of its comparative seclusion into the light of public discussion and criticism. When so many lives hung on the supply of nurses, people were aroused to a new sense of their dependence on the products of nursing schools, and many of them learned for the first time of the hopelessly limited resources which nursing educators have had to work with in the training of these indispensable servants. Whatever the future may bring it is unlikely that nursing schools will willingly sink back again into their old isolation, or that they will accept unquestionably the financial status which the older system imposed on them.
>
> *Stewart, 1921, p. 6*

Miss Stewart firmly believed that the educational status of nursing schools was in some ways better at the end of the war than it had been at the beginning.

Numerous studies were initiated, but only a few exerted a profound influence on the development of nursing. These specific studies are briefly reviewed with particular attention given to the recommendations that came forth.

382

Nursing and Nursing Education in the United States (The Goldmark Report, 1923)

Following World War I, attention was focused as never before on the issues of public health. In 1919 the Rockefeller Foundation invited representative men and women to a conference to consider the status of public health nursing in the United States. The consensus of opinion was that the usual program in basic schools of nursing did not adequately prepare nurses for community health practice. A committee was subsequently appointed and financed by the Rockefeller Foundation to study public health nursing education. Dr. C.A. Winslow, professor of public health at Yale, was appointed chair; Josephine Goldmark, a social worker and author, was appointed secretary and chief investigator. It soon became evident that the scope of the study was too narrow, that the subject of nursing and nursing education needed to be investigated as a whole. The work was expanded and the Committee for the Study of Nursing Education began

> to survey the entire field occupied by the nurse and other workers of related type; to form a conception of the tasks to be performed and the qualifications necessary for their execution; and on the basis of such a study of function to establish sound minimum education standards for each type of nursing service for which there appears to be a vital need.
>
> *Committee for the Study of Nursing Education, 1923*

Representatives of twenty-three schools of nursing and forty-nine public health agencies in various sections of the country were surveyed. After three years a preliminary report was released in 1922 followed by the final report published in 1923, commonly known as the Goldmark Report but sometimes called the Winslow-Goldmark Survey. The conclusions clearly echoed the statements that had been made by the nursing leaders of the day. Each of the ten conclusions was significant, but the following stand out:

> *Conclusion I:* ... That as soon as may be practicable, all agencies, public or private, employing public health nurses, should require as a prerequisite for employment the basic hospital training, followed by a post-graduate course including both class work and field work, in public health nursing.

□ □ □

> *Conclusion IV:* That steps should be taken through state legislation for the definition and licensure of a subsidiary grade of nursing service, the subsidiary type of worker to serve under practicing physicians in the care of mild and chronic illness and convalescence, and possibly to assist under the direction of the trained nurse in certain phases of hospital and visiting nursing.

□ □ □

> *Conclusion VII:* Superintendents, supervisors, instructors, and public health nurses should in all cases receive special additional training beyond the basic nursing course.

□ □ □

> *Conclusion X:* That the development of nursing service adequate for the care of the sick and for the conduct of the modern public

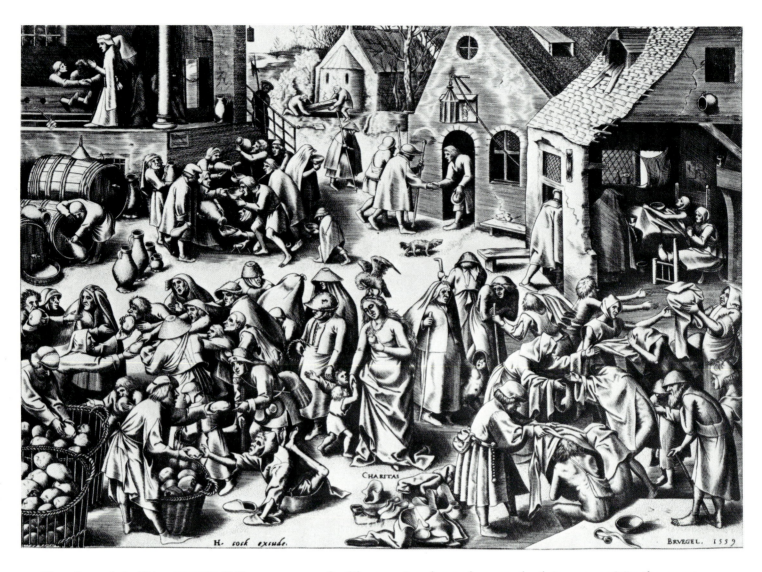

Pieter Bruegel the Elder, CHARITY, *1559.*
Engraving. Museum Boymans-van
Beuningen, Rotterdam, Netherlands.

health campaign demands as an absolute prerequisite the securing of funds for the endowment of nursing education of all types; and that it is of primary importance, in this connection, to provide reasonably generous endowment for university schools of nursing.

Committee for the Study of Nursing Education, 1923

A direct outcome of the study was the establishment of the Yale University School of Nursing (1923), financed by the Rockefeller Foundation. Under the leadership of Annie W. Goodrich and her associate, Effie J. Taylor, who succeeded her, this school successfully demonstrated the importance of an independently endowed and professional school of nursing. Other endowed schools followed at Vanderbilt University, the University of Toronto, and Frances Payne Bolton at Western Reserve University.

Studies by the Committee on the Grading of Nursing Schools

The Committee on the Grading of Nursing Schools was composed of representatives of nursing, medical, and hospital organizations as well as a few educational and lay members. Dr. William Darrach, a well-known surgeon, was the chairman. Dr. May Ayres Burgess, an educator, psychologist, and statistician, directed the study. The committee was officially established in November 1925 to grade and classify schools of nursing, to study the work of nurses, and to define the duties within the scope of nursing. The study was partially financed by outside sources, but nurses themselves donated $115,000 over a five-year period.

Nurses, Patients, and Pocketbooks (1928). The first report that focused on the supply and demand of nursing service, *Nurses, Patients, and Pocketbooks,* was published in 1928. The original purpose of the committee that wrote this report, the grading of nursing schools, was postponed because it was determined that grading needed to be based on and accompanied by careful inquiry into nursing education and employment. The committee thus decided on a five-year program that would be divided into three separate projects: a study of supply and demand for nursing service, a job analysis of what nurses did and how they should be prepared to function, and the actual grading of nursing schools based on the facts of the other two projects. A questionnaire was used to collect information relevant to this first project, and conclusions were based on replies from hospitals, patients, nurses, physicians, and public health directors.

The report covered a wide and interesting group of problems and vividly demonstrated the economic conflict between nurses and their employers and between student service and school of nursing objectives. Specific findings included the following: educational requirements for entrance into nursing schools were minimal; most nursing schools were of poor educational quality; nursing schools existed merely to provide service to hospitals; a serious overproduction of graduate nurses had led to chronic unemployment; salaries and working conditions were extremely poor. These findings were a serious indictment of nursing education and showed its failure to meet existing social needs for nursing service. After the findings were published, the American Medical Association withdrew from the committee without expressing a clear reason for its action.

In general, the conclusions of this committee agreed with those of the Committee on Nursing and Nursing Education in the United States and with the comments and criticisms of nursing leaders. One immediate measure recommended was the replacement of student nurses in hospitals by graduate nurses. In addition, two important resolutions were unanimously adopted by the committee:

1. No hospital should be expected to bear the cost of nursing education out of funds collected for the care of the sick. The education of nurses is as much a public responsibility as is the education of physicians, public school teachers, librarians, ministers, lawyers, and other students planning to engage in professional public service, and the cost of such education should come, not out of a hospital budget, but from private or public funds.

2. The fact that a hospital is faced with serious financial difficulties should have no bearing upon whether or not it will conduct a school of nursing. The need of a hospital for cheap labor should not be considered a legitimate argument for

maintaining such a school. The decision as to whether or not a school of nursing should be conducted in co-operation with a given hospital should be based solely upon the kinds and amounts of educational experience which that hospital is prepared to offer.

Committee on the Grading of Nursing Schools, 1928, pp. 447–448

An Activity Analysis of Nursing (1934). The project concerned with job analysis and the teaching of nursing was conducted at the committee's request by Ethel Johns, a nurse editor and consultant, and Blanche Pfefferkorn, a nurse and director of studies at the National League of Nursing Education. An attempt was made to document the exact functions of nurses in different occupational categories, to describe exactly what nurses actually did. The report clearly and concisely indicated what the patient, the physician, the hospital, and the general public expected of nursing.

Nursing Schools Today and Tomorrow (1934). In the final publication of the committee, *Nursing Schools Today and Tomorrow,* the essentials for a professional program of education were outlined. It contained the facts necessary for reform in schools of nursing and became a vehicle to influence public opinion in favor of nursing. Conditions that would not be tolerated in any nursing school were also specified. Recommendations on professional standards were emphasized and stressed:

> a collegiate level of education; an enriched curriculum, with more and better theory and less and better practice; a better-prepared student body and faculty comparable with those in other professional schools; an organization better fitted to safeguard the professional status and freedom of the school, "dominated by neither hospital nor treasury, nor nursing traditions"; and funds adequate to provide for such a school.
>
> *Stewart, 1943, pp. 214–215*

Finally, the grading committee strongly recommended that the National League of Nursing Education undertake the accreditation of nursing schools.

Curriculum Studies and Reports

From 1914 to 1919 Isabel M. Stewart served as secretary of the Curriculum Committee of the League (originally called the Education Committee) and was its chairman from 1920 to 1937. Three important studies emerged from this committee. The first was the *Standard Curriculum for Schools of Nursing,* published in 1917. "The purpose of this study was to bring about greater uniformity in the programs of nursing schools and to help in improving the content and quality of the teaching as well as other conditions affecting the education of nurses" (Stewart, 1943, p. 211). The body of this study contained a systematic plan for the education of nurses and outlined specific courses along with their objectives, content, and methods; lists of bibliographies, equipment, and schedules completed the scheme.

Within a few years the second study was begun, and it resulted in the publication of *Curriculum for Schools of Nursing* in 1927. The word *standard* was dropped to avoid the notion that it was a requirement to be adopted by schools of nursing. This study was essentially a revision and expansion of the first. A job analysis technique was used to outline the functions and qualifications of the nurse, which constituted the practical objectives of the nursing school curriculum. Miss Nutting and Miss Stewart did most of the writing for these volumes, although the actual conduction of the studies was done by the entire committee.

In 1935 Isabel Stewart urged that another revision be done to meet the current trends in nursing education necessary to comply with community needs.

> She called for a cooperative research project that would encourage participation by many people. She hoped that, through widespread involvement, schools that had been too dependent on the League's curriculum outlines might learn to build their own curriculums by taking materials from the common stock and adapting them to their different situations and stages of development. She desired a serious analysis of the philosophy of nursing education, goals to be aimed for and values to be conserved, the kind of services nurses should be prepared to give to society, the kind of individuals nursing schools should select for preparation, and the kind of preparation needed to fit them for living and serving.
>
> *Christy, 1969c, p. 47*

The project proved to be one of the most far-reaching and ambitious efforts undertaken in this area. It included the participation of representatives of all the professional organizations, allied professions, and the community. The project called for a review and reevaluation, not only of existing curricula but of the traditional philosophies underlying them. Under the direction of Miss Stewart, curriculum committees were organized in all of the state leagues of nursing education, with state subcommittees and local committees under these. Miss Stewart prepared all the materials relevant to the various phases of the work for presentation to her central committee. These in turn were sent back to the state leagues, state subcommittees, and local committees. The project was a *process of sharing* in which participating individuals and groups were educated through their involvement. R. Louise McManus, Miss Stewart's successor at Teachers College, emphasized the project's significance:

> I have always thought of it as one of the first major, mass studies in nursing. But more than that, it was mass education, because many people who didn't know what a curriculum *was* before that, had an opportunity to participate in the construction of the curriculum—and *learn* what it was.
>
> It was "operation bootstrap" for the profession and Miss Stewart did a masterly job. Through the materials that she prepared for the various committees she really educated the mass of nursing educators across the country.
>
> *McManus, cited in Christy, 1969c, p. 47*

The report published by the League in 1937, *A Curriculum Guide for Schools of Nursing,* was the product of the scholarly mind and wise leadership of Isabel Stewart.

Isabel Maitland Stewart (1878–1963) was American nursing's most influential spokeswoman in the area of education for forty-five years. It was Miss Stewart who developed the first course dealing specifically with the teaching of nursing at Teachers College. Eventually this course was expanded and developed into an entire program for the preparation of teachers of nursing. Isabel Stewart's reputation as a curriculum expert became so well established that in later years she was known as "Miss Curriculum" (Stewart, 1961, p. 184).

Miss Stewart was born in Fletcher, Ontario, a village near the city of Chatham. Her Canadian background is particularly significant in that she became part of a nucleus of three Canadian nurses who shaped the destiny of nursing education:

> Many American nurses do not realize the debt we owe to our Canadian sisters. Three of our greatest leaders were born in Canada but spent most of their most productive years contributing to nursing and nursing education in the United States. The first, M. Adelaide Nutting, . . . was born in Waterloo, Quebec; Isabel Hampton Robb . . . came from Welland, Ontario. The third, Isabel M. Stewart, was born in Ontario also, and one might speculate on what differences there might have been in the developments in both American and Canadian nursing had these three not migrated to the United States. . . . Isabel Stewart, particularly, following in the footsteps of her mentor, M. Adelaide Nutting, had great impact on American nursing education.
>
> *Christy, 1969c, p. 44*

Isabel Stewart was one of nine children, all of whom were encouraged to engage in educational pursuits. Beginning her career as a schoolteacher in Canada, she soon turned to nursing and graduated from Winnipeg General Hospital in 1903. Her pursuit of further education led her to Teachers College, where she earned several degrees. Miss Stewart became an assistant to Professor M. Adelaide Nutting and eventually succeeded her as director of the college's Division of Nursing Education, a position she held for twenty-two years. Although best known for her accomplishments as chairman of the Curriculum Committee of the League, Isabel Stewart was also an active research investigator who planned and implemented studies that led to a wealth of useful information for nursing education and practice. Until her death in 1963, she remained an active participant in nursing activities. Throughout her lifetime she filled the roles of scholar, author, educator, researcher, administrator, and leader with distinction.

Isabel Stewart's interests were wide and varied. She was deeply interested in education in all aspects, particularly the education of women. Her study of history strengthened her belief that women could not rise to the full demands of any vocation or profession without education and knowledge of the social conditions and needs of their day. Thus the fullest development of nursing was not possible without emancipation from the conditions of subjection under which women and nurses had suffered for so many years.

Early in her professional career Miss Stewart began her contributions to nursing organizations, which provided her with an essential vehicle for improvement of professional training and curriculum in schools of nursing throughout the country. She belonged to many

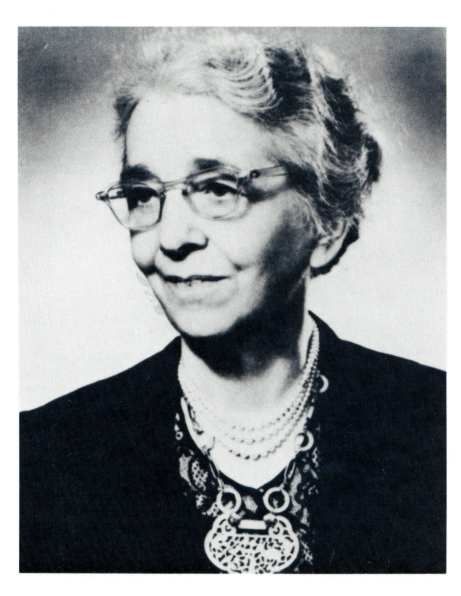

Portrait of ISABEL STEWART. *Donahue Collection.*

nursing organizations, both national and international, in which she became a prominent figure. In these organizations she worked on a multitude of committees. A prolific writer, she published numerous works through which she interpreted modern trends in both general and nursing education. Two of these publications stand out as particularly important and were directly linked to her intense love of history: *A Short History of Nursing,* first published in 1920 and written with Lavinia L. Dock, and *The Education of Nurses* (1943). An examination of the latter work can lead to an important conclusion. It was written by an individual who had the outstanding ability to select significant facts, who had the rare vision, insight, and imagination to demonstrate relationships and interpret them to professional workers. *The Education of Nurses* was the closest thing to a philosophy of nursing education ever written.

As the years went by, Miss Stewart feared for the loss of the humanitarian aspects that had long been a vital force in nursing. Recognizing that a definite decline in the study of this area was occurring, she commented:

> I feel very strongly these days that we are failing to develop the social and humanistic side of nursing—the spirit of nursing as we used to call it—and all that goes to the *balancing* of the scien-

tific and technical aspects—it would mean a restudy of that whole area dealing with the philosophy and history of nursing and the social sciences, and the strengthening of our cultural roots, both in nursing schools (basic) and in the preparation of graduate nurses for developing this phase of nursing.

I am distressed to realize that we are doing less in this field today than we did a few years ago and there seems to be very little interest in it. Miss [Maude] Muse spoke of it the other day and she feels much as I do. It is a part of the sickness of our civilization that we have *overstressed* the scientific and technical side and have neglected the other aspects of our work and education.

Letter from Isabel M. Stewart
to Lillian A. Hudson, c. 1940–1947

Nursing for the Future (1948)

The study called *Nursing for the Future* was initiated in connection with the postwar planning of the National Nursing Council. A grant of $28,000 was given to the council by the Carnegie Corporation in 1947 for the investigation of nursing practice and the preparation required for it. Esther Lucile Brown, a social anthropologist and director of the Department of Studies in the Professions at the Russell Sage Foundation, was authorized to conduct this study to determine the "needs of society" for nursing. Her data were obtained firsthand as she personally visited fifty geographically representative schools in the country, held three regional workshop conferences with nursing directors (representing 1250 schools), and met with individual nurses, physicians, hospital administrators, and others involved with nursing. A large number of far-reaching recommendations were published in this report, which is also known as *The Brown Report.* One of the strongest proposals was

> that effort be directed to building basic schools of nursing in universities and colleges, comparable in number to existing medical schools, that are sound in organizational and financial structure, adequate in facilities and faculty, and well-distributed to serve the needs of the entire country.
>
> *Brown, 1948, p. 178*

The report was endorsed in principle by the boards of directors of the six national nursing organizations in existence. However, many physicians and hospital administrators were openly hostile to the recommendations.

Nursing Schools at the Mid-Century (1950)

A Joint Committee on Implementing the Brown Report was established by the NLNE in 1948 (it was renamed the National Committee for the Improvement of Nursing Services in 1949). Early work of this committee consisted of the collection of factual information about nursing school programs and the interim classification of schools. This was to precede the development of a more comprehensive accreditation system and program. A questionnaire was used, and the hope was to obtain information from *all* schools of nursing (96% return rate) in the United States. Each of the participating schools was evaluated according to long-accepted criteria by the profession. The schools were classified according to a total score obtained by the weighting of the various criteria of administrative policies, financial organization, faculty, curriculum, clinical field, library, student selection and provisions for student welfare, and student performance on state board examinations. In 1950 the findings were published in *Nursing Schools at the Mid-Century* and provided a method for schools of nursing to evaluate their programs.

Canadian Studies

Through the initiative of the Canadian Nurses Association, a joint committee of this association and the Canadian Medical Association was established in 1929 to undertake a nationwide study of nursing education in Canada. The study was conducted by Dr. George M. Weir, a well-known educator and sociologist in the Department of Education of the University of British Columbia. The *Survey of Nursing Education in Canada* (1932), also known as *The Weir Report*, pointed out serious weaknesses that existed in the hospital schools. Important reforms were recommended: a higher educational standard; increased affiliations between schools; increased employment of graduate nurses; student tuition; and qualified instructors. The survey also recommended that "no hospital having fewer than 75 beds, exclusive of cots and bassinets, and a daily average of at least 50 patients, be recognized as competent to conduct an approved Training School" (Gibbon and Mathewson, 1947, p. 375).

Following the release of this report, the Canadian Nurses Association organized a National Curriculum Committee, which published *The Proposed Curriculum for Schools of Nursing in Canada* in 1936. This project was conducted by a special committee and chaired by Marion Lindeberg, director of the Department of Nursing Education at McGill University. The findings were similar to those in the United States and led to the closing of a number of smaller training schools. The study and the later *Supplement* became valuable guides to assist with the establishment of a sounder educational foundation for nursing in Canada.

*M*an's role in the grim business of war has been fully portrayed in art and literature. The exhausting strain, the danger, the suffering and the brutal death which are his portion, have all been given eloquent expression. . . . But the heroic part taken by women, in the terrible ordeal of war, is only faintly heard and little noted. The mute anguish transcending tears, the infinite sacrifice and the high courage which are theirs, are voiceless amid the full throated cannon's roar, nor do they inscribe a record by fire and sword. . . .

To only a few, among all the world's many gallant women, is reserved the solemn privilege of being a part of the great forces locked in battle, and of being numbered among those elect of earth who, as participants, directly govern the course of history. The nurse, because of her special training and the high calling to which her life is dedicated, brings to the battlefield indispensable attributes which she alone possesses. Voluntarily she comes in response to the utmost need of the men with shattered bodies whose cry is for the compassionate touch of a woman's hand. . . . She endures all of the ordeal borne by womanhood and in addition she shares with man his bitter lot upon the field of battle.

Julia O. Flikke